A Clinician's Guide to Angioplasty

A Clinician's Guide to Angioplasty

Edited by Casey Judd

hayle
medical

New York

Hayle Medical,
750 Third Avenue, 9th Floor,
New York, NY 10017, USA

Visit us on the World Wide Web at:
www.haylemedical.com

© Hayle Medical, 2018

ISBN: 978-1-63241-478-6

Cataloging-in-Publication Data

   A clinician's guide to angioplasty / edited by Casey Judd.
      p. cm.
   Includes bibliographical references and index.
   ISBN 978-1-63241-478-6
   1. Angioplasty. 2. Blood-vessels--Surgery. I. Judd, Casey.
RD598.5 .C55 2018
617.413--dc23

Table of Contents

Preface

Angioplasty is a surgical procedure which restores arteries and veins to its normal functioning. It is meant to treat arterial atherosclerosis and is a minimally invasive procedure. This book on angioplasty discusses the various techniques that are involved in it such as stenting and balloon septostomy. Coronary angioplasty and peripheral angioplasty are the most common disorders for which treatment is sought. A number of latest researches have been included in this book to keep the readers up-to-date with the global concepts in this area of study. For someone with an interest and eye for detail, this book covers the most significant topics in the field of angioplasty.

The researches compiled throughout the book are authentic and of high quality, combining several disciplines and from very diverse regions from around the world. Drawing on the contributions of many researchers from diverse countries, the book's objective is to provide the readers with the latest achievements in the area of research. This book will surely be a source of knowledge to all interested and researching the field.

In the end, I would like to express my deep sense of gratitude to all the authors for meeting the set deadlines in completing and submitting their research chapters. I would also like to thank the publisher for the support offered to us throughout the course of the book. Finally, I extend my sincere thanks to my family for being a constant source of inspiration and encouragement.

Editor

Inpatient Coronary Angiography and Revascularisation following Non-ST-Elevation Acute Coronary Syndrome in Patients with Renal Impairment: A Cohort Study Using the Myocardial Ischaemia National Audit Project

Catriona Shaw[1,2]*, **Dorothea Nitsch**[3], **Retha Steenkamp**[1], **Cornelia Junghans**[4], **Sapna Shah**[5], **Donal O'Donoghue**[6], **Damian Fogarty**[7], **Clive Weston**[8], **Claire C. Sharpe**[2]

1 UK Renal Registry, Southmead Hospital, Bristol, United Kingdom, 2 Department of Renal Sciences, Division of Transplantation Immunology and Mucosal Biology, Kings College London, London, United Kingdom, 3 London School of Hygiene and Tropical Medicine, London, United Kingdom, 4 Department of Epidemiology and Public Health, University College London, London, United Kingdom, 5 Department of Renal Medicine, Kings College Hospital, London, United Kingdom, 6 Department of Renal Medicine, Salford Royal NHS Foundation Trust, Salford, United Kingdom, 7 Department of Renal Medicine, Belfast Health and Social Care Trust, Belfast, Northern Ireland, United Kingdom, 8 Myocardial Ischaemia National Audit Project, College of Medicine, Swansea University, Swansea, Wales, United Kingdom

Abstract

Background: International guidelines support an early invasive management strategy (including early coronary angiography and revascularisation) for non-ST-elevation acute coronary syndrome (NSTE-ACS) in patients with renal impairment. However, evidence from outside the UK suggests that this approach is underutilised. We aimed to describe practice within the NHS, and to determine whether the severity of renal dysfunction influenced the provision of angiography and modified the association between early revascularisation and survival.

Methods: We performed a cohort study, using multivariable logistic regression and propensity score analyses, of data from the Myocardial Ischaemia National Audit Project for patients presenting with NSTE-ACS to English or Welsh hospitals between 2008 and 2010.

Findings: Of 35 881 patients diagnosed with NSTE-ACS, eGFR of $<$60 ml/minute/1.73 m^2 was present in 15 680 (43.7%). There was a stepwise decline in the odds of undergoing inpatient angiography with worsening renal dysfunction. Compared with an eGFR$>$90 ml/minute/1.73 m^2, patients with an eGFR between 45–59 ml/minute/1.73 m^2 were 33% less likely to undergo angiography (adjusted OR 0.67, 95% CI 0.55–0.81); those with an eGFR$<$30/minute/1.73 m^2 had a 64% reduction in odds of undergoing angiography (adjusted OR 0.36, 95%CI 0.29–0.43). Of 16 646 patients who had inpatient coronary angiography, 58.5% underwent inpatient revascularisation. After adjusting for co-variables, inpatient revascularisation was associated with approximately a 30% reduction in death within 1 year compared with those managed medically after coronary angiography (adjusted OR 0.66, 95%CI 0.57–0.77), with no evidence of modification by renal function (p interaction = 0.744).

Interpretation: Early revascularisation may offer a similar survival benefit in patients with and without renal dysfunction, yet renal impairment is an important determinant of the provision of coronary angiography following NSTE-ACS. A randomised controlled trial is needed to evaluate the efficacy of an early invasive approach in patients with severe renal dysfunction to ensure that all patients who may benefit are offered this treatment option.

Editor: Joshua M. Hare, University of Miami Miller School of Medicine, United States of America

Funding: The authors have no support or funding to report.

Competing Interests: The authors have declared that no competing interests exist.

* E-mail: catriona.shaw@nbt.nhs.uk

Introduction

Thirty to forty percent of patients presenting with NSTE-ACS have renal impairment [1]. Compared with patients with preserved renal function those with impairment have a 2–5 fold greater risk of death after NSTE-ACS; those with most severe renal impairment being at highest risk [2]. The projected annual cost to the National Health Service (NHS) of additional cardiovascular events occurring in patients with chronic kidney disease (12 000 myocardial infarctions and 7 000 strokes per year) is £174–178 million [3].

Generally an 'early invasive' approach after NSTE-ACS – characterised by routine coronary angiography, followed where possible by early percutaneous or surgical revascularisation – has been demonstrated to improve patient survival [4]. Yet patients with renal impairment were under-represented in the clinical trials that showed this benefit [5]. Current European and American guidelines advise early angiography after NSTE-ACS *irrespective* of renal function [6,7]. However, several reports from outside the UK suggest that patients with renal dysfunction are significantly less likely to undergo angiography or subsequent revascularisation [1,8–10]. Reasons for this discrepancy, between guidelines and practice, are likely to be complex. Remaining uncertainty as to whether renal dysfunction negates the benefit associated with early revascularisation may contribute.

We used data from the Myocardial Ischaemia National Audit Project (MINAP) to describe and quantify use of an early invasive approach after NSTE-ACS in those with normal and those with impaired renal function in NHS clinical practice. We investigated the association between inpatient coronary angiography and death. Furthermore, for patients undergoing inpatient angiography, we investigated whether renal dysfunction at the time of presentation modified the association between revascularisation and death within 1 year.

Methods

Study Population

Care of patients presenting with ACS to all acute NHS hospitals in England and Wales are monitored through MINAP [11–13]. Briefly, each patient entry contains prospectively collected information on aspects of diagnosis, investigation and management. The project uses highly secure electronic systems of data entry and transmission, and allows linkage with the NHS Central Register for mortality tracking. Assurance of data quality involves continual monitoring of key fields and an annual validation exercise. MINAP is supported by the British Cardiovascular Society under the auspices of the National Institute for Cardiovascular Outcomes Research (NICOR) and is commissioned and funded by the Healthcare Quality Improvement Partnership.

Anonymised data from an adult population with a diagnosis of NSTE-ACS admitted to hospital between 1st Jan 2008 and 31st March 2010 were used. The diagnosis of NSTE-ACS was made by the local clinician using their judgement of presenting symptoms and requiring elevated blood troponin concentration, with or without electrocardiographic changes consistent with ischaemia. Patients with ST elevation were excluded from this analysis.

Study Exposures

The first single serum creatinine (μmol/l) within 24 hours of admission was used to estimate the glomerular filtration rate (eGFR) in ml/minute/1.73 m^2 using the equation developed by the Chronic Kidney Disease Epidemiology Collaboration (CKD EPI) [14]. All creatinine values were assumed not to have been calibrated by isotope dilution mass spectrometry and therefore were multiplied by a 0.95 standardisation factor. Renal function was initially categorised as eGFR>90 ml/minute/1.73 m^2, eGFR 60–90 ml/minute/1.73 m^2, eGFR 45–59 ml/minute/1.73 m^2, eGFR 30–44 ml/minute/1.73 m^2, eGFR 15–29 ml/minute/1.73 m^2 and <15 ml/minute/1.73 m^2 for the descriptive analysis [15]. As relatively low numbers of patients with an eGFR 15–29 ml/minute/1.73 m^2 and <15 ml/minute/1.73 m^2 underwent inpatient coronary angiography or inpatient revascularisation the two eGFR categories were combined for subsequent analyses (eGFR<30 ml/minute/1.73 m^2).

Inpatient revascularisation was defined as inpatient percutaneous coronary intervention (PCI) or coronary artery bypass grafting (CABG). Patients were categorised as medically managed following inpatient coronary angiography if i) PCI or CABG was planned after discharge, or ii) the patient refused such interventions, or iii) the procedures were neither planned nor performed during the index admission.

Study Outcomes

The primary study outcomes were performance of inpatient coronary angiography – dichotomised as performed or not performed – and all-cause death within one year of presentation. Patients who died on the day of admission were excluded from analyses.

Confounder Variables

Demographic factors included age (10 year categories), sex, ethnicity, hospital of admission and self- reported smoking status. The Index of Multiple Deprivation was included. This index reflects information on the seven domains of income: employment; health and disability; education, skills and training; barriers to housing and services; living environment; and crime [16]. Comorbidities included a history of hypertension, previous angina, previous myocardial infarction, hyperlipidaemia, peripheral vascular disease, cerebrovascular disease, chronic obstructive airways disease, congestive cardiac failure, diabetes mellitus, previous PCI and previous CABG. Haemoglobin (g/dl) recorded within 24 hours of admission and peak troponin were also used.

We lacked direct measurements of left ventricular function. Surrogates for reduced function included a history of congestive cardiac failure or previous myocardial infarction. Systolic blood pressure (SBP) and heart rate at the time of admission are validated prognostic markers in ACS and thought to be representative of the degree of acute left ventricular dysfunction [17]. The first SBP (mmHg) recorded after admission to hospital was used. If the patient presented with a treatable tachyarrhythmia, the first stable SBP after treatment was used. The heart rate (beats/minute) was recorded from the first ECG after admission to hospital, whilst in a stable cardiac rhythm. The ECG appearances at presentation were included (normal, left bundle branch block, ST segment depression, T wave changes only, other abnormality).

Statistical Analyses

All statistical analyses were done using STATA version 11.2.

Confounder exposure associations were cross-tabulated both in the full study population and in the subgroup of patients undergoing inpatient coronary angiography. The frequency and proportions of missing data within each variable were tabulated and distributions of population characteristics for participants included in the complete case analysis were compared with individuals who were excluded due to incomplete data on the *a priori* variables.

Univariable and then multivariable logistic regression models adjusted for all study covariables were used to estimate the odds ratio for the association between eGFR category and undergoing inpatient coronary angiography. Robust standard errors were used to account for clustering at hospital level.

Logistic regression models were also used to assess the association between inpatient coronary angiography and all-cause death. As it was expected that in some cases those that did not undergo inpatient angiography would vary substantially in their baseline characteristics compared with those that did, a propensity score was estimated to help ensure adequate overlap between the distributions of confounders in the two treatment groups [18]. The analysis was repeated restricting to a sub group of the cohort with improved balance in baseline co-variables. The propensity score was the conditional probability that an individual had inpatient coronary angiography and was obtained for each individual by fitting a logistic regression model with outcome inpatient coronary

Table 1. Selected covariates stratified by eGFR category at time of presentation in 35 881 adults presenting with non-ST-elevation acute coronary syndrome (all data is presented as numbers with column percentage unless otherwise stated).

	eGFR (ml/minute/1.73 m^2)					
	>90	60–90	45–59	30–44	15–29	<15
	N = 6 482	N = 13 719	N = 6 990	N = 5 452	N = 2 665	N = 573
Demographic						
Male gender	4781(73.8)	9223(67.2)	4010(57.4)	2749(50.4)	1326(49.8)	336(58.6)
Age, median (IQR)	58(50–66)	72(63–80)	79(72–85)	83(77–88)	84(78–88)	80(73–86)
Past Medical History						
Hypertension	2680(41.4)	7089(51.7)	4161(59.5)	3375(61.9)	1671(62.7)	387(67.5)
Stroke	333(5.1)	1276(9.3)	950(13.6)	883(16.2)	439(16.5)	107(18.7)
PVD	241(3.7)	591(4.3)	442 (6.3)	390(7.2)	235(8.8)	71(12.4)
Treated hyperlipidaemia	2243(34.6)	4805(35.0)	2449(35.0)	1866(34.2)	854(32.1)	177(30.9)
CCF	128(2.0)	723(5.3)	688(9.8)	917(16.8)	584(21.9)	106(18.5)
Previous MI	1382(21.3)	3964(28.9)	2662(38.1)	2394(43.9)	1318(49.5)	256(44.7)
Previous PCI	787(12.1)	1488(10.9)	727(10.4)	549(10.1)	227(8.5)	52(9.1)
Previous CABG	362(5.6)	1121(8.2)	695(9.9)	536(9.8)	256(9.6)	57(10.0)
Diabetes Mellitus	1150(17.7)	2727(19.9)	1748(25.0)	1735 (31.8)	965(36.2)	235(41.0)
Current smoker	2820(43.5)	2948(21.5)	950(13.6)	520(9.5)	237(8.9)	59(10.3)
Diagnostics						
Haemoglobin (g/dl), median (IQR)	14.2(13.0–15.2)	13.8(12.4–15.0)	13.0(11.7–14.1)	12.0(10.9–13.5)	11.3(10.0–12.6)	10.6(9.5–12.0)
Peak Troponin, median(IQR)	0.7(0.2–3.1)	0.7(0.2–3.3)	0.8(0.2–3.9)	0.9(0.2–4.1)	1.2(0.3–5.3)	1.7(0.4–8.2)
Systolic blood pressure (mmHg), mean (sd)	143(26)	144(28)	142(29)	140(30)	135(31)	137(33)
Heart rate (beats/min), median (IQR)	77(66–90)	78(66–93)	82(69–99)	85(71–101)	85(71–100)	86 (71–100)
IP Coronary angiography	4720(72.8)	7445(54.3)	2613(37.4)	1366(25.1)	416(15.6)	86(15.0)
IP revascularisation	2992(46.2)	4422(32.2)	1370(19.6)	697(12.8)	205(7.7)	46(8.0)
IP PCI	2758(42.5)	3977(29.0)	1208(17.3)	609(11.2)	183(6.9)	44(7.7)
IP CABG	234(3.6)	445(3.2)	162(2.3)	88(1.6)	22(0.8)	2(0.3)

Abbreviations: IMD score = score of deprivation; PVD = peripheral vascular disease; CCF = congestive cardiac failure; MI = myocardial infarction; PCI = percutaneous coronary intervention; CABG = coronary artery bypass graft; eGFR = estimated glomerular filtration rate; IP - inpatient; IQR = interquartile range; sd = standard deviation.

angiography with all the pre-specified co-variables included. All of the pre-specified co-variables were considered *a priori* confounders.

Diagnostic coronary angiography is a pre-requisite for being considered for revascularisation. The analysis to evaluate whether renal dysfunction modified patient survival after inpatient coronary revascularisation compared with medical management was therefore limited to individuals who underwent inpatient coronary angiography. Again a propensity score was estimated to help ensure adequate overlap between the distributions of confounders in the two treatment groups. The propensity score was the conditional probability that an individual had inpatient revascularisation, and was obtained for each individual by fitting a logistic regression model with outcome inpatient revascularisation with all the pre-specified co-variables. After estimation of the conditional propensity score one patient from the medically managed group was excluded as they could not be matched due to a very low propensity score. Improved balance in the distribution in the co-variables between the two treatment groups was achieved (Appendix S1). Multivariable logistic regression analysis was subsequently carried out using robust standard errors with outcome death or alive within one year. Evidence of effect modification between eGFR category and inpatient revascularisation or medical management on the odds of death within one year was tested (Wald test). Evidence of effect modification between

gender and inpatient revascularisation or medical management was also tested [19]. The interaction terms were maintained in the model at a threshold of p<0.01. Results are presented as multivariable adjusted odds ratios with 95% confidence intervals.

Sensitivity Analyses

Logistic regression with the propensity score included as the single co-variable was conducted. Robust standard errors and bootstrapping methods (50 repetitions) were used.

To evaluate possible bias introduced by patients who died early after admission to hospital the analyses were repeated using a cohort limited to individuals who survived five days or more.

Secondary preventative medications including aspirin, clopidogrel, ACE inhibitors, beta-blockers and statins have been shown to influence outcome after NSTE-ACS [20–23]. Whether these medications were prescribed at time of discharge was included in the multivariable model evaluating the association between inpatient revascularisation and death within one year.

Sensitivity analysis using datasets derived using multiple imputation was also conducted [24].

Ethical Approval

Ethics committee (11/L0/0246), Kings College Hospital Research and Development (KCH11-081), and MINAP Academic Group approvals were obtained prior to commencement of the analysis.

Results

Renal Impairment at the Time of Presentation with NSTE-ACS and Subsequent Inpatient Coronary Angiography

GFR could not be estimated for 18.2% (16 632/91 342) due to missing data on creatinine, gender, age or ethnicity (Appendix S2). Data was missing regarding coronary angiography in 4.5%, management strategy (inpatient revascularisation or medical management) in 18.3% and for mortality in <1% of patients. 15.8% of individuals excluded from the complete case analysis due to incomplete data died compared with 19.0% of those included (Appendix S3). Complete data on all co-variables was available in 35 881 cases. Approximately 40% (n = 15 680/35 881) had an eGFR<60 ml/minute/1.73 m^2, and 9.0% (n = 3 238) an eGFR< 30 ml/minute/1.73 m^2 (Table 1). The median age was 75 years, and 22 425 (62.5%) were male. Individuals with impaired renal function tended to be older, with a higher co-morbid profile, and more likely to die within 1 year (Table 1, Figure 1).

Inpatient coronary angiography was performed in 16 646 (46.4%) of the cohort. Patients who had inpatient coronary angiography were more likely to be male, younger and have fewer co-morbid conditions than those who did not (Table 2). Death within 1 year occurred in 30.6% patients who did not undergo inpatient coronary angiography compared with 5.7% in those that did. 72.8% of individuals with normal renal function (an eGFR> 90 ml/minute/1.73 m^2) underwent inpatient coronary angiography compared with 15.5% of those with an eGFR<30 ml/ minute/1.73 m^2 (Table 1).

After adjusting for all other comorbidities and covariables, there was a stepwise reduction in the odds of undergoing inpatient coronary angiography with increasing severity of renal impairment; a reduction of 33% in patients with eGFR 45–59 ml/ minute/1.73 m^2 (adjusted OR 0.67, 95% CI 0.55–0.81), 42% in those with an eGFR between 30–44 ml/minute/1.73 m^2 (adjusted OR 0.58, 95% CI 0.48–0.70), and 64% in those with eGFR< 30 ml/minute/1.73 m^2 (adjusted OR 0.36, 95% CI 0.29–0.43) compared with patients with an eGFR>90 ml/minute/1.73 m^2 (Table 3).

Renal Impairment at the Time of Presentation with NSTE-ACS and the Association between Inpatient Coronary Angiography and Death within 1 Year

In patient coronary angiography was associated with a survival benefit in each eGFR category (Table 4). In those with an eGFR 60–90 ml/minute/1.73 m^2 inpatient coronary angiography was associated with a reduction in the estimated odds of death of 70% (adjusted OR 0.29, 95% CI 0.25–0.33) and by 54% in those with an eGFR<30 ml/minute/1.73 m^2 (adjusted OR 0.46, 95%CI 0.36–0.58). On restricting the analysis to a subgroup with improved balance in the distribution of baseline characteristics based on estimated propensity score (N = 16 617), the estimated survival benefit observed did not change, except in those with an eGFR<30 ml/minute/1.73 m^2 in whom the estimated survival benefit was more conservative (adjusted OR 0.59, 95% CI 0.37–0.96) (data not shown).

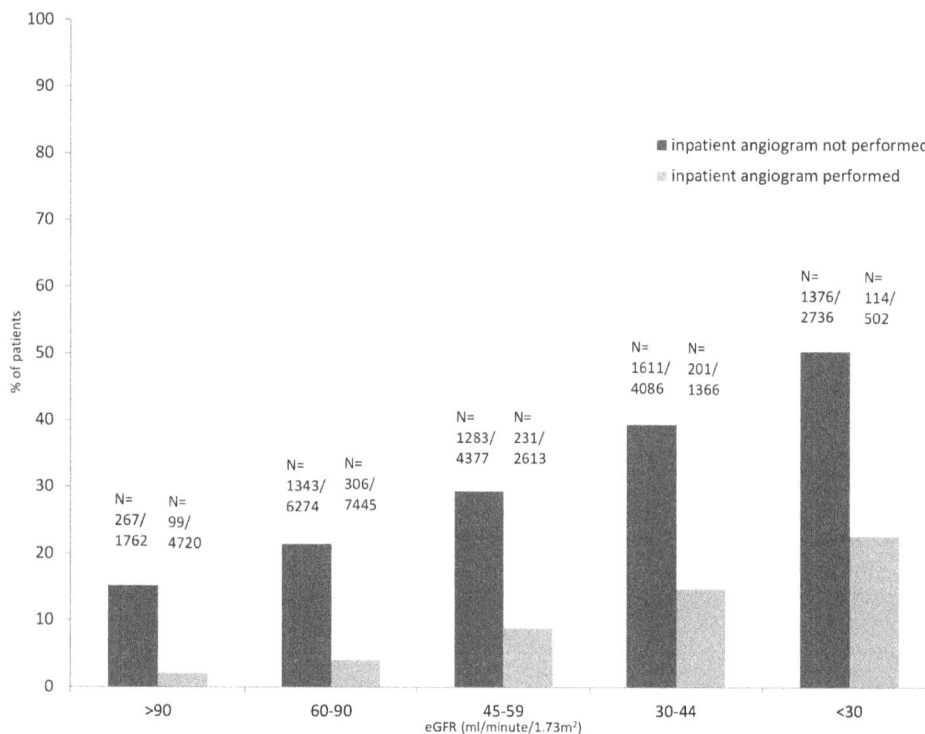

Figure 1. Percentage of patients that died within 1 year after non-ST-elevation acute coronary syndrome. Percentage of patients that died within 1 year after non-ST-elevation acute coronary syndrome stratified by category of estimated glomerular filtration rate at the time of presentation and whether inpatient coronary angiography was performed. *Abbreviations eGFR = estimated glomerular filtration rate; *this analysis included 35 881 patients presenting with NSTE-ACS.

Table 2. Selected covariates stratified by whether inpatient coronary angiography was performed or not, in 35 881 adults presenting with non-ST-elevation acute coronary syndrome (all data is presented as numbers with column percentage unless otherwise stated).

	IP Coronary angiography not performed	IP Coronary angiography performed
	N = 19 235	N = 16 646
Demographic		
Male gender	10 821 (56.3)	11 604 (69.7)
Age in years, median (IQR)	81 (72–87)	68 (56–76)
Past Medical History		
Hypertension	10 631 (55.3)	8 732 (52.5)
Stroke	2 842 (14.8)	1 146 (6.9)
PVD	1 228 (6.4)	7 42 (4.5)
Treated hyperlipidaemia	5 717 (29.7)	6 677 (40.1)
CCF	2 466 (12.8)	680 (4.1)
Previous MI	7 586 (39.4)	4 309 (26.4)
Previous PCI	1 559 (8.3)	2 231 (13.4)
Previous CABG	1 736 (9.0)	1 291 (7.8)
Diabetes Mellitus	5 030 (26.2)	3 530 (21.2)
Current smoker	2 912 (15.1)	46 22 (27.8)
Diagnostics		
Haemoglobin (g/dl), median (IQR)	12.6 (11.0–14.0)	14.0 (12.8–15.0)
Peak Troponin, median (IQR)	0.8 (0.2–3.7)	0.8 (0.2–3.6)
eGFR (ml/minute/1.73 m^2)		
>90	1 762 (9.2)	4 720 (28.4)
60–90	6 274 (32.6)	7 445 (44.7)
45–59	4 377 (22.8)	2 613 (15.7)
30–44	4 086 (21.2)	1 366 (8.2)
15–29	2 249 (11.7)	416 (2.5)
<15	487 (2.5)	86 (0.5)
Systolic blood pressure (mmHg), mean (sd)	140 (29)	145 (27)
Heart rate (beats/min), median (IQR)	84 (70–100)	76 (65–90)

Abbreviations: IP = inpatient; IMD score = score of deprivation; PVD = peripheral vascular disease; CCF = congestive cardiac failure; MI = myocardial infarction; PCI = percutaneous coronary intervention; CABG = coronary artery bypass graft; eGFR = estimated glomerular filtration rate; IQR = interquartile range; sd = standard deviation.

Table 3. Results of the multivariable logistic regression analysis in 35 881 individuals with non-ST-elevation acute coronary syndrome for the association between eGFR and inpatient coronary angiography.

eGFR (ml/minute/1.73 m^2)	Age & gender adjusted OR (95% CI)	P-value (Wald)	Multivariable Adjusted OR (95% CI)*	P-value (Wald)
>90	1		1	
60–90	0.81 (0.71–0.93)	0.003	0.81 (0.70–0.94)	0.006
45–59	0.58 (0.48–0.70)	<0.001	0.67 (0.55–0.81)	<0.001
30–44	0.42 (0.35–0.51)	<0.001	0.58 (0.48–0.70)	<0.001
<30	0.21 (0.18–0.26)	<0.001	0.36 (0.29–0.43)	<0.001

*Multivariable model adjusted for age, ethnicity, gender, IMD score, systolic blood pressure, heart rate, haemoglobin, peak troponin, ECG diagnosis, history of angina, hyperlipidaemia, hypertension, peripheral vascular disease, cerebrovascular disease, chronic obstructive airways disease, congestive cardiac failure, previous percutaneous coronary intervention, previous coronary artery bypass graft, previous myocardial infarction, diabetes, current smoking status and hospital.
Abbreviations: OR = odds ratio; CI = confidence interval; eGFR = estimated glomerular filtration rate.

Table 4. Results of the multivariable logistic regression analysis in 35 881 individuals with non-ST-elevation acute coronary syndrome for the association between inpatient coronary angiography and all-cause death.

eGFR (ml/minute/1·73 m^2)	Inpatient angiography status	Multivariable Adjusted OR (95% CI)*	P-value (Wald)
>90	Inpatient angiography not performed	1	
	Inpatient angiography	0.21 (0.17–0.27)	<0.001
60–90	Inpatient angiography not performed	1	
	Inpatient angiography	0.29 (0.25–0.33)	<0.001
45–59	Inpatient angiography not performed	1	
	Inpatient angiography	0.37 (0.32–0.43)	<0.001
30–44	Inpatient angiography not performed	1	
	Inpatient angiography	0.41 (0.34–0.48)	<0.001
<30	Inpatient angiography not performed	1	
	Inpatient angiography	0.46 (0.36–0.58)	<0.001

*p-interaction (Wald test) between eGFR category and inpatient coronary angiography and mortality: <0.001.
*Multivariable model adjusted for age, ethnicity, gender, IMD score, systolic blood pressure, heart rate, haemoglobin, peak troponin, ECG diagnosis, history of angina, hyperlipidaemia, hypertension, peripheral vascular disease, cerebrovascular disease, chronic obstructive airways disease, congestive cardiac failure, previous percutaneous coronary intervention, previous coronary artery bypass graft, previous myocardial infarction, diabetes, current smoking status and hospital.
Abbreviations: OR = odds ratio; CI = confidence interval; eGFR = estimated glomerular filtration rate.

Renal Impairment at the Time of Presentation with NSTE-ACS and the Association between Inpatient Revascularisation and Death within 1 Year

Of 16 646 patients who had inpatient coronary angiography, 9 732 (58.5%) underwent inpatient revascularisation (Figure 2). On the basis of the propensity score, there was good overlap in the distribution of baseline characteristics between the group that underwent inpatient revascularisation and those who underwent angiography only (Appendix S1). Only 16% of patients with severe renal dysfunction at presentation (eGFR<30 ml/min/1.73 m^2) underwent inpatient coronary angiography and could be considered for early revascularisation. However, of the 502 patients in this renal category that did have diagnostic angiography, nearly 50% underwent subsequent inpatient revascularisation (Table 5). The adjusted odds of undergoing inpatient revascularisation did not vary depending on eGFR category (data not shown).

538 deaths (7.8%) occurred within a year in those patients managed medically after inpatient coronary angiography compared with 413 deaths (4.2%) amongst patients who had inpatient revascularisation. After adjusting for co-variables, inpatient revascularisation was associated with a reduction in the odds of death within 1 year of approximately 30% (adjusted OR 0.66, 95%CI 0.57–0.77) (Table 6). When stratified by eGFR category there was a trend that the relative survival benefit of inpatient revascularisation may be less in those with an eGFR<30 ml/minute/1.73 m^2 (adjusted OR 0.80, 95% CI 0.52–1.24) compared with the other eGFR categories (eGFR 60–90 ml/minute/1.73 m^2 adjusted OR 0.63, 95% CI 0.49–0.81). However the confidence intervals between eGFR categories overlapped and there was no statistical evidence of modification by severity of renal dysfunction on the association between inpatient revascularisation and death (p-interaction = 0.744) (Table 6 and 7). There was weak evidence of effect modification by gender on this association with a trend to a lower adjusted odds of death in women (p-interaction = 0.060).

Sensitivity Analysis

Results of the logistic regression model adjusted for the propensity score as a single co-variable demonstrated a similar reduction in the odds for death within 1 year associated with inpatient revascularisation (adjusted OR 0.68, 95% CI 0.58–0.80, Table 6).

Limiting the analysis to 5-day survivors did not alter the associations observed (Appendix S4a, 4b and 4c).

We repeated the analysis excluding 116 patients who had declined revascularisation. No change in the associations found in our main analysis was observed (data not shown).

Inclusion of aspirin, clopidogrel, ACE inhibitors, beta-blockers or statins prescribed at discharge in the model did not change the adjusted odds for death associated with inpatient revascularisation within 1 year (adjusted OR 0.68, 95% CI 0.57–0.80), with no evidence of modification by severity of renal dysfunction (p-interaction = 0.711).

After multiple imputation, the adjusted odds ratios were marginally more conservative (Appendix S5a and 5b; data not shown for the analysis of the association between inpatient coronary angiography and death).

Discussion

In this study of over 35 000 individuals with NSTE-ACS in England and Wales, admitted to NHS hospitals between 2008 and 2010, we have demonstrated that renal dysfunction is common and that patients with renal impairment are much less likely to undergo inpatient diagnostic coronary angiography than patients with normal renal function. This association was maintained after adjusting for differences in numerous baseline characteristics and comorbidities and was observed across the range of renal impairment, including those patients with moderate renal dysfunction (eGFR 30–59 ml/minute/1.73 m^2). Inpatient coronary angiography was associated with an improved survival. In those patients with moderate renal dysfunction that did undergo inpatient angiography, nearly 50% of patients then underwent

Table 5. Selected covariates stratified by management strategy in 16 646 adults who underwent inpatient coronary angiography presenting with non-ST-elevation acute coronary syndrome.

	In patient Medical Management	In Patient Revascularisation
	N = 6 914	N = 9 732
Demographic		
Male gender	4 552 (65.8)	7 052 (72.5)
Age in years, median (IQR)	69 (60–77)	66 (57–75)
Past Medical History		
Hypertension	3 784 (54.7)	4 948 (50.8)
Stroke	563 (8.1)	583 (6.0)
PVD	359 (5.2)	383 (3.9)
Treated hyperlipidaemia	2 709 (39.2)	3 968 (40.8)
CCF	369 (5.3)	311 (3.2)
Previous MI	2 050 (29.7)	2 340 (24.0)
Previous PCI	912 (13.2)	1 319 (13.6)
Previous CABG	618 (8.9)	673 (6.9)
Diabetes Mellitus	1 594 (23.1)	1 936 (19.9)
Current smoker	1 656 (24.0)	2 966 (30.5)
Diagnostics		
Haemoglobin (g/dl), median (IQR)	13.8 (12.5–15.0)	14.0 (13.0–15.0)
Peak Troponin, median(IQR)	0.9 (0.2–4.0)	0.8 (0.2–3.3)
eGFR (ml/minute/1.73 m^2)		
>90	1 728 (25.0)	2 992 (30.7)
60–90	3 023 (43.7)	4 422 (45.4)
45–59	1 243 (18.0)	1 370 (14.1)
30–44	669 (9.7)	697 (7.2)
15–29	211 (3.1)	205 (2.1)
<15	40 (0.6)	46 (0.5)
Systolic blood pressure (mmHg), mean (sd)	144 (27)	145 (28)
Heart rate (beats/min), median (IQR)	79 (67–93)	76 (65–88)

Abbreviations: PVD = peripheral vascular disease; CCF = congestive cardiac failure; MI = myocardial infarction; PCI = percutaneous coronary intervention; CABG = coronary artery bypass graft; eGFR = estimated glomerular filtration rate; IQR = interquartile range; sd = standard deviation.
All data is presented as numbers with column percentage unless otherwise stated. Where percentages do not equal 100% this is due to rounding.

revascularisation with a similar survival benefit as seen in patients with preserved renal function.

The majority of patients (84%) with severe renal dysfunction (eGFR<30 ml/min/1.73 m^2) did not undergo inpatient diagnostic angiography. Therefore it is unclear whether, amongst this large group without inpatient diagnostic angiography, early revascularisation in those with suitable coronary lesions would have imparted a survival benefit.

Our finding that patients with renal dysfunction are less likely to undergo early coronary angiography than patients with preserved renal function is supported by several other analyses from different health care systems [1,8–10,25]. We suspect that the reasons are complex, reflecting both individual patient and clinician level factors as well as organisational factors spanning community and hospital level care. Patients with renal dysfunction are more likely to present with atypical clinical features [25,26] and not necessarily directly to cardiologists. Clinical uncertainty as to the interpretation of troponin measurements in patients with renal impairment can compound diagnostic difficulties [27]. Concerns regarding the risk of acute kidney injury (AKI), in particular

related to contrast-induced AKI, or a presumed increased risk of bleeding complications are also likely to influence management decisions [6,28]. However, recent work suggests the risks of AKI associated with coronary angiography after ACS are overstated [9]. In addition, routine coronary angiography as part of renal transplant work-up in patients with advanced renal impairment is not associated with an accelerated decline in renal function [29]. As many patients with NSTE-ACS undergo angiography on a semi-urgent basis there are opportunities for clinicians to ensure adequate hydration and optimal angiographic practices that reduce the risk of AKI. In a previous study from the GRACE collaboration the most commonly reported reason for foregoing an early-invasive management strategy in those with renal impairment was insufficient risk (37.7%), while concerns over comorbidity (12.5%) and bleeding (7.2%) were minor in comparison [30]. However, the median GRACE score of those patients deemed 'low risk' was paradoxically high. Misrepresentation of risk and resultant denial of early-invasive management may contribute to worse outcomes in patients with renal dysfunction

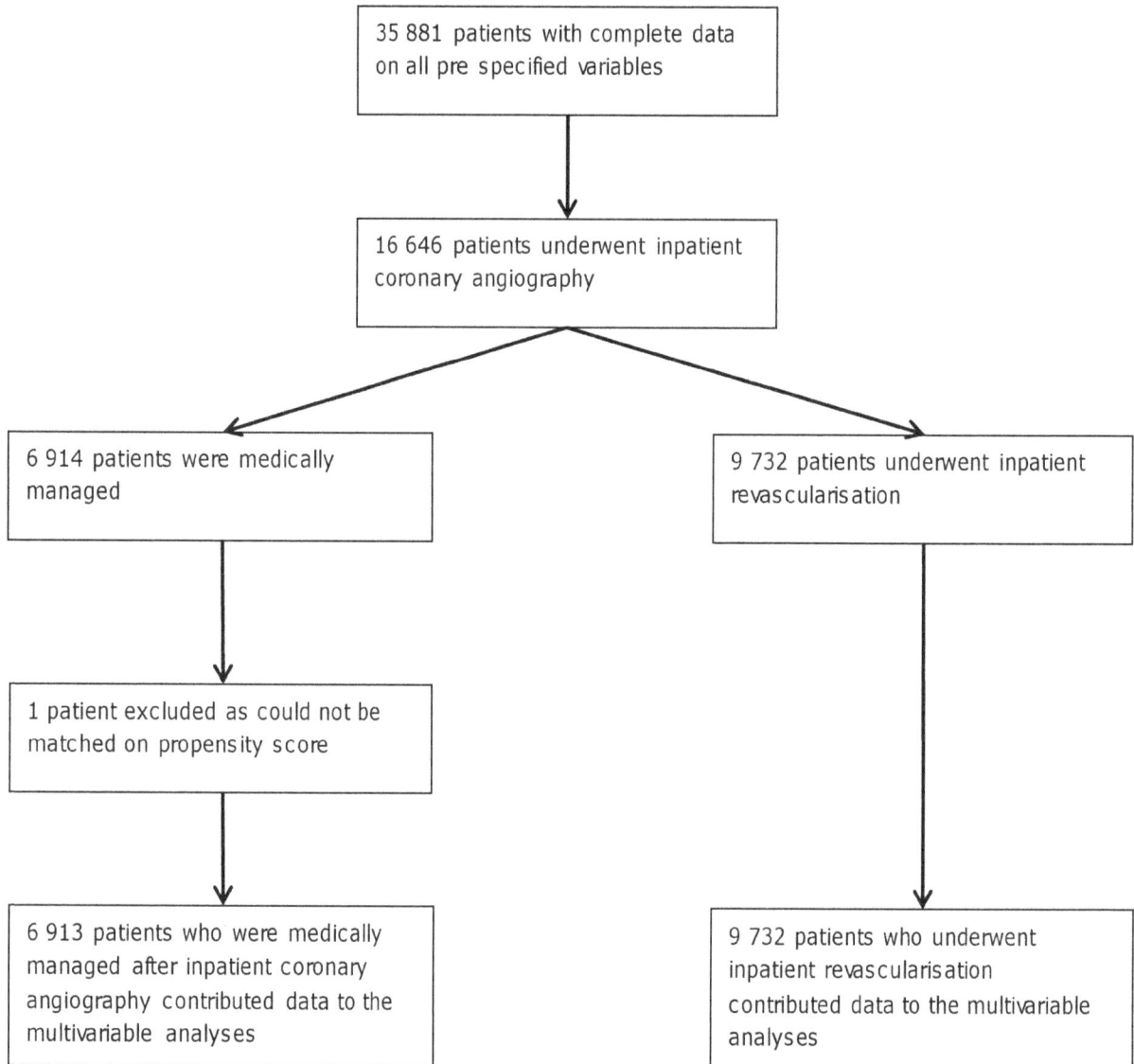

Figure 2. Number of patients in the complete case analysis contributing to various stages of the analysis.

Table 6. Results of the adjusted logistic regression analysis in 16 645 individuals with non-ST-elevation acute coronary syndrome for the association between inpatient revascularisation and mortality compared with individuals who were medically managed after inpatient coronary angiography.

Management Strategy	Age & gender adjusted OR (95% CI)	P-value (Wald)	Multivariable Adjusted OR (95% CI)*	P-value (Wald)	Propensity score adjusted OR (95% CI)	P-value (Wald)
Medical Mx	1		1		1	
In patient Revascularisation	0.60(0.52–0.70)	<0.001	0.66(0.57–0.77)	<0.001	0.68(0.58–0.80)	<0.001

*p-interaction (Wald test) between eGFR category and inpatient revascularisation and mortality: 0.744.
Multivariable Model adjusted for age, ethnicity, gender, IMD score, eGFR, systolic blood pressure, heart rate, haemoglobin, peak troponin, ECG diagnosis, history of angina, hyperlipidaemia, hypertension, peripheral vascular disease, cerebrovascular disease, chronic obstructive airways disease, congestive cardiac failure, previous percutaneous coronary intervention, previous coronary artery bypass graft, previous myocardial infarction, diabetes, current smoking status and hospital.
Propensity Score estimated using age, ethnicity, gender, IMD score, eGFR, systolic blood pressure, heart rate, haemoglobin, peak troponin ECG diagnosis, history of angina, hyperlipidaemia, hypertension, peripheral vascular disease, cerebrovascular disease, chronic obstructive airways disease, congestive cardiac failure, previous percutaneous coronary intervention, previous coronary artery bypass graft, previous myocardial infarction, diabetes, current smoking status.
Abbreviations: Medical Mx = medical management; OR = odds ratio; CI = confidence interval; eGFR = estimated glomerular filtration rate.

Table 7. Results of the adjusted logistic regression analysis in 16 645 individuals with non-ST-elevation acute coronary syndrome for the association between inpatient revascularisation and mortality compared with individuals who were medically managed after inpatient coronary angiography stratified by category of renal dysfunction.

eGFR (ml/minute/1.73 m²)	Management Strategy	Multivariable Adjusted OR (95% CI)*	P-value (Wald)
>90	Medical Mx	1	
	In patient Revascularisation	0.55(0.36–0.85)	0.008
60–90	Medical Mx	1	
	In patient Revascularisation	0.63(0.49–0.81)	<0.001
45–60	Medical Mx	1	
	In patient Revascularisation	0.69(0.51–0.95)	0.020
30–45	Medical Mx	1	
	In patient Revascularisation	0.68(0.49–0.94)	0.021
<30	Medical Mx	1	
	In patient Revascularisation	0.80(0.52–1.24)	0.320

*p-interaction (Wald test) between eGFR category and inpatient revascularisation and mortality: 0.744.
Multivariable Model adjusted for age, ethnicity, gender, IMD score, eGFR, systolic blood pressure, heart rate, haemoglobin, peak troponin, ECG diagnosis, history of angina, hyperlipidaemia, hypertension, peripheral vascular disease, cerebrovascular disease, chronic obstructive airways disease, congestive cardiac failure, previous percutaneous coronary intervention, previous coronary artery bypass graft, previous myocardial infarction, diabetes, current smoking status and hospital.
Propensity Score estimated using age, ethnicity, gender, IMD score, eGFR, systolic blood pressure, heart rate, haemoglobin, peak troponin ECG diagnosis, history of angina, hyperlipidaemia, hypertension, peripheral vascular disease, cerebrovascular disease, chronic obstructive airways disease, congestive cardiac failure, previous percutaneous coronary intervention, previous coronary artery bypass graft, previous myocardial infarction, diabetes, current smoking status.
Abbreviations: Medical Mx = medical management; OR = odds ratio; CI = confidence interval; eGFR = estimated glomerular filtration rate.

[30], and in other high risk groups in whom the same treatment paradox has been observed [31–33].

Earlier major clinical trials have compared a routine early invasive strategy with a selective invasive strategy after NSTE-ACS, rather than outcomes after revascularisation specifically [4,34–36]. Patients with renal impairment have been under-represented in these studies [5] and no direct RCT evidence regarding an early invasive strategy, or specifically outcomes after revascularisation, are available in patients with renal impairment. A systematic review and meta-analysis of individual level data from five RCTs that had recorded information on renal function suggested that the benefits of an early invasive strategy are preserved in patients with renal impairment, with a trend in reduction of risk of death and non-fatal re-infarction at one year (in patients with chronic kidney disease (CKD) stages 3–5 i.e. an eGFR<60 ml/minute/1.73 m², a pooled estimate risk ratio 0.76 (95% CI 0.49–1.17) was reported) [37]. Among the studies included in that meta-analysis the mean age ranged from 59–66 years, 14–28% had diabetes and mortality rates in the 'conservative' arms were 2.5–10%. Patients with CKD accounted for 19.4% (1 453/7 481) with the majority having an eGFR 30–60 ml/minute/1.73 m² (80%). Our real world ACS cohort was quite different to those in the RCTs. In our study, the median age was 75 years, 40% had an eGFR at time of presentation of <60 ml/minute/1.73 m² and at one year 30% of those who did not undergo inpatient coronary angiography had died.

Our analysis of the outcomes associated with inpatient coronary angiography will have included people in the comparison group (those that did not have inpatient coronary angiography) that would have been excluded from the randomised trials, and would therefore not have been considered for revascularisation, thus suggesting a possibly overoptimistic benefit of an early invasive approach. Some of the benefit observed in our comparison of those receiving and those not receiving inpatient angiography may also reflect other management differences between the groups, such as more aggressive antiplatelet or adjunctive medical therapies in the group in our cohort who underwent inpatient coronary angiography [1]. Thus, to further evaluate whether renal function modified outcomes after inpatient revascularisation we restricted the analysis to those in whom a clinical decision to consider revascularisation had been taken following inpatient coronary angiography.

Previous registry-based analyses have reported varied results. Data from the SWEDEHEART registry suggested that early revascularisation improved 1-year survival in patients with NSTE-ACS and mild-to-moderate renal insufficiency [8]. However, the observed benefit declined with lower renal function, and there was a trend toward harm in those with an eGFR<15 ml/minute/1.73 m² or on dialysis (HR 1.61 95% CI 0.84–3.09). The wide confidence interval reflects the low number of patients in this eGFR category (n = 278, with 41 patients undergoing early revascularisation) making it hard to draw firm conclusions. In our study there was no statistical evidence of modification by eGFR category on the survival benefit associated with inpatient revascularisation, a finding supported by a study from the GRACE collaboration [30].

None of our analyses suggest that inpatient angiography or subsequent revascularisation was associated with harm in patients with renal dysfunction, though the fear of this may be influencing clinical judgement and decision making. Consistent with previous studies, the main barrier to revascularisation appears to be the decision to undertake inpatient coronary angiography [30]. The few patients with eGFR<30 ml/min/1.73 m² that do undergo diagnostic angiography may represent a highly select subset of patients with severe renal impairment in whom an early invasive approach is likely to be of most benefit. However, the efficacy of a routine early invasive approach in individuals presenting with this severity of renal dysfunction currently remains essentially undefined.

Our cohort from a national ACS registry provides the most comprehensive account of current clinical practice in England and Wales in terms of the relationships between renal function, early angiography and revascularisation and patient outcomes after NSTE-ACS, and adds further contemporary data to the available research in this field. We have taken account of a range of confounders and have conducted multiple sensitivity analyses, including using datasets derived from multiple imputation, the results of which have supported the findings of our main analyses. However, there are limitations. Most importantly, this is an observational study and not a randomised controlled trial. Confounding may be present although we aimed to minimise this by incorporating a propensity score methodology and a wide range of baseline characteristics. We did not have a direct measure of true kidney function and used eGFR based on the CKD-EPI formula. As only a single creatinine was available for each patient we were unable to evaluate the components of chronic kidney disease or acute kidney injury. Our conclusions therefore refer to renal function at the time of presentation. However, given that historical creatinine values may not always be available to practising clinicians when they make decisions regarding angiography or revascularisation we argue that the findings of this analysis are relevant to clinical practice. Currently, identification of patients on dialysis or those with a renal transplant is not possible within the MINAP dataset. Very few individuals with an eGFR<30 ml/minute/1.73 m^2 contributed to the analysis focussed on inpatient revascularisation and survival as so few had an inpatient coronary angiogram, so it is very likely that individuals on dialysis were excluded. We did not have details of coronary anatomy. After coronary angiography some patients will be treated medically because no treatable culprit lesion is present and others because revascularisation carries unacceptable risk or is unlikely to be successful. Having this information would enable a much more detailed description of the differences between patients with various degrees of renal function, and a deeper understanding of management strategies used and patient outcomes. We lacked information on other important characteristics that stratify risk (in patients who are not offered a routine invasive approach), for example the results of stress tests and measurements of left ventricular function. Nor did we have information on clinical events in hospital, such as further myocardial infarction, which may have influenced clinical decision making. While we were able to categorise patients into those with and those without angiography (and subsequent revascularisation) we lacked information regarding delay from admission to intervention. To evaluate the risk of potential survivor bias we undertook sensitivity analyses restricted to those who survived more than five days, but this is an important limitation. Other outcomes such as cardiac specific mortality, in-hospital mortality and length of stay would be valuable additional information. As mentioned above, our analysis may also have lacked power to detect evidence of modification by category of renal dysfunction on outcomes by management

strategy due to the relatively low numbers of individuals with severe renal impairment contributing to that analysis.

Our analyses from MINAP provide further evidence that patients with renal dysfunction are much less likely to undergo inpatient coronary angiography than individuals with preserved renal function which is not explained by associated comorbidity. Inpatient coronary angiography was associated with improved survival across all categories of renal dysfunction. After inpatient angiography, relative outcomes following revascularisation were not modified by severity of renal dysfunction. As in previous studies however low patient numbers with severe renal dysfunction limit the ability to draw firm conclusions.

There is a discrepancy between the care advised in clinical guidelines regarding an early invasive strategy in patients with renal dysfunction and NSTE-ACS, and care delivered in clinical practice. Further research is required to understand why this variation exists and determine whether there are missed opportunities for quality improvement. In patients with severe renal impairment or those on dialysis a RCT is required to definitively evaluate the efficacy and optimal timing of early angiography and subsequent revascularisation after NSTE-ACS.

Supporting Information

Appendix S1 Distribution of the conditional propensity scores for undergoing inpatient revascularisation after inpatient coronary angiography.

Appendix S2 Frequency of missing data in the non-ST-elevation acute coronary syndrome dataset.

Appendix S3 Key covariates in the patients included in the complete case analysis and patients that were excluded due to incomplete data.

Appendix S4 Comparison between the results of the complete case analysis and the analysis restricted to patients who survived for 5 days or more.

Appendix S5 Comparison between the results of the complete case analysis and the analysis using 10 datasets derived using multiple imputation.

Author Contributions

Conceived and designed the experiments: C. Shaw JS DN C. Sharpe. Analyzed the data: C. Shaw RS. Wrote the paper: C. Shaw. Commented on drafts and approved the final version of the paper and are in agreement with submission to PLOS ONE: DN RS CJ SS DO'D DF CW C. Sharpe.

References

1. Fox CS, Muntner P, Chen AY, Alexander KP, Roe MT, et al. (2010) Use of Evidence-Based Therapies in Short-Term Outcomes of ST-Segment Elevation Myocardial Infarction and Non–ST-Segment Elevation Myocardial Infarction in Patients With Chronic Kidney Disease: A Report From the National Cardiovascular Data Acute Coronary Treatment and Intervention Outcomes Network Registry. Circulation 121: 357–365.

2. Go AS, Chertow GM, Fan D, McCulloch CE, Hsu C-y (2004) Chronic Kidney Disease and the Risks of Death, Cardiovascular Events, and Hospitalization. New England Journal of Medicine 351: 1296–1305.

3. Kerr M, Bray B, Medcalf J, O'Donoghue DJ, Matthews B (2012) Estimating the financial cost of chronic kidney disease to the NHS in England. Nephrology Dialysis Transplantation 27 (Suppl 3): 373–80.

4. Fox KAA, Clayton TC, Damman P, Pocock SJ, de Winter RJ, et al. (2010) Long-Term Outcome of a Routine Versus Selective Invasive Strategy in Patients With Non–ST-Segment Elevation Acute Coronary SyndromeA Meta-Analysis of Individual Patient Data. Journal of the American College of Cardiology 55: 2435–2445.

5. Coca S, Krumholz HM, Garg AX, Parikh CR (2006) Under representation of renal disease in randomized controlled trials of cardiovascular disease. JAMA 296: 1377–1384.

6. Hamm CW, Bassand JP, Agewall S, Bax J, Boersma E, et al. (2011) ESC Guidelines for the management of acute coronary syndromes in patients presenting without persistent ST-segment elevation: The Task Force for the management of acute coronary syndromes (ACS) in patients presenting without

persistent ST-segment elevation of the European Society of Cardiology (ESC). European Heart Journal 32(23): 2999–3054.

7. Jneid H, Anderson JL, Wright RS, Adams CD, Bridges CR, et al. (2012) ACCF/AHA Focused Update of the Guideline for the Management of Patients With Unstable Angina/Non–ST-Elevation Myocardial Infarction (Updating the 2007 Guideline and Replacing the 2011 Focused Update): A Report of the American College of Cardiology Foundation/American Heart Association Task Force on Practice Guidelines. Circulation 126: 875–910.

8. Szummer K, Lundman P, Jacobson SH, Schön S, Lindbäck J, et al. (2009) Influence of Renal Function on the Effects of Early Revascularization in Non-ST-Elevation Myocardial Infarction: Data From the Swedish Web-System for Enhancement and Development of Evidence-Based Care in Heart Disease Evaluated According to Recommended Therapies (SWEDEHEART). Circulation 120: 851–858.

9. James MT, Tonelli M, Ghali WA, Knudtson ML, Faris P, et al. (2013) Renal outcomes associated with invasive versus conservative management of acute coronary syndrome: propensity matched cohort study. BMJ 347: f4151.

10. Blicher TM, Hommel K, Olesen JB, Torp-Pedersen C, Madsen M, et al. (2013) Less use of standard guideline-based treatment of myocardial infarction in patients with chronic kidney disease: a Danish nation-wide cohort study. European Heart Journal 34: 2916–2923.

11. Herrett E, Smeeth L, Walker L, Weston C (2010) The Myocardial Ischaemia National Audit Project (MINAP). Heart 96: 1264–1267.

12. Birkhead J, Pearson M, Norris RM, Rickards AF, Georgiou A (2002) The National Audit of Myocardial Infarction: a new development in the audit process. Journal of Clinical Excellence 4: 379–385.

13. Birkhead JS (2000) Responding to the requirements of the National Service Framework for coronary disease: a core data set for myocardial infarction. Heart 84: 116–117.

14. Levey AS, Stevens LA, Schmid CH, Zhang Y, Castro F III, et al. (2009) A New Equation to Estimate Glomerular Filtration Rate. Annals of Internal Medicine 150: 604–612.

15. Kidney Disease: Improving Global Outcomes (KDIGO) CKD Work Group (2013) KDIGO Clinical Practice Guideline for the Evaluation and Management of Chronic Kidney Disease. Kidney inter., Suppl.; 3: 1–150.

16. Department for Communities and Local Government (2010) The English Indices of Deprivation.

17. Eagle KA, Lim MJ, Dabbous OH Pieper KS, Goldberg RJ, et al. (2004) A validated prediction model for all forms of acute coronary syndrome: Estimating the risk of 6-month postdischarge death in an international registry. JAMA 291(22): 2727–2733.

18. Rosenbaum PR, Rubin DB (1983) The central role of the propensity score in observational studies for causal effects. Biometrika 70: 41–55.

19. Hoenig MR, Aroney CN, Scott IA (2010) Early invasive versus conservative strategies for unstable angina and non-ST elevation myocardial infarction in the stent era. Cochrane Database of Systematic Reviews.

20. Flather MD, Yusuf S, Køber L, Pfeffer M, Hall A, et al. (2000) Long-term ACE-inhibitor therapy in patients with heart failure or left-ventricular dysfunction: a systematic overview of data from individual patients. The Lancet 355: 1575–1581.

21. Cannon CP, Braunwald E, McCabe CH, Rader DJ, Rouleau JL, et al. (2004) Intensive versus Moderate Lipid Lowering with Statins after Acute Coronary Syndromes. New England Journal of Medicine 350: 1495–1504.

22. López Sendó J, Swedberg K, McMurray J, Tamargo J, Maggioni AP, et al. (2004) Expert consensus document on β-adrenergic receptor blockers: The Task Force on Beta-Blockers of the European Society of Cardiology. European Heart Journal 25: 1341–1362.

23. Antithrombotic Trialists' Collaboration (2002) Collaborative meta-analysis of randomised trials of antiplatelet therapy for prevention of death, myocardial infarction, and stroke in high risk patients. BMJ 324: 71–86.

24. Rubin DB (1987) Multiple Imputation for Nonresponse in Surveys; John Wiley and Sons.

25. Fox KAA, Anderson FA, Dabbous OH, Steg PG, López Sendón J, et al. (2007) Intervention in acute coronary syndrome: do patients undergo intervention on the basis of their risk characteristics? The Global Registry of Acute Coronary Events (GRACE). Heart 93: 177–182.

26. Herzog CA (2003) How to Manage the Renal Patient with Coronary Heart Disease: The Agony and the Ecstasy of Opinion-Based Medicine. Journal of the American Society of Nephrology 14: 2556–2572.

27. Kanderian AS, Francis GS (2006) Cardiac troponins and chronic kidney disease. Kidney Int 69: 1112–1114.

28. Wickenbrock I, Perings C, Maagh P, Quack I, Bracht M, et al. (2009) Contrast medium induced nephropathy in patients undergoing percutaneous coronary intervention for acute coronary syndrome: differences in STEMI and NSTEMI. Clinical Research in Cardiology 98: 765–772.

29. Kumar N, Dahri L, Brown W, Duncan N, Singh S, et al. (2009) Effect of Elective Coronary Angiography on Glomerular Filtration Rate in Patients with Advanced Chronic Kidney Disease. Clinical Journal of the American Society of Nephrology 4: 1907–1913.

30. Wong JA, Goodman SG, Yan RT, Wald R, Bagnall AJ, et al. (2009) Temporal management patterns and outcomes of non-ST elevation acute coronary syndromes in patients with kidney dysfunction. European Heart Journal 30: 549–557.

31. Lee CH, Tan M, Yan AT, Fitchett D, Grima EA, et al. (2008) Use of cardiac catheterization for non–st-segment elevation acute coronary syndromes according to initial risk: Reasons why physicians choose not to refer their patients. Archives of Internal Medicine 168: 291–296.

32. Yan AT, Yan RT, Tan M, Fung A, Cohen EA, et al. (2007) Management patterns in relation to risk stratification among patients with non–st elevation acute coronary syndromes. Archives of Internal Medicine 167: 1009–1016.

33. Chertow GM, Normand SLT, McNeil BJ (2004) "Renalism": Inappropriately Low Rates of Coronary Angiography in Elderly Individuals with Renal Insufficiency. Journal of the American Society of Nephrology 15: 2462–2468.

34. Damman P, Hirsch A, Windhausen F, Tijssen JGP, de Winter RJ (2010) 5-Year Clinical Outcomes in the ICTUS (Invasive versus Conservative Treatment in Unstable coronary Syndromes) Trial: A Randomized Comparison of an Early Invasive Versus Selective Invasive Management in Patients With Non–ST-Segment Elevation Acute Coronary Syndrome. Journal of the American College of Cardiology 55: 858–864.

35. Boden WE, ORourke RA, Crawford MH, Blaustein AS, Deedwania PC, et al. (1998) Outcomes in Patients with Acute Non–Q-Wave Myocardial Infarction Randomly Assigned to an Invasive as Compared with a Conservative Management Strategy. New England Journal of Medicine 338: 1785–1792.

36. Cannon CP, Weintraub WS, Demopoulos LA, Vicari R, Frey MJ, et al. (2001) Comparison of Early Invasive and Conservative Strategies in Patients with Unstable Coronary Syndromes Treated with the Glycoprotein IIb/IIIa Inhibitor Tirofiban. New England Journal of Medicine 344: 1879–1887.

37. Charytan DM, Wallentin L, Lagerqvist B, Spacek R, De Winter RJ, et al. (2009) Early Angiography in Patients with Chronic Kidney Disease: A Collaborative Systematic Review. Clinical Journal of the American Society of Nephrology 4: 1032–1043.

2

Socioeconomic Status Correlates with the Prevalence of Advanced Coronary Artery Disease in the United States

Bronislava Bashinskaya[1,2], Brian V. Nahed[3], Brian P. Walcott[3]*, Jean-Valery C. E. Coumans[3], Oyere K. Onuma[1]

1 Massachusetts General Hospital and Department of Medicine (Cardiology Division), Harvard Medical School, Boston, Massachusetts, United States of America, 2 Boston University, Boston, Massachusetts, United States of America, 3 Massachusetts General Hospital and Department of Surgery (Neurosurgery Division), Harvard Medical School, Boston, Massachusetts, United States of America

Abstract

Background: Increasingly studies have identified socioeconomic factors adversely affecting healthcare outcomes for a multitude of diseases. To date, however, there has not been a study correlating socioeconomic details from nationwide databases on the prevalence of advanced coronary artery disease. We seek to identify whether socioeconomic factors contribute to advanced coronary artery disease prevalence in the United States.

Methods and Findings: State specific prevalence data was queried form the United States Nationwide Inpatient Sample for 2009. Patients undergoing percutaneous coronary angioplasty and coronary artery bypass graft were identified as principal procedures. Non-cardiac related procedures, lung lobectomy and hip replacement (partial and total) were identified and used as control groups. Information regarding prevalence was then merged with data from the Behavioral Risk Factor Surveillance System, the largest, on-going telephone health survey system tracking health conditions and risk behaviors in the United States. Pearson's correlation coefficient was calculated for individual socioeconomic variables including employment status, level of education, and household income. Household income and education level were inversely correlated with the prevalence of percutaneous coronary angioplasty (-0.717; -0.787) and coronary artery bypass graft surgery (-0.541; -0.618). This phenomenon was not seen in the non-cardiac procedure control groups. In multiple linear regression analysis, socioeconomic factors were significant predictors of coronary artery bypass graft and percutaneous transluminal coronary angioplasty ($p<0.001$ and $p=0.005$, respectively).

Conclusions: Socioeconomic status is related to the prevalence of advanced coronary artery disease as measured by the prevalence of percutaneous coronary angioplasty and coronary artery bypass graft surgery.

Editor: Giuseppe Biondi-Zoccai, Sapienza University of Rome, Italy

Funding: The authors have no support or funding to report.

Competing Interests: The authors have declared that no competing interests exist.

* E-mail: walcott.brian@mgh.harvard.edu

Introduction

Despite preventive measures and aggressive therapy, coronary artery disease (CAD) is responsible for one out of every six deaths in the United States [1]. An estimated 785,000 individuals have a new myocardial infarction every year and more than half have a recurrent attack [1]. It is well known that a multitude of modifiable risk factors contribute to coronary artery disease. These factors include cholesterol levels, smoking status, hypertension, obesity, psychosocial status, consumption of fruits, vegetables, alcohol, physical activity, smoking status, and many more [2] [3]. Modification of these risk factors, presumably as a result of preventive outpatient care, can have dramatic effects on the primary prevention of CAD. This has been seen in studies on the effects of cholesterol modification with HMG-CoA Reductase inhibitors [4–6] in addition to the non-pharmacologic effects of diet, exercise, and smoking abstinence [7].

Healthcare in the United States is not universally equitable leading to disparities in access to preventive and primary care.

Modifiable CAD risk factors such as cigarette smoking [8], hyperlipidemia [9,10], and diabetes [1,11] have been shown to be disproportionately linked to socioeconomic factors. A study examining these risk factors specifically as they relate to cardiovascular disease has determined that while longitudinal improvements are being made, not all sub-populations in society are equally benefiting. Disparities related to education and income based sub-populations associated with these risk factors are increasingly worse [12,13]. For example, African-American adults have among the highest rates of hypertension in the world (>43%) [1]. These ultimately summate into differences in cardiovascular disease that are recognizable at a geographic (state) level [14].

Socioeconomic factors influence the prevalence of well-established CAD risk factors, and likely influence the prevalence of advanced CAD. Using a disease prevalence approach rather than risk factor analysis, we aim to identify the significance of distinct populations based on income, education level, and employment status as they relate to advanced CAD. This is of significant

Table 1. ICD-9-CM codes grouped according to clinical classifications software.

CCS Code	Procedure	ICD-9-CM Codes
36	Lung resection; lobectomy or pneumonectomy	3220 3221 3222 3223 3224 3225 3226 3227 3229 323 3230 3239 324 3241 3249 325 3250 3259
44	Coronary artery bypass graft (CABG)	3610 3611 3612 3613 3614 3615 3616 3617 3619 362 363 3631 3632 3633 3634 3639
45	Percutaneous transluminal coronary angioplasty (PTCA)	0066 1755 3601 3602 3605
153	Hip replacement; total and partial	0070 0071 0072 0073 0074 0075 0076 0077 0085 0086 0087 8151 8152 8153 8169

importance given the recent focus on improvement with healthcare utilization and quality.

Methods

This study was determined exempt from the Massachusetts General Hospital Institutional Review Board given the de-identified nature of the dataset. To protect confidentiality of patients, the dataset provided suppressed reporting when values were based on 10 or fewer discharges or when fewer than two hospitals in the state were reporting. Survey data was previously obtained via telephone interview from adults 18 years or older who gave verbal consent for de-identified participation. Only one adult was interviewed per household and participants were not compensated.

State specific prevalence data from the US Nationwide Inpatient Sample was queried from the most recent available year, 2009. Weighted national estimates were provided from the Agency for Healthcare Research and Quality (AHRQ), Health-care Cost and Utilization Project's Nationwide Inpatient Sample (NIS) for 2009, based on data collected by individual states and provided to the AHRQ. The total number of weighted discharges in the U.S. is based on the NIS total of = 39,434,956. Statistics based on estimates with a relative standard error (standard error/weighted estimate) greater than 0.30 were excluded. Statistics were

only based on hospitals that meet the definition of "community hospital" - nonfederal, short-term, general and other specialty hospitals, including public hospitals and academic medical centers. Excluded from the analysis were federal, rehabilitation, and psychiatric hospitals, as well as alcoholism/chemical dependency treatment facilities.

The principal procedure was defined as the definitive treatment during the hospital admission (not diagnostic or exploratory). The unit of identification was the discharge: if a particular procedure occurred multiple times during the same discharge, it was only counted once. State-specific prevalence data was then used for further analysis.

Coronary artery bypass graft (CABG) and percutaneous transluminal coronary angioplasty (PTCA) were identified as principal procedures using clinical classifications software (CCS) of ICD-9-CM codes 44 and 45, respectively [15]. Additional procedures, including lung resection and hip replacement (partial and total) were identified as control groups. [Table 1] Information regarding prevalence and in-hospital mortality for each procedure was merged with data from the Behavioral Risk Factor Surveillance System (BRFSS), the largest, on-going telephone health survey system tracking health conditions and risk behaviors in the United States. Statistical analysis of the distribution of results was performed with Prism 5 and InStat for Mac (GraphPad Software, Inc). First, a univariate analysis was performed to evaluate

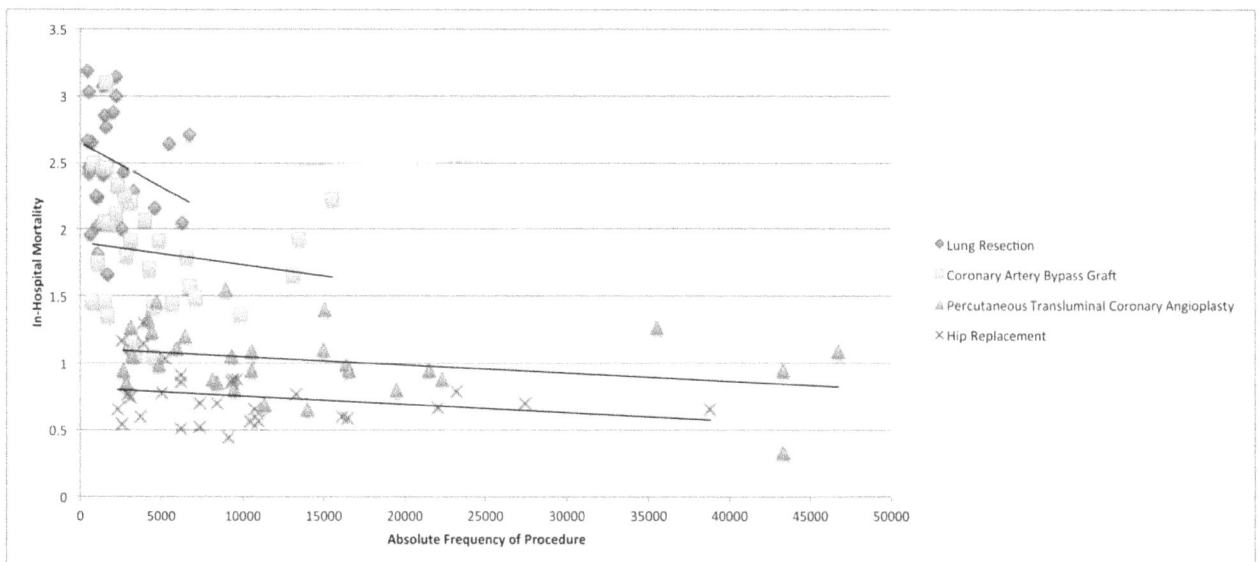

Figure 1. In-hospital morality decreases with increasing absolute frequency of a procedure.

Table 2. States with data available for analysis.

Arizona
Arkansas
California
Colorado
Florida
Illinois
Iowa
Kansas
Kentucky
Maine
Maryland
Massachusetts
Michigan
Minnesota
Missouri
Nebraska
Nevada
New Jersey
New Mexico
New York
North Carolina
Oklahoma
Oregon
South Carolina
Tennessee
Texas
Utah
Washington
West Virginia
Wisconsin

outcomes (population-adjusted procedure prevalence) and the individual socioeconomic variables including employment status, level of education, and household income. A correlation coefficient was calculated independently, without considering the other variables. For the variable of "unemployed for greater than one year", homemakers, students, retired persons, self-employed persons, and those unable to work were excluded. Value ranges of 0–0.09, 0.1–0.3, 0.31–0.5, and 0.51–1.0 were considered to have no, small, medium, and strong correlations, respectively. Next, a multiple linear regression model was constructed to account for all three socioeconomic variables and the population-adjusted prevalence for each procedure. Significance was pre-defined at $p < 0.05$.

Results

Thirty states provided adequate data for interpretation. [Table 2] There was a small to medium negative correlation with prevalence of procedure and in-hospital mortality for all procedures in a state-by-state analysis (Pearson's correlation coefficient (r) range -0.137 to -0.303). [Figure 1] That is, as the absolute frequency of each procedure increased, the in-hospital mortality decreased.

For lung resection (CCS 36), there were a total of 58,176 discharges available for analysis with a mean in-hospital mortality of 2.51%. There was no correlation with the population adjusted prevalence and the percentage of adults unemployed for greater than one year ($r = 0.045$). However, there were small negative correlations with both household income greater than \$ 50,000 USD and having more than a high school education and the population adjusted prevalence ($r = -0.130$ and -0.188, respectively).

For coronary artery bypass graft (CCS 44), there were a total of 135,139 discharges available for analysis with a mean in-hospital mortality of 1.82%. There was a small negative correlation with the population adjusted prevalence and the percentage of adults unemployed for greater than one year ($r = -0.167$). Importantly, there were strong negative correlations with both household income greater than \$ 50,000 USD and having more than a high school education and the population adjusted prevalence ($r = -0.717$ and -0.787, respectively). [Figures 2, 3, 4]

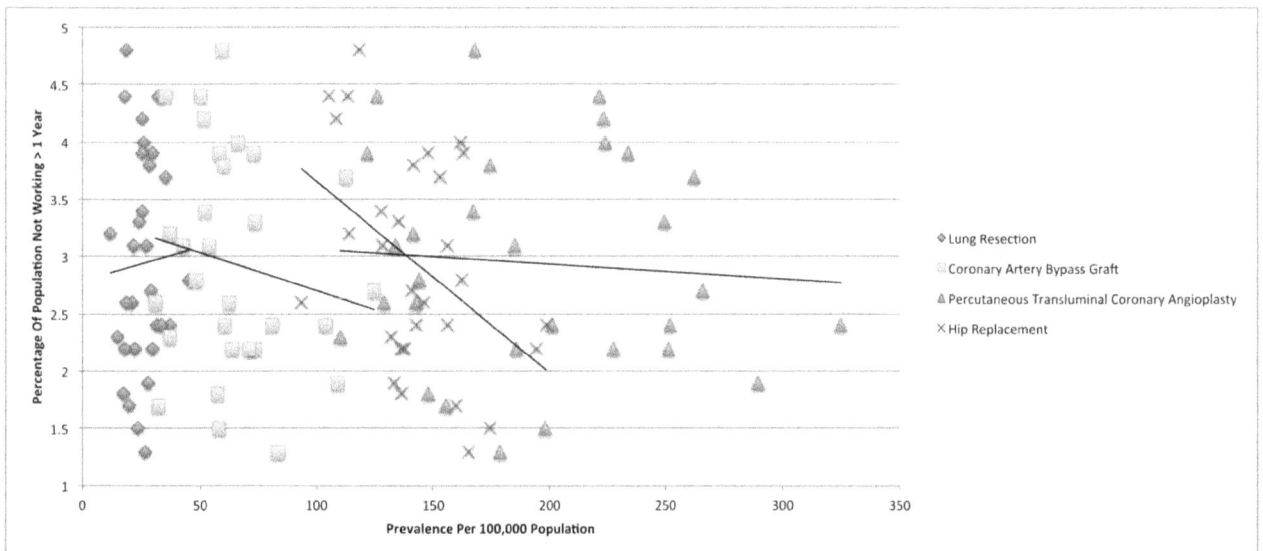

Figure 2. Unemployment for greater than one year is not associated with advanced coronary artery disease.

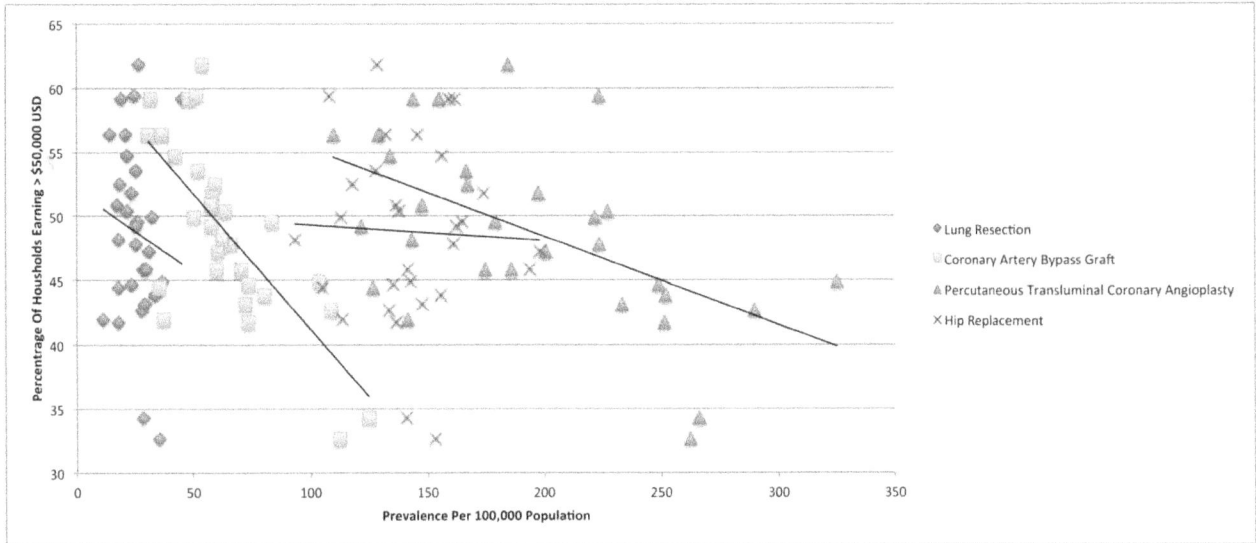

Figure 3. Income is strongly correlated with the prevelance of advanced coronary artery disease.

For percutaneous transluminal coronary angioplasty (CCS 45), there were a total of 428,186 discharges available for analysis with a mean in-hospital mortality of 1.02%. There was no correlation with the population adjusted prevalence and the percentage of adults unemployed for greater than one year (r = 0.076). There were strong negative correlations with both household income greater than $ 50,000 USD and having more than a high school education and the population adjusted prevalence (r = −0.541 and −0.618, respectively).

For hip replacement (CCS 153), there were a total of 303,741 discharges available for analysis with a mean in-hospital mortality of 0.75%. There was a medium negative correlation with the population adjusted prevalence and the percentage of adults unemployed for greater than one year (r = −0.431). However, there was no discernable correlation with either household income

greater than $ 50,000 USD or having more than a high school education and the population adjusted prevalence (r = −0.042 and −0.002, respectively). A summary of the Pearson's correlation coefficient calculations for all procedures is provided in Table 3.

Finally, a multiple linear regression analysis was performed with all three socioeconomic variables for each procedure. [Table 4] Socioeconomic factors were significant predictors of coronary artery bypass graft and percutaneous transluminal coronary angioplasty (p<0.001 and p = 0.005 for overall model, respectively).

Discussion

Some disease processes can be analyzed with sufficient sensitivity and specificity on a large scale by identifying procedures

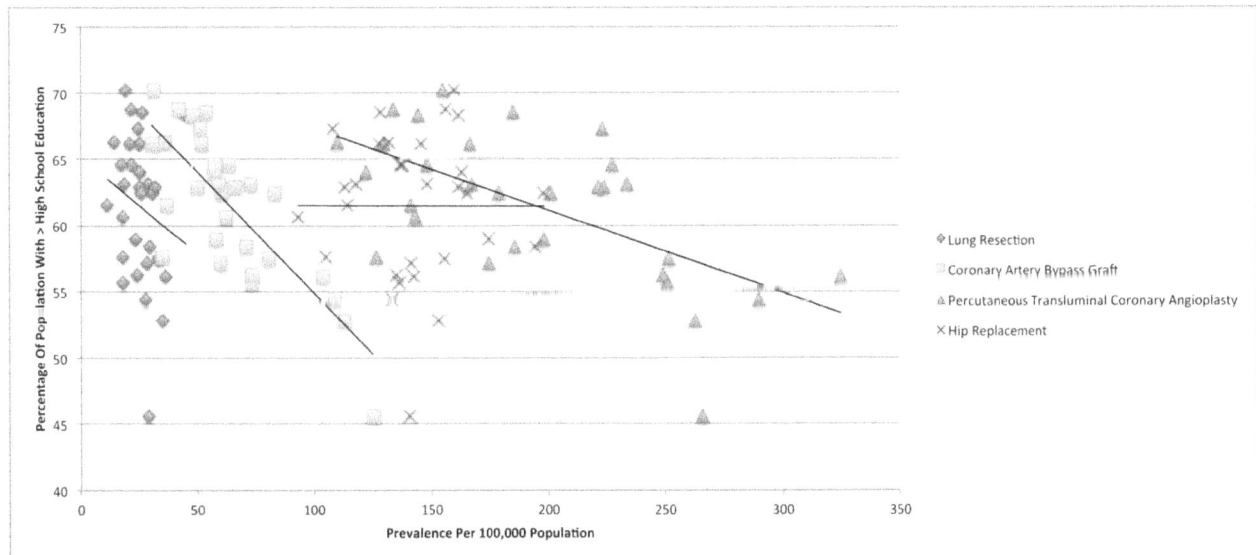

Figure 4. Education level is strongly correlated with the prevalence of advanced coronary artery disease.

Table 3. Relationship between individual socioeconomic variables and the prevalence of different procedures.

	Employment	Education	Income
Lung resection; lobectomy or pneumonectomy	0.045	−0.130	−0.188
Coronary artery bypass graft (CABG)	−0.167	**−0.717****	**−0.787****
Percutaneous transluminal coronary angioplasty (PTCA)	0.076	**−0.541****	**−0.618****
Hip replacement; total and partial	−0.431	−0.042	−0.002

**Strong correlation, Pearson's correlation coefficient.
A correlation matrix was established for various procedures (column 1) and socioeconomic factors (columns 2–4). A Pearson's correlation coefficient was established for each relationship. A negative value indicates a negative correlation. Value ranges of 0–0.09, 0.1–0.3, 0.31–0.5, and 0.51–1.0 were considered to have no, small, medium, and strong correlations, respectively. CABG and PTCA had a strong negative correlation with both education and income.
Socioeconomic Factors Key.
Employment = unemployed for greater than one year.
Education = having more than a high school education.
Income = household income greater than $ 50,000 USD.

related to their advanced stage. For example, early diagnosis and aggressive treatment of *Helicobacter pylori* infection has led to decreased incidence of advanced gastrointestinal ulcer hemorrhage or bowel perforation, and as result fewer surgical procedures related to this diagnosis [16]. Alternatively, improved diagnosis and aggressive treatment may lead to increased frequency of procedures secondary to efficacy as with surgical procedures for ischemic stroke [17].

In this manuscript, we used well-established surrogates for advanced coronary artery disease, coronary artery bypass graft and percutaneous transluminal coronary angioplasty, and investigated their relationship with socioeconomic factors [18–20].

The number of cardiac revascularization procedures was inversely related to highest education levels of the patients. This

coincides with an established body of evidence that the highest formal education level corresponds to known risk factors for heart disease, such as obesity [21], diabetes [22], and hypertension [23]. Education level is also an established and well known correlate of non-cardiac related conditions, such as cancer [24], rheumatoid arthritis [25], cerebrovascular disease [23], and back pain [26]. Education level is an important marker of socioeconomic status not only because it describes the educational attainment that may confer a better understanding and self-management of preventative health measures, but it also indirectly relates to earning potential (household income) and employment status that can both influence ones ability to obtain routine healthcare.

Coronary artery disease often results from a culmination of multiple patient-centered factors such as diet and exercise [27].

Table 4. Multiple linear regression analysis of socioeconomic factors.

Procedure	Variable	Regression Coefficient	95% Confidence Interval	Goodness of Model Fit (R-squared)	Overall Model Significance (P value)
Lung resection; lobectomy or pneumonectomy	Education	−0.491	−1.63, 0.64	0.047	0.732
	Income	0.218	−0.68, 1.12		
	Employment	0.567	−2.49, 3.62		
Coronary artery bypass graft (CABG)	Education	−2.774	−5.10, −0.45	0.641	**<0.001 ****
	Income	−0.509	−2.35, 1.33		
	Employment	−3.708	−9.96, 2.54		
Percutaneous transluminal coronary angioplasty (PTCA)	Education	−6.331	−13.39, 0.73	0.390	**0.005****
	Income	0.169	−5.42, 5.76		
	Employment	−2.708	−21.71, 16.29		
Hip replacement; total and partial	Education	1.711	−1.79, 5.21	0.221	0.086
	Income	−1.450	−4.22, 1.32		
	Employment	−12.201	−21.62, −2.79		

**Significant.
A multiple linear regression analysis was performed for each procedure (column 1) and three socioeconomic factors (column 2). Individual regression coefficients are identified (column 3), along with their respective 95% confidence intervals (column 4). The goodness of model fit (column 5) is the percent of the variation explained by the model. The P value (column 6) represents the significance of each regression model as a whole, incorporating education, income, and employment as variables. This model was significant in describing the relationship of the three socioeconomic variables and the prevalence of CABG and PTCA. No causal mechanism can be identified with any regression analysis technique.

Lifestyle choices such as diet and activity level influence cardiovascular disease risk factors such as hypertension and diabetes mellitus and in turn the development of coronary atherosclerosis [28–32]. Education, both in the classroom setting and via a healthcare provider are likely to influence patient compliance with healthy lifestyle choices as they relate to cardiovascular disease prevention. This provides some explanation to the strong negative correlation of education and the decreased prevalence of coronary artery disease.

Another finding of this study was that income levels correlate with the prevalence of advanced coronary artery disease. Household income levels have previously been associated with health insurance status, medical care use, health, and employment [33]. In a complex interplay of these factors, household income provides a summative metric to compare groups. We chose a value much higher than the defined poverty level in an effort to compensate for the anticipated costs of a balanced diet and healthcare coverage. Even at the generous mark of $ 50,000 USD, a strong correlation was present. It should be noted that no accounting could be made for household size in relationship to income level, as this data does not exist in the accessed databases.

Additional factors that likely influence the development of advanced cardiovascular disease include biological differences in certain ethnic and gender groups not accounted for in this study, such as factors that alter the interaction between prothrombotic factors and atherosclerosis [13]. It has been shown that living in a disadvantaged neighborhood is a risk factor for coronary heart disease, even after controlling for income and education [34].

The strength of this study includes the use of two well-established national databases that encompass hundreds of thousands of people, enabling a robust comparison between study and control groups. Limitations include the geographic reporting at the state level that make regional differences at the neighborhood or even city level difficult to account for. There also exist state-to-state differences in practice patterns between CABG and PTCA. In one of the largest studies of regional discrepancies in treatment modalities for acute myocardial infarction cardiac revascularization, state specific CABG rates varied from 9.3% to 13.1% [35]. The state specific rates for PTCA associated with acute myocardial intervention varied much more widely, ranging from 16.8 to 36.0% [35]. State specific factors may influence whether one is more likely to undergo CABG or PCTA for acute myocardial infarction, however no data currently exist regarding the prevalence of these procedures in all settings.

Inherent to national databases is the potential for geographical biases with respect to aggressiveness of intervention. For example, a patient with multiple medical comorbidities in poor clinical condition may be considered a candidate for CABG in one state but perhaps not in another. These differences are difficult to quantify from a population-based standpoint and are best addressed with prospective, intention to treat analysis. These databases also lack information on the degree of severity of the coronary artery blockage and do not capture clinical data points such as time interval from symptom onset to treatment. All data recorded in national databases are subject to various coding anomalies. We attempted to eliminate this bias by focusing exclusively on the principal diagnosis (that is the major determinant of reimbursement rates) with the assistance of CCS grouping that systematically and compressively identifies key ICD-9-CM procedure codes. Additionally, not all states participate in the BRFSS, limiting the analysis to the data of 30 states. This study is expected to generally underestimate differences in health status, as the amount of undiagnosed disease in those without *any* access to care is impossible to report.

Conclusions

Socioeconomic factors are associated with the prevalence of advanced coronary artery disease, as defined by the geographic prevalence of percutaneous transluminal coronary angioplasty and coronary artery bypass graft surgery. Additional investigation is needed to better define and mitigate the role of socioeconomic factors on the burden of coronary artery disease.

Author Contributions

Conceived and designed the experiments: BB JVC BPW. Performed the experiments: BB OKO JVC BPW. Analyzed the data: BB JVC OKO BVN BPW. Wrote the paper: BB OKO BVN JVC BPW.

References

1. Lloyd-Jones D, Adams RJ, Brown TM, Carnethon M, Dai S, et al. (2010) Heart disease and stroke statistics–2010 update: a report from the American Heart Association. Circulation 121: e46–e215.
2. Wilson PW, D'Agostino RB, Levy D, Belanger AM, Silbershatz H, et al. (1998) Prediction of coronary heart disease using risk factor categories. Circulation 97: 1837–1847.
3. Yusuf S, Hawken S, Ounpuu S, Dans T, Avezum A, et al. (2004) Effect of potentially modifiable risk factors associated with myocardial infarction in 52 countries (the INTERHEART study): case-control study. Lancet 364: 937–952.
4. Shepherd J, Cobbe SM, Ford I, Isles CG, Lorimer AR, et al. (1995) Prevention of coronary heart disease with pravastatin in men with hypercholesterolemia. West of Scotland Coronary Prevention Study Group. N Engl J Med 333: 1301–1307.
5. Colhoun HM, Betteridge DJ, Durrington PN, Hitman GA, Neil HA, et al. (2004) Primary prevention of cardiovascular disease with atorvastatin in type 2 diabetes in the Collaborative Atorvastatin Diabetes Study (CARDS): multicentre randomised placebo-controlled trial. Lancet 364: 685–696.
6. Downs JR, Clearfield M, Weis S, Whitney E, Shapiro DR, et al. (1998) Primary prevention of acute coronary events with lovastatin in men and women with average cholesterol levels: results of AFCAPS/TexCAPS. Air Force/Texas Coronary Atherosclerosis Prevention Study. JAMA 279: 1615–1622.
7. Stampfer MJ, Hu FB, Manson JE, Rimm EB, Willett WC (2000) Primary prevention of coronary heart disease in women through diet and lifestyle. N Engl J Med 343: 16–22.
8. Barbeau EM, Krieger N, Soobader MJ (2004) Working class matters: socioeconomic disadvantage, race/ethnicity, gender, and smoking in NHIS 2000. Am J Public Health 94: 269–278.
9. Paeratakul S, Lovejoy JC, Ryan DH, Bray GA (2002) The relation of gender, race and socioeconomic status to obesity and obesity comorbidities in a sample of US adults. Int J Obes Relat Metab Disord 26: 1205–1210.
10. Linn S, Fulwood R, Rifkind B, Carroll M, Muesing R, et al. (1989) High density lipoprotein cholesterol levels among US adults by selected demographic and socioeconomic variables. The Second National Health and Nutrition Examination Survey 1976–1980. Am J Epidemiol 129: 281–294.
11. Connolly V, Unwin N, Sherriff P, Bilous R, Kelly W (2000) Diabetes prevalence and socioeconomic status: a population based study showing increased prevalence of type 2 diabetes mellitus in deprived areas. J Epidemiol Community Health 54: 173–177.
12. Kanjilal S, Gregg EW, Cheng YJ, Zhang P, Nelson DE, et al. (2006) Socioeconomic status and trends in disparities in 4 major risk factors for cardiovascular disease among US adults, 1971–2002. Arch Intern Med 166: 2348–2355.
13. Anand SS, Yusuf S, Vuksan V, Devanesen S, Teo KK, et al. (2000) Differences in risk factors, atherosclerosis, and cardiovascular disease between ethnic groups in Canada: the Study of Health Assessment and Risk in Ethnic groups (SHARE). Lancet 356: 279–284.
14. Walcott BP, Nahed BV, Kahle KT, Redjal N, Coumans JV (2011) Determination of geographic variance in stroke prevalence using Internet search engine analytics. Neurosurg Focus 30: E19.
15. Elixhauser A, Healthcare Cost and Utilization Project (U.S.) (1996) Most frequent diagnoses and procedures for DRGs, by insurance status. Rockville, Md. Silver Spring, MD: U.S. Dept. Health and Human Services, Public Health Service. Available from AHCPR Publications Clearinghouse. iii, 132 p.
16. Bashinskaya B, Nahed BV, Redjal N, Kahle KT, Walcott BP (2011) Trends in Peptic Ulcer Disease and the Identification of Helicobacter Pylori as a Causative

Organism: Population-based Estimates from the US Nationwide Inpatient Sample. J Glob Infect Dis 3: 366–370.

17. Walcott BP, Kuklina EV, Nahed BV, George MG, Kahle KT, et al. (2011) Craniectomy for malignant cerebral infarction: prevalence and outcomes in US hospitals. PLoS One 6: e29193.

18. Eagle KA, Guyton RA, Davidoff R, Edwards FH, Ewy GA, et al. (2004) ACC/AHA 2004 guideline update for coronary artery bypass graft surgery: a report of the American College of Cardiology/American Heart Association Task Force on Practice Guidelines (Committee to Update the 1999 Guidelines for Coronary Artery Bypass Graft Surgery). Circulation 110: e340–437.

19. Fischman DL, Leon MB, Baim DS, Schatz RA, Savage MP, et al. (1994) A randomized comparison of coronary-stent placement and balloon angioplasty in the treatment of coronary artery disease. Stent Restenosis Study Investigators. N Engl J Med 331: 496–501.

20. Ryan TJ, Faxon DP, Gunnar RM, Kennedy JW, King SB, 3rd, et al. (1988) Guidelines for percutaneous transluminal coronary angioplasty. A report of the American College of Cardiology/American Heart Association Task Force on Assessment of Diagnostic and Therapeutic Cardiovascular Procedures (Subcommittee on Percutaneous Transluminal Coronary Angioplasty). Circulation 78: 486–502.

21. Zhang Q, Wang Y (2004) Trends in the association between obesity and socioeconomic status in U.S. adults: 1971 to 2000. Obes Res 12: 1622–1632.

22. Wamala SP, Lynch J, Horsten M, Mittleman MA, Schenck-Gustafsson K, et al. (1999) Education and the metabolic syndrome in women. Diabetes Care 22: 1999–2003.

23. Gillum RF, Mussolino ME (2003) Education, poverty, and stroke incidence in whites and blacks: the NHANES I Epidemiologic Follow-up Study. J Clin Epidemiol 56: 188–195.

24. Albano JD, Ward E, Jemal A, Anderson R, Cokkinides VE, et al. (2007) Cancer mortality in the United States by education level and race. J Natl Cancer Inst 99: 1384–1394.

25. Callahan LF, Pincus T (1988) Formal education level as a significant marker of clinical status in rheumatoid arthritis. Arthritis Rheum 31: 1346–1357.

26. Dionne CE, Von Korff M, Koepsell TD, Deyo RA, Barlow WE, et al. (2001) Formal education and back pain: a review. J Epidemiol Community Health 55: 455–468.

27. Curry WT, Jr., Barker FG, 2nd (2009) Racial, ethnic and socioeconomic disparities in the treatment of brain tumors. J Neurooncol 93: 25–39.

28. Cowie CC, Rust KF, Ford ES, Eberhardt MS, Byrd-Holt DD, et al. (2009) Full accounting of diabetes and pre-diabetes in the U.S. population in 1988–1994 and 2005–2006. Diabetes Care 32: 287–294.

29. Satia JA, Galanko JA, Siega-Riz AM (2004) Eating at fast-food restaurants is associated with dietary intake, demographic, psychosocial and behavioural factors among African Americans in North Carolina. Public Health Nutr 7: 1089–1096.

30. Shea S, Misra D, Ehrlich MH, Field L, Francis CK (1992) Predisposing factors for severe, uncontrolled hypertension in an inner-city minority population. N Engl J Med 327: 776–781.

31. Morland K, Wing S, Diez Roux A, Poole C (2002) Neighborhood characteristics associated with the location of food stores and food service places. Am J Prev Med 22: 23–29.

32. Unger JB, Reynolds K, Shakib S, Spruijt-Metz D, Sun P, et al. (2004) Acculturation, physical activity, and fast-food consumption among Asian-American and Hispanic adolescents. J Community Health 29: 467–481.

33. Hadley J (2003) Sicker and poorer–the consequences of being uninsured: a review of the research on the relationship between health insurance, medical care use, health, work, and income. Med Care Res Rev 60: 3S–75S; discussion 76S–112S.

34. Diez Roux AV, Merkin SS, Arnett D, Chambless L, Massing M, et al. (2001) Neighborhood of residence and incidence of coronary heart disease. N Engl J Med 345: 99–106.

35. Saleh SS, Hannan EL, Ting L (2005) A multistate comparison of patient characteristics, outcomes, and treatment practices in acute myocardial infarction. Am J Cardiol 96: 1190–1196.

3

Temporal Trends of System of Care for STEMI: Insights from the Jakarta Cardiovascular Care Unit Network System

Surya Dharma[1]*, Bambang Budi Siswanto[1], Isman Firdaus[1], Iwan Dakota[1], Hananto Andriantoro[1], Alexander J. Wardeh[2], Arnoud van der Laarse[3], J. Wouter Jukema[3,4]

1 Department of Cardiology and Vascular Medicine, Faculty of Medicine, University of Indonesia, National Cardiovascular Center Harapan Kita, Jakarta, Indonesia, 2 Department of Cardiology, M.C. Haaglanden, The Hague, The Netherlands, 3 Department of Cardiology, Leiden University Medical Center, Leiden, the Netherlands, 4 Interuniversity Cardiology Institute the Netherlands, Utrecht, the Netherlands

Abstract

Aim: Guideline implementation programs are of paramount importance in optimizing acute ST-elevation myocardial infarction (STEMI) care. Assessment of performance indicators from a local STEMI network will provide knowledge of how to improve the system of care.

Methods and Results: Between 2008–2011, 1505 STEMI patients were enrolled. We compared the performance indicators before (n = 869) and after implementation (n = 636) of a local STEMI network. In 2011 (after introduction of STEMI networking) compared to 2008–2010, there were more inter-hospital referrals for STEMI patients (61% vs 56%, p<0.001), more primary percutaneous coronary intervention (PCI) procedures (83% vs 73%, p = 0.005), and more patients reaching door-to-needle time ≤30 minutes (84.5% vs 80.2%, p<0.001). However, numbers of patients who presented very late (>12 hours after symptom onset) were similar (53% vs 51%, NS). Moreover, the numbers of patients with door-to-balloon time ≤90 minutes were similar (49.1% vs 51.3%, NS), and in-hospital mortality rates were similar (8.3% vs 6.9%, NS) in 2011 compared to 2008–2010.

Conclusion: After a local network implementation for patients with STEMI, there were significantly more inter-hospital referral cases, primary PCI procedures, and patients with a door-to-needle time ≤30 minutes, compared to the period before implementation of this network. However, numbers of patients who presented very late, the targeted door-to-balloon time and in-hospital mortality rate were similar in both periods. To improve STEMI networking based on recent guidelines, existing pre-hospital and in-hospital protocols should be improved and managed more carefully, and should be accommodated whenever possible.

Editor: Renate B. Schnabel, University Heart Center, Germany

Funding: The authors have no support or funding to report.

Competing Interests: The authors have declared that no competing interests exist.

* E-mail: drsuryadharma@yahoo.com

Introduction

The recent 2012 European Society of Cardiology (ESC) guideline on ST-segment elevation myocardial infarction (STEMI) stressed the importance of networking for the management of acute myocardial infarction (AMI) [1]. In an earlier report, we emphasized the concept of a trained health system network in order to decrease the mortality rate of STEMI patients. The mission of such a network is how to increase the use of acute reperfusion treatment in the pre-hospital and hospital settings, using a pharmaco-invasive strategy in Jakarta, Indonesia [2].

After the initial introduction of the network, we analyzed the effectiveness of the system to improve the network protocols using a registry that we set up in 2008 as an integral part of modern health care [3,4]. We analyzed the quality of care and performance indicators of our local acute coronary syndrome registry, to further improve the STEMI system of care in Jakarta, Indonesia.

Methods

Data was collected from the Jakarta Acute Coronary Syndrome (JAC) registry database which included 1505 patients admitted with acute STEMI in the Emergency Department of the National Cardiovascular Center Harapan Kita (NCCHK), Jakarta, Indonesia from 2008 to 2011 (Figure 1). The NCCHK acts as a national referral hospital and the main receiving center in Jakarta with 24 hours cardiovascular services including primary PCI capabilities. Initial diagnosis was made on the basis of presence of typical chest pain and ST segment elevation (≥0.1 mV) in two or more contiguous leads on the admission ECG.

All demographic, clinical and laboratory variables were obtained from a standardized STEMI registry form. Raised body

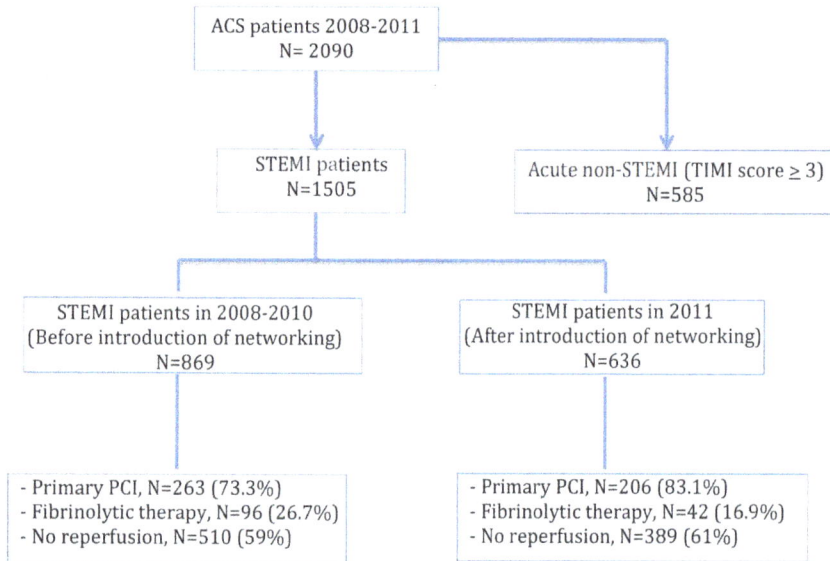

Figure 1. Patient distribution in the Jakarta Acute Coronary Syndrome registry. ACS = acute coronary syndrome, STEMI = ST-elevation myocardial infarction, PCI = percutaneous coronary intervention, TIMI = Thrombolysis in Myocardial Infarction.

mass index (BMI) was defined as a BMI>25 kg/m^2. Diabetes mellitus was diagnosed in patients with a history of oral antidiabetic or insulin medication or fasting blood glucose >125 mg/dl at study entrance; hypertension was diagnosed by the Joint National Committee VII criteria on hypertension or if currently taking antihypertensive treatment; dyslipidemia was diagnosed in patients with a history of lipid lowering medication or a fasted total cholesterol level >200 mg/dl, or LDL >130 mg/dl, or HDL<40 mg/dl, or triglyceride >150 mg/dl, and a positive family history of premature coronary artery disease (CAD) if CAD had developed before the age of 65 years in a first degree relative.

We compared the profiles of STEMI patients before the introduction of the STEMI networking (between 2008–2010) with those after introduction of the network (in 2011). Reperfusion therapy was given according to the recommendations of the ESC and American College of Cardiology/American Heart Association guidelines. The JAC registry and the analysis of the registry described in this manuscript have been approved by the institutional review board (IRB) committee of the Department of Cardiology and Vascular Medicine, Faculty of Medicine, University of Indonesia, National Cardiovascular Center Harapan Kita. There is no informed consent because data were analyzed anonymously and waived by the IRB committee.

Study endpoint

Study endpoints are the performance indicators in two time periods: before and after the implementation of the network, such as the number of inter-hospital referral cases, number of primary PCI procedures, number of patients who presented very late (>12 hours after onset of chest pain), and the time delay between admission to the hospital and actual reperfusion (door-to-balloon time and door-to-needle time).

Statistical methods

Continuous variables are presented as mean values ± standard deviation (SD) or median (minimum-maximum) if not fitting a normal distribution. Categorical variables were expressed as percentages or proportions. Normally distributed variables were

compared by Student t-test and skewed distribution data by Mann-Whitney U-test. Categorical variables were tested by chi-square test. A p value<0.05 was considered significant. All statistical analyses were performed with SPSS version 17.0 (SPSS Inc., Chicago, IL, USA).

Results

The median age of the STEMI patients was 55 years (ranging from 24 to 96 years) and the majority was male (86%). As reported earlier [2], hypertension was the most common risk factor (54%) in our STEMI population and the risk factors did not differ between the two periods. The source of referral was mostly from another hospital (58.3%) (Table 1).

The number of inter-hospital referrals for STEMI patients has significantly increased in 2011 compared to 2008–2010 (61.2% vs 56.2%, p<0.001), but numbers of patients with STEMI who presented very late were similar (53.1% vs 51.2%, p = 0.466). There was a significant increase of primary PCI in 2011 (83.1% vs 73.3% p = 0.005) (Table 2). For patients who received fibrinolytic therapy, the numbers of patients with a door-to-needle time ≤30 minutes was higher in 2011 than in 2008–2010 (84.5% vs 80.2%, p<0.001). For patients who underwent primary PCI, the number of patients with a door-to-balloon time <90 minutes had not improved (49.1% vs 51.3%, p = 0.364) (Table 3). In-hospital mortality had not changed between 2011 and 2008–2010 (8.3% vs 6.9%, p = 0.303).

Discussion

The Jakarta Cardiovascular Care Unit Network system was built to improve the system of care of AMI in Jakarta, Indonesia, serving about 11 million people with living in a density of 15,000 people/km^2 [2]. The effectiveness of the system can be monitored by recording the performance indicators in STEMI patients, such as number of patients receiving acute reperfusion treatment (numbers of primary PCI and fibrinolytic therapy), time from door to reperfusion, and number of patients who presented very late [4,5].

Table 1. Demographic data and hospitalization information of STEMI patients (N = 1505).

Variables	Description
Age, years	55 (24–96)
Gender, N (%)	
Female	214 (14,2%)
Male	1291 (85.7%)
Source of referral, N (%)	
Walk in/ambulance	502 (33.3%)
Primary physician	56 (3.7%)
Inter-hospital	878 (58.3%)
Intra-hospital	70 (4.6%)
Risk factor profile	
Raised BMI (>25 kg/m²)	320 (21.2%)
Carotid artery stenosis	3 (0.2%)
Family history of known CAD	368 (24.4%)
Dyslipidemia	580 (38.5%)
Hypertension	813 (54%)
Diabetes Mellitus	434 (29%)
Current smoker	698 (46.3%)

BMI = body mass index, CAD = coronary artery disease.

After the introduction of the network, there was a growing awareness of the primary physician in the primary hospital, as is shown by the increased numbers of STEMI patients referred from another hospital.

In the receiving center, the number of patients receiving primary PCI has increased after the application of the network, which might suggest that the pre-hospital protocol to make an accurate diagnosis of AMI has improved. However, the proportion of patients who received PCI with a door-to-balloon time ≤90 minutes, as recommended by the guideline, had not improved between the two periods. It has shown earlier that when PCI-related time delay increases, the mortality benefit decreases [6–8]. Moreover, the 2012 ESC guideline on management of STEMI patients [1] has strengthen the importance of shortening the time delay for primary PCI, and recommends a door-to-balloon time <60 minutes in a PCI-capable hospital.

The numbers of patients receiving fibrinolytic therapy have decreased in 2011, although more patients had reached a door-to-needle time ≤30 minutes compared to the 2008–2010 period before the network was introduced. It should be noted that fibrinolytic therapy of STEMI patients was given in the in-hospital setting. If the estimated first medical contact to balloon time is >120 minutes, we wish to start, in the near future, fibrinolytic therapy in the pre-hospital setting, as recommended by the guideline [1]. Local authorities have to collaborate in training all health care providers on how to perform fibrinolytic therapy according to a standard protocol.

Finally, the proportion of patients with STEMI who presented very late (>12 hours) had not improved between the two periods. As late presentation is associated with high mortality [2], we should get the patients to the hospitals that provide reperfusion

Table 2. STEMI profile based on network application period.

Variables	2008–2010 (before implementation of AMI networking) N = 869	2011 (after implementation of AMI networking) N = 636	P value
Age, years	55 (24–85)	55 (29–96)	0.407
Male, N (%)	735 (84%)	556 (87%)	0.242
Referral status			
Walk in/ambulance	281 (32.3%)	221 (34.7%)	
Primary physician	43 (4.9%)	13 (2.0%)	
Inter-hospital	488 (56.2%)	390 (61,2%)	<0.001
Intra hospital	57 (6.6%)	13 (2.0%)	
Risk Factors			
Hypertension	457 (52.6%)	356 (56%)	0.339
Family History of known CAD	199 (22.9%)	169 (26.6%)	0.224
Dyslipidemia	305 (35.1%)	275 (43.2%)	0.202
Diabetes Mellitus	236 (27.2%)	198 (31.1%)	0.190
Current Smoker	399 (45.9%)	299 (47%)	0.806
Onset of infarction			
≤12 hours	422 (48.8%)	299 (46.9%)	0.466
>12 hours	442 (51.2%)	338 (53.1%)	
Reperfusion strategy			
Primary PCI	263 (73.3%)	206 (83.1%)	0.005
Fibrinolytic therapy	96 (26.7%)	42 (16.9%)	

Data are presented as numbers and percentages. PCI = percutaneous coronary intervention.

Table 3. Characteristics of STEMI patients before and after implementation of Jakarta Cardiovascular Care Unit Network System.

Variables	2008–2010 (before implementation of MI networking)	2011 (after implementation of MI networking)	P value
	N = 869	N = 636	
Location of MI			
Anterior	530 (61%)	376 (59.1%)	0.464
Non anterior	339 (39%)	260 (40.9%)	
Killip class			
I	598 (69.2%)	429 (68.5%)	
II	223 (25.8%)	151 (24.1%)	0.047
III	25 (2.9%)	17 (2.7%)	
IV	18 (2.1%)	29 (4.6%)	
DTN≤30 minutes	77 (80.2%)	120 (84.5%)	<0.001
DTB≤90 minutes	135 (51.3%)	105 (49.1%)	0.364
In-hospital mortality	60 (6.9%)	53 (8.3%)	0.303

Data are presented as numbers and percentages. MI = myocardial infarction, DTN = door-to-needle time, DTB = door-to-balloon time.

therapy earlier. The in-hospital mortality has not changed in the two periods, which may be expected as the proportions of patients with door-to-balloon <90 minutes and patients who presented very late (>12 hours) have not changed between the two periods. For that purpose we have to analyse how to improve patient delay by recognizing the symptoms earlier and system delay by using electrocardiography (ECG) transmission and improving availability of ambulances.

Based on the results of the performance indicators before and after network introduction, the pre-hospital and in-hospital protocols should be improved. In pre-hospital protocols improvements to be implemented include: 1) the use of pre-hospital triage forms. We have made two models of a pre-hospital triage form and an ambulance communication chart form (Figures S1 and S2). These forms should be filled by the healthcare providers in the pre-hospital setting; 2) the 12-lead ECG should be recorded in all patients with suspected AMI and should be transmitted to our center as the host of the network. Pre-hospital 12-lead ECG plays an important role in a system of care for STEMI patients [9–11]. Currently, we are using a fax machine for ECG transmission but this system has several limitations, such as the unavailability of a fax machine in the ambulance. Therefore, we should transmit the ECG by a telephone- or, internet-based system; 3) a routine educational course should be attended to improve the skill and knowledge of the primary physician and nurses who are working in the emergency department or ambulance. To improve the in-hospital protocols of the receiving center, several improvements to implement are: 1) all administration processes related to reperfusion treatment should be managed in the emergency department as an integrated health care system; 2) as the host of the network, we have installed a catheterization laboratory in the emergency department that may contribute to reduce the time delay to reperfusion treatment; 3) for STEMI patients in whom the diagnosis has been made in the pre-hospital setting, the patients should be send directly to the cath-lab, by-passing the emergency department.

An intensive collaboration should be made between Indonesian Heart Association, Indonesian Heart Foundation and the local government of Jakarta in order to: 1) provide an education to the community about recognizing earlier signs and symptoms of a

heart attack; 2) not to fear of coming to hospital; and 3) find the best solution for financial issues related to reperfusion therapy.

Prior AMI guideline implementation programs have improved patient care and patient's outcome [12–14]. However, the widespread dissemination of evidence-based medicine in daily practice is still lacking and a significant number of patients remain undertreated [15–19]. Therefore, the integrated STEMI care program we developed and implemented will include pre-hospital and in-hospital care. As preliminary data looks promising, we must keep improving all points of the health care system.

Study limitations

This single center registry should be combined with the registries of other receiving centers in the city to know the real STEMI profile in Jakarta. However, our center is the cardiac referral hospital in Jakarta with the highest case load, thus characteristics of the patients in our National Cardiovascular Center Harapan Kita registry will reflect the STEMI profile in Jakarta very well. Furthermore, this study provides preliminary data with comparatively low power.

Conclusion

For STEMI patients, the introduction of a regional AMI network has significantly increased the number of inter-hospital referral cases and the number of patients who underwent acute reperfusion procedures in the receiving center, with more patients who reached door-to-needle time <30 minutes. However, the proportion of patients who presented very late, the door-to-balloon time, and the in-hospital mortality have not improved. The receiving and referral center protocols have to be adapted to increase the quality of care of AMI patients in Jakarta.

Supporting Information

Figure S1 The pre-hospital triage of AMI patients in Jakarta Cardiovascular Care Unit Network System. An internet-based ECG transmission system (Heart line) is located in the Emergency Department of the National Cardiovascular Center Harapan Kita Hospital with 24 hours service. Diagnosis and choice of reperfusion therapy will be decided through the

Heart line. The choice of fibrinolytic agent is either Streptokinase or Alteplase. In post-fibrinolytic patients, rescue PCI will be performed if fibrinolysis has failed. After a successful fibrinolytic therapy, coronary angiography will be performed within 3–24 hours. EMS = emergency medical service, BP = blood pressure, HR = heart rate, RR = respiratory rate, SR = sinus rhythm, SB = sinus bradycardia, ST = sinus tachycardia, AF = atrial fibrillation, SVT = supra-ventricular tachycardia, VT = ventricular tachycardia, VF = ventricular fibrillation, AV = atrioventricular, NCCHK = national cardiovascular center Harapan Kita, RBBB = right bundle branch block, LBBB = left bundle branch block, PPCI = primary percutaneous coronary intervention, FMC = first medical contact, p.o = per os (oral).

Figure S2 The communication form and fibrinolytic check list for the emergency medical service/ambulance staff. STEMI = ST-segment elevation myocardial infarction, non STE ACS = non-ST elevation acute coronary syndrome, CNS = central nervous system, AV = arteriovenous, BP = blood pressure, NCCHK = National Cardiovascular Center Harapan Kita.

Author Contributions

Conceived and designed the experiments: SD. Performed the experiments: SD. Analyzed the data: SD BBS IF ID HA AJW AVDL JWJ. Wrote the paper: SD BBS IF ID HA AJW AVDL JWJ. Designed the study: JWJ.

References

1. Steg Ph G, James SK (2012) On behalf of the Task Force for The 2012 European Society of Cardiology Guideline on management of acute myocardial infarction in patients presenting with ST segment elevation. Eur Heart J 33: 2569–2619.
2. Dharma S, Juzar DA, Firdaus I, Soerianata S, Wardeh AJ, et al (2012) Acute myocardial infarction system of care in the third world. Neth Heart J 20:254–259.
3. Danchin N (2009) System of care for ST-segment elevation myocardial infarction. Impact of different models on clinical outcomes. JACC Cardiovasc Interv 2:901–908.
4. Liem SS, van der Hoeven BL, Oemrawsingh PV, Bax JJ, van der Bom JG, et al (2007) MISSION!: Optimization of acute and chronic care for patients with acute myocardial infarction. Am Heart J 153:e1–e11.
5. Eagle KA, Montoye CK, Riba AL, DeFranco AC, Parrish R, et al (2005) Guideline-based standardized care is associated with substantially lower mortality in Medicare patients with acute myocardial infarction: the American College of Cardiology's Guidelines Applied in Practice (GAP) Projects in Michigan. J Am Coll Cardiol 46:1242–1248.
6. Cannon CP, Gibson M, Lambrew CT, Shoultz DA, Levy D, et al (2000) Relationship of symptom-onset-to-balloon time and door-to-balloon time with mortality in patients undergoing angioplasty for acute myocardial infarction. JAMA 283:2941–2947.
7. Nallamothu BK, Bates ER (2003) Percutaneous coronary intervention versus fibrinolytic therapy in acute myocardial infarction: is timing (almost) everything? Am J Cardiol 92:824–826.
8. De Luca G, Suryapranata H, Ottervanger JP, Antman EM (2004) Time delay to treatment and mortality in primary angioplasty for acute myocardial infarction. Circulation 109:1223–1225.
9. Rokos IC, French WJ, Koenig WJ, Stratton SJ, Nighswonger B, et al (2009) Integration of prehospital electrocardiograms and ST-elevation myocardial infarction receiving center (SRC) networks: impact on door to balloon times across 10 independent regions. JACC Cardiovasc Interv 2:339–343.
10. Kudenchuk PJ, Maynard C, Cobb LA, Wirkus M, Martin JS, et al (1998) Utility of the prehospital electrocardiogram in diagnosing acute coronary syndromes: the Myocardial Infarction Triage and Intervention (MITI) Project. J Am Coll Cardiol 32:17–27.
11. Diercks DB, Kontos MC, Chen AY, Pollack CV, Wiviott SD, et al (2009) Utilization and impact of prehospital electrocardiograms for patients with acute ST-segment elevation myocardial infarction: data from the NCDR (National Cardiovascular Data Registry) ACTION (Acute Coronary Treatment and Intervention Outcomes Network) Registry. J Am Coll Cardiol 53:161–166.
12. Labresh KA, Ellrodt AG, Gliklich R, Liljestrand J, Peto R (2004) Get with the guidelines for cardiovascular secondary prevention: pilot results. Arch Intern Med 164:203–209.
13. Eagle KA, Montoye CK, Riba AL, DeFranco AC, Parrish R, et al (2005) Guideline based standardized care is associated with substantially lower mortality in Medicare patients with acute myocardial infarction: the American College of Cardiology's Guidelines Applied in Practice (GAP) Projects in Michigan. J Am Coll Cardiol 46:1242–1248.
14. Fonarow GC, Gawlinski A, Moughrabi S, Tilisch JH (2001) Improved treatment of coronary heart disease by implementation of a Cardiac Hospitalization Atherosclerosis Management Program (CHAMP). Am J Cardiol 87:819–822.
15. Burwen DR, Galusha DH, Lewis JM, Bedinger MR, Radford MJ, et al (2003) National and state trends in quality of care for acute myocardial infarction between 1994–1995 and 1998–1999: the Medicare health care quality improvement program. Arch Intern Med 163:1430–1439.
16. Hasdai D, Behar S, Wallentin L, Danchin N, Gitt AK, et al (2002) A prospective survey of the characteristics, treatments and outcomes of patients with acute coronary syndromes in Europe and the Mediterranian basin; the Euro Heart Survey of Acute Coronary Syndromes (Euro Heart Survey ACS). Eur Heart J 23:1190–1201.
17. Barron HV, Bowlby LJ, Breen T, Rogers WJ, Canto JG, et al (1998) Use of reperfusion therapy for acute myocardial infarction in the United States: data from the National Registry of Myocardial Infarction 2. Circulation 97:1150–1156.
18. Nallamothu BK, Bates ER, Herrin J, Wang Y, Bradley EH, et al (2005) Times to treatment in transfer patients undergoing primary percutaneous coronary intervention in the United States: National Registry of Myocardial Infarction (NRMI) ¾ analysis. Circulation 111:761–767.
19. EUROASPIRE I and II Group (2001) Clinical reality of coronary prevention guidelines: a comparison of EUROASPIRE I and II in nine countries. European Action on Secondary Prevention by Intervention to Reduce Events. Lancet 357:995–1001.

4

Small Dense Low Density Lipoprotein Particles Are Associated with Poor Outcome after Angioplasty in Peripheral Artery Disease

Vincenzo Jacomella[1][*][♪], Philipp A. Gerber[2][♪], Kathrin Mosimann[1], Marc Husmann[1], Christoph Thalhammer[1], Ian Wilkinson[3], Kaspar Berneis[2], Beatrice R. Amann-Vesti[1]

1 Clinic for Angiology, University Hospital Zurich, Zurich, Switzerland, 2 Clinic for Endocrinology, University Hospital Zurich, Zurich, Switzerland, 3 Clinical Pharmacology Unit, University of Cambridge, Cambridge, United Kingdom

Abstract

Purpose: In patients suffering from symptomatic peripheral artery disease (PAD), percutaneous revascularization is the treatment of choice. However, restenosis may occur in 10 to 60% in the first year depending on a variety of factors. Small dense low density lipoprotein (sdLDL) particles are associated with an increased risk for cardiovascular events, but their role in the process of restenosis is not known. We conducted a prospective study to analyze the association of sdLDL particles with the outcome of balloon angioplasty in PAD. The composite primary endpoint was defined as improved walking distance and absence of restenosis.

Methods: Patients with angiographically documented PAD of the lower extremities who were scheduled for lower limb revascularization were consecutively recruited for the study. At baseline and at three month follow-up triglyceride, total cholesterol, LDL size and subclasses and HDL cholesterol and ankle-brachial index (ABI) were measured. Three months after the intervention duplex sonography was performed to detect restenosis.

Results: Sixty-four patients (53% male) with a mean age of 68.6 ± 9.9 years were included. The proportion of small- dense LDL particles (class III and IV) was significantly lower ($33.1\pm11.0\%$ vs. $39.4\pm12.1\%$, p = 0.038) in patients who reached the primary end-point compared with those who did not. Patients with improved walking distance and without restenosis had a significantly higher LDL size at baseline (26.6 ± 1.1 nm vs. 26.1 ± 1.1 nm, p = 0.046) and at follow-up (26.7 ± 1.1 nm vs. 26.2 ± 0.9 nm, p = 0.044) than patients without improvement.

Conclusions: Small-dense LDL particles are associated with worse early outcome in patients undergoing percutaneous revascularization for symptomatic PAD.

Editor: Yin Tintut, Los Angeles, United States of America

Funding: The authors have no funding or support to report.

Competing Interests: The authors have declared that no competing interests exist.

* Email: vincenzo.jacomella@usz.ch

♪ These authors contributed equally to this work.

Introduction

Peripheral artery disease (PAD) has a prevalence of up to 20% in the elderly population [1]. The majority of patients are asymptomatic [2]; therefore, early modification of risk factors is mandatory to reduce the high rate of morbidity and mortality associated with PAD [3].

Up to 10–35% of PAD patients are symptomatic [2], with reduced quality of life due to pain and impaired mobility. The presence of chronic wounds and critical ischemia may compromise limb viability. Revascularization with angioplasty is an approved therapeutic option to improve quality of life in patients with intermittent claudication, and the treatment of choice in critical limb ischemia. However, despite new devices and techniques, restenosis is still a major problem, occurring in 10 to 60% of cases

after an initially technically successful angioplasty. The rate of restenosis depends on a variety of factors, such as severity of the PAD (i.e. claudication versus critical limb ischemia), the lesion type (occlusion versus stenosis), the quality of both run-in and run-off vessels, the length of the lesions but also on cardiovascular risk factors [2,4,5], such as diabetes, hyperlipidemia, hypertension and smoking.

Earlier publications have outlined the importance of low density lipoprotein (LDL) size as a predictor of cardiovascular events and progression of coronary artery disease [6]. The presence of small, dense LDL (sdLDL) particles is an established cardiovascular risk factor by the national Cholesterol Education Program Adult treatment Panel III. sdLDL particle size is a predictive marker for cardiovascular mortality in PAD patients [7], but its role in the process of restenosis and clinical outcome in patients undergoing percutaneous revascularization is unclear. Therefore, we conducted a prospective study to investigate the potential role of sdLDL particle as a predictor of early restenosis and adverse clinical outcome after angioplasty with or without stenting.

Methods

Study design and patients

In this prospective, single-center, observational study, the effect of sdLDL particles on restenosis and clinical outcome after endovascular lower limb revascularization in PAD patients was investigated.

Patients with atherosclerotic PAD, Fontaine I–III of the lower limb, with or without a history of peripheral vascular intervention or vascular surgery, who were scheduled for an intervention, were consecutively recruited. Exclusion criteria were cardiac arrhythmia, chronic inflammatory vascular disorders or failed revascularization, defined as a more than 50% residual stenosis confirmed angiographically or by duplex ultrasound after the procedure. All examinations were performed at the study center (Clinic for Angiology, University Hospital Zurich).

After baseline investigation patients underwent peripheral angioplasty with plain balloon angioplasty, with or without stenting (without drug-coated balloon or stent). The decision to implant a stent was left to the operator, but patients receiving a drug-eluting stent were excluded.

At baseline, body mass index (BMI), total cholesterol, LDL cholesterol, HDL cholesterol, triglycerides, LDL-phenotype and ankle-brachial index (ABI) were recorded. Details of other risk factors and medication were recorded, and walking capacity was evaluated using a walking questionnaire (SF-35). At three months follow-up, LDL-phenotype and ABI were determined. A Duplex ultrasound examination to detect restenosis of the target lesion was performed, and walking capacity was assessed with a questionnaire (SF-35).

The primary endpoint was defined as improved walking distance and absence of restenosis.

The local ethics committee ("Kantonale Ethikkommission Zürich") approved the study and all patients gave written informed consent.

Laboratory measurements

Triglycerides, total cholesterol and lipoprotein cholesterol values were measured by enzymatic procedures (Abbott ABA 200 instrument). HDL cholesterol was determined by the dextran sulphate-magnesium precipitation procedure. Low-density lipoprotein cholesterol was calculated with the Friedewald formula [8]. To assess LDL particles size and distribution, non-denaturing polyacrylamide gradient gel electrophoresis (GGE) of plasma was performed at 10–14°C in 2–16% polyacrylamide gradient gels. Gels were subjected to electrophoresis for 24 h at 125 V in tris borate buffer (pH 8.3) as described elsewhere [9]. Gels were fixed and stained for lipids in a solution containing Oil Red O in 60% ethanol at 55°C. Gels were placed on a light source and photographed using a Luminescent Image Analyzer, LAS-3000 of Fujifilm. Migration distance for each absorbance peak was determined and the molecular diameter corresponding to each peak was calculated from a calibration curve generated from the migration distance of size standards of known diameter, which includes carboxylated latex beads (Duke Scientific, Palo Alto, CA), thyroglobulin and apoferritin (HMW Std, Pharmacia, Piscataway, NJ) having molecular diameter of 38.0 nm, 17.0 nm and 12.2 nm, respectively, and lipoprotein calibrators of previously determined particle size. LDL subclass distribution (LDL I (272–285 nm), IIA

(265–272 nm), IIB (256–265 nm), IIIA (247–256 nm), IIIB (242–247 nm), IVA (233–242 nm) and IVB (220–233 nm)) as percentage of total LDL was calculated.

Ankle-brachial index and Duplex ultrasound

Ankle-brachial arterial pressure index was assessed with the patient in the supine position. Systolic ankle blood pressure of the posterior and anterior tibial artery, and the peroneal artery on both legs was obtained by hand-held 6 MHz Doppler probe (Kranzbühler, Logidop 2, Pilger Medical Electronics, Switzerland). ABI was calculated as the ratio of the highest ankle systolic blood pressure divided by the highest brachial systolic blood pressure for each leg. The ABI of the treated leg was taken as the study parameter.

Patency of the revascularized segment was assesed at three months follow-up visit with duplex ultrasound (DUS), primary patency was maintained until restenosis (>50% diameter reduction) defined by a peak systolic velocity (PSV) ratio >2.4 was documented by DUS.

Revascularization procedure

All patients were treated according to guidelines with thrombocyte antiaggregation and/or anticoagulation, statins, and antihypertensive therapy if indicated.

In addition to best medical treatment, patients were treated with balloon angioplasty, stent implantation was additionally performed at the discretion of the interventionalist. Medication remained unchanged except for clopidogrel given for a period of 28 days in case of stent implantation.

Statistical analysis

Data are presented as means ± SD, or values and percentages. For the analysis of categorical data, the χ^2 and Fisher's exact test were applied. For comparison of continuous variables in two independent groups, the Mann–Whitney U test was used. A generalized linear model was used for the testing of correlations. A value of $p<0.05$ was considered significant.

Results

Patient characteristics

A total of 64 patients were included in the study (53.1% males, mean age 68.6±9.9 years). Baseline data are summarized in Table 1. Mean ABI was 0.71±0.20. Antiplatelet/anticoagulation medication at baseline included acetylsalicylic acid (90.6%), clopidogrel (53.1%), low molecular weight heparin (14.1%) and oral anticoagulation with phenprocoumon (6.3%). Lipid-lowering agents (statins) were used in 90.6% of patients. Antihypertensive medication included diuretics (37.5%), beta-blocker (32.8%), calcium channel blockers (29.7%), ACE inhibitors (31.3%), angiotensin II receptor antagonists (26.6%) and aldosterone receptor antagonists (6.3%).

Most patients were classified as Fontaine stage IIb (50%) and IIa (21%). Only 6% and 1.2% were staged Fontaine stage I or III, respectively. Fotaine stages were defined as follows: Stage I - asymptomatic, incomplete blood vessel obstruction, stage II - mild claudication pain in limb, stage IIA - Claudication at a distance of greater than 200 metres, stage IIB - Claudication distance of less than 200 metres, stage III - rest pain, mostly in the feet, stage IV - necrosis and/or gangrene of the limb.

Outcome

The combined endpoint of improved walking distance without occurrence of restenosis was reached in 24 (37.5%) patients with a

Table 1. Baseline characteristics of study population (n = 64).

Characteristic	Mean/proportion
Age (years)	69±10
Sex male/female (%)	53/47
BMI (kg/m^2)	25.2±4.3
Total cholesterol (mmol/l)	4.6±1.1
HDL cholesterol (mmol/l)	1.3±0.6
LDL cholesterol (mmol/l)	2.4±0.9
Triglycerides (mmol/l)	2.1±1.4
Coronary artery disease (%)	28
Cerebrovascular disease (%)	31
Renal insufficiency (%)	22
Arterial Hypertension (%)	83
Diabetes mellitus (%)	30
Smoker	
Current (%)	48
Ever (%)	80

Values are given in absolute numbers (mean±SD) or as percentage.

significant improvement of ABI from 0.70±0.20 to 0.93±1.80 (p<0.002). Restenosis or reocclusion of the treated lesion occurred in 11 patients. The use of stents (in 39.1% of patients) did not influence the combined endpoint (reached in 33.3% of patients without stent implantation and in 44% of patients with stent implantation, p = 0.44).

LDL size

At baseline, mean LDL particle size was 26.3±1.1 nM, and did not differ at follow-up (26.4±1.0 nM, ns). LDL particle size was significantly higher in women than in men at both time points (baseline: 26.6±1.1 nM vs. 26.0±1.1 nM, follow-up: 26.6±0.8 nM vs. 26.1±1.1 nM, p<0.05). There was no correlation between LDL size and age, but there was a negative correlation with BMI at follow-up (p = 0.006), and a trend towards a negative correlation at baseline (p = 0.07).

LDL size at baseline and at follow-up was different between patients achieving the primary end-point and those who did not. Patients with improved walking distance and without restenosis had a significantly higher LDL size at baseline (26.6±1.1 nM vs. 26.1±1.1 nM, p = 0.046) and at follow-up (26.7±1.1 nM vs. 26.2±0.9 nM, p = 0.044, figure 1) than those who did not improve or restenosed.

LDL particle subclasses

The distribution of different LDL subclasses among patients which improvement compared to those without improvement at three months follow-up is shown in figure 2. The proportion of small dense LDL particles (class III and IV) was significantly lower in patients who reached the primary end-point compared to those who did not. These differences were seen at baseline (33.1±11.0% vs. 39.4±12.1%, p = 0.038) and at follow-up (39.8±8.2% vs. 46.8±10.1%, p = 0.008). If the components of the primary endpoint were analyzed separately, a tendency was detected towards a lower proportion of small dense LDL particles in patients without restenosis (compared to those with restenosis) at baseline (36.4±11.6% vs. 40.8±13.2%, p = 0.30) and at follow-up (43.1±10.2% vs. 48.1±8.6%, p = 0.09), and a significant differ-

ence was seen in patients with improved walking distance (compared to those without improvement) at baseline (33.6±11.3% vs. 39.5±12%, p = 0.04) and at follow-up (40.9±9.1% vs. 46.4±10%, p = 0.04).

Using a generalized linear model, the effect of different cardiovascular risk factors was assessed. The proportion of small, dense LDL particles at follow-up was still significantly lower in patients who met the end-point after adjustment for gender, smoking status and the diagnoses of arterial hypertension, dyslipidemia or diabetes mellitus (p = 0.03, table 2).

Other cardiovascular risk factors

In addition to the assessment with a generalized linear model, the individual effect of baseline cardiovascular risk factors – in particular conventional risk factors – other than LDL size was further assessed by analyzing differences between the two outcome groups.

Age was not different in patients who reached the primary end-point compared to those who did not (67.5±10.5 vs. 69.3±9.5, p = 0.69), as was BMI (25.4±4.7 vs. 25.1±4.0 kg/m^2, p = 0.92) and gender (female gender 58.3% vs. 40.0%, p = 0.20). Further, there was no difference in the concentration of total cholesterol (4.7±1.0 mM vs. 4.5±1.2 mM, p = 0.57), HDL cholesterol (1.4±0.6 mM vs. 1.2±0.5 mM, p = 0.38), LDL cholesterol (2.5±0.6 mM vs. 2.3±1.0 mM, p = 0.07) or triglycerides (1.7±0.9 vs. 2.4±1.7 mM, p = 0.23). Statin therapy was installed in 90.6% of patients at baseline, and started in the remaining 9.4% (6 patients) at the time of admission. The primary outcome did not differ significantly between patients with and without statin therapy (p = 0.19).

Discussion

The results of this study show that patients with a successful outcome after percutaneous revascularization of PAD have a larger LDL particles size compared to patients who fail to show a

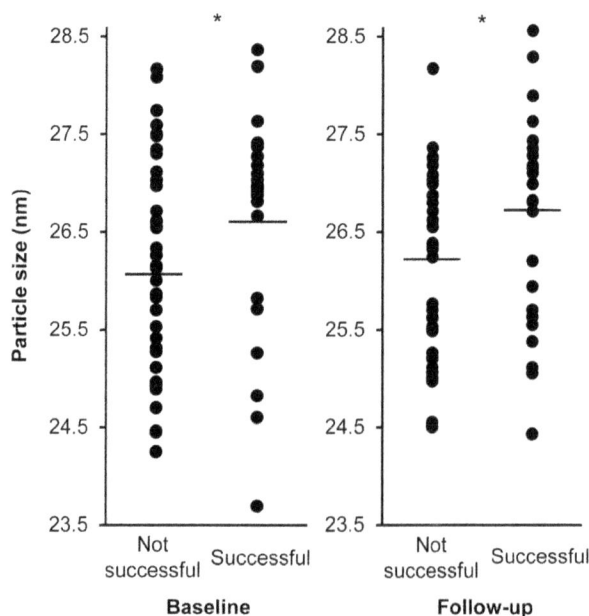

Figure 1. LDL particle size in non-successful (restenosis and/or absence of clinical improvement) vs successful revascularization, * p<0.05.

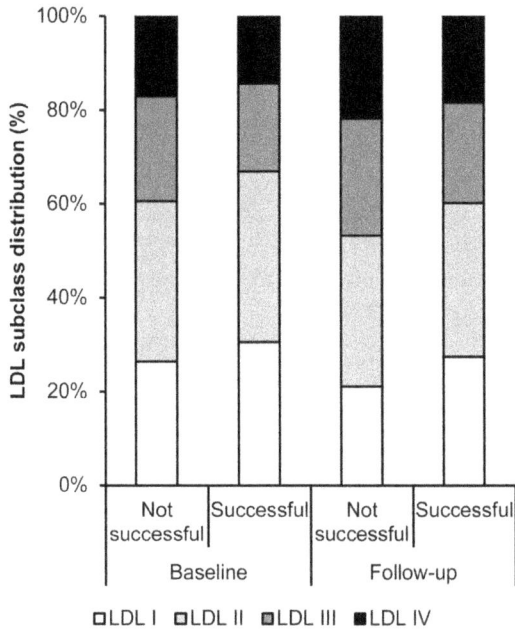

Figure 2. Relative distribution of the different LDL size subclasses (from LDL I = large to LDL IV = small) within the two outcome groups.

particles are absorbed better by the arterial tissue [13]. In addition, there is probably a greater affinity with the proteoglycans of connective tissue [14] and greater exposure to oxidative processes [15]. Furthermore, a correlation of small dense LDL particles with progressing atherosclerosis has been shown in many studies. Increased intima media thickness is associated with a smaller LDL particle size. In addition to these cross-sectional association studies [16,17], we collected also prospective data showing a predictive value of the amount of small dense LDL particles at baseline regarding progression of intima media thickness during a follow-up of two years in patients with dysglycemia [18].

Angioplasty causes a mechanical vascular injury with induction of an inflammatory reaction. It is characterized by inflammatory cell infiltration, release of growth factors, medial smooth muscle cell (SMC) modulation and proliferation [19]. Therefore, it is conceivable that all these mechanisms, which lead to neointimal proliferation, are accelerated by the presence of sdLDL particles.

In contrast to sdLDL particles, there was no association of LDL cholesterol levels with the primary endpoint, therefore LDL cholesterol seems not able to predict the outcome of endovascular intervention. This is probably due to the fact that rigorous LDL cholesterol control with statins is installed in patients suffering from PAD. Further, the independence of LDL cholesterol levels and sdLDL particles is underlined by studies describing different effects of certain therapies on LDL cholesterol and sdLDL [20].

The GGE method for determination of LDL particle size and classification has been shown to be reliable, with a high agreement when compared to other methods. However, it should be mentioned that there are also other methods as nuclear magnetic resonance or ion mobility with comparable precision. Further, newer methods have been developed that are convenient to use and may help to establish the use of LDL particle size outside the academic research [21]

The strength of this study is that the data were prospectively assessed in a well-defined cohort of patients with PAD undergoing revascularization. Further, due to the single center design of the study, it was possible that all clinical and biochemical measurements were performed at the same place and by the same investigators, therefore limiting possible inter-observer biases. This was of particular importance with respect to the measurement of LDL size and assessment of restenosis rate. A limitation is the relatively small sample size.

In summary, the presence of high amounts of small dense LDL particles is a negative predictor regarding successful outcome of peripheral angioplasty. Therefore, measurement of this parameter should be considered in patients undergoing balloon angioplasty. Further, therapies targeting LDL particle size and the proportion

clinical improvement or who develop restenosis of the treated vessel. This suggests that small LDL particle size may be used as a predictor of poor outcome after peripheral angioplasty.

A correlation between some lipid markers such as lipoprotein (a) or other serum lipid subfractions and restenosis rate after angioplasty of the peripheral or coronary arteries has already been shown [10]. However, to our knowledge this is the first study investigating the impact of the LDL particle size with respect to restenosis and clinical outcome in claudicants.

Patients with PAD have a high level of small LDL-particles [11], and are more prone to cardiovascular events [6]. In patients with coronary stent implantation, an increase in LDL particle size during follow-up is associated with reduced incidence of in-stent restenosis [12]. Here we show an association with baseline (and follow-up) LDL particle size, but not with its changes during follow-up.

The reasons for the atherogenicity of small LDL particle are varied and not completely understood, it is thought that the small

Table 2. Multiple linear regression was performed to assess the effect of the amount of small dense LDL particles as well as gender, smoking status and the diagnoses of arterial hypertension, dyslipidemia or diabetes mellitus on the primary outcome

Parameter	Coefficient	95% Confidence Interval		p-Value
		Lower	Upper	
sdLDL particles (%)	−0.014	−0.026	−0.001	0.03
Female Gender	0.075	−0.156	0.306	0.53
Smoker	0.001	−0.225	0.227	0.99
Hypertension	−0.142	−0.440	0.156	0.35
Dyslipidemia	0.057	−0.189	0.304	0.65
Diabetes	−0.129	−0.380	0.122	0.31

of sdLDL particles might be considered in patients with high amounts of sdLDL particles in the future to improve clinical outcome after vascular intervention.

References

1. Criqui MH (2001) Peripheral arterial disease–epidemiological aspects. Vasc Med 6: 3–7.
2. Norgren L, Hiatt WR, Dormandy JA, Nehler MR, Harris KA, et al. (2007) Inter-Society Consensus for the Management of Peripheral Arterial Disease (TASC II). Journal of vascular surgery: official publication, the Society for Vascular Surgery [and] International Society for Cardiovascular Surgery, North American Chapter 45 Suppl S: S5–67.
3. Hiatt WR (2001) Medical treatment of peripheral arterial disease and claudication. The New England journal of medicine 344: 1608–1621.
4. Maca TH, Ahmadi R, Derfler K, Ehringer H, Gschwandtner ME, et al. (2002) Influence of lipoprotein(a) on restenosis after femoropopliteal percutaneous transluminal angioplasty in Type 2 diabetic patients. Diabetic medicine: a journal of the British Diabetic Association 19: 300–306.
5. Kugler CF, Rudofsky G (2003) The challenges of treating peripheral arterial disease. Vascular medicine 8: 109–114.
6. Austin MA, Breslow JL, Hennekens CH, Buring JE, Willett WC, et al. (1988) Low-density lipoprotein subclass patterns and risk of myocardial infarction. JAMA: the journal of the American Medical Association 260: 1917–1921.
7. Berneis K, Rizzo M, Spinas GA, Di Lorenzo G, Di Fede G, et al. (2009) The predictive role of atherogenic dyslipidemia in subjects with non-coronary atherosclerosis. Clinica chimica acta; international journal of clinical chemistry 406: 36–40.
8. Friedewald WT, Levy RI, Fredrickson DS (1972) Estimation of the concentration of low-density lipoprotein cholesterol in plasma, without use of the preparative ultracentrifuge. Clin Chem 18: 499–502.
9. Krauss RM, Burke DJ (1982) Identification of multiple subclasses of plasma low density lipoproteins in normal humans. J Lipid Res 23: 97–104.
10. Giovanetti F, Gargiulo M, Laghi L, D'Addato S, Maioli F, et al. (2009) Lipoprotein(a) and other serum lipid subfractions influencing primary patency after infrainguinal percutaneous transluminal angioplasty. Journal of endovascular therapy: an official journal of the International Society of Endovascular Specialists 16: 389–396.
11. Rizzo M, Pernice V, Frasheri A, Berneis K (2008) Atherogenic lipoprotein phenotype and LDL size and subclasses in patients with peripheral arterial disease. Atherosclerosis 197: 237–241.
12. Kim JS, Kim MH, Lee BK, Rim SJ, Min PK, et al. (2008) Effects of increasing particle size of low-density lipoprotein on restenosis after coronary stent implantation. Circ J 72: 1059–1064.
13. Bjornheden T, Babyi A, Bondjers G, Wiklund O (1996) Accumulation of lipoprotein fractions and subfractions in the arterial wall, determined in an in vitro perfusion system. Atherosclerosis 123: 43–56.
14. Galeano NF, Al-Haideri M, Keyserman F, Rumsey SC, Deckelbaum RJ (1998) Small dense low density lipoprotein has increased affinity for LDL receptor-independent cell surface binding sites: a potential mechanism for increased atherogenicity. Journal of lipid research 39: 1263–1273.
15. Tribble DL, Rizzo M, Chait A, Lewis DM, Blanche PJ, et al. (2001) Enhanced oxidative susceptibility and reduced antioxidant content of metabolic precursors of small, dense low-density lipoproteins. The American journal of medicine 110: 103–110.
16. Berneis K, Jeanneret C, Muser J, Felix B, Miserez AR (2005) Low-density lipoprotein size and subclasses are markers of clinically apparent and non-apparent atherosclerosis in type 2 diabetes. Metabolism 54: 227–234.
17. Hayashi Y, Okumura K, Matsui H, Imamura A, Miura M, et al. (2007) Impact of low-density lipoprotein particle size on carotid intima-media thickness in patients with type 2 diabetes mellitus. Metabolism 56: 608–613.
18. Gerber PA, Thalhammer C, Schmied C, Spring S, Amann-Vesti B, et al. (2013) Small, Dense LDL Particles Predict Changes in Intima Media Thickness and Insulin Resistance in Men with Type 2 Diabetes and Prediabetes – A Prospective Cohort Study. PLoS ONE 8: e72763.
19. Simon DI (2012) Inflammation and Vascular Injury. Circulation Journal 76: 1811–1818.
20. Berneis K, Rizzo M, Berthold HK, Spinas GA, Krone W, et al. (2010) Ezetimibe alone or in combination with simvastatin increases small dense low-density lipoproteins in healthy men: a randomized trial. Eur Heart J 31: 1633–1639.
21. Hirano T, Ito Y, Saegusa H, Yoshino G (2003) A novel and simple method for quantification of small, dense LDL. J Lipid Res 44: 2193–2201.

Author Contributions

Conceived and designed the experiments: VJ BRA KM PAG. Performed the experiments: VJ KM PAG. Analyzed the data: BRA KB CT IW MH. Contributed reagents/materials/analysis tools: BRA MH KB CT. Wrote the paper: BRA VJ PAG IW MH CT.

5

Stent Thrombosis is the Primary Cause of ST-Segment Elevation Myocardial Infarction following Coronary Stent Implantation: A Five Year Follow-Up of the SORT OUT II Study

Søren Lund Kristensen[1,2]*, Anders M. Galløe[1], Leif Thuesen[3], Henning Kelbæk[4], Per Thayssen[5], Ole Havndrup[1], Peter Riis Hansen[2], Niels Bligaard[6], Kari Saunamäki[4], Anders Junker[5], Jens Aarøe[7], Ulrik Abildgaard[2], Jørgen L. Jeppesen[8]

1 Department of Cardiology, Copenhagen University Hospital Roskilde, Roskilde, Denmark, 2 Department of Cardiology, Copenhagen University Hospital Gentofte, Hellerup, Denmark, 3 Department of Medicine, Aarhus University Hospital Herning, Herning, Denmark, 4 The Heart Centre, Copenhagen University Hospital Rigshospitalet, Copenhagen, Denmark, 5 Department of Cardiology, Odense Universy Hospital, Odense, Denmark, 6 Department of Cardiology, Copenhagen University Hospital Bispebjerg, Copenhagen, Denmark, 7 Department of Cardiology, Aalborg University Hospital, Aalborg, Denmark, 8 Department of Medicine, Copenhagen University Hospital Glostrup, Glostrup, Denmark

Abstract

Background: The widespread use of coronary stents has exposed a growing population to the risk of stent thrombosis, but the importance in terms of risk of ST-segment elevation myocardial infarctions (STEMIs) remains unclear.

Methods: We studied five years follow-up data for 2,098 all-comer patients treated with coronary stents in the randomized SORT OUT II trial (mean age 63.6 yrs. 74.8% men). Patients who following stent implantation were readmitted with STEMI were included and each patient was categorized ranging from definite- to ruled-out stent thrombosis according to the Academic Research Consortium definitions. Multivariate logistic regression was performed on selected covariates to assess odds ratios (ORs) for definite stent thrombosis.

Results: 85 patients (4.1%), mean age 62.7 years, 77.1% men, were admitted with a total of 96 STEMIs, of whom 60 (62.5%) had definite stent thrombosis. Notably, definite stent thrombosis was more frequent in female than male STEMI patients (81.8% vs. 56.8%, p = 0.09), and in very late STEMIs (p = 0.06). Female sex (OR 3.53 [1.01–12.59]) and clopidogrel (OR 4.43 [1.03–19.01]) was associated with increased for definite stent thrombosis, whereas age, time since stent implantation, use of statins, initial PCI urgency (STEMI [primary PCI], NSTEMI/unstable angina [subacute PCI] or stable angina [elective PCI]), and glucose-lowering agents did not seem to influence risk of stent thrombosis.

Conclusion: In a contemporary cohort of coronary stented patients, stent thrombosis was evident in more than 60% of subsequent STEMIs.

Editor: Pierfrancesco Agostoni, University Medical Center Utrecht, Netherlands

Funding: Boston Scientific and Cordis, a Johnson & Johnson company, supported the completion of the primary SORT OUT II study and event detection for a follow-up period of five years. They had no role in the design of the current substudy and did not provide support for its completion.

Competing Interests: The authors received funding from Boston Scientific and Cordis.

* Email: slk@heart.dk

Introduction

Stent thrombosis is a rare but serious complication following coronary stenting, associated with a high risk of acute coronary artery closure, ST-segment elevation myocardial infarction (STEMI) and sudden cardiac death [1,2]. Up until recently, a growing number of patients has been treated with coronary stents, leaving them exposed to the risk of stent thrombosis [3]. This was reflected in a recent study of consecutive STEMI patients, where the number of STEMIs resulting from stent thrombosis nearly doubled (6% to 11%) in the period from 2003–10 [4].

Despite these findings, information on the percentage of STEMIs caused by stent thrombosis is sparse, and most studies on the topic are hampered by short follow-up [5]. The primary goal of the present study was to evaluate the prevalence of stent thrombosis in patients presenting with STEMI after percutaneous coronary intervention (PCI) during long term follow-up, and additionally, to identify clinical predictors of stent thrombosis in these subjects. For these analyses, we examined data from 2098 patients treated with coronary stents in the SORT OUT II trial [5].

Methods

Study population

The Danish Organization on Randomized Trials with clinical Outcome (SORT OUT) is an independent clinical cardiovascular research collaboration among the five Danish centers performing coronary stent implantations. In the present study we used follow-up data from the SORT OUT II trial, which in the period 2004–2006, randomized 2098 patients eligible for percutaneous coronary intervention (PCI), to one of the first two commercially available drug-eluting stents; the sirolimus-eluting Cypher stent (Cordis/Johnson & Johnson, Florida) or the paclitaxel-eluting Taxus stent (Boston Scientific Group, Massachusetts).[5] Each citizen in Denmark is provided with a unique and permanent civil registration number, and by use of this number all in- and outpatient hospital admissions, deaths and emigrations are reported to national registries and identifiable from these sources.

We assessed all SORT OUT II participants irrespective of randomization as there were no short- or long-term differences in the risk of major adverse cardiovascular events and stent thrombosis when comparing the two stents [5,6]. The SORT OUT II cohort was followed from stent implantation until death, migration, or five years from study inclusion. Patients hospitalized with one (or more) STEMI(s) during follow-up comprised the present study cohort.

Outcome – stent thrombosis probability

All STEMI admissions following SORT OUT II study inclusion were identified by case notes, electrocardiogram (ECG) findings, and cardiac biomarkers. Each STEMI was then categorized as definite-, probable-, possible- or ruled out stent thrombosis, according to the classification defined by the Academic Research Consortium (ARC) [7].

Categorization of stent thrombosis probability was based on detailed records of hospital admission, including case notes, ECG findings, and angiographic findings. Information on out-of hospital deaths were obtained from general practitioners' records and outpatients coronary artery angiographies were evaluated from the records and/or by inspection of copies of the angiographic recordings. Classification as definite stent thrombosis demanded either angiographic or autopsy confirmation. In order to resemble a real-life scenario of stent thrombosis risk in coronary stented patients admitted with STEMI, we also included information on non-randomized stents unrelated to the SORT OUT II study in our stent thrombosis evaluation. Finally, we merged probable- and possible stent thrombosis into one group (possible stent thrombosis) and further we stratified the STEMIs in three groups according to time passed since stent implantation; early (0–30 days), late (31–365 days) and very late stent thrombosis (>365 days). All the above outcomes, including ECGs and angiograms, and also the specific causes of cardiac and non- cardiac deaths, were adjudicated by the independent SORT OUT II adjudication committee, as described in details elsewhere [5]. The basis of the cause of death adjudication was the main underlying disease causing death. In most cases, the cause of death was cancer (n = 67), and in these cases, patients were adjudicated not to have stent thrombosis.

Medical treatment

From patient records, we assessed each patients use of the following medications at time of STEMI (ATC codes); aspirin (B01AC06, N02BA01), clopidogrel (B01AC04), vitamin K antagonists (B01AA), angiotensin-converting enzyme inhibitors (ACE-Is)/angiotensin receptor blockers (ARBs) (C09), beta-blockers (C07), loop diuretics (C03C), proton-pump inhibitors (A02BC), calcium channel antagonists (C08), nitrates (C01DA) and glucose-lowering agents (A10). All patients in SORT OUT II were prescribed 12 months of dual antiplatelet treatment (low dose aspirin and clopidogrel) and monotherapy with aspirin onwards after PCI. We did not have information on the overall compliance in the SORT OUT II cohort, but a prior registry-based Danish study on post-MI treatment adherence showed that approximately 80% were treated with dual antiplatelet therapy for one year following PCI [8]. Among the 31 SORT OUT II patients who were admitted with a STEMI within 12 months of initial stent implantation, none were treated with vitamin K antagonists, 18 (58.1%) received the recommended dual antiplatelet therapy, 10 (32.3%) were treated with aspirin monotherapy and the remaining 3 (9.6%) patients received no antithrombotic therapy.

Statistics

Baseline characteristics for the study population were summarized as means with standard deviations for continuous variables and frequencies and percentages for categorical variables. For descriptive statistics we used Chi-square tests for categorical data and Kruskall-Wallis test for non-parametric data. We fitted a multivariate logistic regression model to estimate odds ratios (ORs) for the probability of definite stent thrombosis, as compared to possible or ruled out stent thrombosis among patients subsequently admitted with STEMI. The model included adjustments for; sex, age (divided into inter-quartile ranges [IQR]), time since PCI (categorized as early [<30 days], late [31–364 days] or very late [>365 days]), initial PCI urgency (elective vs. subacute or primary [acute] PCI), and pharmacological treatment with aspirin, clopidogrel, and antidiabetics. As a sensitivity analysis, we included cases of unexplained death (n = 52), which according to ARC criteria corresponds to probable stent thrombosis if death occurs within 30 days of PCI, and possible stent thrombosis if more than 30 days after PCI. In the sensitivity analysis, we estimated odds ratios for definite *or* probable stent thrombosis as opposed to definite stent thrombosis alone in the primary analysis.

Ethics

The SORT OUT II study was conducted in accordance with the second Helsinki declaration and the local biomedical research committee (Health Research Ethical Committee of the Capital Region, Denmark) approved the study. Trial registration: clinicaltrials.gov, identifier: NCT00388934. All study participants provided written informed consent.

Results

Within 5 years of coronary stent implantation, we identified 85 patients (4.1%) who were admitted with a total of 96 STEMIs (Figure 1). Definite stent thrombosis was confirmed in 60 STEMIs (62.5%) whereas 14 STEMIs (13.5%) were classified as probable or possible stent thrombosis and in the remaining 22 STEMIs (24.0%) stent thrombosis was ruled out i.e. lesions were not related to a prior stented area (de novo lesions). In 13 patients the categorization as definite- or possible stent thrombosis was related to a non-randomized stent, i.e. stent(s) that were implanted before or after the patient was randomized in the SORT OUT II trial. General characteristics of the STEMI population stratified by stent thrombosis probability are summarized in Table 1. The mean age was 62.7 (SD 11.0) years and 77.1% were men. Notably, STEMI resulting from definite stent thrombosis appeared to be more common in women than in men (81.8% vs. 56.8%, p = 0.09), and more than a year after stent implantation (p = 0.06), whereas we found no relation between initial PCI indication at randomization and stent thrombosis probability (p = 0.56). A total of 11 patients suffered a second STEMI during follow-up, of whom five had definite stent thrombosis, five had recurring definite stent thrombosis, and one had a de novo lesion. The cumulative number of STEMI and definite stent thrombosis cases according to time passed since study inclusion is shown in Figure 2. We compared the use of cardiovascular medication at time of STEMI stratified by the presence of stent thrombosis, and observed no significant differences, except for the use of dual anti-platelet therapy which was higher in the definite stent thrombosis group (p = 0.03). Use of glucose-lowering agents also seemed more frequent in patients with definite stent thrombosis but the difference was non-significant (p = 0.15). In a multivariate logistic regression model (Figure 3) female sex was associated with a significantly increased risk of definite stent thrombosis (OR 3.73 [95% CI 1.04–13.41]), as well as use of clopidogrel (OR 4.46 [1.03–19.34]). There was a non-significant indication towards a protective effect of aspirin use (OR 0.43 [0.09–2.01]), and no association to age, initial PCI urgency, time since PCI and glucose-lowering agents. Of note, from a total of 256 deaths which occurred during 5 year follow-up, 52 patients (3 within 30 days of PCI) died of unexplained causes (Figure 1). We did not include these cases of unexplained death in our primary analysis, although we included them in a sensitivity analysis. In this sensitivity analysis where we examined the risk of definite *or* probable stent thrombosis, odds ratios were consistent with findings of the primary analysis, although ongoing use clopidogrel was no longer associated with a significantly increased risk of (definite and probable) stent thrombosis (not shown).

Discussion

In this study of a large population of all-comers treated with coronary stents, the number of patients re-admitted with STEMI within five year of follow-up was low. However, in more than 60% of STEMIs patients had definite stent thrombosis. The majority of stent thrombosis occurred very late (>365 days after initial stent implantation). Thus, our data imply that secondary preventions strategies work reasonably well to prevent STEMI culprits in non-PCI treated segments of the coronary vasculature, but also that implanted stents endure as vulnerable areas of the coronary arteries.

In a multivariate analysis comparing STEMIs with and without evidence of stent thrombosis, we failed to find an association between initial PCI urgency (elective vs. subacute or acute) and stent thrombosis. This together with the somewhat surprising finding of an association between stent thrombosis and DAPT was in contrast to a previous study of stent thrombosis predictors [2,9,10]. In fact, the association between DAPT and definite stent thrombosis was primarily observed in patients (n = 65) who suffered a STEMI more than 12 months after stent implantation. Among these patients, 13 received DAPT, of whom 12 presented with STEMIs caused by definite stent thrombosis. It is likely that the latter patients were considered by treating physicians to be at higher risk as DAPT had been continued beyond the recommended 12 months, albeit that as indicated in Table 1, there were no apparent differences in measured potential risk factors for stent thrombosis, e.g. index PCI urgency (acute coronary syndrome vs. stable angina) or diabetes prevalence as measured by treatment with glucose-lowering drugs.

We also observed a trend towards a protective effect of ongoing aspirin treatment, and a significantly elevated OR for definite stent thrombosis in female STEMI subjects. We have no obvious explanation for the higher risk of stent thrombosis in females and the finding warrants confirmation from other studies.

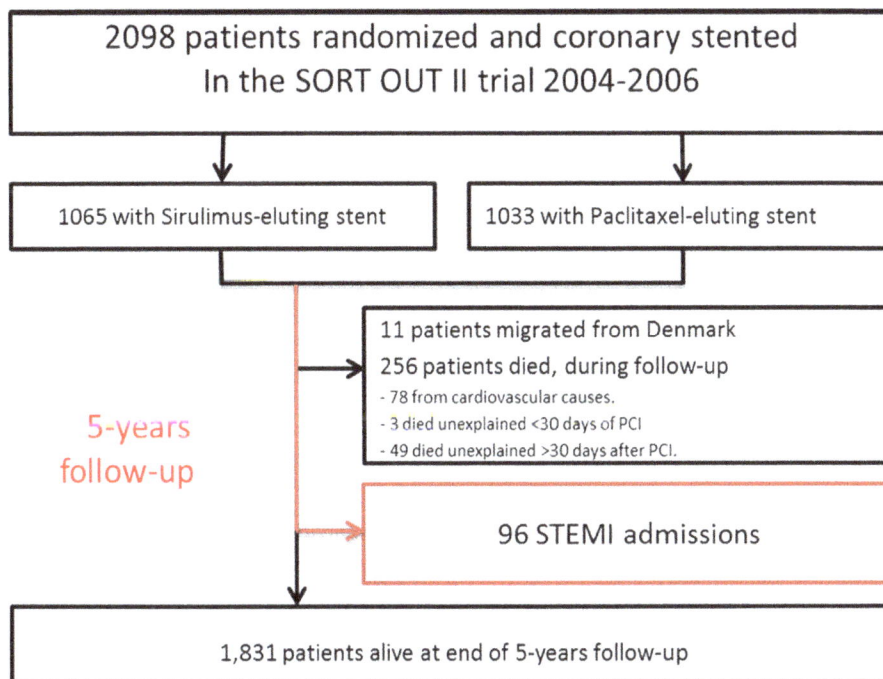

Figure 1. Flowchart of the STEMI-subgroup study population. STEMI – ST segment elevation myocardial infarction.

Cumulative incidence of STEMI and definite stent thrombosis

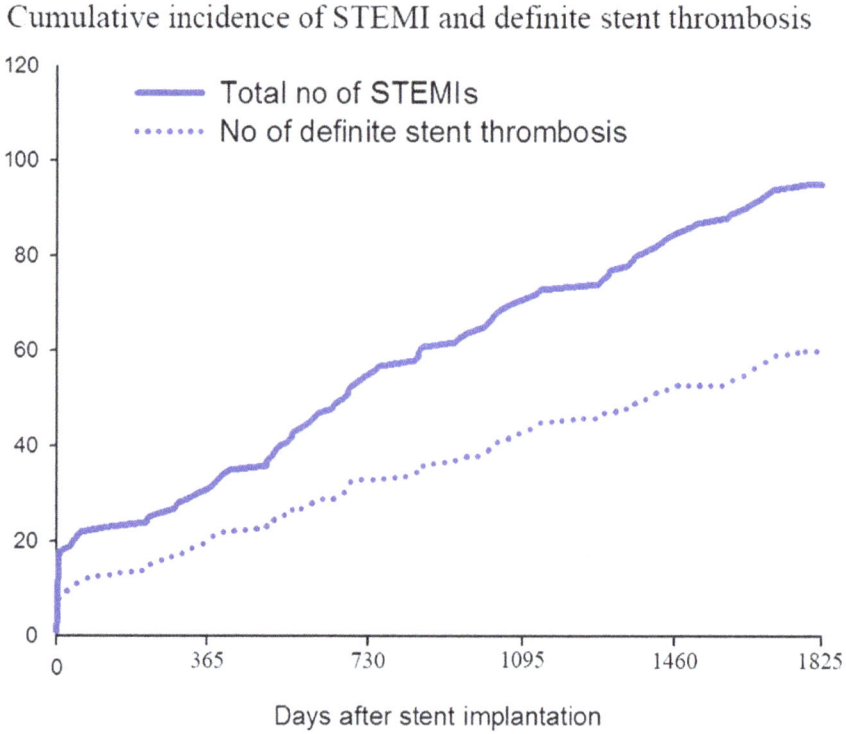

Figure 2. Fraction of STEMI's caused by definite stent thrombosis according to time from stent implantation. STEMI - ST segment elevation myocardial infarction.

We chose not to include cases of unexplained death in our primary analysis as our intention was to focus on definite stent thrombosis alone, and a more clinical perspective of previously coronary stented patients admitted with STEMI. However, we included cases of unexplained deaths in a sensitivity analysis and found results comparable to those of the primary analysis. Our finding of definite-, probable- or possible stent thrombosis in 7.4% of the study subjects after 5-year follow-up corresponded quite well with a large meta-analysis, although the median follow-up in that analysis was 22 months [10]. Indeed, in the current study we demonstrated that the rate of stent thrombosis continued at a relatively constant rate beyond the first two years after stent implantation.

Studies of first generation drug-eluting stents in clinical practice with unselected patients demonstrated higher rates of stent thrombosis compared to the randomized trials, which emphasized the importance of dual antiplatelet treatment after implantation of drug-eluting stents [1,10–12]. The comprehensive meta-analysis by Palmerini et al. further showed that the majority of studies, similar to SORT OUT II, found non-inferiority when comparing the sirolimus and paclitaxel eluting stents.

Studies comparing prognosis after stent thrombosis induced STEMI vs. de novo induced lesion STEMI have shown higher

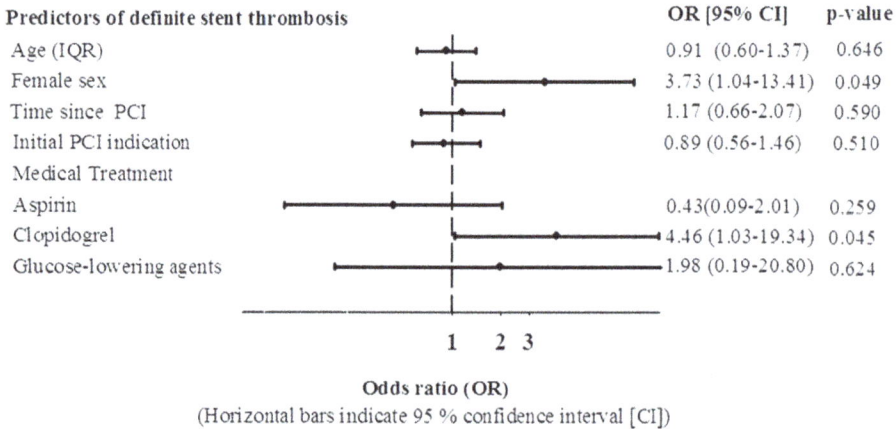

Figure 3. Odds ratios for definite stent thrombosis according to presence of selected covariates. STEMI - ST segment elevation myocardial infarction, OR – Odds ratio, CI – confidence interval.

Table 1. General characteristics of patients at time of admission for STEMI.

	Total	Definite stent thrombosis	Probable or possible stent thrombosis	No stent thrombosis	P-value
No. of STEMIs (%)	96 (100)	60 (62.5)	13 (13.5)	23 (24.0)	
Age, mean (SD)/years	62.7 (11.0)	62.3 (12.0)	61.6 (11.0)	64.1 (8.3)	0.42
Male, (%)	74 (77.1)	42 (56.8)	11 (14.9)	21 (28.4)	0.09
Female (%)	22 (22.9)	18 (81.8)	2 (9.1)	2 (9.1)	
Initial PCI urgency (%)					0.56
Primary PCI	24 (25.0)	14 (23.3)	2 (15.4)	8 (34.8)	
Subacute*	36 (37.5)	22 (36.6)	7 (53.8)	7 (30.4)	
Elective	36 (37.5)	24 (40.0)	4 (30.8)	8 (34.8)	
Days to STEMI/ST (%)					0.06
Early (0–30)	18 (18.8)	9 (15.0)	1 (7.7)	8 (34.8)	
Late (31–365)	13 (13.5)	11 (18.4)	0 (0)	2 (8.7)	
Very late (>365)	65 (67.7)	40 (66.6)	12 (92.3)	13 (56.5)	
Medical treatment (%)					
Aspirin	86 (89.6)	53 (88.3)	12 (92.3)	21 (91.3)	0.87
Clopidogrel	20 (20.8)	17 (28.3)	0 (0)	3 (13.0)	0.03
Dual antiplatelet therapy	20 (20.8)	17 (28.3)	0 (0)	3 (13.0)	0.03
Vitamin K antagonists	6 (6.3)	4 (6.7)	0 (0)	2 (8.7)	0.71
Statins	76 (79.2)	46 (76.7)	11 (84.6)	19 (82.6)	0.73
ACE-I/ARBs	44 (45.8)	30 (50.0)	4 (30.8)	10 (43.5)	0.44
Beta-blockers	64 (66.7)	40 (66.7)	8 (61.5)	16 (69.6)	0.89
Diuretics	30 (31.3)	19 (31.7)	4 (30.8)	7 (30.4)	0.99
Protein pump inhibitors	19 (19.8)	14 (23.3)	2 (15.4)	3 (13.0)	0.52
Ca-antagonists	17 (17.7)	9 (15.0)	3 (23.1)	5 (21.7)	0.67
Nitrates	15 (15.6)	12 (20.0)	1 (7.7)	2 (8.7)	0.31
Glucose-lowering agents	10 (10.4)	9 (15.0)	0 (0)	1 (4.3)	0.15

ST = stent thrombosis, ACE-I = Angiotensin-converting enzyme inhibitors, ARBs = angiotensin receptor blockers. PPI = Proton pump inhibitors. Dual antiplatelet therapy = clopidogrel and aspirin.
*Subacute PCI – patients with NSTEMI or unstable angina pectoris.

risk in regards of mortality, risk of recurrent myocardial infarction and post-PCI rates of major adverse cardiovascular events following stent thrombosis [13–15]. Along this line, a 7-year outcome with fractional flow reserve (FFR)-guided PCI, showed a significantly reduced risk for recurrent MI when PCI were deferred by FFR vs. performed due to PCI [16]. This reduced risk might be due to potential PCI-related damage or atherosclerotic disease being more advanced in previously stented segments. The LEADERS trial, which compared biolimus- and sirolimus-eluting stents showed a significant reduction in very late stent thrombosis (>1 year) for the biolimus-stent [17]. Contrarily, the SORT OUT V study which was a similar comparison of the biolimus and sirolimus stents, found no improvement in regard of a combined endpoint of cardiac death, myocardial infarction and stent thrombosis [18]. Interestingly, a significantly increased risk of definite stent thrombosis was observed among patients treated with the biolimus-stent, which may indicate that the risk of stent thrombosis and its marked contribution to subsequent STEMI cases observed in the present study remains relevant for patients treated with newer generations of drug-eluting stents.

Conclusions

In a large unselected PCI population treated with coronary stents, the incidence of subsequent STEMIs was low within five years of follow-up. However, stent thrombosis was present in more than 60% of STEMIs in these patients with one or more previously implanted stents, and the risk of stent thrombosis was higher beyond the first year following stent implantation. Continued focus on reduction of stent thrombosis, particularly beyond the first year after PCI is warranted.

Acknowledgments

The SORT OUT II study investigators: Niels Bligaard, M.D., Leif Thuesen, M.D., Henning Kelbæk, M.D., Per Thayssen, M.D., Jens Aarøe, M.D., Peter R. Hansen, M.D., Jens F. Lassen, M.D., Kari Saunamäki, M.D., Anders Junker, M.D., Jan Ravkilde, M.D., Ulrik.

Abildgaard, M.D., Hans H. Tilsted, M.D., Thomas Engstrøm, M.D., Jan S. Jensen, M.D., Hans E. Bøtker, M.D., Søren Galatius M.D., Carsten T. Larsen, M.D., Steen D. Kristensen, M.D., Lars R.Krusell, M.D., Steen Z. Abildstrøm, M.D., Evald H Christiansen M.D., Ghita Stephansen, R.N, Jørgen L. Jeppesen M.D., Anders M. Galløe, M.D.

Author Contributions

Conceived and designed the experiments: SLK AG JJ. Performed the experiments: AG LT HK PT PRH NB KS AJ JA UA. Analyzed the data: SLK AG JJ. Contributed reagents/materials/analysis tools: AG LT HK PT OH PRH NB KS AJ JA UA JJ. Contributed to the writing of the manuscript: SLK AG JJ LT KS PRH UA OH.

References

1. Iakovou I, Schmidt T, Bonizzoni E, Ge L, Sangiorgi GM, et al. (2005) Incidence, predictors, and outcome of thrombosis after successful implantation of drug-eluting stents. JAMA 293: 2126–30.
2. D'Ascenzo F, Bollati M, Clementi F, Castagno D, Lagerqvist B, et al. (2012) Incidence and predictors of coronary stent thrombosis: Evidence from an international collaborative meta-analysis including 30 studies, 221,066 patients, and 4276 thromboses. Int J Cardiol 2: 575–84.
3. Riley RF, Don CW, Powell W, Maynard C, Dean LS. (2011) Trends in coronary revascularization in the United States from 2001 to 2009: recent declines in percutaneous coronary intervention volumes. Circ Cardiovasc Qual Outcomes 4: 193–7.
4. Brodie BR, Hansen C, Garberich RF, Browning JA, Tobbia P, et al. (2012) ST-segment elevation myocardial infarction resulting from stent thrombosis: an enlarging subgroup of high-risk patients. J Am Coll Cardiol 60: 1989–91.
5. Galloe AM, Thuesen L, Kelbaek H, Thayssen P, Rasmussen K, et al. (2008) Comparison of paclitaxel- and sirolimus-eluting stents in everyday clinical practice: the SORT OUT II randomized trial. JAMA 299: 409–16.
6. Bligaard N, Thuesen L, Saunamaki K, Thayssen P, Aaroe J, et al. (2014) Similar five-year outcome with paclitaxel- and sirolimus-eluting coronary stents. Scand Cardiovasc J 48: 148–55.
7. Cutlip DE, Windecker S, Mehran R, Boam A, Cohen DJ, et al. (2007) Clinical end points in coronary stent trials: a case for standardized definitions. Circulation 115: 2344–51.
8. Lindhardsen J, Ahlehoff O, Gislason GH, Madsen OR, Olesen JB, et al. (2012) Initiation and adherence to secondary prevention pharmacotherapy after myocardial infarction in patients with rheumatoid arthritis: a nationwide cohort study. Ann Rheum Dis 71: 1496–501.
9. van Werkum JW, Heestermans AA, Zomer AC, Kelder JC, Suttorp MJ, et al. (2009) Predictors of coronary stent thrombosis: the Dutch Stent Thrombosis Registry. J Am Coll Cardiol 53: 1399–409.
10. Palmerini T, Biondi-Zoccai G, Della Riva D, Stettler C, Sangiorgi D, et al. (2012) Stent thrombosis with drug-eluting and bare-metal stents: evidence from a comprehensive network meta-analysis. Lancet 379: 1393–402.
11. Daemen J, Wenaweser P, Tsuchida K, Abrecht L, Vaina S, et al. (2007) Early and late coronary stent thrombosis of sirolimus-eluting and paclitaxel-eluting stents in routine clinical practice: data from a large two-institutional cohort study. Lancet 369: 667–78.
12. Moreno R, Fernandez C, Hernandez R, Alfonso F, Angiolillo DJ, et al. (2005) Drug-eluting stent thrombosis: results from a pooled analysis including 10 randomized studies. J Am Coll Cardiol 45: 954–9.
13. Chechi T, Vecchio S, Vittori G, Giuliani G, Lilli A, et al. (2008) ST-segment elevation myocardial infarction due to early and late stent thrombosis a new group of high-risk patients. J Am Coll Cardiol 51: 2396–402.
14. Ergelen M, Gorgulu S, Uyarel H, Norgaz T, Aksu H, et al. (2010) The outcome of primary percutaneous coronary intervention for stent thrombosis causing ST-elevation myocardial infarction. Am Heart J 159: 672–6.
15. Parodi G, Memisha G, Bellandi B, Valenti R, Migliorini A, et al.(2009) Effectiveness of primary percutaneous coronary interventions for stent thrombosis. Am J Cardiol 103: 913–6.
16. Li J, Elrashidi MY, Flammer AJ, Lennon RJ, Bell MR, et al. (2013) Long-term outcomes of fractional flow reserve-guided vs. angiography-guided percutaneous coronary intervention in contemporary practice. Eur Heart J 34: 1375–83.
17. Serruys PW, Farooq V, Kalesan B, de Vries T, Buszman P, et al. (2013) Improved Safety and Reduction in Stent Thrombosis Associated With Biodegradable Polymer-Based Biolimus-Eluting Stents Versus Durable Polymer-Based Sirolimus-Eluting Stents in Patients With Coronary Artery Disease: Final 5-Year Report of the LEADERS (Limus Eluted From A Durable Versus ERodable Stent Coating) Randomized, Noninferiority Trial. JACC Cardiovasc Interv 6: 777–89.
18. Christiansen EH, Jensen LO, Thayssen P, Tilsted HH, Krusell LR, et al. (2013) Biolimus-eluting biodegradable polymer-coated stent versus durable polymer-coated sirolimus-eluting stent in unselected patients receiving percutaneous coronary intervention (SORT OUT V): a randomised non-inferiority trial. Lancet 381: 661–9.

6

Systematic Testing of Literature Reported Genetic Variation Associated with Coronary Restenosis: Results of the GENDER Study

Jeffrey J. W. Verschuren[1], Stella Trompet[1,2,6], Iris Postmus[2,6], M. Lourdes Sampietro[3,7],
Bastiaan T. Heijmans[4,6], Jeanine J. Houwing-Duistermaat[5], P. Eline Slagboom[4,6], J. Wouter Jukema[1,6,7,8]*

1 Department of Cardiology, Leiden University Medical Center, Leiden, The Netherlands, 2 Department of Gerontology and Geriatrics, Leiden University Medical Center, Leiden, The Netherlands, 3 Department Human Genetics, Leiden University Medical Center, Leiden, The Netherlands, 4 Molecular Epidemiology, Leiden University Medical Center, Leiden, The Netherlands, 5 Department of Medical Statistics and Bioinformatics, Leiden University Medical Center, Leiden, The Netherlands, 6 Netherlands Consortium for Healthy Ageing, Leiden, The Netherlands, 7 Interuniversity Cardiology Institute of the Netherlands (ICIN), Utrecht, The Netherlands, 8 Durrer Center for Cardiogenetic Research, Amsterdam, The Netherlands

Abstract

Background: Coronary restenosis after percutaneous coronary intervention still remains a significant problem, despite all medical advances. Unraveling the mechanisms leading to restenosis development remains challenging. Many studies have identified genetic markers associated with restenosis, but consistent replication of the reported markers is scarce. The aim of the current study was to analyze the joined effect of previously in literature reported candidate genes for restenosis in the GENetic DEterminants of Restenosis (GENDER) databank.

Methodology/Principal Findings: Candidate genes were selected using a MEDLINE search including the terms 'genetic polymorphism' and 'coronary restenosis'. The final set included 36 genes. Subsequently, all single nucleotide polymorphisms (SNPs) in the genomic region of these genes were analyzed in GENDER using set-based analysis in PLINK. The GENDER databank contains genotypic data of 2,571,586 SNPs of 295 cases with restenosis and 571 matched controls. The set, including all 36 literature reported genes, was, indeed, significantly associated with restenosis, p = 0.024 in the GENDER study. Subsequent analyses of the individual genes demonstrated that the observed association of the complete set was determined by 6 of the 36 genes.

Conclusion: Despite overt inconsistencies in literature, with regard to individual candidate gene studies, this is the first study demonstrating that the joint effect of all these genes together, indeed, is associated with restenosis.

Editor: Yan Gong, College of Pharmacy, University of Florida, United States of America

Funding: This work was funded by grants from the Interuniversity Cardiology Institute of the Netherlands (ICIN) http://www.icin.nl/, the European Community Framework FP7 Programme under grant agreement [n° HEALTH-F2-2009-223004; http://cordis.europa.eu/projects/90569_en.html], the Center for Medical Systems Biology (CMSB) [http://www.cmsb.nl], a center of excellence approved by the Netherlands Genomics Initiative/Netherlands Organisation for Scientific Research (NWO), and the Netherlands Consortium for Healthy Ageing (NCHA) [http://www.healthy-ageing.nl]. JWJ is an established clinical investigator of the Netherlands Heart Foundation (2001D032) [http://www.hartstichting.nl/]. The funders had no role in study design, data collection and analysis, decision to publish or the preparation of the manuscript.

Competing Interests: The authors have declared that no competing interests exist.

* E-mail: j.w.jukema@lumc.nl

Introduction

Restenosis is a complex disease for which the causative mechanisms have not yet been fully identified. Despite medical advances, restenosis still remains a significant complication after percutaneous coronary intervention (PCI).[1] Identification of risk factors and underlying mechanisms could not only be useful in risk stratification of patients, they also contribute to our understanding of this condition. In addition, these factors could provide evidence on which to base individually tailored treatment and aid in the development of novel therapeutic modalities.[2] Unraveling the mechanisms leading to restenosis development remains challenging. Genetic susceptibility is known to play a role in the individuals risk of developing this complication.[1] Many studies have focused on

identification of genetic markers associated with restenosis. Over the last decades genetic research has developed from candidate gene approaches [3–5] to multiplex arrays [6] and finally to genome wide association studies (GWAS).[7] Genetic variation in large array of plausible candidate genes have been associated with restenosis, however, consistent replication of the reported markers is scarce.[1] Possible explanations for this lack of consistency are the small sample size of many (especially relative more dated) studies, phenotype heterogeneity and lack of proper replication cohorts.

Currently more and more GWAS are being performed, investigating many diseases, including cardiovascular diseases.[8,9] An advantage of GWAS is the hypothesis-free approach of this method, enabling identification of new genetic loci associated with the disease of interest. With respect to restenosis, a disadvantage of

Table 1. Demographic, clinical and lesion characteristics of the study population.

	Cases (n = 295)	Controls (n = 571)	p-value
Age (years)	62.8±10.6	62.4±10.9	0.59
BMI (kg.m^{-2})	26.7±3.6	27.1±3.7	0.20
Male sex	213 (72)	421 (74)	0.63
Diabetes	58 (20)	119 (21)	0.68
Hypercholesterolemia	179 (61)	341 (60)	0.79
Hypertension	138 (47)	211 (37)	0.005
Current smoker	68 (23)	148 (26)	0.36
Family history of MI	117 (40)	210 (37)	0.41
Previous MI	119 (40)	246 (43)	0.44
Stable angina	188 (64)	400 (68)	0.06
Multivessel disease	155 (53)	248 (43)	0.01
Restenotic lesion	23 (8)	48 (8)	0.76
Total occlusion	57 (19)	97 (17)	0.40
Type C lesion	95 (38)	154 (27)	0.11
Stenting	199 (68)	385 (67)	0.99

Values were given as n (%) or mean ± SD. Patients using anti-diabetic medication or insulin at study entry were considered to be diabetics. Hypertension was defined as a blood pressure of either above 160 mmHg systolic or 90 mmHg diastolic. Hypercholesterolaemia was defined as total cholesterol concentrations of above 5 mmol/L. BMI: body mass index, MI: myocardial infarction. P-values are determined by Pearsons Chi-Square (discrete variables) or unpaired 2-sided t-test (continuous variables).

the GWAS approach is that due to the complexity of the disease the effect size of individual genetic markers is likely to be small and therefore hard to detect. Moreover, the availability of (large) replication cohorts is very limited. In 2011, the first GWAS on restenosis in the GENetic DEterminants of Restenosis (GENDER) study identified a new susceptibility locus on chromosome 12.[7] The fact that this GWAS only identified this previously unknown locus does not mean that genetic variation in the previously proposed candidate genes does not affect restenosis development. It merely indicates that the influence of other individual markers is probably too small to detect in the GWAS setting. Especially for the complex traits, a more appropriate approach to interpret GWAS data is to analyze the combined effect of a single nucleotide polymorphism (SNP) set, grouped per pathway or gene region.[10]

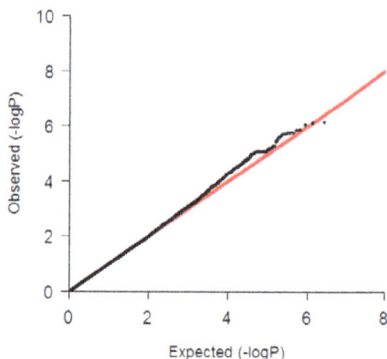

Figure 1. Q-Q plot for the GWAS after imputation on clinical restenosis in the GENDER study population. Lambda = 1.027.

To date, investigation into a possible joined effect of multiple genetic markers for restenosis has not been performed.

The goal of the current study is to investigate whether the last decade of research on genetics of restenosis has led to a set of genes that is associated with restenosis in a set-based analysis using the available genotypic data of the GENDER databank.

Methods

Gene Selection

Candidate genes previously associated with restenosis were selected after a search of literature of papers published up to November 2011. Genes were identified searching MEDLINE using keywords as 'genetic polymorphism', 'candidate gene', 'restenosis' and 'percutaneous coronary intervention'. Selection criteria included a sample size of >250 patients and the observation of a significant association of a SNP with restenosis. The final set included 36 genes. All available SNPs from the GENDER GWAS databank within a 10-Kb window around these genes were analyzed.

Study Population

The design of GENDER and the genome-wide association study (GWAS), which has been performed in a subset of this study population, have both been described previously.[7,11] In brief, GENDER included 3,104 consecutive unrelated symptomatic patients treated successfully by PCI for angina. The study protocol conforms to the Declaration of Helsinki and was approved by the ethics committees of each participating institution. Written informed consent was obtained from each participant before the PCI procedure. During a follow-up period of 9 months, the endpoint clinical restenosis, defined as renewed symptoms requiring target vessel revascularization (TVR) either by repeated PCI or CABG, by death from cardiac causes or myocardial infarction not attributable to another coronary event than the target vessel, was recorded. During follow-up, 346 patients developed clinical restenosis. Blood samples were collected at the index procedure for DNA isolation. The GWAS was performed in 325 cases of restenosis and 630 controls matched by gender, age, and some possible confounding clinical variables for restenosis in the GENDER study such as total occlusion, diabetes, current smoking and residual stenosis. Genotyping was performed using the Illumina Human 610-Quad Beadchips following the manufacturer's instructions. After genotyping, samples and genetic markers were subjected to a stringent quality control protocol. The final dataset consisted of 866 individuals (295 cases, 571 controls) and 556,099 SNPs that passed all quality control criteria, together covering 89% of the common genetic variation in the European population.[7,12] Imputation was performed with MACH software based on the HapMap II release 22 CEU build 36 using the default settings.[13] This program infers missing genotypes based on the known genotypic data of the samples together with haplotypes from a reference population provided by HapMap taken into account the degree of linkage disequilibrium (LD). After subsequent quality control, we excluded SNPs for further analyses with a call rate lower than 95% (n = 3335) or with a significant deviation from Hardy–Weinberg equilibrium (HWE) in controls (P<0.00001) (n = 79). The final GENDER Biobank dataset consisted of 866 (295 cases, 571 controls) individuals and 2,571,586 SNPs.

Statistical Analysis

The statistical analyses were performed using the set-based test of PLINK v1.07.[14] During this test, first a single SNP analysis of

Table 2. Candidate genes and the studies that reported their association with restenosis.

Candidate gene			Literature based study characteristics and results					
Gene	Entrez nr	Location	Study size	% of cases	Follow-up (mo)	Top SNP	Effect size (95% CI)[a]	Ref
adrenergic beta-2-receptor (ADRB2)	154	5q31–q32	3104	9.8	9	rs1042713	HR 1.33 (1.06–1.68)	[6]
advanced glycosylation end product-specific receptor (AGER)	177	6p21.3	267	UK	6–9	rs1800624	↓	[24]
			297	25.9	6	rs2070600	NS	[25]
angiotensin II receptor, type 1 (AGTR1)	184	3q24	272	29.8	6	rs5186	NS	[26]
			3104	9.8	9	rs5186	OR 1.85 (1.28–2.66)	[27]
Butyrylcholinesterase (BCHE)	590	3q26.1–q26.2	461	23.2	6	rs1803274	OR 5.5 (1.6–21.4)	[28]
chemokine (C–C motif) ligand 11 (CCL11)	6356	17q21.1–q21.2	3104	9.8	9	rs4795895	HR 0.73 (0.58–0.93)	[6]
CD14	929	5q31.1	129	24	6	rs2569190	RR 3.8 (1.2–11.6)	[29]
			3104	9.8	9	rs2569190	HR 0.74 (0.55–0.99)	[6]
cyclin-dependent kinase inhibitor 1B (p27, Kip1) (CDKN1B)	1027	12p13.1-p12	433	11.3	12	rs34330	NS	[30]
			2309	8.8	9	rs36448499	HR 0.61 (0.40–0.93)	[31]
collagen, type III, alpha 1 (Col3A1)	1281	2q31	527	9.1	6	rs1800255	OR 4.2 (1.4–11.2)	[32]
colony stimulating factor 2 (CSF2)	1437	5q31.1	3104	9.8	9	rs25882	HR 0.76 (0.61–0.94)	[6]
chemokine (C-X3-C motif) receptor 1 (CX3CR1)	1524	3p21.3	365	25.5	6	rs3732379	OR 2.4 (1.3–4.2)	[33]
cytochrome b-245, alpha polypeptide (CYBA)	1535	16q24	730	35.8	6	rs4673	OR 0.5 (0.3–0.8)	[34]
cytochrome P450, family 2, subfamily C, polypeptide 19 (CYP2C19)	1557	10q24	928	19.1	12	rs12248560	↓	[35]
fibrinogen beta chain (FGB)	2244	4q28	527	9.1	6	rs1800790	OR 2.7 (1.2–6.2)	[32]
			2257	8.8	9	rs1800790	NS	[36]
coagulation factor V (F5)	2153	1q23	3104	9.8	9	rs6025	HR 0.40 (0.19–0.85)	[37]
glutathione peroxidase 1 (GPX1)	2876	3p21.3	461	23.2	6	rs1050450	OR 2.1 (1.2–3.8)	[28]
interleukin 10 (IL10)	3586	1q31–q32	162	39.5	UK	rs1800871	HR 0.39 (0.16–0.94)	[38]
			1850	17.6	12		NS	[39]
			3104	9.8	9	rs3024498	HR 2.0 (1.4–2.8)	[40]
interleukin 1 receptor antagonist (IL1RN)	3557	2q14.2	183	46.4	12	VNTR	HR 5.24 (1.63–16.81)	[41]
			779	43.9	6	VNTR	NS	[42]
			1850	20.3	12	rs419598	OR 0.73 (0.58–0.92)	[3]
insulin receptor (INSR)	3643	19p13.3–p13.2	461	23.2	6	7,067,365C>A	OR 1.9 (1.2–3.1)	[28]
integrin, beta 2 (ITGB2)	3689	21q22.3	1207	21.2	12	rs235326	OR 0.71 (0.55–0.92)	[4]
lipoprotein lipase (LPL)	4023	8p22	3104	9.8	9	rs328	OR 0.62 (0.44–0.86)	[43]
matrix metallopeptidase 12 (MMP12)	4321	11q22.3	527	9.1	6	rs2276109	OR 3.9 (1.0–12.4)	[32]
matrix metallopeptidase 9 (MMP9)	4318	20q11.2–q13.1	461	23.2	6	rs2664538	OR 2.0 (1.0–3.9)	[28]
methylenetetrahydrofolate reductase (NAD(P)H) (MTHFR)	4524	1p36.3	260	36.9	6	rs1801133	OR 3.58 (1.51–8.46)	[44]
			800	18.9	12	rs1801133	NS	[45]
nitric oxide synthase 3 (NOS3)	4846	7q36	205	29.3	6	rs2070744	OR 2.06 (1.08–3.94)	[46]
			901	10.2	9	rs1799983	HR 1.67 (1.09–2.54)	[47]
			1556	20.8	12	rs1799983	NS	[48]
purinergic receptor P2Y, G-protein coupled, 12 (P2RY12)	64805	3q24–q25	2062	8.4	9	Haplotype of 5 SNPs	HR 1.6 (1.2–2.0)	[49]
serpin peptidase inhibitor, clade E, member 1 (SERPINE1)	5054	7q21.3–q22	1850	20.3	12	rs1799899	NS	[50]
			3104	9.8	9	rs1799899	HR 1.26 (1.07–1.49)	[37]

Table 2. Cont.

Candidate gene			Literature based study characteristics and results					
Gene	Entrez nr	Location	Study size	% of cases	Follow-up (mo)	Top SNP	Effect size (95% CI)[a]	Ref
K(lysine) acetyltransferase 2B (KAT2B, PCAF)	8850	3p24	3104	9.8	9	rs2948080	HR 0.80 (0.67–0.97)	[51]
peroxisome proliferator-activated receptor gamma (PPARG)	5468	3p25	565	28.7	6	rs3856806	↓	[52]
			935	18.3	12	rs3856806	NS	[53]
c-ros oncogene 1, receptor tyrosine kinase (ROS1)	6098	6q22	461	23.2	6	rs529038	HR 1.8 (1.1–2.8)	[28]
thrombomodulin (THBD)	7056	20p11.2	730	35.8	6	rs1042579	OR 2.1 (1.3–3.53)	[34]
thrombospondin 4 (THBS4)	7060	5q13	628	UK	6–10	rs1866389	OR 2.67 (1.04–6.80)	[54]
thrombopoietin (THPO)	7066	3q27	527	9.1	6	rs6141	OR 2.4 (1.1–5.3)	[32]
tumor necrosis factor (TNF)	7124	6p21.3	1850	17.6	12	rs1800629	NS	[39]
			3104	9.8	9	rs361525	HR 0.60 (0.37–0.98)	[5]
tumor protein p53 (TP53)	7157	17p13.1	132	0	UK	rs1042522	↑	[55]
			433	11.3	12	rs1042522	NS	[30]
			779	43.9	6	Haplotype of 3 SNPs	OR 0.58 (0.40–0.83)	[56]
uncoupling protein 3 (UCP3)	7352	11q13.4	527	9.1	6	rs1800849	OR 5.2 (1.9–13.0)	[32]
vitamin D receptor (VDR)	7421	12q13.11	3104	9.8	9	Haplotype of rs 11568820 and rs4516035	HR 0.72 (0.57–0.93)	[57]

[a]The direction of the association between genetic variation and the risk of restenosis, when effect size is not available; ↓ protective effect, ↑ deleterious effect. Entrez nr; unique gene ID number used in NCBI database. Abbreviations: UK, unknown; NS, not significant; OR, odds ratio; HR, hazard ratio; RR, relative risk; Ref, reference.

all SNPs within the set is performed. Subsequently a mean SNP statistic is calculated from the single SNP statistics of a maximum amount of independent SNPs below a certain p-value threshold. If SNPs are not independent and the LD (expressed in R^2) is above a certain threshold, the SNP with the lowest p-value in the single SNP analysis is selected. This analysis is repeated in a certain amount of permutations of the phenotype. An empirical p-value for the SNP set is computed by calculating the number of times the test statistic of the simulated SNP sets exceeds that of the original SNP set. For the analysis of this study, the parameters were set to p-value threshold <0.05, R^2 threshold <0.1, maximum number of SNPs = 5 and 10,000 permutations.

Initially, the set including all 36 genes is tested as a whole for the association with restenosis. Subsequent analysis of the individual genes will be justified only when the complete set is significantly associated with the endpoint.

Results

Patient characteristics are presented in Table 1. No significant differences were found between cases and controls regarding the known risk factors for restenosis (age, diabetes, smoking, stenting and previous restenosis). Hypertension and multivessel disease were more common in the cases compared to the controls.

In Figure 1 the QQ-plot of the GENDER GWAS after imputation is shown, demonstrating that no genomic inflation has occurred in this analysis (lambda = 1.027). The complete set of 36 genes, previously associated with restenosis in literature, contained 2,581 SNPs. A detailed description of the individual studies and candidate genes can be found in Table 2. The largest gene was

chemokine (C-X3-C motif) receptor 1 (CX3CR1) of 316.54 kb, contributing 384 SNPs (14.8%), and glutathione peroxidase 1 (GPX1) was with 1.18 kb the smallest gene, only contributing 8 SNPs (0.3%). Analysis of the complete set using the set-based test demonstrated a significant association with clinical restenosis, with an empirical p-value of 0.024.

To determine which genes are mainly responsible for this association we subsequently investigated the association of the individual gene based sets. Six of the 36 genes were demonstrated to have an empirical p-value below 0.05 (Table 3). In order of descending p-values the associated genes are; angiotensin II receptor type 1 (AGTR, p = 0.028), glutathione peroxidase 1 (GPX1, p = 0.025), K(lysine) acetyltransferase 2B (KAT2B, also known as PCAF, p = 0.023), matrix metallopeptidase 12 (MMP12, p = 0.019), fibrinogen beta chain (FGB, p = 0.013) and vitamin D receptor (VDR, p = 0.012). Detailed information on the individual SNPs in these genes is depicted in Table 4. The SNP with the lowest individual p-value was rs11574027 in the VDR gene, p = 1.4E-04. In the complete GWAS analysis, which has been published in 2011 [7], this SNP ranked 116th. The strongest association in that analysis was found with a SNP in an intergenic region on chromosome 12, p = 1.0E-06.

Logistic regression models with and without the 11 SNPs described in Table 4 demonstrated that together these SNPs explained 9.0% (R Square improved from 0.008 to 0.098) of the occurrence of clinical restenosis in this cohort.

As a final analysis we removed the 6 significantly associated genes from the complete set. Subsequent analysis of the subset of the other 30 genes did not demonstrate a remaining joined effect, p = 0.65 after 10,000 permutations.

Table 3. Results of individual gene set-based analysis of genes previously associated with restenosis.

Gene	Chr	Start (bp)	End (bp)	Size (kb)	SNPs	Sign. SNPs	Indep. SNPs	P-value
ADRB2	5	148 186 349	148 188 381	2.03	32	8	2	0.088
AGER	6	32 256 724	32 260 001	3.28	37	1	1	0.228
AGTR1	3	149 898 348	149 943 480	45.13	100	5	1	**0.028**
BCHE	3	166 973 387	167 037 944	64.56	101	8	2	0.314
CCL11	17	29 636 800	29 639 312	2.51	18	0	0	1.000
CD14	5	139 991 501	139 993 439	1.94	22	4	2	1.000
CDKN1B	12	12 761 576	12 766 569	4.99	13	0	0	1.000
Col3A1	2	189 547 344	189 585 717	38.37	97	2	2	0.649
CSF2	5	131 437 384	131 439 757	2.37	28	0	0	0.965
CX3CR1	3	39 279 990	39 596 531	316.54	384	3	1	0.358
CYBA	16	87 237 199	87 244 958	7.76	14	1	1	0.182
CYP2C19	10	96 512 453	96 602 660	90.21	43	1	1	1.000
FGB	4	155 703 596	155 711 686	8.09	25	2	1	**0.013**
F5	1	167 747 816	167 822 393	74.58	200	1	1	1.000
GPX1	3	49 369 615	49 370 795	1.18	8	1	1	**0.024**
IL10	1	205 007 571	205 012 462	4.89	30	5	1	**0.053**
IL1RN	2	113 601 609	113 608 063	6.45	62	0	0	0.991
INSR	19	7 063 266	7 245 011	181.75	172	20	5	0.263
ITGB2	21	45 130 299	45 165 303	35.00	57	6	4	0.663
LPL	8	19 841 058	19 869 049	27.99	75	14	5	1.000
MMP12	11	102 238 675	102 250 922	12.25	36	3	3	**0.019**
MMP9	20	44 070 954	44 078 606	7.65	23	10	3	0.067
MTHFR	1	11 768 374	11 788 702	20.33	61	1	1	1.000
NOS3	7	150 319 080	150 342 608	23.53	20	0	0	0.987
P2RY12	3	152 538 066	152 585 234	47.17	121	0	0	1.000
SERPINE1	7	100 556 303	100 558 421	2.12	27	0	0	0.863
KAT2B	3	20 056 528	20 170 898	114.37	144	19	4	**0.023**
PPARG	3	12 304 349	12 450 854	146.51	144	14	5	1.000
ROS1	6	117 716 223	117 853 711	137.49	206	1	1	0.631
THBD	20	22 974 271	22 978 301	4.03	22	0	0	1.000
THBS4	5	79 366 747	79 414 861	48.11	61	3	2	0.292
THPO	3	185 572 467	185 578 626	6.16	16	1	1	0.165
TNF	6	31 651 329	31 654 089	2.76	41	2	2	0.370
TP53	17	7 512 445	7 531 642	19.20	17	1	1	0.120
UCP3	11	73 388 958	73 397 778	8.82	34	1	1	0.183
VDR	12	46 521 589	46 585 081	63.49	93	2	2	**0.012**

Chromosome and genomic region based on HapMap Rel 28 Phase II+III. P-value based on permutation (10,000). Abbreviations: SNPs, number of SNPs in genomic region including 10 kb window; Sign.SNPs, number of SNPs with p<0.05; Indep.SNPs, number of significant and independent SNPs, considering threshold of $R^2<0.1$.

Discussion

With this study we aimed at clarifying the ambiguities regarding genetic predisposition for developing restenosis after PCI. We show that the joined effect of the complete spectrum of candidate genes, so far proposed to be involved in the restenotic process, results in a significant association with restenosis. This association is determined by six individual genes. Analyzing a subset containing the 30 genes not associated with the endpoint on an individual basis, did not show a remaining joined effect, making the involvement of genetic variation in these genes on restenosis development more unlikely.

The six associated genes span a wide range of different functions underlining the complexity of the disease. When examining the biological pathways with involvement of these genes, only the VDR and KAT2B genes share a common pathway. The genes are both involved in the Vitamin D receptor pathway described by BioCarta.[15] This pathway mainly involves the transcriptional regulating capacities of this receptor and is involved in controlling cellular growth, differentiation and apoptosis. Since these processes are all thought to be important contributors to the restenotic process, this indeed is a plausible pathway to be involved in restenosis development.[1].

Table 4. Significantly associated SNPs of the 6 top genes.

Gene	SNP	Chr	bp	Function	Alleles	MAF case	MAF control	OR	p-value	Origin	Imputation quality
AGTR1	rs5182	3	149942085	Exon, synonymous	T/C	0.43	0.50	0.75	0.0040	Genotyped	–
FGB	rs1044291	4	155712802	3′UTR	T/C	0.38	0.30	1.40	0.0028	Imputed	0.970
GPX1	rs8179164	3	49372288	Promoter	A/T	0.02	0.04	0.42	0.0077	Imputed	0.993
MMP12	rs12808148	11	102238373	Downstream	C/T	0.16	0.09	1.82	0.00021	Imputed	0.953
	rs17099726	11	102257062	Promoter	G/T	0.03	0.06	0.54	0.032	Imputed	0.957
KAT2B	rs6776870	3	20126544	Intron	G/C	0.14	0.21	0.62	0.00064	Imputed	0.999
	rs2929404	3	20069570	Intron	T/C	0.21	0.15	1.49	0.0026	Imputed	0.981
	rs17796904	3	20096353	Intron	T/C	0.16	0.12	1.43	0.012	Genotyped	–
	rs4858767	3	20141941	Intron	G/C	0.29	0.34	0.79	0.037	Imputed	0.994
VDR	rs11574027	12	46573640	Intron	T/G	0.03	0.007	4.19	0.00014	Genotyped	–
	rs11574077	12	46539194	Intron	G/A	0.07	0.04	1.60	0.029	Genotyped	–

SNP, single nucleotide polymorphism; Chr, chromosome; bp, base pair; MAF, minor allele frequency in control group; OR, odds ratio. The imputation quality indicates the average posterior probability for the most likely genotype generated by MACH, ranging from 0–1.

The rationale of set-based analysis is to overcome the marginally weak effect of single SNPs by analyzing a set of SNPs, since these SNPs could jointly have strong genetic effects. Most studies utilizing the candidate gene approach analyzed only one or at most a few SNPs within the gene of interest. The likelihood that exactly those SNPs are the causal or associated SNPs is of course small. A broader approach, like this set-based analysis, is therefore more likely to detect an associated gene by combining multiple SNPs with a possible marginal individual effect.[16,17] For the current study we used the PLINK software [14], although multiple statistical programs are available for this type of analysis. Gui et al. compared 7 tests analyzing the WTCCC Crohn's Disease dataset.[18] One of their overall conclusions was that the set-based test in PLINK was the most powerful algorithm. Another study, applying PLINK set-based test, Global test, GRASS and SNP ratio test, for the analysis of three pathways regarding human longevity observed similar results with the different tests.[19].

For the current study we analyzed the data using a threshold of linkage disequilibrium defined by $R^2 \geq 0.1$. The standard setting in PLINK is a R^2 of 0.5. In our opinion this threshold is too high for the intended analysis for this study. A higher threshold will include more SNPs in higher LD, which would be unfavorable, since we were interested in independent loci contributing to the risk of restenosis. By decreasing this threshold, only SNPs were selected that had a R^2 below 0.1, and thus independent of each other.

Although hypertension and multivessel disease were more frequent in cases compared to controls we decided not to correct for these variables. In the complete GENDER population these variables were not independent predictors for restenosis development [11], so the differences in the current subpopulation likely resulted by chance during the selection process. Also, other studies provide no convincing data that hypertension is related to restenosis [1]. It is therefore unlikely that previous associations of some of the current candidates genes (VDR, FGB, AGTR1 and GPX1) with hypertension[20–23], have influenced our results, although this cannot be completely excluded.

A limitation of the current study could be that we analyzed imputed genotypic data, which introduces some amount of uncertainty. However, since we were interested in the combined effect of SNPs, an extensive genomic coverage was paramount for this analysis. Only analyzing the genotyped GWAS data would have resulted in the coverage of some of the smaller genes by only 1 or 2 SNPs. Therefore we decided that the more extensive genomic coverage of the imputed dataset outweighed the small introduction of possible error. A second limitation is that the analyses were only performed in the GENDER population. Availability of other populations with thorough genetic data on restenosis is however very limited. To our knowledge, the GWAS on restenosis in the GENDER population is the first, and only, examining this endpoint on a genome wide scale. Finally, the conclusions of this study are only based on genetic analyses. Functional studies should be performed to elucidate the biological consequences of these findings.

In conclusion, with these results we demonstrate that the efforts in unraveling the genetic factors influencing the risk of restenosis of the last years has resulted in a set of genes that joint together is indeed likely to be associated with restenosis, despite the overt inconsistencies of the individual studies. Confirmation of the association of these genes with the occurrence of restenosis after PCI helps our understanding of the genetic etiology of the disease. Future additional research strategies, like biological pathway analysis of GWAS data or even (exome) sequencing, might help us find the missing heritability of restenosis after PCI and increase our knowledge of the biological mechanistic background of restenosis development. This knowledge could subsequently result in identification of new treatment targets or development of novel preventive measure or risk stratification models.

Author Contributions

Conceived and designed the experiments: JJWV ST IP MLS BTH JJH-D EPS JWJ. Performed the experiments: JJWV ST MLS. Analyzed the data: JJWV ST. Contributed reagents/materials/analysis tools: ST IP MLS BTH JWJ. Wrote the paper: JJWV ST IP BTH JWJ.

References

1. Jukema JW, Verschuren JJ, Ahmed TA, Quax PH (2012) Restenosis after PCI. Part 1: pathophysiology and risk factors. Nat Rev Cardiol 9: 53–62.

2. Jukema JW, Ahmed TA, Verschuren JJ, Quax PH (2012) Restenosis after PCI. Part 2: prevention and therapy. Nat Rev Cardiol 9: 79–90.

3. Kastrati A, Koch W, Berger PB, Mehilli J, Stephenson K, et al. (2000) Protective role against restenosis from an interleukin-1 receptor antagonist gene polymorphism in patients treated with coronary stenting. J Am Coll Cardiol 36: 2168–2173.

4. Koch W, Bottiger C, Mehilli J, von BN, Neumann FJ, et al. (2001) Association of a CD18 gene polymorphism with a reduced risk of restenosis after coronary stenting. Am J Cardiol 88: 1120–1124.

5. Monraats PS, Pires NM, Schepers A, Agema WR, Boesten LS, et al. (2005) Tumor necrosis factor-alpha plays an important role in restenosis development. FASEB J 19: 1998–2004.

6. Monraats PS, Pires NM, Agema WR, Zwinderman AH, Schepers A, et al. (2005) Genetic inflammatory factors predict restenosis after percutaneous coronary interventions. Circulation 112: 2417–2425.

7. Sampietro ML, Trompet S, Verschuren JJ, Talens RP, Deelen J, et al. (2011) A genome-wide association study identifies a region at chromosome 12 as a potential susceptibility locus for restenosis after percutaneous coronary intervention. Hum Mol Genet 20: 4748–4757.

8. O'Donnell CJ, Nabel EG (2011) Genomics of cardiovascular disease. N Engl J Med 365: 2098–2109.

9. Keating BJ, Tischfield S, Murray SS, Bhangale T, Price TS, et al. (2008) Concept, design and implementation of a cardiovascular gene-centric 50 k SNP array for large-scale genomic association studies. PLoS One 3: e3583.

10. Ma L, Han S, Yang J, Da Y (2010) Multi-locus test conditional on confirmed effects leads to increased power in genome-wide association studies. PLoS One 5: e15006.

11. Agema WR, Monraats PS, Zwinderman AH, de Winter RJ, Tio RA, et al. (2004) Current PTCA practice and clinical outcomes in The Netherlands: the real world in the pre-drug-eluting stent era. Eur Heart J 25: 1163–1170.

12. Sampietro ML, Pons D, de Knijff P, Slagboom PE, Zwinderman A, et al. (2009) A genome wide association analysis in the GENDER study. Neth Heart J 17: 262–264.

13. Li Y, Willer CJ, Ding J, Scheet P, Abecasis GR (2010) MaCH: using sequence and genotype data to estimate haplotypes and unobserved genotypes. Genet Epidemiol 34: 816–834.

14. Purcell S, Neale B, Todd-Brown K, Thomas L, Ferreira MA, et al. (2007) PLINK: a tool set for whole-genome association and population-based linkage analyses. Am J Hum Genet 81: 559–575.

15. Biocarta website. Biocarta pathway. Available: http://www.biocarta.com/pathfiles/h_vdrpathway.asp. Accessed 2012 Mar 1.

16. Fridley BL, Biernacka JM (2011) Gene set analysis of SNP data: benefits, challenges, and future directions. Eur J Hum Genet 19: 837–843.

17. Torkamani A, Topol EJ, Schork NJ (2008) Pathway analysis of seven common diseases assessed by genome-wide association. Genomics 92: 265–272.

18. Gui H, Li M, Sham PC, Cherny SS (2011) Comparisons of seven algorithms for pathway analysis using the WTCCC Crohn's Disease dataset. BMC Res Notes 4: 386.

19. Deelen J, Uh HW, Monajemi R, van HD, Thijssen PE, et al. (2011) Gene set analysis of GWAS data for human longevity highlights the relevance of the insulin/IGF-1 signaling and telomere maintenance pathways. Age (Dordr) In press. 10.1007/s11357-011-9340-3 [doi].

20. Swapna N, Vamsi UM, Usha G, Padma T (2011) Risk conferred by FokI polymorphism of vitamin D receptor (VDR) gene for essential hypertension. Indian J Hum Genet 17: 201–206.

21. Kolz M, Baumert J, Gohlke H, Grallert H, Doring A, et al. (2009) Association study between variants in the fibrinogen gene cluster, fibrinogen levels and hypertension: results from the MONICA/KORA study. Thromb Haemost 101: 317–324.

22. Niu W, Qi Y (2010) Association of the angiotensin II type I receptor gene +1166 A>C polymorphism with hypertension risk: evidence from a meta-analysis of 16474 subjects. Hypertens Res 33: 1137–1143.

23. Mansego ML, Solar GM, Alonso MP, Martinez F, Saez GT, et al. (2011) Polymorphisms of antioxidant enzymes, blood pressure and risk of hypertension. J Hypertens 29: 492–500.

24. Falcone C, Emanuele E, Buzzi MP, Ballerini L, Repetto A, et al. (2007) The-374T/A variant of the rage gene promoter is associated with clinical restenosis after coronary stent placement. Int J Immunopathol Pharmacol 20: 771–777.

25. Shim CY, Park S, Yoon SJ, Park HY, Kim HT, et al. (2007) Association of RAGE gene polymorphisms with in-stent restenosis in non-diabetic Korean population. Cardiology 107: 261–268.

26. Gross CM, Perrot A, Geier C, Posch MG, Hassfeld S, et al. (2007) Recurrent in-stent restenosis is not associated with the angiotensin-converting enzyme D/I, angiotensinogen Thr174Met and Met235Thr, and the angiotensin-II receptor 1 A1166C polymorphism. J Invasive Cardiol 19: 261–264.

27. Wijpkema JS, van Haelst PL, Monraats PS, Bruinenberg M, Zwinderman AH, et al. (2006) Restenosis after percutaneous coronary intervention is associated with the angiotensin-II type-1 receptor 1166A/C polymorphism but not with polymorphisms of angiotensin-converting enzyme, angiotensin-II receptor, angiotensinogen or heme oxygenase-1. Pharmacogenet Genomics 16: 331–337.

28. Oguri M, Kato K, Hibino T, Yokoi K, Segawa T, et al. (2007) Genetic risk for restenosis after coronary stenting. Atherosclerosis 194: e172–e178.

29. Shimada K, Miyauchi K, Mokuno H, Watanabe Y, Iwama Y, et al. (2004) Promoter polymorphism in the CD14 gene and concentration of soluble CD14 in patients with in-stent restenosis after elective coronary stenting. Int J Cardiol 94: 87–92.

30. Tiroch K, Koch W, Mehilli J, Bottiger C, Schomig A, et al. (2009) P27 and P53 gene polymorphisms and restenosis following coronary implantation of drug-eluting stents. Cardiology 112: 263–269.

31. van Tiel CM, Bonta PI, Rittersma SZ, Beijk MA, Bradley EJ, et al. (2009) p27kip1-838C>A single nucleotide polymorphism is associated with restenosis risk after coronary stenting and modulates p27kip1 promoter activity. Circulation 120: 669–676.

32. Oguri M, Kato K, Hibino T, Yokoi K, Segawa T, et al. (2007) Identification of a polymorphism of UCP3 associated with recurrent in-stent restenosis of coronary arteries. Int J Mol Med 20: 533–538.

33. Niessner A, Marculescu R, Kvakan H, Haschemi A, Endler G, et al. (2005) Fractalkine receptor polymorphisms V249I and T280M as genetic risk factors for restenosis. Thromb Haemost 94: 1251–1256.

34. Horibe H, Yamada Y, Ichihara S, Watarai M, Yanase M, et al. (2004) Genetic risk for restenosis after coronary balloon angioplasty. Atherosclerosis 174: 181–187.

35. Tiroch KA, Sibbing D, Koch W, Roosen-Runge T, Mehilli J, et al. (2010) Protective effect of the CYP2C19 *17 polymorphism with increased activation of clopidogrel on cardiovascular events. Am Heart J 160: 506–512.

36. Monraats PS, Rana JS, Zwinderman AH, de Maat MP, Kastelein JP, et al. (2005)-455G/A polymorphism and preprocedural plasma levels of fibrinogen show no association with the risk of clinical restenosis in patients with coronary stent placement. Thromb Haemost 93: 564–569.

37. Pons D, Monraats PS, de Maat MP, Pires NM, Quax PH, et al. (2007) The influence of established genetic variation in the haemostatic system on clinical restenosis after percutaneous coronary interventions. Thromb Haemost 98: 1323–1328.

38. Martinez-Rios MA, Pena-Duque MA, Fragoso JM, Delgadillo-Rodriguez H, Rodriguez-Perez JM, et al. (2009) Tumor necrosis factor alpha and interleukin 10 promoter polymorphisms in Mexican patients with restenosis after coronary stenting. Biochem Genet 47: 707–716.

39. Koch W, Tiroch K, von BN, Schomig A, Kastrati A (2003) Tumor necrosis factor-alpha, lymphotoxin-alpha, and interleukin-10 gene polymorphisms and restenosis after coronary artery stenting. Cytokine 24: 161–171.

40. Monraats PS, Kurreeman FA, Pons D, Sewgobind VD, de Vries FR, et al. (2007) Interleukin 10: a new risk marker for the development of restenosis after percutaneous coronary intervention. Genes Immun 8: 44–50.

41. Marculescu R, Mlekusch W, Exner M, Sabeti S, Michor S, et al. (2003) Interleukin-1 cluster combined genotype and restenosis after balloon angioplasty. Thromb Haemost 90: 491–500.

42. Zee RY, Fernandez-Ortiz A, Macaya C, Pintor E, Fernandez-Cruz A, et al. (2003) IL-1 cluster genes and occurrence of post-percutaneous transluminal coronary angioplasty restenosis: a prospective, angiography-based evaluation. Atherosclerosis 171: 259–264.

43. Monraats PS, Rana JS, Nierman MC, Pires NM, Zwinderman AH, et al. (2005) Lipoprotein lipase gene polymorphisms and the risk of target vessel revascularization after percutaneous coronary intervention. J Am Coll Cardiol 46: 1093–1100.

44. Chung SL, Chiou KR, Charng MJ (2006) 677TT polymorphism of methylenetetrahydrofolate reductase in combination with low serum vitamin B12 is associated with coronary in-stent restenosis. Catheter Cardiovasc Interv 67: 349–355.

45. Koch W, Ndrepepa G, Mehilli J, Braun S, Burghartz M, et al. (2003) Homocysteine status and polymorphisms of methylenetetrahydrofolate reductase are not associated with restenosis after stenting in coronary arteries. Arterioscler Thromb Vasc Biol 23: 2229–2234.

46. Gomma AH, Elrayess MA, Knight CJ, Hawe E, Fox KM, et al. (2002) The endothelial nitric oxide synthase (Glu298Asp and 786T>C) gene polymorphisms are associated with coronary in-stent restenosis. Eur Heart J 23: 1955–1962.

47. Pons D, Monraats PS, Zwinderman AH, de Maat MP, Doevendans PA, et al. (2009) Metabolic background determines the importance of NOS3 polymorphisms in restenosis after percutaneous coronary intervention: A study in patients with and without the metabolic syndrome. Dis Markers 26: 75–83.

48. Gorchakova O, Koch W, von BN, Mehilli J, Schomig A, et al. (2003) Association of a genetic variant of endothelial nitric oxide synthase with the 1 year clinical outcome after coronary stent placement. Eur Heart J 24: 820–827.

49. Rudez G, Pons D, Leebeek F, Monraats P, Schrevel M, et al. (2008) Platelet receptor P2RY12 haplotypes predict restenosis after percutaneous coronary interventions. Hum Mutat 29: 375–380.

50. Bottiger C, Koch W, Lahn C, Mehilli J, von BN, et al. (2003) 4G/5G polymorphism of the plasminogen activator inhibitor-1 gene and risk of restenosis after coronary artery stenting. Am Heart J 146: 855–861.

51. Pons D, Trompet S, de Craen AJ, Thijssen PE, Quax PH, et al. (2011) Genetic variation in PCAF, a key mediator in epigenetics, is associated with reduced

vascular morbidity and mortality: evidence for a new concept from three independent prospective studies. Heart 97: 143–150.

52. Neugebauer P, Goldbergova-Pavkova M, Kala P, Bocek O, Jerabek P, et al. (2009) Nuclear receptors gene polymorphisms and risk of restenosis and clinical events following coronary stenting. Vnitr Lek 55: 1135–1140.

53. Koch W, Jung V, von BN, Schomig A, Kastrati A (2004) Peroxisome proliferator-activated receptor gamma gene polymorphisms and restenosis in diabetic patients after stenting in coronary arteries. Diabetologia 47: 1126–1127.

54. Rittersma SZ, Boekholdt SM, Koch KT, Geuzebroek R, Bax M, et al. (2004) Thrombospondin gene polymorphisms and the risk of angiographic coronary in-stent restenosis. Am J Med 116: 499–500.

55. Kojima S, Iwai N, Tago N, Ono K, Ohmi K, et al. (2004) p53Arg72Pro polymorphism of tumour suppressor protein is associated with luminal narrowing after coronary stent placement. Heart 90: 1069–1070.

56. Zee RY, Cook NR, Kim CA, Fernandez-Cruz A, Lindpaintner K (2004) TP53 haplotype-based analysis and incidence of post-angioplasty restenosis. Hum Genet 114: 386–390.

57. Monraats PS, Fang Y, Pons D, Pires NM, Pols HA, et al. (2010) Vitamin D receptor: a new risk marker for clinical restenosis after percutaneous coronary intervention. Expert Opin Ther Targets 14: 243–251.

7

Bindarit Inhibits Human Coronary Artery Smooth Muscle Cell Proliferation, Migration and Phenotypic Switching

Marcella Maddaluno[1,9], **Gianluca Grassia**[1,9], **Maria Vittoria Di Lauro**[1], **Antonio Parisi**[1], **Francesco Maione**[1], **Carla Cicala**[1], **Daniele De Filippis**[1], **Teresa Iuvone**[1], **Angelo Guglielmotti**[2], **Pasquale Maffia**[1,3], **Nicola Mascolo**[1]*, **Armando Ialenti**[1]*

1 Department of Experimental Pharmacology, University of Naples Federico II, Naples, Italy, 2 Angelini, ACRAF, S.Palomba-Pomezia, Rome, Italy, 3 Institute of Infection, Immunity and Inflammation, College of Medical, Veterinary and Life Sciences, University of Glasgow, Glasgow, United Kingdom

Abstract

Bindarit, a selective inhibitor of monocyte chemotactic proteins (MCPs) synthesis, reduces neointimal formation in animal models of vascular injury and recently has been shown to inhibit in-stent late loss in a placebo-controlled phase II clinical trial. However, the mechanisms underlying the efficacy of bindarit in controlling neointimal formation/restenosis have not been fully elucidated. Therefore, we investigated the effect of bindarit on human coronary smooth muscle cells activation, drawing attention to the phenotypic modulation process, focusing on contractile proteins expression as well as proliferation and migration. The expression of contractile proteins was evaluated by western blot analysis on cultured human coronary smooth muscle cells stimulated with TNF-α (30 ng/mL) or fetal bovine serum (5%). Bindarit (100–300 μM) reduced the embryonic form of smooth muscle myosin heavy chain while increased smooth muscle α-actin and calponin in both TNF-α- and fetal bovine serum-stimulated cells. These effects were associated with the inhibition of human coronary smooth muscle cell proliferation/migration and both MCP-1 and MCP-3 production. The effect of bindarit on smooth muscle cells phenotypic switching was confirmed *in vivo* in the rat balloon angioplasty model. Bindarit (200 mg/Kg/day) significantly reduced the expression of the embryonic form of smooth muscle myosin heavy chain, and increased smooth muscle α-actin and calponin in the rat carodid arteries subjected to endothelial denudation. Our results demonstrate that bindarit induces the differentiated state of human coronary smooth muscle cells, suggesting a novel underlying mechanisms by which this drug inhibits neointimal formation.

Editor: Olivier Kocher, Harvard Medical School, United States of America

Funding: A.I. received the project grants (004FA11072; 004FA10204) from Angelini for this study. The funders had no role in study design, data collection and analysis, decision to publish, or preparation of the manuscript. The authors discussed with the funders the study design and decision to publish.

Competing Interests: This study was funded by Angelini, the employer of author Angelo Guglielmotti. Bindarit is an Angelini product. There are no further patents, products in development or marketed products to declare.

* E-mail: ialenti@unina.it (AI); nicoladomenicocferd.mascolo@unina.it (NM)

9 These authors contributed equally to this work.

Introduction

Vascular smooth muscle cell (VSMC) proliferation and migration are key events in intimal hyperplasia occurring in vascular restenosis [1]. After vascular injury, VSMCs exhibit marked differences in morphology, migration, and proliferation rate compared with normal medial cells. Additionally, the highly proliferative VSMCs undergo a shift from a differentiated (contractile) to a dedifferentiated (synthetic, noncontractile) state. This process, called phenotypic modulation, is characterized by the loss of expression of the VSMC-specific genes, such as smooth muscle α-actin (α-SMA) and calponin, as well as a selective upregulation of the embryonic form of smooth muscle myosin heavy chain (SMemb) [2,3]. The phenotypic switching is accompanied by increased expression of extracellular matrix proteins, cytokines and chemokines [2,4,5].

The pro-inflammatory CC chemokine, monocyte chemoattractant protein 1 (MCP-1)/CCL2, plays a pivotal role in intimal hyperplasia via macrophages recruitment and VSMC activation

[5,6]. It has been demonstrated that MCP-1 induces human VSMC proliferation [7], migration [8], and regulates the functional switch of these cells from the contractile to the synthetic phenotype [9].

Bindarit is an anti-inflammatory agent that inhibits MCP-1/CCL2, MCP-3/CCL7 and MCP-2/CCL8 synthesis [10], acting through the down-regulation of NF-kB pathway [11], that shows potent anti-inflammatory activity in animal models of both acute and chronic inflammation [12–15]. We have previously demonstrated that oral administration of bindarit inhibits neointimal formation in rodent models of vascular injury by reducing both VSMC proliferation/migration and neointimal macrophage content, effects associated with the inhibition of MCP-1/CCL2 production [16]. Recently, we also demonstrated the efficacy of bindarit on in-stent stenosis in the preclinical porcine coronary stent model [17]. Importantly, a double-blind, randomized, placebo-controlled phase II clinical trial, with the aim of investigating the effect of bindarit in human coronary restenosis, showed that bindarit induced a significant reduction of in-stent late loss [18]. However, the mechanisms underlying the efficacy of bindarit in controlling neointimal formation/restenosis have not been fully elucidated. Therefore, we investigated the effect of bindarit on human coronary VSMC activation, drawing attention to the phenotypic modulation process, focusing on contractile proteins expression as well as proliferation and migration. In addition, we also investigated the effect of bindarit *in vivo* on phenotypic modulation of VSMCs in rat carotid arteries subjected to vascular injury.

Methods

Treatments

Bindarit,   2-methyl-2-[[1-(phenylmethyl)-1H-indazol-3-yl]-methoxy] propanoic acid (MW 324.38) was synthesised by

Angelini (Angelini Research Center - ACRAF, Italy). Pharmaco-kinetic studies in rodents show that bindarit is well absorbed when administered by oral route and it has a mean half-life of about 9 h (Product data sheet, Angelini Research Center).

Animals were treated with bindarit, suspended in 0.5% methylcellulose aqueous solution, at the dose of 100 mg/Kg given orally, by gastric gavage, twice a day [16]. Rats were treated with bindarit from 2 days before angioplasty up to 28 days after. In each experiment control animals received an equal volume of methylcellulose (0.5 mL/100 g). The concentrations of bindarit used for *in vitro* experiments have previously been found to be effective in inhibiting MCP-1 production in rat VSMCs as well as cell proliferation and migration [16].

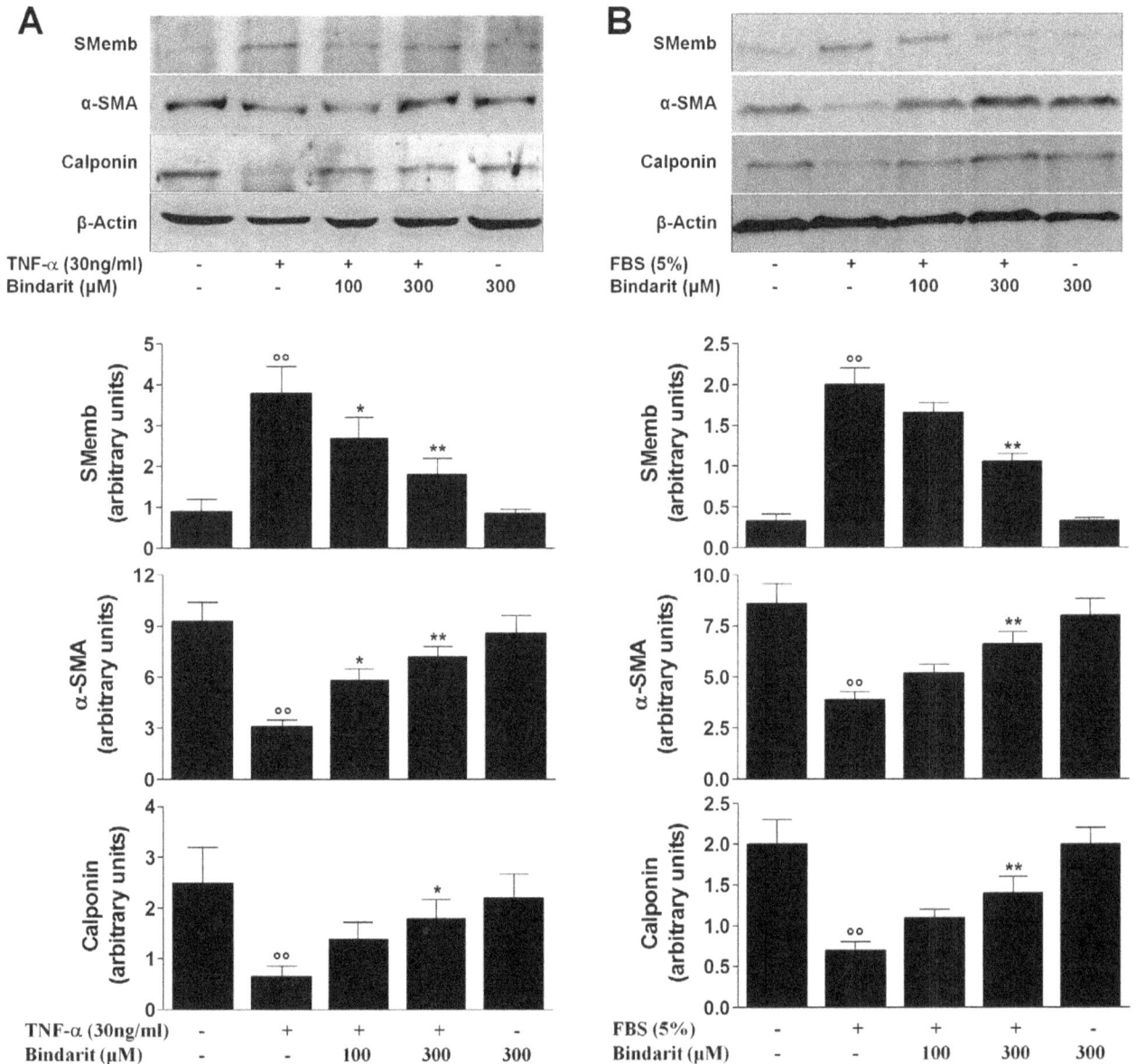

Figure 1. Effect of bindarit on contractile proteins expression in CASMCs. Representative Western blots and relative densitometric analysis showing the effects of bindarit (100 and 300 μM) on contractile proteins expression levels modulated by (**A**) TNF-α (30 ng/mL) or (**B**) FBS (5%). Results are expressed as mean ± SEM of three separate experiments run in triplicate. °°P<0.01 *vs* unstimulated cells; *P<0.05, **P<0.01 *vs* untreated cells.

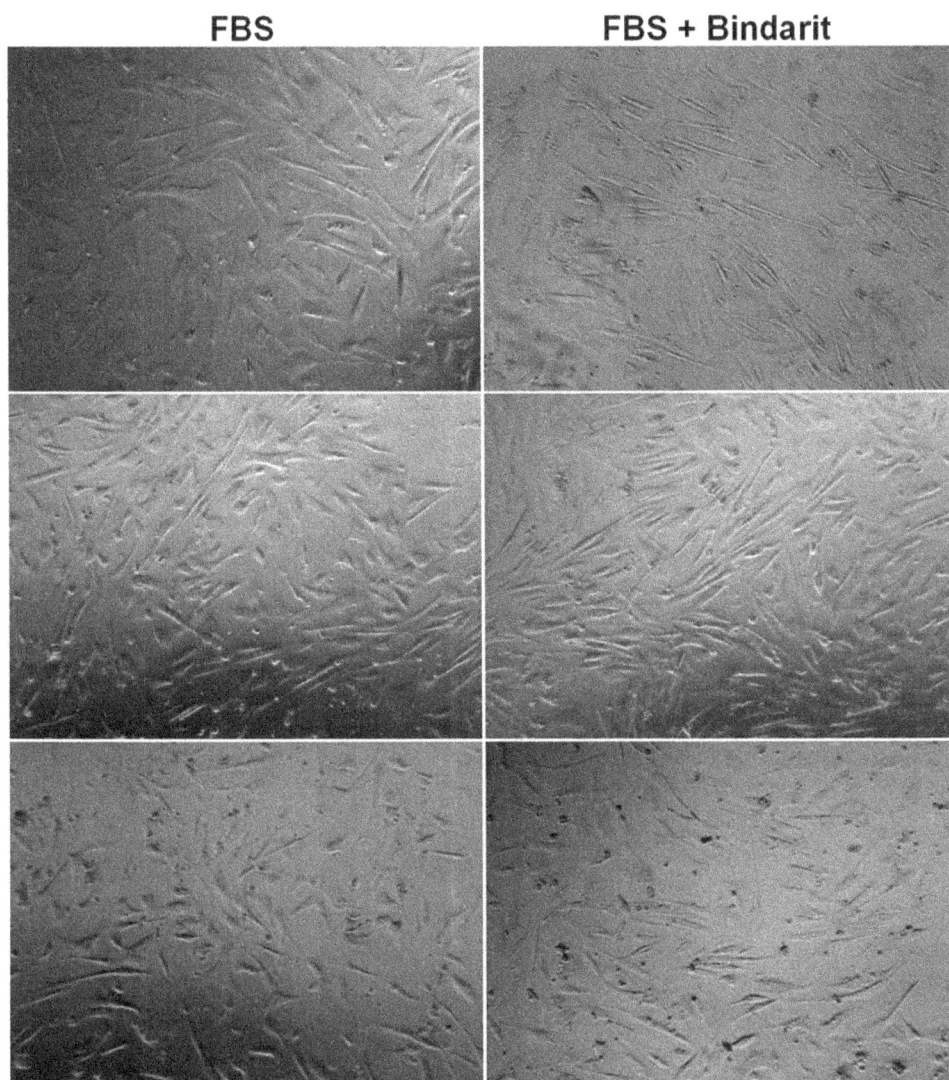

Figure 2. Effect of bindarit on morphological changes induced by FBS in CASMCs. Phase-contrast photomicrographs of CASMCs cultured in medium with 5% FBS for 48 hours with or without bindarit (300 μM).

Cell Culture

Human coronary artery smooth muscle cells (CASMCs) were purchased from Lonza (lot numb: 6F4008 and 16737) [19], grown in Smooth Muscle Basal Medium (SmBM; Lonza) supplemented with 0.5 mg/mL hEGF, 5 mg/mL insulin, 1 mg/mL hFGF, 50 mg/mL gentamicin/amphotericin-B, 5% fetal bovine serum (FBS, Lonza) and used between passages 3–8 for all experiments. Before initiation of the assays, to achieve cell quiescence, CASMCs in exponential growth were switched into SmBM supplemented with 0.1% FBS in the absence of growth factors for 48 hours.

Total Cellular Extracts

CASMCs were cultured in 24 multi-well plates until 90% confluence; after the induction of quiescence, cells were stimulated with tumor necrosis factor-α (TNF-α, 30 ng/mL) or FBS (5%) in presence or absence of bindarit (100–300 μM). After 48 hours cells were washed two times with ice cold PBS and 30 μL/well of lysis buffer (50 mM Tris-HCl, 1% Triton,

1 mM Na_3VO_4, 1 mM EDTA, 0.2 mM PMSF, 25 μg/mL Leupeptin, 10 μg/mL Aprotinin, 10 mM NaF, 150 mM NaCl, 10 mM β-glycerophosphate, 5 mM pyrophosphate, H_2O) were added. Protein concentration was determined by the Bio-Rad protein assay kit (Bio-Rad).

Western Blot Analysis on CASMCs

CASMCs lysates (20 μg) were separated by Sodium Dodecyl Sulphate - PolyAcrylamide Gel Electrophoresis (SDS-PAGE), transferred onto nitrocellulose membranes (Millipore) and probed with a primary antibody against human α-SMA (1:5000, Sigma-Aldrich), calponin (1:5000, Sigma-Aldrich) or MYH9/10 (SMemb, 1:2000, Santa Cruz). The membranes were washed three times with 0.5% Triton in PBS and incubated with anti-mouse immunoglobulins coupled to peroxidase (1:1000; DAKO). The immunocomplexes were visualised by the enhanced chemi-luminescence (ECL) method, results were analyzed by ImageJ densitometry software and normalized to β-actin.

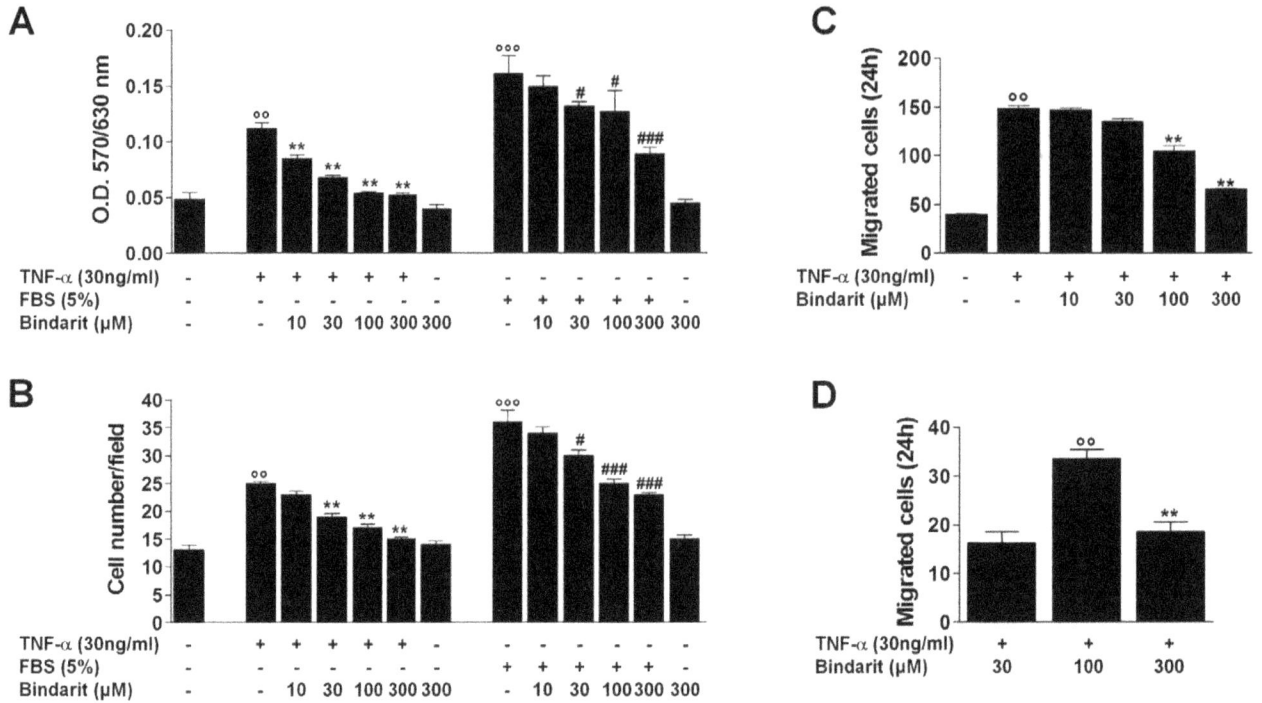

Figure 3. Effect of bindarit on CASMC proliferation, migration and invasion. CASMC proliferation assessed by MTT assay (**A**) and by cell counting expressed as number of cells per field (**B**). Effect of bindarit on CASMC migration (**C**) and invasion (**D**). Results are expressed as mean ± SEM of three separate experiments run in triplicate. $^{\circ\circ}P<0.01$, $^{\circ\circ\circ}P<0.001$ vs unstimulated cells; $**P<0.01$ vs TNF-α-stimulated cells; $^{\#}P<0.05$, $^{\#\#\#}P<0.001$ vs FBS-stimulated cells.

Evaluation of CASMC Morphological Changes

CASMCs were used after the induction of quiescence in 48-well plastic culture plates at the density of 1×10^4 cells/well. Cells were stimulated with FBS (5%) in presence or absence of bindarit (300 μM). After 48 hours cells were photographed at a magnification of ×200 and the images were stored in the image analysis system (LAS, Leica).

Cell Proliferation Study

The cell proliferation assay was carried out using the MTT method. CASMCs were plated on 24-well plastic culture plates at the density of 1.5×10^4 cells/well. After the induction of quiescence, cells were stimulated with TNF-α (30 ng/mL, Provitro) or FBS (5%) for 48 hours in the presence or absence of bindarit (10–300 μM). 0.5 mg/ml of MTT in Phosphate Buffered Saline (PBS) were added and, after 3 hours, a solution containing 50% N,N'-dirnethylformamide and 20% SDS (pH 4.8) was used for the solubilisation of the formazan dye. Absorbance values at 570 nm were determined the next day with an Enzyme-linked immunosorbent assay (ELISA) assay reader (Bio-Rad), using 630 nm as the reference wavelength.

CASMC proliferation was also evaluated as cell duplication by directly counting the cell number. Briefly, 1×10^4 cells were seeded onto 24-well plastic culture plates and allowed to adhere overnight. After the induction of quiescence, the cells were stimulated with TNF-α (30 ng/mL) or FBS (5%) in presence or absence of bindarit (10–300 μM). After 72 hours, medium was removed, cells were fixed with methanol and stained with 4',6-diamidino-2-phenylindole (DAPI). Proliferation was evaluated as cell duplication by counting the number of cells in 8 random fields of each well at ×100 magnification.

Chemotactic Migration and Invasion

CASMC migration was evaluated using a modified Boyden chamber (Corning 24 mm Transwell with 8.0 μm pore polycarbonate membrane insert) coated with rat-tail collagen I (Sigma-Aldrich). Biocoat Matrigel invasion chambers (with 8.0 μm pore) were used according to the manufacturer's instructions for invasion studies (Becton-Dickinson). Briefly, starved CASMCs were trypsinized and pre-treated or not with bindarit (10–300 μM) for 2 hours. Three ×10^4 cells were plated in the upper chamber in 500 μL of 0.1% FBS medium with or without bindarit. The lower chamber was filled with 600 μL of 0.1% FBS medium in the absence (unstimulated cells) or presence of TNF-α (30 ng/mL). After 24 hours the migrated cells were fixed and stained with haematoxylin. Cell migration was quantified by counting the number of cells (magnification ×200) per insert.

Gelatin Zymography

CASMCs were cultured in 96-well culture plates in 10% FBS medium until 90% confluence. After the induction of quiescence, cells were stimulated with TNF-α (30 ng/mL) in the presence or absence of bindarit (300 μM). After 24 hours the media were collected, clarified by centrifugation and subjected to electrophoresis in 8% SDS-PAGE containing 1 mg/mL gelatin. After electrophoresis the gels were re-natured by washing with 2.5% Triton X-100, to remove SDS, and by incubation for 24 h at 37°C in 50 mM Tris buffer containing 200 mM NaCl and 20 mM $CaCl_2$, pH 7.4. The gels were stained with 0.5% Coomassie brilliant blue R-250 (Sigma) in 10% acetic acid and 45% methanol and destained with 10% acetic acid and 45% methanol. Bands of gelatinase activity appeared as transparent areas against a blue

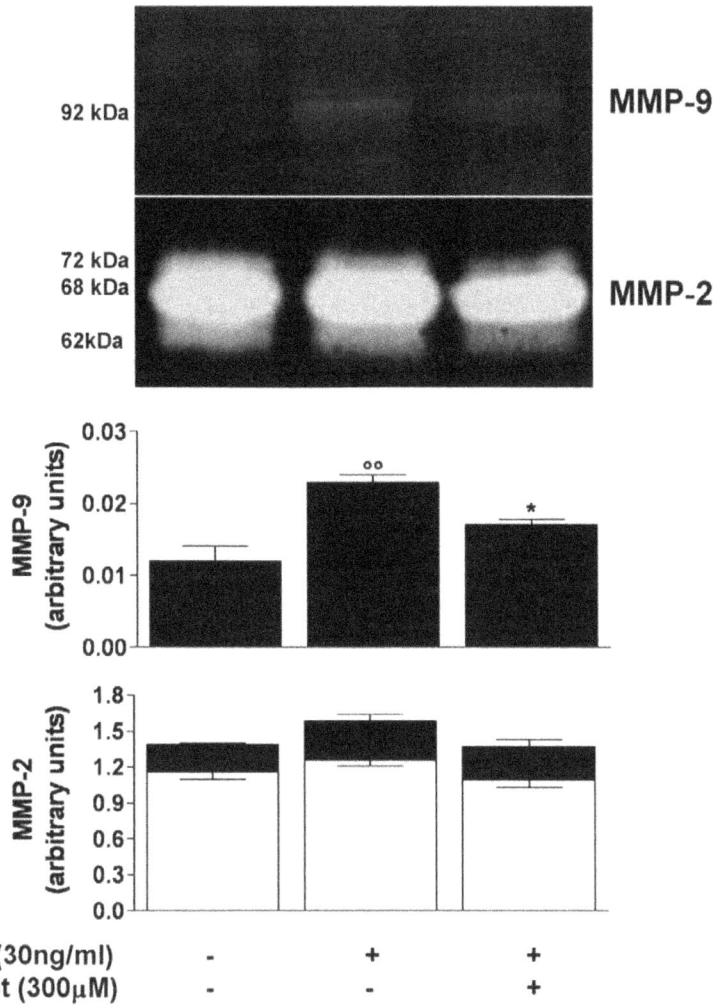

Figure 4. Effect of bindarit on matrix metalloproteinase-2 and matrix metalloproteinase 9 activity. Representative gel zymography of conditioned medium from TNF-α (30 ng/mL)-stimulated CASMCs and relative densitometric analysis showing the effect of bindarit (300 μM) on MMP-9 activated form and both MMP-2 latent (white columns) and activated (black columns) forms. Results are expressed as mean ± SEM of 3 experiments. °°P<0.01 vs unstimulated cells; °P<0.05 vs TNF-α-stimulated cells.

background. Gelatinase activity was then evaluated by quantitative densitometry.

Enzyme-linked Immunosorbent Assay (ELISA)

CASMCs were used after the induction of quiescence in 48-well plastic culture plates at the density of 1×10^4 cells/well. Cells were stimulated with TNF-α (30 ng/mL) in presence or absence of bindarit (10–300 μM). After 6, 12, 24 and 48 hours media were collected, centrifuged at 2000×g for 10 min at 4°C and supernatants were immediately frozen at −80°C until used for MCP-1 (OptEIA, BD) or MCP-3 (Quantikine Human CCL7/MCP-3 Immunoassay, R&D Systems) measurement by ELISA.

Animals

Male Wistar rats (Harlan Laboratories) weighing 200–300 g were used for the present study. Animals were maintained on a 12/12 h light/dark cycle with free access to food and water at the Department of Experimental Pharmacology, University of Naples Federico II (Permit Number: 064F). All procedures were performed according to Italian ministerial authorization (DL

116/92) and European regulations on the protection of animals used for experimental and other scientific purposes.

Rat Carotid Balloon Angioplasty

Rats were anaesthetized with an intraperitoneal injection of ketamine (100 mg/Kg) (Gellini International) and xylazine (5 mg/Kg) (Sigma). Endothelial denudation of the left carotid artery was performed by using a balloon embolectomy catheter (2F, Fogarty, Edwards Lifesciences) according to the procedure well validated in our laboratories [20]. Rats were euthanized 7, 14 and 28 days after angioplasty. Carotid arteries were collected and processed as described below.

Morphometric Analysis

Carotid arteries from rats were fixed by perfusion with phosphate-buffered saline (PBS; pH 7.2) followed by PBS containing 4% formaldehyde through a cannula placed in the left ventricle. Paraffin-embedded sections were cut (6 mm thick) from the approximate middle portion of the artery and stained with haematoxylin and eosin to demarcate cell types. Ten

Table 1. Effect of bindarit on MCP-1 production by TNF-α- or FBS-stimulated CASMCs.

	MCP-1 (ng/mL)		
	6 h	12 h	24 h
unstimulated cells	0.1±0.01	0.4±0.04	2.1±0.02
bindarit 300 μM	0.1±0.01	0.4±0.02	2.0±0.03
TNF-α 30 ng/ml	1.6±0.07°°	3.0±1.09°°	13.1±0.12°°
+ bindarit 10 μM	1.5±0.01	2.4±0.04**	11.5±0.15**
+ bindarit 30 μM	1.4±0.01*	2.1±0.02**	10.8±0.10**
+ bindarit 100 μM	1.3±0.02**	1.8±0.05**	10.3±0.29**
+ bindarit 300 μM	1.1±0.06**	1.5±0.05**	8.0±0.05**
FBS 5%	1.5±0.22	5.5±0.26+++	23.5±1.89+++
+ bindarit 10 μM	1.5±0.29	4.7±0.61	22.5±1.56
+ bindarit 30 μM	1.4±0.64	3.4±0.75	15.8±2.18#
+ bindarit 100 μM	1.3±0.74	2.6±0.55##	10.5±0.87###
+ bindarit 300 μM	1.0±0.34	2.5±0.30##	8.8±1.32###

Results are expressed as mean ± SEM of three separate experiments run in triplicate.
°°$P<0.01$, +++$P<0.001$ vs unstimulated cells; *$P<0.05$, **$P<0.01$ vs TNF-α-stimulated cells; #$P<0.05$, ##$P<0.01$, ###$P<0.001$ vs FBS-stimulated cells.

Table 2. Effect of bindarit on MCP-3 production by TNF-α-stimulated CASMCs.

	MCP-3 (pg/mL)		
	6 h	12 h	24 h
unstimulated cells	70.0±8.00	164.3±40.31	211.3±44.49
bindarit 300 μM	90.3±9.40	178.3±53.35	210.3±52.61
TNF-α 30 ng/ml	116.9±25.71	501.0±78.48°°	714.3±87.83°°°
+ bindarit 10 μM	113.3±16.13	428.0±46.46	671.3±99.47
+ bindarit 30 μM	114.7±18.17	438.0±69.79	477.7±34.80
+ bindarit 100 μM	110.0±20.30	286.0±49.00	440.3±31.84
+ bindarit 300 μM	104.3±21.53	164.7±10.81*	151.3±6.36***

Results are expressed as mean ± SEM of three separate experiments run in triplicate.
°°$P<0.01$, °°°$P<0.001$ vs unstimulated cells; *$P<0.05$, **$P<0.01$, ***$P<0.001$ vs TNF-α-stimulated cells.

sections from each carotid artery were reviewed and scored under blind conditions. The cross-sectional areas of media and neointima were determined by a computerized analysis system (LAS, Leica). The neointimal and medial areas were computed as follows: neointimal area = internal elastic lamina (IEL) minus lumen area; medial area = external elastic lamina area minus IEL area.

Total Extracts from Rat Carotid Arteries

Total extracts were prepared from liquid nitrogen frozen pooled carotid arteries (n = 2), crushed into powder, in a mortar with a pestle,and resuspended in 150 μl of lysis buffer (20 mM HEPES, 0.4 mM NaCl, 1.5 mM MgCl2, 1 mM EGTA, 1 mM EDTA, 1% Triton X-100, and 20% glycerol) containing protease inhibitors (1 mM DTT, 0.5 mM PMSF, 15 mg/mL Try-inhibitor, 3 mg/mL pepstatin-A, 2 mg/mL leupeptin, and 40 mM benzamidine) [20,21]. After centrifugation at 13000×g at 4°C for 30 min, supernatants were collected and stored at −80°C until the assays. Protein concentration was determined by the Bio-Rad protein assay kit (Bio-Rad). MCP-1 levels were quantified by ELISA as described in Supplementary methods in Methods S1.

Western Blot Analysis on Rat Carotid Arteries

The levels of Proliferating Cell Nuclear Antigen (PCNA), α-SMA, calponin and SMemb were evaluated in total extracts from rat carotid arteries prepared, separated by SDS-PAGE and transferred to nitrocellulose membranes as described above. After incubation with a primary antibody against PCNA (1:2000, Sigma-Aldrich), α-SMA (1:5000), calponin (1:3000) or SMemb (1:2000), the membranes were washed and incubated with anti-mouse immunoglobulins coupled to peroxidase (1:2000). The immunocomplexes were visualised by the ECL chemiluminescence method and results were normalized to glyceraldehyde-3-phosphate dehydrogenase (GAPDH).

Immunohistochemistry

Paraffin sections (6 μm) from rat carotid arteries (7, 14 and 28 days after angioplasty, or naïve animals) were deparaffinised and endogenous peroxidase activity was blocked by incubating with 0.3% H_2O_2 following antigenic recovery. The sections were incubated with the primary antibody against α-SMA (1:100), calponin (1:50) or SMemb (1:200) diluted in blocking buffer/0.3% Triton X-100 (MP Biomedicals) in PBS overnight before being washed in TNT wash buffer (Tris–HCl, pH 7.5, 0.15 M NaCl, and 0.05% Tween 20; Sigma). Sections incubated with isotype matched antibodies were used as negative controls. Subsequently, sections were incubated with biotinylated anti-mouse (1:500, DakoCytomation) diluted in blocking buffer 0.3% Triton X-100, washed in TNT wash buffer, treated with horseradish peroxidise labelled streptavidin, and exposed to diaminobenzidine chromogen with haematoxylin counterstain. The sections were photographed and the images were stored in the image analysis system (LAS, Leica).

Statistical Analysis

Results are expressed as mean ± SEM of n animals for *in vivo* experiments and mean ± SEM of multiple experiments for in vitro assays. The Student *t* test was used to compare 2 groups or ANOVA (2-tailed probability value) was used with the Dunnett post hoc test for multiple groups using GraphPad Instat 3 software (San Diego, CA). The level of statistical significance was 0.05 per test.

Results

Effect of Bindarit on Contractile Proteins Expression in CASMCs

CASMCs were stimulated with TNF-α (30 ng/mL) or FBS (5%) for 48 hours and the lysates from these cells were subjected to Western blot analysis. As shown in Figure 1, bindarit significantly reduced the expression of SMemb in both TNF-α-stimulated cells (by 29% $P<0.05$ and 53% $P<0.01$, at 100 and 300 μM respectively) and FBS-stimulated cells (by 20% $P<0.01$ at 300 μM). The differentiated state of CASMCs induced by bindarit was also confirmed by the significant increased expression of α-SMA in both TNF-α-stimulated cells (by 87% $P<0.05$ and 132% $P<0.01$, at 100 and 300 μM respectively) and FBS-stimulated cells (by 69% $P<0.01$ at 300 μM). Treatment with bindarit at 300 μM

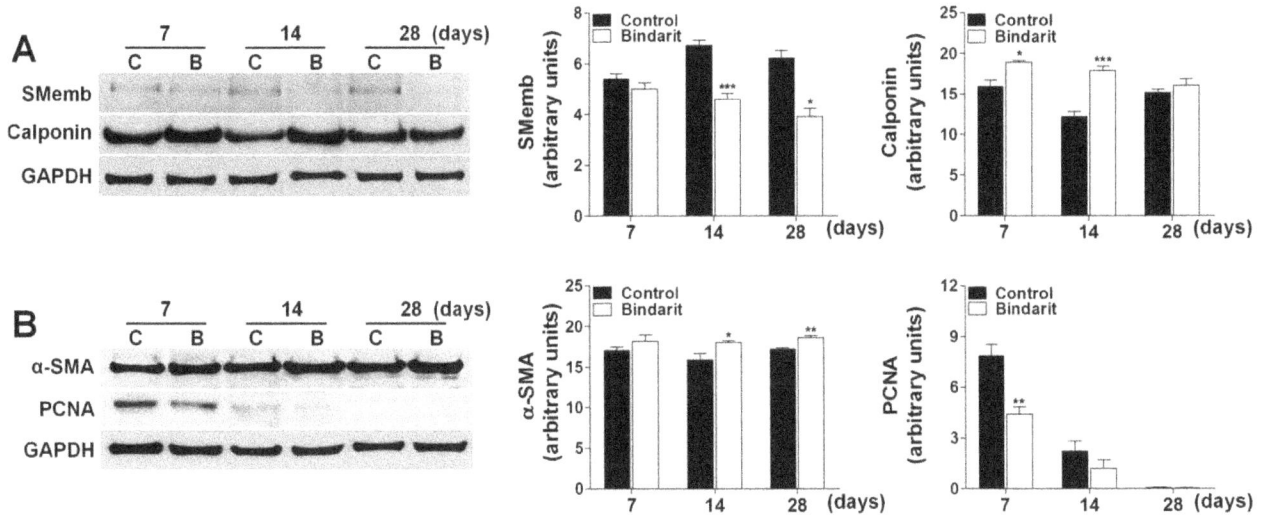

Figure 5. Effect of bindarit on contractile protein expression in rat carotid arteries. A and **B**. Representative Western blots and relative densitometric analysis showing the effect of the oral administration of bindarit (200 mg/Kg/day) on SMemb, calponin, α-SMA and PCNA expression levels in rat carotid arteries at days 7, 14 and 28 days after injury. Results are expressed as mean ± SEM, where n = 4 pools. *$P<0.05$, **$P<0.01$ and ***$P<0.001$ vs control group.

also significantly increased calponin expression when compared with both TNF-α-stimulated cells by 172% ($P<0.05$) and FBS-stimulated cells by 100% ($P<0.01$).

Effect of Bindarit on Morphological Changes Induced by FBS in CASMCs

In addition to VSMC-specific protein expression we examined VSMC morphology. After 48 hours of stimulation with FBS (5%) the CASMCs were characterized by a flattened morphology as result of the dedifferentiation to a synthetic phenotype (Figure 2). Bindarit (300 μM) induced an elongated spindle-shaped phenotype, typical of a differentiated state (Figure 2).

Effect of Bindarit on CASMC Proliferation

VSMCs plasticity exhibited in response to vascular injury, is characterized by both loss of VSMC-specific proteins expression and the increase in the proliferation.

As shown in Figure 3A, bindarit at 10, 30, 100, and 300 μM significantly ($P<0.01$) inhibited TNF-α (30 ng/mL)-induced CASMC proliferation by 24%, 39%, 52% and 54%, respectively. Similar inhibitory effects of bindarit were observed in FBS (5%)-stimulated CASMCs (Figure 3A).

We also evaluated CASMC proliferation by directly counting the cells (Figure 3B). Bindarit, which was ineffective at 10 μM, significantly ($P<0.01$) inhibited the TNF-α-induced CASMC number increase by 24%, 32% and 40%, at 30, 100, and 300 μM respectively. Similar inhibitory effects of bindarit were observed when FBS was used as stimulant (Figure 3B). Bindarit alone (300 μM) had no effect on cell proliferation/viability (Figure 3A and 3B).

Effect of Bindarit on CASMC Migration and Invasion

The higher proliferation rate of dedifferentiated VSMCs is accompanied by increased mitogen-mediated migration. Therefore, we evaluated the effect of bindarit (10–300 μM) on TNF-α-induced VSMC chemotaxis. Bindarit significantly ($P<0.01$) inhibited chemotactic migration at 100 and 300 μM by 30% and 55%, respectively (Figure 3C). Moreover, bindarit (300 μM)

significantly ($P<0.01$) reduced CASMC invasion by 50% through the Matrigel barrier which mimics extracellular matrix (Figure 3D). Bindarit alone (300 μM) had no effect on both migration and invasion (data not shown).

Effect of Bindarit on Matrix Metalloproteinase-2 and Matrix Metalloproteinase 9 Activity

Subconfluent cultures of CASMCs were exposed to TNF-α (30 ng/mL) for 24 hours in the presence or absence of bindarit (300 μM) to assess gelatinase production. Gelatin zymography of control supernatants showed the constitutive release of the latent form of matrix metalloproteinase 2 (MMP-2), visualized as a bands at 72 kDa and 68 kDa. Neither the stimulation with TNF-α, nor the treatment with bindarit significantly modified the release of the active form (62 kDa) (Figure 4). The stimulation with TNF-α significantly ($P<0.01$) induced the release of MMP-9 (92 kDa) which was significantly ($P<0.05$) inhibited by bindarit (Figure 4).

Effect of Bindarit on MCP-1 and MCP-3 Production

The effect of bindarit on MCP-1 and MCP-3 production by CASMCs was determined by ELISA. As shown in table 1, stimulation of CASMCs with TNF-α (30 ng/mL) or FBS (5%) caused a time-dependent increase of MCP-1 levels compared with unstimulated cells. Bindarit (10–300 μM) caused a significant concentration-related inhibition of MCP-1 production. As shown in table 2, bindarit (30–300 μM) significantly reduced MCP-3 production in TNF-α (30 ng/mL) stimulated CASMCs. FBS (5%) had no effect on MCP-3 production (data not shown). Bindarit alone (300 μM) did not significantly affect basal MCP-1 or MCP-3 levels (table 1 and 2).

Effect of Bindarit on Neointimal Formation in Rat Carotid Arteries

We have previously demonstrated the efficacy of bindarit in reducing balloon-induced neointimal formation in rats, 2 weeks after angioplasty [15]. Here we confirm previously results and extend our observation to the entire time course of neoitimal development, correlating vascular response to injury to contractile

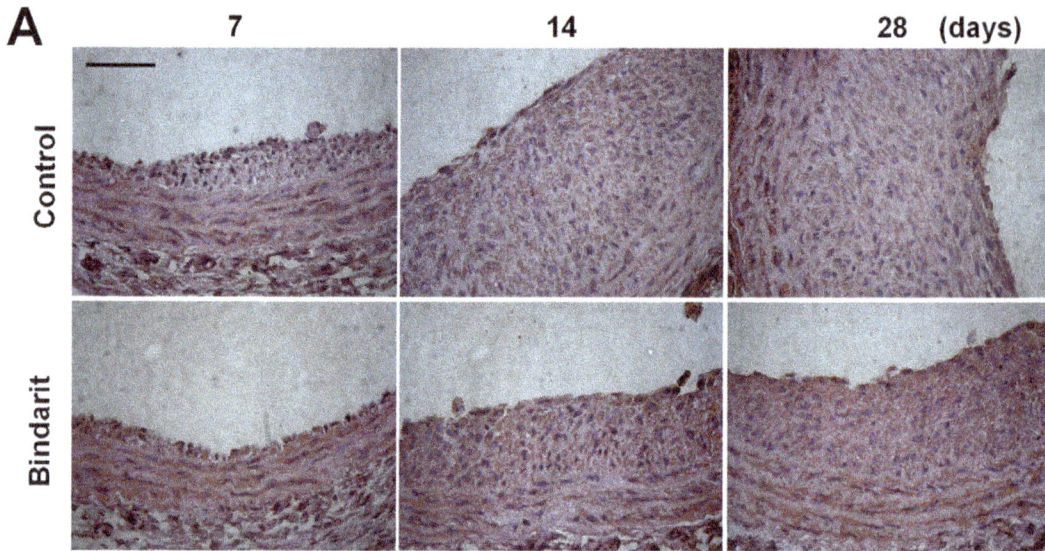

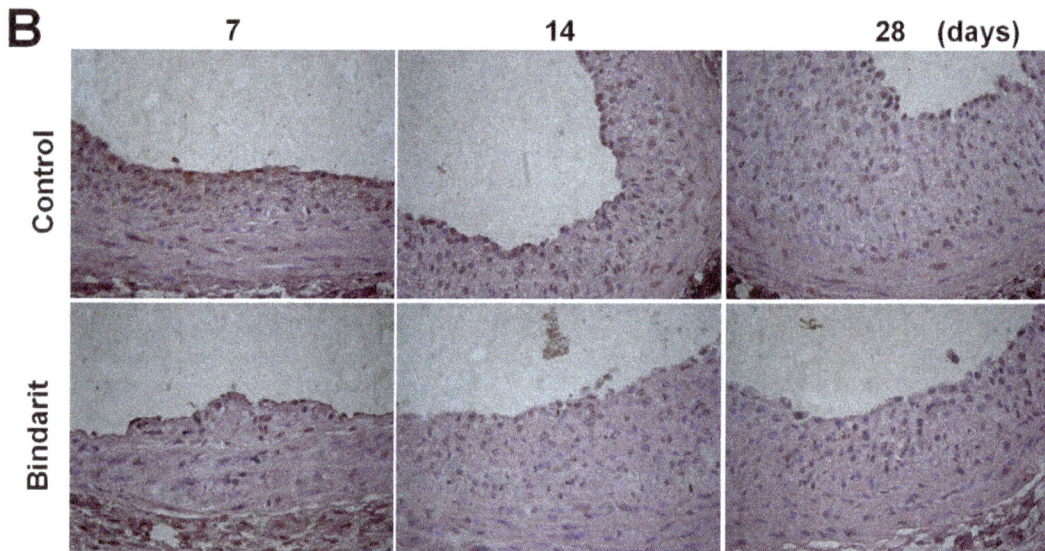

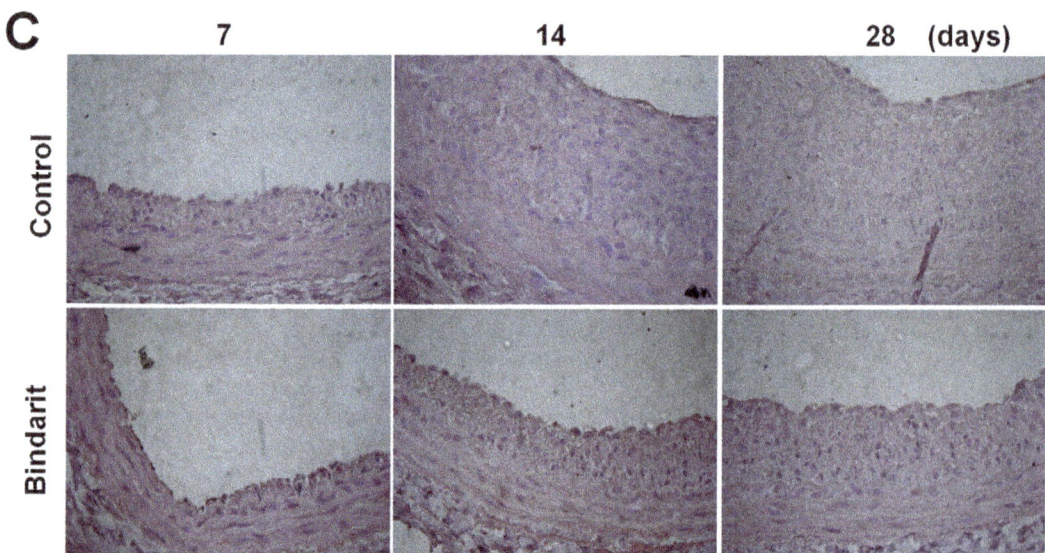

Figure 6. Effect of bindarit on contractile proteins localization in rat carotid arteries. Immohistochemical localization of α-SMA (**A**), SMemb (**B**) and calponin (**C**) expression in rat carotid arteries 7, 14 and 28 days after angioplasty. Bar = 100 μm.

protein expression. The oral administration of bindarit significantly ($P<0.001$) inhibited the neointimal growth at 14 and 28 days by 21% and 29% respectively (Supplementary data, Table S1). Similarly, bindarit reduced neointima/media ratio (see Supplementary results in Methods S1 and Table S1). Moreover bindarit significantly ($P<0.001$) induced an increase in lumen area at 14 and 28 days by 26% and 63%, respectively (Supplementary data, Table S1). These effects were associated with a significant reduction of MCP-1 levels in injured carotid arteries of rats treated with bindarit (Supplementary results in Methods S1 and Table S2).

Effect of Bindarit on Contractile Proteins Expression in Rat Carotid Arteries

As shown in Figure 5A, treatment with bindarit significantly reduced the expression of SMemb at 14 and 28 days (by 31%, $P<0.001$ and 37% $P<0.05$, respectively) and increased the expression of calponin at 7 and 14 days (by 19%, $P<0.05$ and 47%, $P<0.001$). Bindarit also increased the expression of α-SMA at 14 and 28 days (by 13%, $P<0.05$ and 8%, $P<0.01$, respectively) and, as previously demonstrated [16], reduced the expression of PCNA at 7 days (by 44%, $P<0.01$) (Figure 5B).

Localization of contractile proteins in rat carotid arteries was performed by immunohistochemistry to determine the temporal expression and cellular localization. α-SMA resulted highly expressed in the medial VSMCs of non-injured carotid sections (data not shown), while negative control IgG showed no signal (data not shown). At day 7, medial VSMCs, close to the lumen, started to lose α-SMA staining, as consequence of changes in phenotype. At day 14, VSMCs in the media and neointima, although stained with the anti-α-SMA antibody, showed weaker signal than the medial VSMCs at day 7. At day 28, the α-SMA resulted highly expressed in the medial VSMCs, instead the expression in the neointimal cells resulted still weak or absent. Although bindarit did not modify α-SMA localization, it determined a higher α-SMA expression in both media and neointima, at all time points considered (Figure 6A).

Non-injured carotid sections lacked immunoreactive SMemb (data not shown). In contrast, injured carotid arteries showed a remarkable number of cells in the media and neointima strongly positive for SMemb, at all time points considered, while negative control IgG showed no signal (data not shown). The treatment with bindarit reduced the number of the SMemb-positive cells at day 7 and, more interesting, the SMemb-positive cells resulted absent in the media at day 14 and 28 (Figure 6B).

Immunoreactivity for calponin was visible in the medial VSMCs of non-injured carotid sections (data not shown), while negative control IgG showed no signal (data not shown). At all time points considered, the injured arteries lacked immunoreactive calponin. Intriguingly, at day 7 and day 14, the vessels from bindarit-treated rats showed calponin signal in the medial VSMCs (Figure 6C).

Discussion and Conclusions

VSMC dedifferentiation and phenotype change are thought to be important aspects of vascular wall remodeling during atherosclerosis and neointimal hyperplasia. The present study provides evidence that bindarit induces the differentiated phenotype of VSMCs both *in vitro*, on human coronary VSMCs, and *in vivo*, in the rat carotid balloon angioplasty model. Bindarit differentiation-promoting effect is associated to its ability in suppressing cell

proliferation and migration as well as in reducing MCP-1 and MCP-3 production.

In the arterial wall, VSMCs normally exist in a quiescent, differentiated state, representing the contractile phenotype. During neointimal formation VSMCs became activated and change towards the synthetic phenotype characterised by a high rate of proliferation and chemotactic response, changes in the cytoskeleton composition [2] and increased expression of extracellular matrix proteins, cytokines and chemokines [2,4,5].

It is well known that chemokines mediate VSMC activation during vascular injury [5,6], with MCP-1 [7] and MCP-3 [19] shown to directly induce human VSMC proliferation and MCP-1 shown to induce cell migration [8] and the functional switch from the contractile to the synthetic phenotype [9]. This process is characterized by the downregulation of the differentiation markers such as α-SMA and calponin, concurrent with the upregulation of SMemb, that typifies immature VSMCs [2]. Importantly, it is now well established that differentiation and proliferation are not mutually exclusive and that many factors other than VSMC proliferation status influence the differentiation state. Inhibition of proliferation alone is not sufficient to promote VSMC differentiation [22]. However, anti proliferative agents used for inhibition of experimental neointimal formation, like simvastatin [23], or human restenosis, like rapamycin [24], are also able to induce VSMC differentiated phenotype [24,25].

Bindarit is a selective inhibitor of MCP-1/CCL2, MCP-3/CCL7, and MCP-2/CCL8 synthesis [10] acting through the down-regulation of NF-kB pathway [11]. It is effective in reducing neointimal formation in both non-hyperlipidemic and hyperlipidemic rodent models of vascular injury [16] as well as in a model of coronary in-stent stenosis in the pig [17] having a direct effect on VSMC proliferation/migration and reducing neointimal macrophage content [16,17]. Recently, a phase II clinical trial, has demonstrated the efficacy of bindarit in reducing in-stent late loss [18]. To better understand the effect of bindarit on human VSMC, here we evaluated the phenotypic modulation of CASMC analyzing the contractile proteins (α-SMA, calponin and SMemb) expression. α-SMA is known to be expressed in a wide variety of non-VSMC cell types, under certain circumstances, for this reason we also analyzed calponin, that is univocally expressed by fully differentiated, mature VSMC [2]. We observed that the expression of contractile proteins in CASMCs changed in response to stimulation with FBS and the proinflammatory cytokine TNF-α, with a reduction of α-SMA and calponin, and a concomitant increase of SMemb. These changes were significantly reversed by bindarit. CASMCs grown in presence of FBS exhibited a flattened morphology, feature of the synthetic phenotype. After bindarit treatment cells acquired the elongated and spindle-shaped morphology, typical feature of the contractile phenotype. Further bindarit inhibited CASMC proliferation, migration and invasion through the Matrigel barrier and reduced metalloproteinase (MMP)-9 activity, which is known to be key for VSMC migration into the intimal area [26,27]. Bindarit also reduced the levels of both MCP-1 and MCP-3, data in line with results observed in other species [16,17].

The effect of bindarit on VSMC phenotypic switching was confirmed *in vivo* in the rat carotid arteries subjected to balloon-induced endothelial denudation, an ideal experimental model for studying VSMC behaviour [7]. The inhibition of neointimal formation observed in bindarit treated rats was associated with a modulation of the contractile proteins expression patterns. Indeed, treatment with bindarit reduced the expression of SMemb and increased the expression of α-SMA and calponin after vascular injury.

In conclusion, our study demonstrates that bindarit regulates the contractile proteins expression and phenotype switching of VSMCs. Our data suggest a novel underlying mechanisms by which bindarit can inhibit neointimal formation in human restenosis.

Supporting Information

Table S1 Morphometric analysis of rat carotid arteries 7, 14 and, 28 days after angioplasty. The results are expressed as mean ± SEM (n = 10). *$P<0.05$, ***$P<0.001$ *vs* control group.

Table S2 MCP-1 levels in injured carotid arteries. The results are expressed as mean ± SEM (n = 4). *$P<0.05$, **$P<0.01$ *vs* control group.

Author Contributions

Conceived and designed the experiments: GG MM AI NM AG. Performed the experiments: GG MM MVDL DDF AP FM. Analyzed the data: GG MM AG AI PM CC TI NM MVDL DDF AP FM. Wrote the paper: GG MM AI NM PM AG.

References

1. Marx SO, Totary-Jain H, Marks AR (2011) Vascular smooth muscle cell proliferation in restenosis. Circ Cardiovasc Interv 4: 104–111.
2. Owens GK, Kumar MS, Wamhoff BR (2004) Molecular regulation of vascular smooth muscle cell differentiation in development and disease. Physiol Rev 84: 767–801.
3. Regan CP, Adam PJ, Madsen CS, Owens GK (2000) Molecular mechanisms of decreased smooth muscle differentiation marker expression after balloon injury. J Clin Invest 106: 1139–1147.
4. Charey DJ (1991) Control of growth and differentiation of vascular cells by extracellular matrix proteins. Annu Rev Physiol 53: 161–177.
5. Schober A (2008) Chemokines in vascular dysfunction and remodeling. Arterioscler Thromb Vasc Biol 28: 1950–1959.
6. Schober A, Zernecke A, Liehn EA, von Hundelshausen P, Knarren S, Kuziel WA, et al. (2004) Crucial role of the CCL2/CCR2 axis in neointimal hyperplasia after arterial injury in hyperlipidemic mice involves early monocyte recruitment and CCL2 presentation on platelets. Circ Res. 95: 1125–33.
7. Selzman CH, Miller SA, Zimmerman MA, Gamboni-Robertson F, Harken AH, et al. (2002) Monocyte chemotactic protein-1 directly induces human vascular smooth muscle proliferation. Am J Physiol Heart Circ Physiol 283: H1455–H1461.
8. Parenti A, Bellik L, Brogelli L, Filippi S, Ledda F (2004) Endogenous VEGF-A is responsible for mitogenic effects of MCP-1 on vascular smooth muscle cells. Am J Physiol Heart Circ Physiol. 286: H1978–84.
9. Denger S, Jahn L, Wende P, Watson L, Gerber SH, et al. (1999) Expression of monocyte chemoattractant protein-1 cDNA in vascular smooth muscle cells: induction of the synthetic phenotype: a possible clue to VSMC differentiation in the process of atherogenesis. Atherosclerosis 144: 15–23.
10. Mirolo M, Fabbri M, Sironi M, Vecchi A, Guglielmotti A, et al. (2008) Impact of the anti-inflammatory agent bindarit on the chemokinome: selective inhibition of the monocyte chemotactic proteins. Eur Cytokine Netw 19: 119–22.
11. Mora E, Guglielmotti A, Biondi G, Sassone-Corsi P (2012) Bindarit: an anti-inflammatory small molecule that modulates the NFκB pathway. Cell Cycle 11: 159–69.
12. Perico N, Benigni A, Remuzzi G (2008) Present and future drug treatments for chronic kidney diseases: evolving targets in renoprotection. Nat Rev Drug Discov 7: 936–853.
13. Rulli NE, Guglielmotti A, Mangano G, Rolph MS, Apicella C, et al. (2009) Amelioration of alphavirus-induced arthritis and myositis in a mouse model by treatment with bindarit, an inhibitor of monocyte chemotactic proteins. Arthritis Rheum 60: 2513–2523.
14. Bhatia M, Devi Ramnath RD, Chevali L, Guglielmotti A (2005) Treatment with bindarit, a blocker of MCP-1 synthesis, protects mice against acute pancreatitis. Am J Physiol Gastrointest Liver Physiol 288: G1259–G1265.
15. Bhatia M, Landolfi C, Basta F, Bovi G, Ramnath RD, et al. (2008) Treatment with bindarit, an inhibitor of MCP-1 synthesis, protects mice against trinitrobenzene sulfonic acid-induced colitis. Inflamm Res 57: 464–471.
16. Grassia G, Maddaluno M, Guglielmotti A, Mangano G, Biondi G, et al. (2009) The anti-inflammatory agent bindarit inhibits neointima formation in both rats and hyperlipidaemic mice. Cardiovasc Res 84: 485–93.
17. Ialenti A, Grassia G, Gordon P, Maddaluno M, Di Lauro MV, et al. (2011) Inhibition of in-stent stenosis by oral administration of bindarit in porcine coronary arteries. Arterioscler Thromb Vasc Biol 31: 2448–54.
18. Colombo A, Limbruno U, Lettieri C, Lioy E, Guglielmotti A, et al. (2012) A double blind randomized study to evaluate the efficacy of bindarit in preventing coronary stent restenosis. J Am Coll Cardiol. 59: E11–E11.
19. Maddaluno M, DiLauro MV, Di Pascale A, Santamaria R, Guglielmotti A, et al. (2011) Monocyte chemotactic protein-3 induces human coronary smooth muscle cell proliferation. Atherosclerosis 217: 113–9.
20. Grassia G, Maddaluno M, Musilli C, De Stefano D, Carnuccio R, et al. (2010) The IκB kinase inhibitor nuclear factor-κB essential modulator-binding domain peptide for inhibition of injury-induced neointimal formation. Arterioscler Thromb Vasc Biol 30: 2458–66.
21. Maffia P, Grassia G, Di Meglio P, Carnuccio R, Berrino L, et al. (2006) Neutralization of Interleukin-18 Inhibits Neointimal Formation in a Rat Model of Vascular Injury. Circulation 114: 430–437.
22. Alexander MR and Owens GK (2012) Epigenetic control of smooth muscle cell differentiation and phenotypic switching in vascular development and disease. Annu Rev Physiol. 74: 13–40.
23. Indolfi C, Cioppa A, Stabile E, Di Lorenzo E, Esposito G, et al. (2000) Effects of hydroxymethylglutaryl coenzyme a reductase inhibitor simvastatin on smooth muscle cell proliferation in vitro and neointimal formation in vivo after vascular injury. J Am Coll Cardiol 35: 214–21.
24. Martin KA, Merenick BL, Ding M, Fetalvero KM, Rzucidlo EM, et al. (2007) Rapamycin promotes vascular smooth muscle cell differentiation through insulin receptor substrate-1/phosphatidylinositol 3-kinase/akt2 feedback signaling. J Biol Chem 282: 36112–36120.
25. Wada H, Abe M, Ono K, Morimoto T, Kawamura T, et al. (2008) Statins activate GATA-6 and induce differentiated vascular smooth muscle cells. Biochem Biophys Res Commun 374: 731–736.
26. Newby AC, Zaltsman AB (2000) Molecular mechanisms in intimal hyperplasia. J Pathol 190: 300–309.
27. Bendeck MP, Zempo N, Clowes AW, Galardy RE, Reidy MA (1994) Smooth muscle cell migration and matrix metalloproteinase expression after arterial injury in the rat. Circ Res 75: 539–545.

8

The Impact of SYNTAX Score of Non-Infarct-Related Artery on Long-Term Outcome among Patients with Acute ST Segment Elevation Myocardial Infarction Undergoing Primary Percutaneous Coronary Intervention

Min-I Su[1], Cheng-Ting Tsai[1], Hung-I Yeh[1,2], Chun-Yen Chen[1,2]*

1 Division of Cardiology, Department of Internal Medicine, Mackay Memorial Hospital, Taipei, Taiwan, **2** Mackay Medical College, New Taipei City, Taiwan

Abstract

Objective: We investigated the impact of the severity of stenosis in a non-infarct-related artery (IRA) on the long-term prognosis of patients with ST-segment elevation myocardial infarction (STEMI) undergoing primary percutaneous coronary intervention (PCI).

Methods: Three hundred one consecutive patients (age: 59.7 $\pm$ 13.2 years, 85.5% men) underwent primary PCI during 2009–2012. Receiver operating characteristic curve analysis found the optimal cutoff for non-IRA SYNTAX score (SS) to be 2.5. We divided the patients into two groups according to this cutoff value.

Results: By multivariable analysis, non-IRA SS ($\geq$2.5) was an independent predictor of major adverse cardiac events (hazard ratio [HR]: 2.15, 95% confidence interval [CI]: 1.21–3.79, P = 0.008) and all-cause mortality (HR: 3.49, 95% CI: 1.13–10.8, P = 0.03). However, the prediction of cardiovascular mortality had only borderline significance (HR: 3.29, 95% CI: 0.90–12.08, P = 0.07).

Conclusion: STEMI patients treated with primary PCI and moderate to severe non-IRA stenosis (SS $\geq$2.5) have more subsequent cardiac events. Those populations should be treated with more aggressive preventive and medical management.

Editor: Chiara Lazzeri, Azienda Ospedaliero-Universitaria Careggi, Italy

Funding: The authors have no funding or support to report.

Competing Interests: The authors have declared that no competing interests exist.

* Email: mwplasma@ms9.hinet.net

Introduction

Acute thrombotic occlusion of a coronary artery is the leading cause of ST-segment elevation myocardial infarction (STEMI) [1]. Primary percutaneous coronary intervention (PCI) is currently the preferred therapy for restoring perfusion of the infarct-related artery (IRA), also known as the culprit artery[2], [3]. Between 40 and 65% of patients treated with primary PCI for STEMI have multi-vessel disease (MVD)[4–6], which is an independent predictor of long-term mortality in these patients[7,8]. Studies have indicated that MVD with chronic total occlusion (CTO) is a risk factor associated with a worse outcome in STEMI patients who undergo primary PCI. However, the association between the severity of non-IRA lesions and mortality in STEMI patients has not been elucidated.

The SYNTAX score (SS) is an angiographic scoring tool for systematically quantifying the severity and assessing the charac-

teristics of each coronary lesion[9]. It is used worldwide to predict long-term outcomes in patients with coronary artery disease undergoing elective PCI or coronary artery bypass graft surgery[10,11]. The SS is also useful for predicting short- and long-term outcomes in patients with STEMI who are treated with primary PCI[12–15].

The aim of our study was to quantify and assess the severity of non-IRA lesions calculated by SS, and to determine the impact of the severity of non-IRA in patients presenting with STEMI and treated with primary PCI.

Materials and Methods

Subjects

This study was conducted in accordance with the Declaration of Helsinki and was approved by the Institutional Review Board of Mackay Memorial Hospital. The patient records and information were anonymized and de-identified prior to analysis. Three hundred twenty-three consecutive patients undergoing primary PCI for STEMI at a single tertiary center between August 2009 and December 2012 were included in this analysis. Acute STEMI was defined as typical chest pain lasting for>30 min within the last 12 h, with electrocardiographic findings of ST elevation>1 mm in at least two consecutive leads or new-onset left bundle branch block, and elevation of serum levels of troponin-I or the MB fraction of creatine kinase. The diagnosis was confirmed by coronary angiography in all patients. We excluded from the study patients who reported a previous MI within 6 months, previous coronary artery bypass surgery, symptom onset more than 12 h before, pretreatment with thrombolytic therapy before primary PCI, previous hemodialysis, sepsis, neoplasm, hematological disorders, or acute stroke during the course of their hospital stay. Treatment of complications such as ventricular arrhythmia, cardiogenic shock, and cardiac arrest was administered according to guidelines.

Data Collection and Definitions

Demographic data, disease history (such as hypertension [HTN] or diabetes mellitus [DM]), current tobacco use, coronary angiographic results, and prescribed medications were obtained from the hospital medical registry. The blood total cholesterol, high-density lipoprotein cholesterol, low-density lipoprotein cholesterol (LDL-C), triglyceride (TG), and glycated hemoglobin (HbA1c), and creatinine levels were evaluated on the same day that the patients underwent primary PCI. All blood samples were collected by venipuncture after at least 8 h of fasting. HTN was defined as a history of HTN, a systolic BP of ≥140 mmHg, or a diastolic BP of ≥90 mmHg. Patients were defined as having DM if they had a history of DM, HbA1c levels ≥6.5%, or if they were using oral hypoglycemic agents or insulin. All patients received 300 mg aspirin and 300 mg clopidogrel orally, and were given a bolus of intravenous unfractionated heparin (75–100 U/kg) prior to primary PCI. At the discretion of the attending interventional cardiologist, glycoprotein IIb/IIIa inhibitors were administered as adjunctive therapy. Coronary angiography was performed using a Philip Integris BH 5000 device equipped with the cardiovascular (CV) angiography analysis system CAAS II (Best, Netherlands). The SS was calculated retrospectively by two trained operators who were blinded to the patients' demographics and outcomes. The SS was determined for all coronary lesions with>50% diameter stenosis in a vessel>1.5 mm, based on the SYNTAX Score Calculator 2.1 (www.syntaxscore.com). The pervious studies demonstrated both IRA SS calculated before any intervention preformed and IRA SS calculated after flow restoration were independent predictors of clinical outcomes[13,14], but how to evaluate SS after intervention is inconclusive. Therefore, total SS, SS of the IRA, and SS of non-IRA were all calculated before any intervention preformed in our study. The non-IRA SS was calculated as the sum of the SS in all non-culprit coronary arteries of MVD.

Clinical outcomes

The outcome measure in the current analysis was the time from the date of primary PCI until the first occurrence of a component of the composite endpoint: all-cause death, CV death (caused by MI, refractory heart failure, or ventricular arrhythmia), reinfarction (fatal or non-fatal MI), target lesion revascularization for myocardial ischemia, or stroke. Major adverse CV events (MACE) were defined as the composite of CV death, reinfarction (fatal or non-fatal MI), target vessel revascularization for ischemia, or

stroke. Follow-up for all patients was continued until December 31, 2013.

Statistical Analysis

Results are expressed as mean ± SD or as percentages. Student's t test was used to compare differences between groups for continuous variables, and the chi-square test was employed for categorical data. Receiver operating characteristic (ROC) curve analysis is the most common technique used for assessing diagnostic tests and to identify a cutoff point[16]. In this study, we want to chose the cutoffs by MACE as the outcome measure to discriminate the value of IRA and non-IRA Syntax Score proposed to be used as decisional levels in clinical practice when it is necessary to revascularize the non IRA. According to the ROC curve, we were able to define the cutoff point for the SS for IRA and non-IRA to maximize the clinical sensitivity and specificity of the test. We used the cutoff point as a criterion for the classification of the severity of non-IRA lesions. A Cox proportional hazards model was used to calculate hazard ratios (HRs) to determine the factors contributing to all-cause death, CV death, and MACE. The HRs (95% confidence intervals [CIs]) were adjusted for sex, age, HTN, DM, smoking status, LDL-C level (<100 mg/dL versus ≥100 mg/dL), IRA SS (<10.25 versus ≥10.25), and non-IRA SS (<2.5 versus ≥2.5). Kaplan–Meier survival curves were constructed and compared using the log-rank test. A P-value <0.05 was considered significant. All statistical analyses were performed using SPSS software, version 19 (IBM SPSS Statistics, State of New York) and STATA (version 11.0, College Station, Texas).

Results

Patient characteristics

A total of 323 patients were initially considered for study inclusion. Ten were excluded because no complete diagnostic coronary angiogram was available and another 2 because they had previously undergone coronary bypass grafting. Survival status and follow-up could not be obtained in 10 foreign patients. Overall, a total of 301 consecutive patients were included in our study for analysis. A Mean of SS in IRA and non –IRA was 12. 8 ± 0.4 and 6.2 ± 0.5, respectively. A median of SS in IRA and non –IRA was 11 and 3, respectively. Firstly, we used ROC to determine the appropriate cutoff value for severity of non-IRA lesions that corresponded to MACE (Figure 1). The closer the ROC curve to the upper-left corner, the higher the predictive power for predicting MACE. The optimal cutoff point for non-IRA SS was 2.5, with a sensitivity and specificity for MACE of 68% and 51%, respectively. The optimal cutoff point of IRA SS was 10.25, with a sensitivity and specificity for MACE of 61% and 50%, respectively. The area under the ROC curve (AUC) did not differ between IRA and non-IRA lesions (P = 0.85).

Since we were investigating the association between the severity of non-IRA lesions and clinical outcomes, we divided the patients at the cutoff point for non-IRA SS of 2.5, yielding subgroups with no/mild non-IRA stenosis (SS <2.5) and moderate/severe non-IRA stenosis (SS ≥2.5). Table 1 shows the baseline characteristics of these subgroups. Patients who had moderate/severe non-IRA stenosis were more likely to have HTN as comorbidity (66.5% vs. 47.6%, P = 0.001). Patients with moderate/severe non-IRA stenosis had a higher total SS than those with no/mild non-IRA stenosis (23.8 ± 10.3 vs. 13.7 ± 7, P <0.001). There were no differences in intra-aortic balloon pumping support, use of temporary pacemaker or extracorporeal membrane oxygenation, prescribed medication, Killip classification, IRA SS, or IRA

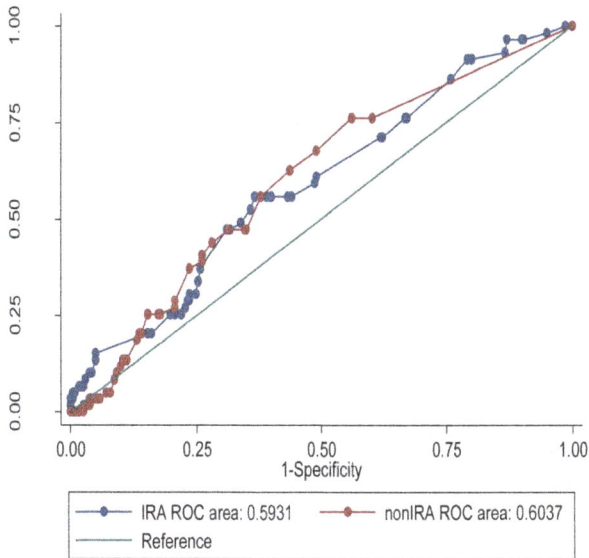

Figure 1. Receiver operating characteristic (ROC) curve analysis and cutoff value for the severity of stenosis of infarcted and non-infarcted related arteries in patients with acute ST-elevation myocardial infarction (STEMI).

location between patients with no/mild non-IRA stenosis and those with moderate/severe non-IRA stenosis. Compared to those with moderate/severe non-IRA stenosis, patients with no/mild non-IRA stenosis had a lower incidence of MACE (13.3% vs. 25.3%, P = 0.009), CV mortality (2.8% vs. 8.3%, P = 0.04), and all-cause mortality (3.5% vs. 10.1%, P = 0.02).

Clinical outcomes

All patients received clinical follow-up with a median duration of 580 days. A total of 80 endpoints occurred during follow-up: 59 (19.6%) new CV events and 21 (7.0%) deaths. Patients who had non-IRA CTO had a higher MACE rate of 8.0 % (versus 6.9 % for those who had no non-IRA CTO; p = 0.834); a higher CV mortality of 8.0% (versus 5.5 % for those who had no non-IRA CTO; p = 0.609); a higher MACE of 24 % (versus 19.2 % for those who had no non-IRA CTO; p = 0.563). The rate of all cause mortality in patients with triple vessel disease (TVD), double vessel disease (DVD) and single vessel disease (SVD) was 12.6%, 5.8%, and 3.6% (p = 0.04) The rate of MACE in patients with TVD, DVD and SVD was10.6%, 4.9% and 2.8% (p = 0.01). The rate of CV mortality patients with TVD, DVD and SVD was 10.6%, 4.9% and 2.8% (p = 0.06). The Cox proportional hazards regression model was used for multivariate analysis of MACE, all-cause mortality, and CV mortality after acute STEMI. The independent variables of the regression model included age, sex (men vs. women), current smoking status, HTN, DM, LDL-C ($\geq$ 100 vs. <100 mg/dL), IRA SS ($\geq$10.25 vs. <10.25) and non-IRA SS ($\geq$2.5 vs. <2.5). The predictors of MACE, all-cause mortality, and CV mortality are shown in Table 2. After adjustment for the parameters mentioned above, non-IRA SS of $\geq$2.5 vs. <2.5 (adjusted HR [AHR]: 2.15, 95% CI: 1.21–3.79, P = 0.008) was an independent predictor of MACE. DM (AHR: 3.04, 95% CI: 1.03–8.99, P = 0.04), an LDL-C level of $\geq$100 vs. <100 mg/dL (AHR: 0.29, 95% CI: 0.10–0.84, P = 0.02), and a non-IRA SS of $\geq$2.5 vs. <2.5 (AHR: 3.49, 95% CI: 1.13–10.8, P = 0.03) were independent predictors of all-cause mortality. DM (AHR: 7.64,

95% CI: 1.63–35.8, P = 0.01) was an independent predictor of CV mortality, but the non-IRA SS of $\geq$2.5 vs. <2.5 (AHR: 3.59, 95% CI: 0.90–12.08, P = 0.07) only showed a trend to predict CV mortality, with borderline statistical significance.

Since we found that non-IRA SS was a shared and strong predictor of MACE, Kaplan–Meier analysis was performed to examine the univariate association between the two subgroups of non-IRA SS scores ($\geq$2.5 vs. <2.5), IRA SS scores ($\geq$10.25 vs. < 10.25), and the outcomes of the cohort (Figure 2). The patients with no/mild non-IRA stenosis (non-IRA SS <2.5) exhibited a significantly lower rate of MACE, all-cause mortality, and CV mortality than those with moderate/severe non-IRA stenosis (SS $\geq$2.5; 81%, 95%, 97% vs. 55%, 86%, 89%, respectively; P < 0.05). However, there was no difference in MACE, all-cause mortality, or CV mortality between patients with IRA SS $\geq$10.25 and those with IRA SS <10.25.

Discussion

Our study demonstrates that the extent of non-IRA stenosis is an independent predictor of long-term all-cause mortality and MACE after adjustment for confounding variables. Our overall primary PCI mortality is in agreement with published data[17]. In our study, 36.5% of patients with MI had non-IRA stenosis: a result similar to those of previous studies[4–8,15,18]. Prior studies in the primary PCI era indicated that MVD was a significant predictor of poor outcomes in patients undergoing primary PCI, compared with single-vessel disease (SVD)[19,20]. Sorajja et al demonstrated that MVD was associated with a higher rate of IRA and non-IRA revascularization in patients with STEMI after primary PCI[18]. Furthermore, the presence of CTO in a non-IRA is associated with worse outcomes in patients undergoing primary PCI for acute STEMI[8,21-23]. In those studies, MVD was an independent factor for CV events, and the severity of non-IRA lesions seemed to play a role in contributing to CV events. In a post hoc analysis of the Harmonizing Outcomes with RevascularIZatiON and Stents in Acute Myocardial Infarction trial, the CV event rate was found to be higher in patients with MVD and non-IRA CTO than in those with SVD[8]. Our study found similar results. However, the contribution of the severity of IRA and non-IRA stenosis to the outcome of STEMI patients treated with primary PCI was not elucidated. Therefore, we considered the IRA and non-IRA SS independently, to investigate which component had an impact on the prognosis. Our analysis demonstrated that patients with moderate/severe non-IRA stenosis (score $\geq$2.5) had a higher incidence of MACE, CV mortality, and all-cause mortality than those with no/mild non-IRA stenosis (score <2.5), but the same result was not found for IRA SS. Our study indicated that patients with moderate/severe non-IRA stenosis might need more aggressive treatment.

The mechanisms underlying the greater frequency of CV events in patients with moderate/severe non-IRA stenosis are multifactorial. First, in our study the patients with moderate/severe non-IRA stenosis had a higher prevalence of comorbidities (such as HTN and DM) compared to those with no/mild non-IRA stenosis. Second, MVD was a significant predictor of a poor outcome after primary PCI, compared with SVD[8,18,19]. Our study showed that there was almost a twofold increase in the relative risk of MACE for those with moderate/severe non-IRA stenosis compared to those with no/mild non-IRA stenosis. In one study, nearly 10% of STEMI patients needed subsequent PCI in the non-IRA during a follow-up of up to 3 years[24]. Third, patients presenting with a higher SS might be exposed to complicated primary PCI procedures, including treatment of

Table 1. Clinical and angiographic characteristics of patients with no- mild non- IRA stenosis and moderate-severe non- IRA stenosis.

	no- mild non- IRA stenosis (N = 143)	moderate-severe non- IRA stenosis (N = 158)	P value
	SYNTAX score<2.5	SYNTAX score≥ 2.5	
Age (years)	58.8 ± 13.6	60.3 ± 12.9	0.32
Gender (men,%)	120 (83.9%)	137(86.7%)	0.46
Smoking status (yes,%)	89 (62.2%)	98 (62.0%)	0.97
HTN(yes,%)	68 (47.6%)	105 (66.5%)	0.001
DM(yes,%)	42 (29.4%)	63 (39.9%)	0.06
VT(yes,%)*	14 (9.8%)	12 (7.6%)	0.50
CPCR(yes,%)*	11 (7.7%)	14 (8.9%)	0.71
TC (mg/dL)	183.3 ± 44.1	176.7 ± 49.2	0.23
TG (mg/dL)	167.8± 153.1	167.8 ± 191.3	1.00
LDL-C (mg/dL)	112.7 ± 32.5	112.7 ± 35.1	1.00
Device use			
IABP(yes,%)	18 (12.6%)	27 (17.1%)	0.27
TPM(yes,%)	8 (5.6%)	14 (8.9%)	0.28
ECMO(yes,%)	1 (0.7%)	3 (1.9%)	0.35
Medication			
GpIIbIIIa	70 (49.3%)	66 (41.5%)	0.18
Enoxaprine	138 (97.2%)	152 (96.2%)	0.46
Aspirin	138 (97.2%)	151 (95.6%)	0.33
Clopidogrel	139 (97.9%)	148 (93.7%)	0.05
ACEI/ARB	129 (90.8%)	135 (85.4%)	0.12
Beta-Blocker	107 (75.4%)	113 (71.6%)	0.40
Statin	128 (90.1%)	133 (84.2%)	0.10
Killip classification			0.46
Killip I	77 (53.8%)	71 (44.9%)	
Killip II	31 (21.7%)	38 (24.1%)	
Killip III	7 (4.9%)	11 (7.0%)	
Killip IV	28 (19.6%)	38 (24.1%)	
IRA location			0.29
Left main	2 (1.4%)	2 (1.3%)	
LAD	80(55.9%)	73(46.2%)	
LCX	7(4.9%)	14 (8.9%)	
RCA	54 (37.8%)	69 (43.7%)	
Total SS	13.7 ± 7	23.8 ± 10.3	<0.001
IRA SS	13.2 ± 7.0	12.4 ± 6.7	0.31
Non IRA SS	0.5 ± 1.9	11.4 ± 8.5	<0.001
Clinical outcomes			
All cause mortality	5 (3.5%)	16 (10.1%)	0.02
CV death	4 (2.8%)	13 (8.3%)	0.04
MACE	19 (13.3%)	40 (25.3%)	0.009
TLR	10 (7.0%)	19 (12.0%)	0.14
Re-infarction	6 (4.2 %)	17 (10.8%)	0.03
stroke	3 (2.1%)	4 (2.5%)	1.00

Abbreviation: HTN: hypertension; DM: diabetes mellitus; VT: ventricular tachycardia; CPCR: cardiopulmonary cerebral resuscitation;TC: total cholesterol; TG: triglyceride; LDL-C: low density lipoprotein cholesterol; IABP: intra aortic balloon pumping ; TPM: temporary pacemaker; ECMO: extracorporeal membrane oxygenation; Gp: Glyoproein; ACEI: angiotensin converting enzyme; ARB: angiotensin receptor blocker; IRA: infarcted related artery; LAD: left descending artery; LCX: left circumflex; RCA: right coronary artery; SS: SYNTAX score; CV: cardiovascular; MACE: major adverse cardiovascular events; TLR: target lesion revascularization.
*: occurred before primary percutaneous coronary intervention.

Table 2. Cox regression analysis for major adverse cardiovascular events, all cause mortality and cardiovascular mortality.

	MACE		All cause mortality		CV mortality	
	hazard ratio (95% CI)	P value	hazard ratio (95% CI)	P value	hazard ratio (95% CI)	P value
Age (years)	1.02 (1.00–1.05)	0.07	1.04 (0.99–1.08)	0.10	1.02 (0.97–1.07)	0.49
gender(men vs women)	0.82(0.35–1.92)	0.65	1.36 (0.39–4.72)	1.00	10.2(0.24– 4.37)	0.98
HTN (yes vs no)	0.76 (0.43–1.34)	0.34	1.29 (0.39–4.18)	0.68	1.26 (0.33–4.82)	0.74
DM (yes vs no)	1.37 (0.78–2.43)	0.28	3.04 (1.03–8.99)	0.04	7.64(1.63–35.8)	0.01
Smoking status (yes vs no)	0.93 (0.50–1.74)	0.83	1.13 (0.36–3.06)	0.83	0.93 (0.27–3.23)	0.90
LDL ($\geq$100 vs <100 mg/dL)	0.61 (0.35–1.05)	0.07	0.29 (0.10–0.84)	0.02	0.44 (0.15–1.35)	0.15
Non-IRA SS ($\geq$2.5 vs <2.5)	2.15(1.21–3.79)	**0.008**	3.49 (1.13–10.8)	**0.03**	3.29 (0.90–12.08)	0.07
IRA SS ($\geq$10.25 vs <10.25)	1.6 (0.93–2.85)	0.08	1.46(0.56–3.83)	0.44	1.57(0.51–4.80)	0.43

Abbreviation as table 1; CI: confidence interval.

bifurcations or left main disease, with a resulting effect on the clinical outcome, and might require repeated revascularization because of ischemia caused by restenotic lesions in areas of high intervention complexity. The explanation for the high late mortality in patients with moderate/severe non-IRA stenosis could be that they are potentially at a higher risk from the initial acute STEMI. The area at risk from the ischemia would be more extensive in patients with moderate/severe non-IRA stenosis than

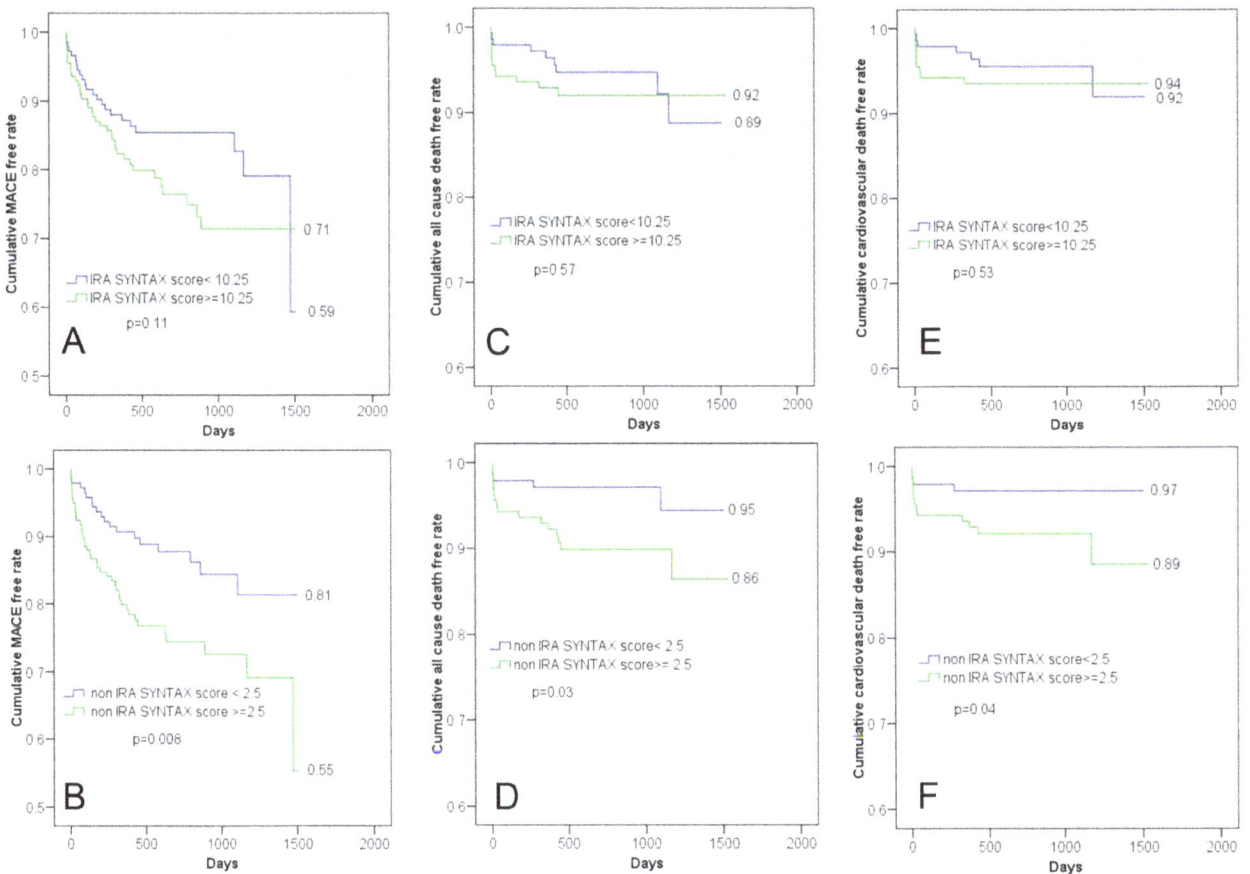

Figure 2. Kaplan–Meier analysis of major adverse cardiovascular events (MACE), all-cause mortality, and cardiovascular mortality in all patients, subdivided according to cutoff levels for non-IRA SS (2.5) and IRA SS (10.25). (A) Cumulative MACE-free rate between patients with IRA SS $\geq$10.25 and <10.25 (B) Statistical significance of the difference in cumulative MACE-free rate between patients with IRA SS $\geq$2.5 and <2.5 (C) Cumulative all-cause mortality-free rate between patients with IRA SS $\geq$10.25 and <10.25 (D) Statistical significance of the difference in cumulative all-cause mortality-free rate between patients with IRA SS $\geq$2.5 and <2.5 (E) Cumulative cardiovascular mortality-free rate between patients with IRA SS $\geq$10.25 and <10.25 (F) Statistical significance of the difference in cumulative cardiovascular mortality-free rate between patients with IRA SS $\geq$2.5 and <2.5.

in those with no/mild non-IRA stenosis. Our findings highlight the fact that non-IRA disease at presentation may not be benign.

The finding that the severity of non-IRA stenosis adds an incremental risk of adverse outcomes in patients with STEMI undergoing primary PCI may have important clinical implications. Based on previous studies, PCI in non-infarct lesions does not show a benefit in terms of reducing death and MI[25,26]. Current guidelines indicate simultaneous treatment of multiple vessels during acute STEMI be performed only in cases of cardiogenic shock[3], whereas staged PCI procedures demonstrate better outcomes in STEMI patients than in those with multiple vessel PCI[27,28]. In contrast, the Preventive Angioplasty in Acute Myocardial Infarction study reported that the primary outcome of cardiac death, MI, or refractory angina was significantly less common in the preventive-PCI group, as compared with optimal medical therapy alone[29]. Therefore, the best strategy for staged revascularization in STEMI with MVD to improve long-term prognosis still needs to be clarified by further clinical trials.

Several limitations of the current study should be mentioned. The main one is that our study was a retrospective observational study from a single center and not a randomized prospective study. The true incidence of CV events could not be estimated from our study. The study used MACE as the outcome measure to discriminate the value of IRA and non-IRA Syntax Score. Since the cutoff is derived by the data themselves, this almost certainly leads to over-estimates of performances such as sensitivity, specificity, positive and negative predictive values. Additionally, our study did not evaluate subsequent revascularization attempts in the non-IRA. Because of the limited sample size and its being a single hospital study, the patients in our study might not be representative of the entire population of acute STEMI patients who undergo primary PCI. In order to confirm our findings, a study with a larger sample of patients is required. However, the results of our analysis should be considered hypothesis generating.

In conclusion, our finding indicate that STEMI patients who are treated with primary PCI and have moderate/severe non-IRA stenosis (score ≥2.5) suffer more subsequent MACE, suggesting that those populations should be treated with more aggressive preventive and medical management.

Author Contributions

Conceived and designed the experiments: MIS CYC. Performed the experiments: CTT HIY CYC. Analyzed the data: MIS CYC. Contributed reagents/materials/analysis tools: HIY. Wrote the paper: MIS CYC.

References

1. Davies MJ, Woolf N, Robertson WB (1976) Pathology of acute myocardial infarction with particular reference to occlusive coronary thrombi. Br Heart J 38: 659–664.
2. Task Force on the management of STseamiotESoC, Steg PG, James SK, Atar D, Badano LP, et al. (2012) ESC Guidelines for the management of acute myocardial infarction in patients presenting with ST-segment elevation. Eur Heart J 33: 2569–2619.
3. O'Gara PT, Kushner FG, Ascheim DD, Casey DE Jr, Chung MK, et al. (2013) 2013 ACCF/AHA guideline for the management of ST-elevation myocardial infarction: executive summary: a report of the American College of Cardiology Foundation/American Heart Association Task Force on Practice Guidelines. Circulation 127: 529–555.
4. Muller DW, Topol EJ, Ellis SG, Sigmon KN, Lee K, et al. (1991) Multivessel coronary artery disease: a key predictor of short-term prognosis after reperfusion therapy for acute myocardial infarction. Thrombolysis and Angioplasty in Myocardial Infarction (TAMI) Study Group. Am Heart J 121: 1042–1049.
5. Moreno R, Garcia E, Elizaga J, Abeytua M, Soriano J, et al. (1998) [Results of primary angioplasty in patients with multivessel disease]. Rev Esp Cardiol 51: 547–555.
6. Kahn JK, Rutherford BD, McConahay DR, Johnson WL, Giorgi LV, et al. (1990) Results of primary angioplasty for acute myocardial infarction in patients with multivessel coronary artery disease. J Am Coll Cardiol 16: 1089–1096.
7. van der Schaaf RJ, Timmer JR, Ottervanger JP, Hoorntje JC, de Boer MJ, et al. (2006) Long-term impact of multivessel disease on cause-specific mortality after ST elevation myocardial infarction treated with reperfusion therapy. Heart 92: 1760–1763.
8. Claessen BE, Dangas GD, Weisz G, Witzenbichler B, Guagliumi G, et al. (2012) Prognostic impact of a chronic total occlusion in a non-infarct-related artery in patients with ST-segment elevation myocardial infarction: 3-year results from the HORIZONS-AMI trial. Eur Heart J 33: 768–775.
9. Sianos G, Morel MA, Kappetein AP, Morice MC, Colombo A, et al. (2005) The SYNTAX Score: an angiographic tool grading the complexity of coronary artery disease. EuroIntervention 1: 219–227.
10. Mohr FW, Morice MC, Kappetein AP, Feldman TE, Stahle E, et al. (2013) Coronary artery bypass graft surgery versus percutaneous coronary intervention in patients with three-vessel disease and left main coronary disease: 5-year follow-up of the randomised, clinical SYNTAX trial. Lancet 381: 629–638.
11. Head SJ, Holmes DR Jr, Mack MJ, Serruys PW, Mohr FW, et al. (2012) Risk profile and 3-year outcomes from the SYNTAX percutaneous coronary intervention and coronary artery bypass grafting nested registries. JACC Cardiovasc Interv 5: 618–625.
12. Yang CH, Hsieh MJ, Chen CC, Wang CY, Chang SH, et al. (2013) The prognostic significance of SYNTAX score after early percutaneous transluminal coronary angioplasty for acute ST elevation myocardial infarction. Heart Lung Circ 22: 341–345.
13. Magro M, Nauta S, Simsek C, Onuma Y, Garg S, et al. (2011) Value of the SYNTAX score in patients treated by primary percutaneous coronary intervention for acute ST-elevation myocardial infarction: The MI SYNTAX-score study. Am Heart J 161: 771–781.
14. Garg S, Sarno G, Serruys PW, Rodriguez AE, Bolognese L, et al. (2011) Prediction of 1-year clinical outcomes using the SYNTAX score in patients with acute ST-segment elevation myocardial infarction undergoing primary percutaneous coronary intervention: a substudy of the STRATEGY (Single High-Dose Bolus Tirofiban and Sirolimus-Eluting Stent Versus Abciximab and Bare-Metal Stent in Acute Myocardial Infarction) and MULTISTRATEGY (Multicenter Evaluation of Single High-Dose Bolus Tirofiban Versus Abciximab With Sirolimus-Eluting Stent or Bare-Metal Stent in Acute Myocardial Infarction Study) trials. JACC Cardiovasc Interv 4: 66–75.
15. Brown AJ, McCormick LM, Gajendragadkar PR, Hoole SP, West NE (2013) Initial SYNTAX Score Predicts Major Adverse Cardiac Events After Primary Percutaneous Coronary Intervention. Angiology.
16. Zou KH, O'Malley AJ, Mauri L (2007) Receiver-operating characteristic analysis for evaluating diagnostic tests and predictive models. Circulation, 115.5: 654–657.
17. Keeley EC, Boura JA, Grines CL (2003) Primary angioplasty versus intravenous thrombolytic therapy for acute myocardial infarction: a quantitative review of 23 randomised trials. Lancet 361: 13–20.
18. Goldstein JA, Demetriou D, Grines CL, Pica M, Shoukfeh M, et al. (2000) Multiple complex coronary plaques in patients with acute myocardial infarction. N Engl J Med 343: 915–922.
19. Sorajja P, Gersh BJ, Cox DA, McLaughlin MG, Zimetbaum P, et al. (2007) Impact of multivessel disease on reperfusion success and clinical outcomes in patients undergoing primary percutaneous coronary intervention for acute myocardial infarction. Eur Heart J 28: 1709–1716.
20. Biondi-Zoccai G, Lotrionte M, Sheiban I (2010) Management of multivessel coronary disease after ST-elevation myocardial infarction treated by primary coronary angioplasty. Am Heart J 160: S28–35.
21. Lexis CP, van der Horst IC, Rahel BM, Lexis MA, Kampinga MA, et al. (2011) Impact of chronic total occlusions on markers of reperfusion, infarct size, and long-term mortality: a substudy from the TAPAS-trial. Catheter Cardiovasc Interv 77: 484–491.
22. Claessen BE, van der Schaaf RJ, Verouden NJ, Stegenga NK, Engstrom AE, et al. (2009) Evaluation of the effect of a concurrent chronic total occlusion on long-term mortality and left ventricular function in patients after primary percutaneous coronary intervention. JACC Cardiovasc Interv 2: 1128–1134.
23. Claessen BE, Hoebers LP, van der Schaaf RJ, Kikkert WJ, Engstrom AE, et al. (2010) Prevalence and impact of a chronic total occlusion in a non-infarct-related artery on long-term mortality in diabetic patients with ST elevation myocardial infarction. Heart 96: 1968–1972.
24. Lemesle G, de Labriolle A, Bonello L, Torguson R, Kaneshige K, et al. (2009) Incidence, predictors, and outcome of new, subsequent lesions treated with percutaneous coronary intervention in patients presenting with myocardial infarction. Am J Cardiol 103: 1189–1195.
25. Parisi AF, Folland ED, Hartigan P (1992) A comparison of angioplasty with medical therapy in the treatment of single-vessel coronary artery disease. Veterans Affairs ACME Investigators. N Engl J Med 326: 10–16.
26. Boden WE, O'Rourke RA, Teo KK, Hartigan PM, Maron DJ, et al. (2007) Optimal medical therapy with or without PCI for stable coronary disease. N Engl J Med 356: 1503–1516.

27. Vlaar PJ, Mahmoud KD, Holmes DR Jr, van Valkenhoef G, Hillege HL, et al. (2011) Culprit vessel only versus multivessel and staged percutaneous coronary intervention for multivessel disease in patients presenting with ST-segment elevation myocardial infarction: a pairwise and network meta-analysis. J Am Coll Cardiol 58: 692–703.

28. Kornowski R, Mehran R, Dangas G, Nikolsky E, Assali A, et al. (2011) Prognostic impact of staged versus "one-time" multivessel percutaneous intervention in acute myocardial infarction: analysis from the HORIZONS-AMI (harmonizing outcomes with revascularization and stents in acute myocardial infarction) trial. J Am Coll Cardiol 58: 704–711.

29. Wald DS, Morris JK, Wald NJ, Chase AJ, Edwards RJ, et al. (2013) Randomized trial of preventive angioplasty in myocardial infarction. N Engl J Med 369: 1115–1123.

9

Pre-Infarction Angina and Outcomes in Non-ST-Segment Elevation Myocardial Infarction: Data from the RICO Survey

Luc Lorgis[1,2], Aurélie Gudjoncik[1,2], Carole Richard[1,2], Laurent Mock[3], Philippe Buffet[1], Philippe Brunel[3], Luc Janin-Manificat[4], Jean-Claude Beer[1], Damien Brunet[3], Claude Touzery[1], Luc Rochette[2], Yves Cottin[1,2], Marianne Zeller[2]*

1 Department of Cardiology, University Hospital, Dijon, France, 2 Laboratory of Cardiometabolic Physiopathology and Pharmacology, INSERM U866, SFR Santé University of Burgundy, Dijon, France, 3 Department of Cardiology, Clinique de Fontaine-lès-Dijon, Fontaine-lès-Dijon, France, 4 Department of Cardiology, CH Beaune, Beaune, France

Abstract

Background: The presence of pre-infarction angina (PIA) has been shown to confer cardioprotection after ST-segment elevation myocardial infarction (STEMI). However, the clinical impact of PIA in non-ST-segment elevation myocardial infarction (NSTEMI) remains to be determined.

Methods and Results: From the obseRvatoire des Infarctus de Côte d'Or (RICO) survey, 1541 consecutive patients admitted in intensive care unit with a first NSTEMI were included. Patients who experienced chest pain <7 days before the episode leading to admission were defined as having PIA and were compared with patients without PIA. Incidence of in-hospital ventricular arrhythmias (VAs), heart failure and 30-day mortality were collected. Among the 1541 patients included in the study, 693 (45%) patients presented PIA. PIA was associated with a lower creatine kinase peak, as a reflection of infarct size (231(109–520) vs. 322(148–844) IU/L, p<0.001) when compared with the group without PIA. Patients with PIA developed fewer VAs, by 3 fold (1.6% vs. 4.0%, p=0.008) and heart failure (18.0% vs. 22.4%, p=0.040) during the hospital stay. Overall, there was a decrease in early CV events by 26% in patients with PIA (19.2% vs. 25.9%, p=0.002). By multivariate analysis, PIA remained independently associated with less VAs.

Conclusion: From this large contemporary prospective study, our work showed that PIA is very frequent in patients admitted for a first NSTEMI, and is associated with a better prognosis, including reduced infarct size and in hospital VAs. Accordingly, protecting the myocardium by ischemic or pharmacological conditioning not only in STEMI, but in all type of MI merits further attention.

Editor: Claudio Moretti, S.G.Battista Hospital, Italy

Funding: This work was supported by the University Hospital of Dijon, Association de Cardiologie de Bourgogne, Conseil Régional de Bourgogne, Fédération Française de Cardiologie, and by grants from the Union Régionale des Caisses d'Assurance Maladie de Bourgogne (URCAM), and the Agence Régionale de Santé (ARS) de Bourgogne. The funders had no role in study design, data collection and analysis, decision to publish, or preparation of the manuscript.

Competing Interests: The authors have declared that no competing interests exist.

* E-mail: marianne.zeller@u-bourgogne.fr

Introduction

Pre-infarction angina (PIA), i.e. angina episodes preceding the onset of acute myocardial infarction (MI), has been suggested in several studies to exert beneficial effects on ST-segment elevation myocardial infarction [1]. In these patients, PIA has been shown to improve the increase in left ventricular wall motion [2], and to induce greater microvascular reflow extent and coronary flow reserve [3]. Moreover, PIA was associated with more rapid reperfusion with thrombolytic therapy [4] and greater degree of ST-segment resolution after primary angioplasty [5]. Several clinical studies reported that PIA both reduces myocardial infarct size [6] and protects against life-threatening ventricular arrhythmias (VAs) [7].

Management of non-ST-segment elevation MI (NSTEMI) patients is a growing clinical challenge, representing nowadays the majority of acute MI in most contemporary registries [8,9]. Moreover, NSTEMI patients have a dramatically high rate of in-hospital cardiovascular complications, almost similar to STEMI population. NSTEMI are also characterized by increased age, and further evidence of co-morbidities such as diabetes, most conditions that are known to reduce the beneficial effects of PIA in STEMI [10,11]. However, the impact of PIA in the setting of NSTEMI patients is currently unknown.

From a large contemporary French survey of acute myocardial infarction, the aim of our study was to analyse the frequency and the potential influence of PIA on cardiovascular outcomes in NSTEMI patients.

Methods

Patients

The design and methods of RICO (obseRvatoire des Infarctus de Côte-d'Or), a French regional survey for acute MI, have been detailed previously [12]. Briefly, since 1st January 2001, the RICO survey collects data from all the consecutive patients admitted for acute myocardial infarction in all public centres (3) or privately funded hospitals (3) of one eastern region of France (Côte d'Or, 500 000 inhabitants). Between 1st January 2001 and 29th February 2008, all the consecutive patients admitted with a first NSTEMI within 24 hours after the onset of symptoms were included in the present study. MI was diagnosed according to European Society of Cardiology and American College of Cardiology criteria [13]. NSTEMI was defined by the absence of persistent ST-segment elevation or new left bundle branch block on the admission ECG. Patients with documented history of MI were excluded from the study.

Data Collection

Data were collected at each site by a trained study coordinator using a standardized case report form. Cases were ascertained by prospective collection of consecutive admissions. Eligible patients are identified during the index admission and medical records are reviewed on an ongoing basis after appropriate consent has been obtained. In addition, hospital listings of discharged patients are systematically reviewed to identify eligible cases with use of the International Classification of Diseases (ICD-9), and corresponding codes in ICD 10. Standardized definitions for MI, patient-related variables and clinical outcomes were used. The present study complied with the Declaration of Helsinki and was approved by the ethics committee of University Hospital of Dijon. Each patient gave written consent before participation.

Data on demographics and risk factors (history of hypertension or treated hypertension, diabetes, hypercholesterolemia, current smoking) were collected prospectively, along with admission characteristics and hemodynamic parameters, such as heart rate and systolic and diastolic blood pressure. Height and body weight were self-reported and body mass index (BMI) was calculated (kg/m^2). Obesity was defined as BMI ≥ 30. Echocardiography was performed at day 2 ± 1 by a local investigator according to the Simpson method using the apical views to calculate left ventricular ejection fraction (LVEF). Treatments administered before and <48 h after hospitalization were also recorded.

The median duration of stay in intensive care unit was also collected. The Global Registry of Acute Coronary Events (GRACE) score, including admission variables including age, heart rate, serum creatinine, systolic blood pressure, Killip class, cardiac arrest, ST-segment deviation, and cardiac markers, was calculated for each patient (www.outcomes-org/grace/acs_risk.cfm) [14]. Blood samples were drawn at admission. Plasma creatinine levels were measured on a Vitros 950 analyzer (Ortho Clinical Diagnostics, Rochester, NY). Cockcroft-Gault formula was used to estimate serum creatinine clearance. C-reactive protein was measured on Dimension Xpand (Dade Behring, Newark, NE) with an immunonephelometry assay. Plasma N-terminal pro B-type natriuretic peptide (NT-proBNP) was determined by ELISA with an Elecsys NT-proBNP sandwich immunoassay on Elecsys 2010 (Roche Diagnostics, Basel, Switzerland). Plasma troponin Ic and creatine kinase peaks were assessed by sampling every eight hours during the first two days after admission (Dimension Vista Intelligent Lab System, Siemens).

Coronary angiography

Of the 1541 patients included in the study, 1437(93%) had coronary angiographic data available. Among these patients, most (i.e. 1400/1437 (97%) underwent coronary angiography during their hospital stay and were included in the angiographic analysis. Significant stenosis was defined as a >50% stenosis in an epicardial vessel.

Outcomes

In-hospital adverse events—i.e. VAs, recurrent MI, cardiogenic shock or death—were recorded. VAs were defined as either sustained ventricular tachycardia (VT) or ventricular fibrillation (VF). VT was defined as a regular wide complex tachycardia of ventricular origin lasting >30 sec or requiring termination due to hemodynamic instability. FV was defined as irregular undulations of varying shape and amplitude on ECG without discrete QRS or T waves that resulted in prompt hemodynamic compromise requiring direct-current cardioversion. Heart failure was defined as a Killip class >1. Recurrent MI was diagnosed by ECG modifications and increased serum troponin.

After hospital discharge, 30-day information on cardiovascular death was acquired by contacting each patient individually, their relatives, or treating physician and by reviewing the hospital records if the patient had been re-hospitalized. Thirty-day follow-up was achieved for most patients (99%).

Definition of pre-infarction angina

Data were prospectively collected on the study form regarding whether patients have ever experienced angina before acute MI. PIA was defined as patients who experienced typical chest pain, chest discomfort or left arm and jaw pain <7 days before the episode leading to admission, lasting less than 20 minutes and having the same character as the admission episode. Patients were categorized into two groups depending on whether or not they experienced PIA.

Statistical analysis

Data are presented as median (25th to 75th percentile) or number (percentage). For continuous variables, we used the Kolmogorov-Smirnov analysis to check the normality of the distribution. They were compared using either Student's t test or Mann and Whitney, as appropriate. Dichotomous variables, expressed as numbers and percents, were compared by the χ^2 test.

Multivariate logistic regression analysis was used to identify independent predictors of PIA on admission. Variables were included in the multivariate model if associated with PIA by univariate analysis (p<0.1), i.e. chronic treatments (aspirin, nitrates and nicorandil), family history of CAD, SBP on admission, obesity and hypertension.

Multivariate logistic regression analysis was used to assess factors potentially associated with the development of in-hospital VAs. The following factors were included: on admission hemodynamic parameters (SBP, heart rate), creatinine clearance, on admission heart failure, female gender, age, and PIA (model 1). In order to analyze the potential role of infarct size on the protective effect of PIA, another model (model 2) was built by adding CK peak to the model 1. Variables entered into the models were chosen based on their significant relationship with VAs in the literature. [15] By using backward selection, only factors with a p value<0.05 were included in the final model. Non-normal variables, such as CK peak, were log-transformed before inclusion in regression analyses. Statistical analyses were performed with SPSS software (SPSS, Inc, Chicago, Ill).

Table 1. Patient characteristics (n (%) or median (interquartile range)).

	No pre-infarction angina N = 848	Pre-infarction angina N = 693	p
Risk factors			
Age, year	69(55–78)	69(57–78)	0.53
Female	282(33)	211(30)	0.26
Obesity	183(22)	190(27)	0.009
Hypertension	455(54)	406(59)	0.06
Diabetes	196(23)	175(25)	0.36
Hypercholesterolemia	372(44)	316(46)	0.53
Current smoking	226(27)	163(24)	0.18
Familial history of CAD	221(26)	220(32)	0.016
Stroke	48(6)	33(5)	0.50
PAD	77(9)	61(9)	0.92
Chronic treatments			
Nicorandil	8(1)	21(3)	0.005
Amiodarone	24(3)	14(2)	0.39
Aspirin	99(12)	153(22)	<0.001
Beta blocker	188(22)	175(25)	0.17
ACE inhibitor	136(16)	113(16)	0.94
Statin	157(19)	138(20)	0.53
Trimetazidine	32(4)	36(5)	0.22
Nitrates	52(6)	93(13)	<0.001
Clinical data on admission			
KILLIP >1	155(18)	112(16)	0.31
LVEF, %	60(50–66)	60 (50–66)	0.93
SBP, mm Hg	141(122–160)	144(129–165)	0.09
DBP, mm Hg	80(70–91)	80(70–93)	0.20
HR, b/min	77(65–90)	78(67–90)	0.49
Anterior wall location	303(36)	235(34)	0.49
Time to admission (min)	195(113–420)	210(110–498)	0.26
GRACE risk score	126(98–155)	129(98–156)	0.94
Biological data			
CRP, mg/L	6.0(2.3–18)	5.4(2.2–14)	0.14
Creatinine clearance, mL/min	72.3(50.9–94.7)	72.6(50–97.6)	0.44
NT-proBNP, pg/mL	736(229–2172)	813(266–2581)	0.26
Glucose, mmol/L	6.55(5.64–8.48)	6.45(5.54–8.37)	0.14
Troponin Ic, peak >100 ULN	328(39)	211(31)	<0.001
CK peak, IU/L	322(148–844)	231(109–520)	<0.001
Angiographic data	**N = 744**	**N = 656**	
Nb diseased vessel			0.001
0	136(18)	73(11)	
1	280(38)	245(37)	
2	182(24)	184(28)	
3 or LM	146(20)	154(23)	
>50% stenosis			
LAD	385(52)	408(62)	<0.001
Cx	346(46)	313(48)	0.651
RC	330(44)	330(50)	0.026
LM	30(4)	49(7)	0.005
Acute treatments			
Vasoactive drug	36(4)	20(3)	0.20

Table 1. Cont.

	No pre-infarction angina N = 848	Pre-infarction angina N = 693	p
Amiodarone	56(7)	33(5)	0.15
Aspirin	771(91)	649(94)	0.059
Beta blocker	659(78)	555(80)	0.29
ACE inhibitor	417(49)	407(59)	<0.001
Statin	545(64)	545(79)	<0.001
PCI	410(48)	402(58)	<0.001

ACE: angiotensin converting enzyme; CABG: coronary artery bypass grafting; CAD: coronary artery disease;CK: creatine kinase; CRP: C-reactive protein; DBP: diastolic blood pressure; HR: heart rate; LVEF: left ventricular ejection fraction; PAD: peripheral artery disease; PCI: percutaneous coronary intervention; SBP: systolic blood pressure. LM: Left main; Cx: Circumflex; RC: Right coronary; LAD: Left anterior descending.

Results

Study population

1541 patients were included in the study, of whom 693 (45%) patients suffered from PIA. The patient characteristics are summarized in Table 1. Median age was 69 (56–78) years. Patients with PIA were more likely to have a familial history of coronary artery disease (32% vs. 26%, p = 0.016) and a higher rate of obesity (27 vs. 22%, p = 0.009) than patients without PIA. There was no difference for the two groups for the other risk factors. PIA patients were more often previously treated with K_{ATP} openers (3% vs. 1%, p = 0.005), nitrates (13% vs. 6%, p<0.001) or aspirin (22% vs. 12%, p<0.001). The mean time from symptom onset to admission was similar for both groups (p = 0.26). Moreover, GRACE risk score, heart failure on admission, MI location and LVEF were similar for the two groups.

PIA was strikingly associated with a lower level of both CK peak (Figure 1), (231(109–520) vs. 322(148–844) IU/L, p<0.001) and troponin Ic peak >100 ULN (211(31%) vs. 328(39%), p<0.001), as a reflection of infarct size. Other biological data, such as CRP, creatinine clearance, NT-proBNP and glycemia on admission were similar for the 2 groups. Within 48 hours after the admission, patients with PIA were more aggressively treated, by either percutaneous coronary intervention (PCI) or acute medications

such as ACE inhibitors or statins. On coronary angiography, patients from the PIA group were characterized by less lack of significant stenosis and more frequent significant stenosis on left anterior descending artery or left main (table 1).

By logistic regression analysis (Table 2), preadmission treatment, such as aspirin, nitrates or nicorandil, and family history of CAD were independently associated with PIA.

Outcomes

Patients who suffered from PIA were markedly less likely, by three fold, to experience VAs during the hospital stay (1.6 vs. 4.0%, p = 0.008) than those without PIA (Figure 2). Moreover, patients with PIA suffered less frequently from heart failure (18.0 vs. 22.4%, p = 0.040). In patients with PIA, there was also a trend toward a decrease in case-fatality at 30 days (3.5 vs. 5.3%, p = 0.106). Overall, a 26% decrease in such short term CV events was reported (19.2% vs. 25.9%, p = 0.002) (Figure 2). The rate of recurrent MI was similar for the 2 groups (p = 0.58).

By multivariate analysis, the presence of PIA was a significant predictor of in-hospital VAs (odds ratio (OR) 0.45; (95% confidence interval (CI): 0.22–0.93; p = 0.03) (model 1, Table 3).

Subgroup analysis showed that beneficial effects of PIA on VAs tended to be observed in most subgroups (i.e. ≥65 (OR 0.47; 95% CI: 0.20–1.06; p = 0.068) and <65 y (OR 0.29; 95% CI: 0.08–1.03; p = 0.056), female (OR 0.24; 95% CI: 0.05–1.07; p = 0.062) and male (OR 0.47; 95% CI: 0.21–1.03; p = 0.060), with dyslipidemia (OR 0.35; 95% CI: 0.11–1.10; p = 0.072) and without (OR 0.43; 95% CI: 0.10–1.03, p – 0.059) and with or without acute treatment such as PCI, ACE inhibitors or statins. Interestingly, the influence of PIA on VAs was lessened in patients with CV risk factors such as hypertension ((OR 0.91; 95% CI: 0.37–2.23; p = 0.845) vs. (OR 0.12; 95% CI: 0.03–0.51; p = 0.004)

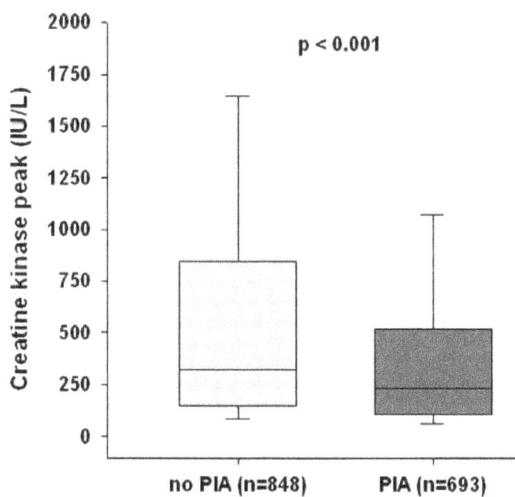

Figure 1. Levels of Creatine Kinase peak (IU/L) during the hospital phase.

Table 2. Multivariate analysis for predictors of pre-infarction angina.

	OR (95% CI)	p
Aspirin	1.89(1.40–2.55)	<0.001
Nitrates	1.99(1.36–2.91)	<0.001
Nicorandil	2.46(1.01–5.95)	0.046
Family history of CAD	1.27(1.00–1.61)	0.049

CAD: coronary artery disease.

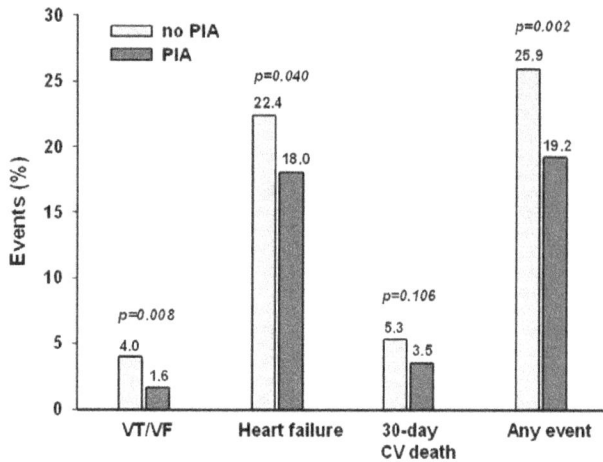

Figure 2. Cardiovascular events (%). *CV: cardiovascular; VT/VF: ventricular tachycardia/ventricular fibrillation.*

Table 3. Multivariate analysis for predictors of in-hospital ventricular arrhythmias.

	Model 1		Model 2	
	OR (95% CI)	p	OR (95% CI)	p
PIA	0.45 (0.22–0.93)	0.030	0.54 (0.26–1.11)	0.100
SBP	0.98 (0.97–1.00)	0.011	0.99 (0.98–1.00)	0.026
HR	1.01 (0.99–1.03)	0.068	1.01 (1.00–1.03)	0.048
CK peak	-	-	2.03 (1.09–3.80)	0.027

CK: creatine kinase; HR: heart rate; PIA: pre-infarction angina; SBP: systolic blood pressure.

without hypertension) or obesity ((OR 0.79; 95% CI: 0.17–3.58; p = 0.758) vs. (OR 0.36; 95% CI: 0.16–0.80; p = 0.012) without obesity), or under chronic use of aspirin ((OR 0.97; 95% CI: 0.16–5.91; p = 0.974) vs. (OR 0.35; 95% CI: 0.16–0.76; p = 0.008 without aspirin) or nitrates ((OR 0.96; 95% CI: 0.13–6.85; p = 0.968) vs. (OR 0.38; 95% CI: 0.17–0.85; p = 0.018) without nitrates). These data suggest that PIA has no additional beneficial effect in patients who have already been protected by such treatment.

Strikingly, when CK peak, as a reflection of infarct size, was added to the model 1, PIA lost its significant association with VAs (OR 0.54; 95% CI: 0.26–1.11; p = 0.10) (model 2, Table 3), suggesting that PIA may limit the development of VAs at least in part through beneficial effects on infarct size. A similar loss of association was found when troponin peak -instead of CK peak- was introduced in the model.

Patients with PIA were more aggressively treated (PCI, CABG, aspirin, statin or ACE inhibitors) that could potentially reduce the incidence of VAs (Table 1). However, logistic regression analysis failed to show any association between these treatments and the incidence of VAs, further suggesting that the beneficial effect of PIA was independent of such treatments (p = 0.955, p = 0.914, p = 0.757, p = 0.967 and p = 0.871 respectively).

Discussion

To the best of our knowledge, this is the first large prospective study to report that pre-infarction angina in patients admitted for a first NSTEMI 1) is very common, occurring in almost 1 in 2 patients, 2) exerts a beneficial effect on short-term outcomes, especially on VAs and is associated with a smaller infarct size. 3) This beneficial effect is less pronounced in patients with CV risk factors such as hypertension or obesity, or under chronic use of CV drugs such as aspirin or nitrates.

Only small sample size study had analysed the impact of PIA in NSTEMI, suggesting decreased in hospital complications. [16] The high rate of PIA observed in our study (>40%) is consistent with the rate reported in STEMI. [6,17] In a recent meta-analysis, PIA was observed in 35% of patients presenting a STEMI. [18] A higher rate of PIA in NSTEMI (vs. STEMI) has also been found in previous studies reporting that patients experiencing PIA were more likely to experience NSTEMI than STEMI. [19,20]. In clinical situations, there is a wide heterogeneity of the timing onset

of PIA before the acute MI, ranging from the first 24 hours to 2 months [1,2]. In agreement with previous works [5,21], our data strongly support a beneficial and protective role of PIA, when experienced within 7 days before the index event. Patients with PIA had similar risk profile than patients without PIA. However, they were more frequently obese, hypertensive and with family history of CAD, consistent with coronary angiographic findings showing a trend for more CAD extent in such group.

Angina occurring before a first STEMI has been suggested to confer multiple cardioprotective effects. TIMI-4 trial showed a significant decrease in hospital death (3 vs. 8%), severe congestive heart failure or shock (1 vs. 7%), and CK peak determining infarct size (119 vs. 154 IU/L) associated with PIA. [22,23] TIMI-9 trial further reported that patients with angina onset within 24 hours of infarction had a lower 30-day cardiac event rate (including death, recurrent MI, heart failure, or shock) than those with onset of angina >24 hours (4% vs 17%) [1]. In-hospital VAs are rather uncommon but major life-threatening complication in acute MI [24,25,26], in particular in NSTEMI [15]. However, only few trials have assessed the impact of PIA on such arrhythmias, limited to out-of-hospital arrhythmias [7] or reperfusion arrhythmias [25]. In our work, PIA was associated with a decreased infarct size -by 28%, as measured by CK peak-, consistent with previous findings [1,4,23]. Our work also showed that conditioning the heart can confer additional benefit over current medical practice procedures. Moreover, our results from multivariate models showing a loss of prognostic capacity of PIA when CK was added to the model, interestingly suggest that PIA may have contributed to the decreased incidence of VAs, via a lower infarct size. However, the underlying mechanisms of the beneficial effects of PIA are not yet clarified.

The PIA-induced development of coronary collateral circulation from the non-ischemic areas has been suggested. Some authors also proposed that increases in pressure due to a subtotal occlusion during short episodes of angina could play an important role by opening and developing coronary collateral vessels, especially in diabetic patients [27]. However, in contrast to experimental studies, the involvement of coronary collateral circulation in the cardioprotective effect of PIA in humans remains controversial. In patients undergoing PCI, an antiarrhythmic effect of preconditioning can occur independently of collateral recruitment [28] Moreover, the protective role of PIA has been observed even in the absence of significant collateral circulation [2,29]. In NSTEMI patients, where coronary arteries are not totally occluded, the involvement of such pathophysiological mechanism in the beneficial effects of PIA may be only modest.

Another potential cardioprotective mechanism relates to experimental ischemic preconditioning. Preconditioning the myocardium during brief episodes of ischemia, before a sustained occlusion, stimulates adenosine receptors, decreases the cellular influx of calcium, leading to a decrease in myocardial energy demands and limiting the extent of myocardial injury. [30] Transient mitochondrial permeability transition pore (mPTP) opening mediates preconditioning-induced protection, via a K+ ATP-dependent channel [31–33]. Experimental preconditioning has been shown to typically reduce infarct size and decrease in ischemia-reperfusion arrhythmias in most animal models. [34–36] Ischemic preconditioning could also induce antiarrhythmic protection in humans [37–41].

Finally, chronic treatment with CV drugs such as aspirin or nitrates, taken before the acute MI, may improve outcomes in patients experiencing PIA. The cardioprotective effect of such chronic preadmission treatments has been indirectly suggested, in a recent retrospective work showing that patients under chronic CV treatments (i.e. aspirin, β-blockers, ACE inhibitors, or statins) before hospital admission were less likely to develop STEMI than NSTEMI. [19] Interestingly, the risk proportionally decreased with the increasing number of medications used before acute MI, underlining the benefit of preventive medication in high-risk patients. Moreover, in the GRACE Study, a history of angina was more common among patients with NSTEMI than among those with STEMI, further lending support for the hypothesis that prior treatment may also modify the disease process and clinical presentation [20]. Nitroglycerin conferred cardioprotection against ischemia through a protein kinase C-dependent pathway [42,43]. Recently, in a large multinational, unselected population over 50.000 MI patients, chronic nitrate use pre-infarction was associated with significantly lower levels of cardiac markers of necrosis, further suggesting a smaller extent of myocardial necrosis

[44]. Hence, in our study, such treatments may have participated at least in part to the beneficial effect associated with PIA.

Our findings on the attenuation of the cardioprotective effect associated with PIA in some subgroups, such as obese or hypertensive patients is consistent with previous works [45,46]. The persistence of myocardial preconditioning in older patients is controversial [10,47]. Our data interestingly suggest that beneficial effects of PIA could be maintained in the older (>65 y) NSTEMI patients.

Conclusion

Our study providing for the first time evidence a beneficial effect associated with PIA in patients presenting a NSTEMI, extent the findings from small proofs-of-concept studies in STEMI patients to all types of MI, on the potential clinical benefit of conditioning the myocardium. Recent randomized trials showed that promising therapeutic intervention i.e. remote ischemic conditioning could exert cardioprotective effect independently of occluded vessels, and suggest mechanisms underlying such benefit at the cellular levels, beyond restoration of perfusion [48]. Accordingly, protecting the myocardium by ischemic or pharmacological conditioning not only in STEMI, but in all type of MI merits further attention.

Acknowledgments

We wish to thank Anne Cécile Lagrost, Florence Bichat and Juliane Berchoud for research assistance and Philip Bastable for English assistance.

Author Contributions

Conceived and designed the experiments: LL MZ YC. Performed the experiments: AG CR LM PB LJ-M J-CB CT PB. Analyzed the data: MZ AG LL. Contributed reagents/materials/analysis tools: MZ DB. Wrote the paper: MZ AG CR LR.

References

1. Kloner RA, Shook T, Antman EM, Cannon CP, Przyklenk K, et al. (1998) Prospective temporal analysis of the onset of preinfarction angina versus outcome: an ancillary study in TIMI-9B. Circulation 97:1042–1045.
2. Noda T, Minatoguchi S, Fujii K, Hori M, Ito T, et al. (1999) Evidence for the delayed effect in human ischemic preconditioning: prospective multicenter study for preconditioning in acute myocardial infarction. J Am Coll Cardiol 34:1966–1974.
3. Colonna P, Cadeddu C, Montisci R, Ruscazio M, Selem AH, et al. (2002) Reduced microvascular and myocardial damage in patients with acute myocardial infarction and preinfarction angina. Am Heart J 144:796–803.
4. Andreotti F, Pasceri V, Hackett DR, Davies GJ, Haider AW, et al. (1996) Preinfarction angina as a predictor of more rapid coronary thrombolysis in patients with acute myocardial infarction. N Engl J Med 334:7–312.
5. Takahashi T, Anzai T, Yoshikawa T, Maekawa Y, Asakura Y, et al. (2002) Effect of preinfarction angina pectoris on ST-segment resolution after primary coronary angioplasty for acute myocardial infarction. Am J Cardiol 90:465–469.
6. Bahr RD, Leino EV, Christenson RH (2000) Prodromal unstable angina in acute myocardial infarction: prognostic value of short- and long-term outcome and predictor of infarct size. Am Heart J 140:126–133.
7. Gheeraert PJ, Henriques JP, De Buyzere ML, De Pauw M, Taeymans Y, et al. (2001) Preinfarction angina protects against out-of-hospital ventricular fibrillation in patients with acute occlusion of the left coronary artery. J Am Coll Cardiol 38:1369–1374.
8. Brieger D, Fox KA, Fitzgerald G, Eagle KA, Budaj A, et al. (2009) Predicting freedom from clinical events in non-ST-elevation acute coronary syndromes: the Global Registry of Acute Coronary Events. Heart 95:888–894.
9. Cambou JP, Simon T, Mulak G, Bataille V, Danchin N (2007) The French registry of Acute ST elevation or non-ST-elevation Myocardial Infarction (FAST-MI): study design and baseline characteristics. Arch Mal Coeur Vaiss 100:524–534.
10. Abete P, Ferrara N, Cacciatore F, Madrid A, Bianco S, et al. (1997) Angina-induced protection against myocardial infarction in adult and elderly patients: a loss of preconditioning mechanism in the aging heart? J Am Coll Cardiol 30:947–954.
11. Ishihara M, Inoue I, Kawagoe T, Shimatani Y, Kurisu S, et al. (2001) Diabetes mellitus prevents ischemic preconditioning in patients with a first acute anterior wall myocardial infarction. J Am Coll Cardiol 38:1007–1011.
12. Zeller M, Steg PG, Ravisy J, Laurent Y, Janin-Manificat L, et al. (2005) Prevalence and impact of metabolic syndrome on hospital outcomes in acute myocardial infarction. Arch Intern Med 165:1192–1198.
13. Alpert JS, Thygesen K, Antman E, Bassand JP (2000) Myocardial infarction redefined-a consensus document of The Joint European Society of Cardiology/ American College of Cardiology Committee for the redefinition of myocardial infarction. J Am Coll Cardiol 36:959–969.
14. Fox KA, Dabbous OH, Goldberg RJ, Pieper KS, Eagle KA, et al. (2006) Prediction of risk of death and myocardial infarction in the six months after presentation with acute coronary syndrome: prospective multinational observational study (GRACE). BMJ 333:1091.
15. Avezum A, Piegas LS, Goldberg RJ, Brieger D, Stiles MK, et al. (2008) Magnitude and prognosis associated with ventricular arrhythmias in patients hospitalized with acute coronary syndromes (from the GRACE Registry). Am J Cardiol 102:1577–1582.
16. Papadopoulos CE, Karvounis HI, Gourasas IT, Parharidis GE, Louridas GE (2003) Evidence of ischemic preconditioning in patients experiencing first non-ST-segment elevation myocardial infarction (NSTEMI). Int J Cardiol 92:209–217.
17. Braunwald E (1996) Acute myocardial infarction the value of being prepared. N Engl J Med 334:51–52.
18. Iglesias-Garriz I, Coloma CG, Fernandez FC, Gomez CO (2005) In-hospital mortality and early preinfarction angina: a meta-analysis of published studies. Rev Esp Cardiol 58:484–490.
19. Bjorck L, Wallentin L, Stenestrand U, Lappas G, Rosengren A (2010) Medication in relation to ST-segment elevation myocardial infarction in patients with a first myocardial infarction: Swedish Register of Information and Knowledge About Swedish Heart Intensive Care Admissions (RIKS-HIA). Arch Intern Med 170:1375–1381.
20. Spencer FA, Santopinto JJ, Gore JM, Goldberg RJ, Fox KA, et al. (2002) Impact of aspirin on presentation and hospital outcomes in patients with acute coronary syndromes (The Global Registry of Acute Coronary Events [GRACE]). Am J Cardiol 90:1056–1061.
21. Jimenez-Navarro M, Jose Gomez-Doblas J, Gomez G, Garcia Alcantara A, Hernandez Garcia JM, et al. (2001) The influence of angina the week before a first myocardial infarction on short and medium-term prognosis. Rev Esp Cardiol 54:1161–1166.

22. Jimenez-Navarro M, Gomez-Doblas JJ, Alonso-Briales J, Hernandez Garcia JM, Gomez G, et al. (2001) Does angina the week before protect against first myocardial infarction in elderly patients? Am J Cardiol 87:11–15.
23. Kloner RA, Shook T, Przyklenk K, Davis VG, Junio L, et al. (1995) Previous angina alters in-hospital outcome in TIMI 4. A clinical correlate to preconditioning? Circulation; 91:37–45.
24. Itoh T, Fukami K, Suzuki T, Aoki H, Ohira K, et al. (2006) Effect of pre-myocardial infarction angina pectoris on post-myocardial infarction arrhythmias after reperfusion therapy. Am J Cardiol; 97:1157–1161.
25. Newby KH, Thompson T, Stebbins A, Topol EJ, Califf RM, et al. (1998) Sustained ventricular arrhythmias in patients receiving thrombolytic therapy: incidence and outcomes. The GUSTO Investigators. Circulation 98:2567–2573.
26. Al-Khatib SM, Granger CB, Huang Y, Lee KL, Califf RM, et al. (2002) Sustained ventricular arrhythmias among patients with acute coronary syndromes with no ST-segment elevation: incidence, predictors, and outcomes. Circulation 106:309–312.
27. Ishihara M, Inoue I, Kawagoe T, Shimatani Y, Kurisu S, et al. (2005) Comparison of the cardioprotective effect of prodromal angina pectoris and collateral circulation in patients with a first anterior wall acute myocardial infarction. Am J Cardiol 95:622–625.
28. Edwards RJ, Redwood SR, Lambiase PD, Tomset E, Rakhit RD, et al. (2002) Antiarrhythmic and anti-ischaemic effects of angina in patients with and without coronary collaterals. Heart 88:604–610.
29. Tomoda H, Aoki N (1999) Comparison of protective effects of preinfarction angina pectoris in acute myocardial infarction treated by thrombolysis versus by primary coronary angioplasty with stenting. Am J Cardiol;84: 621–625.
30. Liu GS, Thornton J, Van Winkle DM, Stanley AW, Olsson RA, et al. (1991) Protection against infarction afforded by preconditioning is mediated by A1 adenosine receptors in rabbit heart. Circulation 84:350–356.
31. Hausenloy D, Wynne A, Duchen M, Yellon D (2004) Transient mitochondrial permeability transition pore opening mediates preconditioning-induced protection. Circulation 109:1714–1717.
32. Murry CE, Jennings RB, Reimer KA (1986) Preconditioning with ischemia: a delay of lethal cell injury in ischemic myocardium. Circulation 74:1124–1136.
33. Yellon DM, Baxter GF (1995) A « second window of protection » or delayed preconditioning phenomenon: future horizons for myocardial protection? J Mol Cell Cardiol 27:1023–1034.
34. Wu ZK, Iivainen T, Pehkonen E, Laurikka J, Tarkka MR (2002) Ischemic preconditioning suppresses ventricular tachyarrhythmias after myocardial revascularization. Circulation 106:3091–3096.
35. Vegh A, Komori S, Szekeres L, Parratt JR (1992) Antiarrhythmic effects of preconditioning in anaesthetised dogs and rats. Cardiovasc Res 26:487–495.
36. Kloner RA, Bolli R, Marban E, Reinlib L, Braunwald E (1998) Medical and cellular implications of stunning, hibernation, and preconditioning: an NHLBI workshop. Circulation 97:1848–1867.
37. Ovize M, Aupetit JF, Rioufol G, Loufoua J, Andre-Fouet X, et al. (1995) Preconditioning reduces infarct size but accelerates time to ventricular fibrillation in ischemic pig heart. Am J Physiol 269:72–79.
38. Airaksinen KE, Huikuri HV (1997) Antiarrhythmic effect of repeated coronary occlusion during balloon angioplasty. J Am Coll Cardiol 29:1035–1038.
39. Pasceri V, Lanza GA, Patti G, Pedrotti P, Crea F, et al. (1996) Preconditioning by transient myocardial ischemia confers protection against ischemia-induced ventricular arrhythmias in variant angina. Circulation 94:1850–1856.
40. Okishige K, Yamashita K, Yoshinaga H, Azegami K, Satoh T, et al. (1996) Electrophysiologic effects of ischemic preconditioning on QT dispersion during coronary angioplasty. J Am Coll Cardiol 28:70–73.
41. Pomerantz BJ, Joo K, Shames BD, Cleveland JC, Banerjee A, et al. (2000) Adenosine preconditioning reduces both pre and postischemic arrhythmias in human myocardium. J Surg Res 90:191–196.
42. Banerjee S, Tang XL, Qiu Y, Takano H, Manchikalapudi S, et al. (1999) Nitroglycerin induces late preconditioning against myocardial stunning via a PKC-dependent pathway. Am J Physiol 277:2488–2494.
43. Leesar MA, Stoddard MF, Dawn B, Jasti VG, Masden R, et al. (2001) Delayed preconditioning-mimetic action of nitroglycerin in patients undergoing coronary angioplasty. Circulation 103:2935–2941.
44. Ambrosio G, Del Pinto M, Tritto I, Agnelli G, Bentivoglio M, et al. (2010) Chronic nitrate therapy is associated with different presentation and evolution of acute coronary syndromes: insights from 52,693 patients in the Global Registry of Acute Coronary Events. Eur Heart J 31:430–438.
45. Takeuchi T, Ishii Y, Kikuchi K, Hasebe N (2011) Ischemic preconditioning effect of prodromal angina is attenuated in acute myocardial infarction patients with hypertensive left ventricular hypertrophy. Circ J 75:1192–1199.
46. Abete P, Cacciatore F, Ferrara N, Calabrese C, de Santis D, et al. (2003) Body mass index and preinfarction angina in elderly patients with acute myocardial infarction. Am J Clin Nutr 78:796–801.
47. Kloner RA, Przyklenk K, Shook T, Cannon CP(1998) Protection Conferred by Preinfarct Angina is Manifest in the Aged Heart: Evidence from the TIMI 4 Trial. J Thromb Thrombolysis 6:89–92.
48. Botker HE, Kharbanda R, Schmidt MR, Bøttcher M, Kaltoft AK, et al. (2010) Remote ischaemic conditioning before hospital admission, as a complement to angioplasty, and effect on myocardial salvage in patients with acute myocardial infarction: a randomised trial. Lancet 375:727–734.

10

Impact of Gender, Co-Morbidity and Social Factors on Labour Market Affiliation after First Admission for Acute Coronary Syndrome. A Cohort Study of Danish Patients 2001–2009

Merete Osler[1,3]*, **Solvej Mårtensson**[1], **Eva Prescott**[2], **Kathrine Carlsen**[1]

1 Research Center for Prevention and Health, Glostrup Hospital, Glostrup, Denmark, **2** Department of Cardiology Y, Bispebjerg Hospital, Copenhagen, Denmark, **3** Institute of Public Health, University of Copenhagen, Copenhagen, Denmark

Abstract

Background: Over the last decades survival after acute coronary syndrome (ACS) has improved, leading to an increasing number of patients returning to work, but little is known about factors that may influence their labour market affiliation. This study examines the impact of gender, co-morbidity and socio-economic position on subsequent labour market affiliation and transition between various social services in patients admitted for the first time with ACS.

Methods: From 2001 to 2009 all first-time hospitalisations for ACS were identified in the Danish National Patient Registry (n = 79,714). For this population, data on sick leave, unemployment and retirement were obtained from an administrative register covering all citizens. The 21,926 patients, aged 18–63 years, who had survived 30 days and were part of the workforce at the time of diagnosis were included in the analyses where subsequent transition between the above labour market states was examined using Kaplan-Meier estimates and Cox proportional hazards models.

Findings: A total of 37% of patients were in work 30 days after first ACS diagnosis, while 55% were on sick leave and 8% were unemployed. Seventy-nine per cent returned to work once during follow-up. This probability was highest among males, those below 50 years, living with a partner, the highest educated, with higher occupations, having specific events (NSTEMI, and percutaneous coronary intervention) and with no co-morbidity. During five years follow-up, 43% retired due to disability or voluntary early pension. Female gender, low education, basic occupation, co-morbidity and having a severer event (invasive procedures) and receiving sickness benefits or being unemployed 30 days after admission were associated with increased probability of early retirement.

Conclusion: About half of patients with first-time ACS stay in or return to work shortly after the event. Women, the socially disadvantaged, those with presumed severer events and co-morbidity have lower rates of return.

Editor: Hamid Reza Baradaran, Iran University of Medical Sciences, Iran (Islamic Republic of)

Funding: The study was funded by the Danish Heart Association (jr nr. 1104-R83-A3441-22623). The funders had no role in study design, data collection and analysis, decision to publish, or preparation of the manuscript.

Competing Interests: The authors have declared that no competing interests exist.

* E-mail: merete.osler@regionh.dk

Introduction

Coronary heart diseases are among the leading causes of morbidity in Western societies. However, during recent years the prognosis has improved considerably, possibly due to the introduction of new invasive and medical treatments [1]. This has led to an increasing number of survivors returning to work after treatment. Established treatments such as percutaneous coronary interventions (PCI) and coronary artery bypass grafting (CABG) as well as patient factors such as gender, age, socio-economic position (SEP) and co-morbidity have been associated with the prognosis of acute coronary syndrome (ACS) [1,2]. These factors also seem to influence the patient's transition from being a patient to returning to normality as maintaining an affiliation to the labour market.

Thus, two reviews have reported that 50–85% of patients in work with myocardial infarction maintain labour market affiliation but this proportion seems to depend on the size of the infarction, and the patient's age and education [3,4]. Similar associations have been found for patients who have had a CABG [3–7] or PCI [7]. These studies have in most cases included small, selected patient groups and incomplete follow-up, particularly because outcome data in many studies were collected by questionnaire. In addition, few had examined the influence of gender and co-morbidity on labour market affiliation after ACS or coronary revascularisation.

One recent study, based on all 63,876 patients aged 30–63 years, who underwent a first CABG or PCI in Sweden between 1994 and 2006, examined sick leave after invasive treatments. This study showed that sick leave following coronary revascularisation was common, especially among women, and was also associated with SEP and co-morbidity [7]. In another population-based study from Finland, return to work was examined by the linkage of the Finnish cardiovascular register with a register for social security benefits for 5,074 patients aged 35–59 who had survived their first myocardial infarction (MI) between 1991 and 1996. This study showed that 58% of men and 56% of women were retained in work two years after their MI, but the authors did not examine whether any other patient or health factors influenced the probability of return to work [8].

Return to work after hospitalisation is in general dependent on gender, concomitant diseases, in particular diabetes, and socio-economic factors. A strong predictor for returning to work after hospitalisation is the occupational status at time of diagnosis. Aside from the recent study from Sweden [7], in the majority of studies conducted so far return to work after ACS, CABG or PCI is only considered for those persons who are in work at the time of diagnosis and thus represents a selected (and probably more healthy) part of the population included in the labour force. Further, in the majority of studies, the outcome has been dichotomised to working/not working. This is, however, a simplification of the occupational consequences of ACS, as in most welfare states not working can be split into different more or less voluntary schemes. Thus, knowledge is lacking on the impact of gender, co-morbidities and SEP on subsequent labour market affiliation and transition between various social services after discharge from hospital in an unselected group of patients surviving their first ACS event.

The aim of this study was therefore to examine the impact of patient's gender, co-morbidity and SEP on subsequent labour market affiliation (in work, unemployed, sick leave and disability or voluntary early retirement) in a cohort of all-Danish patients of working age who had been admitted for the first time for ACS and survived for 30 days thereafter.

Materials and Methods

Ethics statement

The study was based on linking information from four Danish population-based registers: The National Patient Register (NPR), The Danish Prescription Register (DPR), the Integrated Database for Labour Market Research (IDA) and the Register-based Evaluation of Marginalisation (DREAM) [9–11]. The study has been evaluated and approved by the Danish Data Protection Agency [9].

Study population

The study population was derived from the NPR, which provides full histories of diseases leading to hospital admission and outpatient visits since 1979 and 1995, respectively [9]. This information includes dates of admission and discharge and diagnoses coded according to ICD-10 [9]. For this study, all first-time hospitalisations of ACS from the 1 January 2001 to 31 December 2009 were identified (n = 79,714) by the following specific ICD10 codes: I20.0 Unstable angina pectoris; I21.0–I21.3 ST-elevation myocardial infarction (STEMI); 121.4 NSTEMI and I21.9 AMI – Unspecified. ACS diagnoses in the NPR have acceptable coverage and validity, except for unstable angina pectoris [12]. Consequently, this discharge diagnosis should be used with caution. As the outcome under study is labour market participation after ACS, subjects outside the working age of 18–64 years (n = 49,072) and subjects retired due to disability or voluntary early pension before diagnosis (n = 7,706) were excluded from the study. As the majority of fatal events and post-operative

complications occur within the first 30 days after diagnosis, we excluded subjects who died within the first 30 days after diagnosis (n = 1,010). This leads to a study population of 21,926 persons, aged 18–64 years, who were part of the workforce at the time of diagnosis and had survived 30 days after diagnosis.

Outcome variables

The Danish labour market is characterised by a system with a high degree of economic compensation in the case of unemployment or reduced work ability, but also with a high turnover rate. Unemployed persons are warranted economic compensation if they are actively seeking work. During the study period, it was possible to receive a maximum of four years of unemployment benefit. At the end of these four years, or if a person was not qualified for unemployment benefit (i.e. not a member of a union) it was possible to receive social income. If a person was unable to work due to illness or disability, it was possible to receive sickness benefit for a maximum of 52 weeks during a period of two years or to apply for early retirement if the work ability was reduced to a level where it was not possible to hold down a job. This applies to all Danish citizens, independent of job type and insurance status. During the study period the retirement age was 64 years of age.

Transfer payments were obtained from DREAM, covering all citizens in Denmark who have received transfer payments from the state in any given episode since week 32 in 1991 [11]. The register was updated weekly until week 13 in 2011, providing between 65 and up to 568 weeks of follow-up. In this study, 'in work' was defined as not receiving any transfer payments. Transfer income was divided into sickness benefit, unemployment benefit (including social income) and permanent withdrawal from the workforce due to disablement or voluntary early retirement between the age of 60 and 64.

The main outcomes of the study were: 1. permanent withdrawal from the workforce before the age of 64 and thus receiving disability or voluntary early pension; 2. return to work among those who received sickness benefits or were unemployed 30 days after admission for ACS.

Other co-variables

The following explanatory co-morbidity variables were obtained. From the NPR we acquired information on the specific ICD-10 ACS diagnosis as well as date and type of any invasive procedures, coronary angiography (CAG), percutaneous coronary interventions (PCI) and CABG. These variables were used as proxy measures for the severity of the cardiac event. Further information on co-morbidity five years preceding the year of diagnosis was drawn from NPR and DPR. The following diseases were included, compiled and dichotomised to yes/no: chronic obstructive pulmonary disease (COPD), asthma, cancer, diabetes and liver-, kidney-, connective-tissue or psychiatric diseases. The total number of co-morbidities was counted and grouped as 0; 1 to 2, and 3 or more.

Information on SEP was obtained from the IDA, which has been administrated by Statistics Denmark since 1980. The core variables in the database are derived once a year by linkage with Danish administrative registers [10]. Education was computed as the highest level of education registered in IDA and grouped in three categories: basic education (7–9 grade of obligatory schooling); medium education (high-school degree or vocational); higher education (more than high-school degree). Occupation was represented by a variable which specifies the character of employment during the year before diagnosis. The variable was categorised in three job types: at high level (in jobs requiring higher skills, including managers and self-employed with one or

Table 1. Percentage in work, on sick leave and unemployed among patients, aged 18–64 years, admitted first time with acute coronary syndrome, who were part of the workforce at time of diagnosis and survived 30 days thereafter, in relation to gender, co-morbidity and socio-economic factors.

	In work	On sick leave	Unemployed	Chi-square test:p-value*
All (n = 21,926)	37.2	54.9	8.0	
Gender				
Men (n = 16739)	37.0	55.8	7.3	
Women (n = 5187)	38.0	51.7	10.2	p<0.01
Age				
18–29 (n = 344)	54.8	24.1	21.1	
30–39 (n = 2094)	42.9	42.2	14.9	p<0.01
40–49 (n = 6551)	36.3	53.7	10.0	p<0.01
50–59 (n = 11,010)	34.7	59.7	5.8	p<0.01
60–63 (n = 1927)	44.4	51.9	3.7	p<0.01
Cohabitation				
Living with a partner (n = 14,744)	38.1	56.4	5.5	
Single (n = 7011)	34.2	52.6	13.2	p<0.01
Education				
Basic (n = 6392)	30.4	57.9	11.8	
Medium (n = 10,071)	36.0	57.8	6.2	p<0.01
Higher (n = 4734)	47.5	47.5	5.0	p<0.01
Occupation				
Other (n = 2882)	28.6	27.8	43.4	
Wage earners at basic level (n = 12,927)	34.2	62.7	3.1	p<0.01
Wage earners at high level (n = 5997)	46.7	52.3	1.3	p<0.01
ACS diagnosis				
Unstable angina (n = 5475)	55.1	34.4	10.5	
AMI-STEMI (n = 5773)	27.1	65.8	7.1	p<0.01
NSTEMI (n = 4136)	30.5	63.2	6.3	p<0.01
AMI unspecified (n = 6542)	35.3	57.0	7.7	p<0.01
Year of diagnosis				
2001–2003 (n = 7738)	36.3	55.4	8.3	
2004–2006 (n = 7472)	36.0	55.2	8.8	p<0.01
2007–2009 (n = 6716)	39.5	53.2	6.6	p<0.01
Procedures 30 days after admission				
No invasive procedure (n = 5913)	54.0	34.4	11.7	
CAG, only (n = 8777)	33.0	60.0	7.0	p<0.01
PCI (n = 6257)	30.0	63.6	6.2	p<0.01
CABG (n = 802)	12.1	83.3	4.7	p<0.01
Number of co-morbidities				
None (n = 16969)	38.5	54.8	6.8	
1–2 (n = 4256)	31.5	56.4	12.2	p<0.01
3 and more (n = 701)	31.4	51.1	17.5	p<0.01
Work status at time of diagnosis				
In work (n = 11,150)	61.0	38.1	1.0	
Sick leave (n = 8231)	10.0	89.2	0.7	p<0.01
Unemployed (n = 2066)	3.9	21.3	75.8	p<0.01

*Marked category versus first variable category.

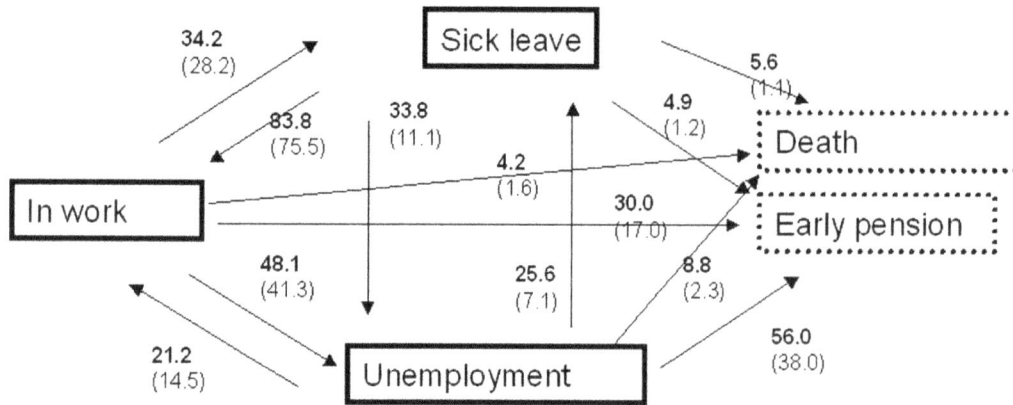

Figure 1. Patients with acute coronary syndrome's transition between various social services. Work, sick leave and unemployment cover persons in the workforce (3 left boxes with bold lines) at baseline for those aged 18–64 years. The lower box with dotted lines refers to early retirement independent of reason (disability or voluntary), which is an irreversible state, where persons are considered to leave the workforce forever (main outcome). Percentages in bold refer to how many patients ever experience the event during follow-up, while percentages in brackets refer to how many experience the transition as the first event after baseline.

more employees), wage earners at basic level (in jobs requiring basic skills) and other (consisting of unemployed, under education or unspecified). Cohabitation status was categorised as single or living with a partner.

Statistical analyses

We used Kaplan-Meier estimation and Cox proportional hazard regression analyses to estimate rate and rate ratios for the two main outcomes early retirement or return to work. Because age is a very strong predictor for the outcomes under study we used age as the underlying time variable. Person-years of follow-up were accumulated from age at 30 days after diagnosis and follow-up was terminated at the age of the event (retirement/ return to work), death or censoring (age 64 or the end of follow-up – the last week of March 2011), whichever came first. We conducted multivariable analyses to evaluate the mutually adjusted effects of each of the covariables (gender, cohabitation status, education, occupation, ACS diagnosis, year of diagnosis, invasive treatment, co-morbidity and work status) on outcomes [13]. We also repeated the analyses in strata for each gender and sub-diagnosis, which did not indicate any specific interactions. Using

Schoenfeld residuals and visual inspection of survival curves, we determined that estimated hazard ratios were constant over the follow-up time. All statistical analyses were carried out in STATA version 12.

Results

Baseline labour market affiliation and transitions

Of the 21,926 included patients, a total of 37% were in work 30 days after first-time admission with an ACS diagnosis, while 55% were on sick leave and 8% were unemployed (Table 1). Table 1 also shows that the probability of being in work was highest among male patients and those who were young, highest educated, living with a partner, had the most uncertain and possibly least severe events (diagnosed with unstable angina, had received no invasive treatment), were diagnosed 2007–2009, had no co-morbidities and were in work before diagnosis.

As persons can change between the different states (in work, sick leave and unemployment) many times during follow-up, all the transitions between the different states are shown in Figure 1. Of those who were working during follow-up, 34% experienced one

Table 2. Workforce participation 30 days, 1 year, 2 years and 5 years after acute coronary syndrome (ACS) in Denmark 2001–2009 among patients, aged 18–64 years, admitted first time with ACS, who were part of the workforce at time of diagnosis and survived 30 days thereafter (n = 21,926).

	30 days after time of diagnosis N (%)	1 year after diagnosis N (%)	2 years after diagnosis N (%)*	5 years after diagnosis N (%)*
Part of the workforce	21926 (100)	21869 (99.7)	19664 (98.4)	15468 (88.0)
In work	8150 (37.2)	8777 (40.1)	8856 (45.0)	10.079 (65.2)
Unemployed	1743 (8.0)	1850 (8.5)	1936 (9.9)	2878 (18.6)
Sick leave	12033 (54.9)	11220 (51.4)	8852 (45.0)	2511 (16.2)
Not part of the workforce	0	35 (0.2)	249 (1.3)	1824 (10.4)
Disability or voluntary early pension	0 (0)	30 (85.7)	231 (92.8)	1751 (96.0)
Old-age pension	0 (0)	5 (14.3)	18 (7.2)	72 (4.0)
Dead	0 (0)	22 (0.1)	66 (0.3)	278 (1.6)

*Does not sum to total due to end of follow-up (n = 1947 after 2 years and n = 4356 after 5 years).

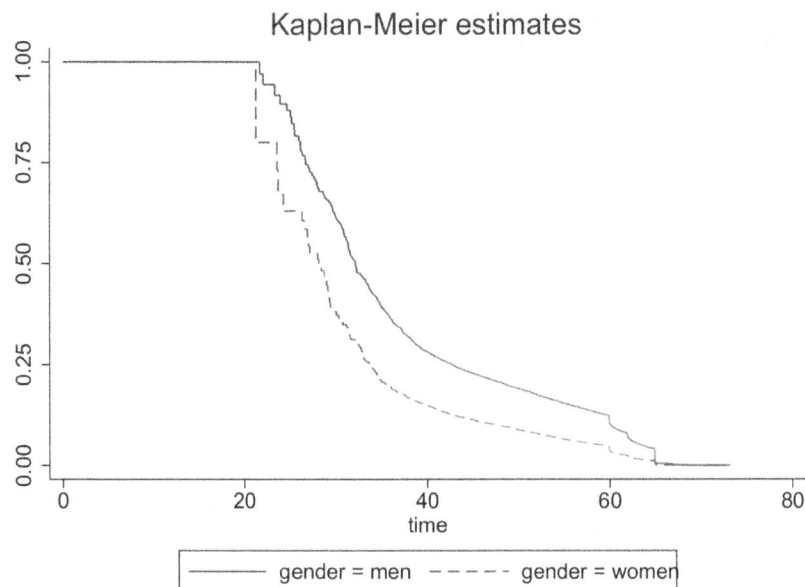

Figure 2. Kaplan-Meier estimates for early retirement after acute coronary syndrome by gender.

or more periods on sick leave and 30% were allocated to disability or voluntary early pension after one or more periods of sick leave and/or unemployment. The proportion in work increased, while the proportion on sick leave decreased during follow-up. Further, the proportion that was still a part of the workforce decreased. Thus, five years after ACS, 88% were still a part of the workforce. Among these, 65% were in work, 19% were unemployed and 16% were on sick leave (Table 2). The majority of patients who had left the labour force were under the age of 64 years and therefore receiving disability or voluntary early pension.

Determinants of early retirement

During follow-up a total of 43% withdrew permanently from the workforce. The mean number of years from 30 days after diagnosis to retirement, death or censoring was 4.1 years (median 3.7 years; range 0.0–10.2). Figure 2 shows the Kaplan-Meier estimates for men and women.

The probability of retirement due to disability or voluntary early pension was highest among women, patients above 50 years of age, those lowest educated, in basic or other jobs, living with a partner, who were on sick leave or unemployed 30 days after admission, who were diagnosed 2007–2009, had received CABG, and with co-morbidity (Table 3, first data column). The most prevalent co-morbidities were psychiatric disease (7.7%), diabetes (6.0%) and COPD (5.9%) and they were all associated with increased probability of early retirement – Hazard Ratio (HR) = 1.72(1.61–1.84), HR = 1.30(1.20–1.70) and 1.25(1.15–1.35), respectively (data not shown).

When age at retirement was taken into account female gender, living single, low education, basic occupation, receiving sickness benefits or being unemployed 30 days after admission, co-morbidity, ACS-diagnosed 2007–2009, unspecific and greater severity of events (being diagnosed with STEMI, NSTEMI and unspecified AMI and receiving invasive treatment) were associated with increased rates of early retirement (Table 3, second data column). When all factors were mutually adjusted, the estimates for cohabitation status, the ACS sub-diagnosis, and treatment attenuated and became insignificant.

Determinants of return to work

Among the 13,776 patients who were unemployed or on sick leave 30 days after the index event, 79% returned to work at least once during follow-up. Mean years of follow-up was 1.3 (median 0.3 years; range 0.0–10.0). Figure 3 provides the Kaplan-Meier estimates for men and women. The probability of returning to work was highest among male patients, below 50 years of age, those living with a partner, highest educated, with higher occupations, being diagnosed 2002–2003, with less severe events (NSTEMI, having PCI), who were on sick leave 30 days after admission, and with no co-morbidity (Table 4). Patients with psychiatric disease, diabetes or COPD were less likely to return to work (HR = 0.39(0.37–0.41); 0.58(0.54–0.62); and 0.62(0.56–0.67), respectively). The same factors were associated with increased rates of return to work when age was taken into account (Table 4, second column). However, the HR for year of diagnosis were reversed. Similar was seen after controlling for potential confounders (Table 4, third column). Compared to the group of persons in work 30 days after diagnosis the mean number of years from inclusion to retirement or censoring was much lower (0.9 years) among unemployed or sick-listed ACS patients.

Discussion

This population-based cohort study showed that around 79% of patients of working age with a first time ACS diagnose either continued working or returned to work once during a mean follow-up of 1.3 years

Most patients experienced some shifts between the mutually exclusive states work, sick leave and unemployment before they reached the irreversible state of early retirement. In total 43% patients left the labour market either due to disability or voluntarily. This proportion of patients who retired early seems to be in accordance with the findings in the Finnish register-based study where 40% of patients with MI aged 35–50 were on a disability pension two years after the event, while 62% and 57% were in work after one and two years, respectively [8]. In the present study, of all ACS patients the percentage in work after one and two years was somewhat lower – 40% and 45%, respectively.

Table 3. The percentage and Hazard Ratio (HR) of disability or voluntary early pension after a mean follow-up of 4.1 years among patients, aged 18–64 years, admitted first time with acute coronary syndrome, who were part of the workforce at time of diagnosis and survived 30 days thereafter, in relation to gender, co-morbidity and socio-economic factors.

	% on disability or voluntary early pension	Crude* HR (95% CI)	Mutually adjusted HR (95% CI)
All (n = 21,926)	42.7		
Gender			
Men (n = 16739)	42.3	1	1
Women (n = 5187)	44.1	1.30(1.24–1.37)	1.30(1.24–1.37)
Age			
18–29 (n = 344)	39.2		
30–39 (n = 2094)	25.6		
40–49 (n = 6551)	19.9	*	*
50–59 (n = 11,010)	52.8		
60–63 (n = 1927)	81.5		
Cohabitation			
Living with a partner (n = 14,744)	44.4	1	1
Single (n = 7011)	38.8	1.08(1.04–1.13)	1.00(0.96–1.05)
Education			
Basic (n = 6392)	46.3	1	1
Medium (n = 10,071)	43.1	0.89(0.85–0.93)	0.97(0.96–1.03)
Higher (n = 4734)	37.8	0.68(0.64–0.72)	0.85(0.83–0.91)
Occupation			
Other (n = 2882)	52.5	1.97(1.84–2.10)	1.57(1.43–1.69)
Wage earners at basic level (n = 12,927)	43.6	1.46(1.39–1.54)	1.32(1.24–1.37)
Wage earners at high level (n = 5997)	36.7	1	1
ACS diagnosis			
Unstable angina (n = 5475)	40.2	1	1
AMI-STEMI (n = 5773)	42.8	1.12(1.06–1.20)	1.01(0.95–1.07)
NSTEMI (n = 4136)	42.7	1.10(1.07–1.17)	0.97(0.93–1.04)
AMI unspecified (n = 6542)	44.7	1.08(1.02–1.14)	1.00(0.94–1.04)
Year of diagnosis			
2001–2003 (n = 7738)	57.8	1	1
2004–2006 (n = 7472)	43.7	1.10 (1.05–1.15)	1.07(1.02–1.12)
2007–2009 (n = 6716)	24.1	1.20 (1.13–1.27)	1.18(1.12–1.26)
Procedures 30 days after admission			
No invasive procedure (n = 5913)	44.4	1	1
CAG, only (n = 8777)	40.6	1.14(1.08–1.20)	1.03(0.98–1.11)
PCI (n = 6257)	42.7	1.13(1.07–1.19)	1.05(0.99–1.13)
CABG (n = 802)	60.0	1.29(1.17–1.42)	1.08(0.75–1.20)
Number of co-morbidities			
None (n = 16969)	39.9	1	1
1–2 (n = 4256)	51.3	1.45 (1.38–1.58)	1.35 (1.28–1.42)
3 and more (n = 701)	58.5	1.62 (1.47–1.79)	1.51 (1.37–1.68)
Work status at time of diagnosis			
In work (n = 11,150)	30.4	1	1
Sick leave (n = 8231)	49.1	3.15(2.92–3.40)	1.90(1.81–2.01)
Unemployed (n = 2066)	56.0	1.98(1.89–2.07)	2.94(2.72–3.19)

*age underlying timescale.

Kaplan-Meier estimates

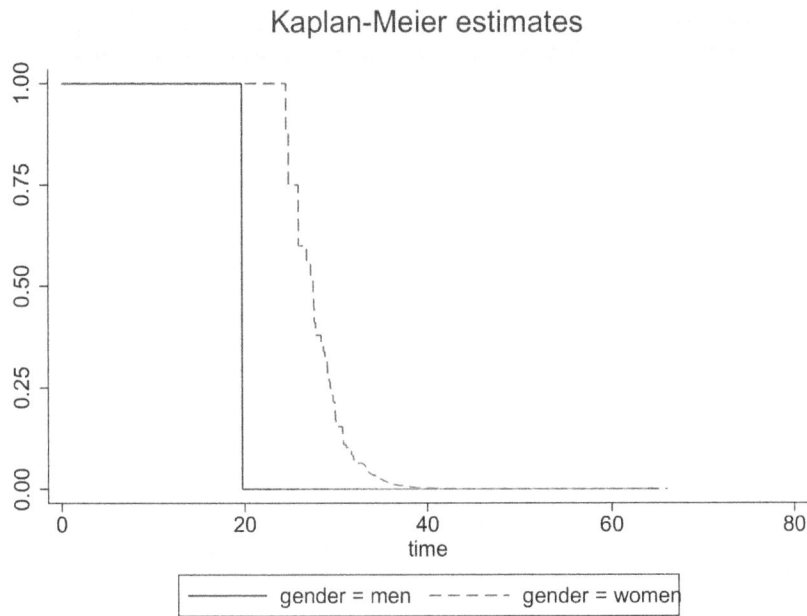

Figure 3. Kaplan-Meier estimates for return to work after acute coronary syndrome by gender.

We also found that the probability of return to work was highest in males, those with high SEP, no co-morbidity, with NSTEMI diagnosis and who had a PCI. Over the last decades, studies have shown that younger women (<70 years) have a poorer prognosis than their male peers [14,15]. Our and the Swedish study on CABG and PCI patients [7] suggest that such a gender difference also applies to women's work affiliation.

Low SEP has predicted lower rates of return to work in most other studies [3–5,7]. This might reflect that high SEP jobs are more flexible with regard to taking changes in work capacity into account and that work ability in low SEP jobs is more affected by ACS than in high SEP jobs. In the present study co-morbidity, in particular major psychiatric diseases (schizophrenia/depression), was prevalent and associated with a lower rate of return to the labour market. The previous studies from Finland and Sweden [5,7] also found that co-morbidity was associated with labour market affiliation, and in both studies this was most evident for diabetes. However, the Finnish study had only included somatic diseases, while the Swedish comprised both somatic and psychiatric co-morbidity.

Fewer have examined the impact of ACS sub-diagnosis and invasive procedures on return to work, since most studies have been restricted to specific diagnosis (mainly MI) or procedures (mainly CABG) [16–18]. In a study from the 1990s Mark et al. found no significant one–year return-to-work rate among 1,252 ACS patients receiving initial percutaneous transluminal coronary angioplasty or CABG versus initial medical therapy [19]. Similarly, in two randomised controlled trials there was no difference in the number of persons returning to work after PCI and CABG [20,21]. Our finding of a more favourable job prognosis for NSTEMI events and PCI-treated patients might reflect that these variables are proxies for the severity of the disease. Further, these patients might get through the event more easily due to more specific treatment regimes.

The number of patients allocated to disability or voluntary early pension differed between the three labour market groups. Those who experienced one or more episodes of unemployment had the highest risk of early retirement pension, while those in work had the lowest. This finding could be caused by the contextual legislation in Denmark where sickness benefit is only assigned for 52 weeks, after which time the person is supposed to return to work or take early retirement pension. The observed increased risk for pension after unemployment could then be caused by the fact that patients with ACS return to work after 52 weeks of sickness benefit and experience that the balance between job demands and perceived work ability is out of adjustment and then have to quit their job. Another explanation lies in the fact that the highest risk factor for unemployment is previous episodes of unemployment, and that unemployed persons in general are known to be less healthy than persons in work, which could point towards an increased risk for early retirement pension among ACS patients who were unemployed before diagnosis.

Strengths and limitations

The primary strength of this study is the large patient population which covers all patients admitted first time with ACS in the period from 2001 to 2009 in Denmark. The patients were identified in the NPR and data from this register is considered to have a high quality for patients with a coronary heart disease diagnosis. Thus, a previous study found a positive predictive value for myocardial infarction in the NPR of around 90% [12,22]. However, the positive predictive value was lower (around 45%) for unstable angina. The information on determinants in the present study is based on data from nationwide registers with high completeness and good validity and missing values are random and not associated with the outcome under study, whereby selection-bias is removed. Variables regarding socio-economic position and affiliation to the labour market are administrative data collected prospectively, why recall bias is eliminated. Our study also has, however, some limitations. First of all we were not able to include more detailed information on work environment, which has been shown to be associated with the possibilities of reductions in work hours and reassignment to other work tasks. We defined return to work as not receiving any transfer payments, which can lead to misclassification of persons leaving

Table 4. The percentage and Hazard Ratio (HR) of return to work among patients, aged 18–64 years, admitted first time with acute coronary syndrome, who were on sick leave or were unemployed 30 days after diagnosis in relation to gender, co-morbidity and socio-economic factors.

	% return to work	Crude HR (95% CI*)	Mutually adjusted HR (95% CI)
All (n = 13776)	79.3		
Gender			
Men (n = 10561)	81.3	1	1
Women (n = 3217)	72.9	0.61(0.60–0.64)	0.66(0.63–0.70)
Age			
18–29 (n = 152)	80.1		
30–39 (n = 1195)	80.3		
40–49 (n = 4170)	81.5	*	*
50–59 (n = 7181)	78.3		
60–63 (n = 1080)	77.1		
Cohabitation		1	1
Living with a partner (n = 9132)	82.3	0.60(0.58–0.63)	0.72(0.70–0.76)
Single (n = 4616)	73.5		
Education			
Basic (n = 4454)	74.6	1	
Medium (n = 6442)	81.0	1.40(1.35–1.47)	1.13(1.08–1.13)
Higher (n = 2488)	85.5	1.85(1.77–1.97)	1.43(1.35–1.52)
Occupation			
Other (n = 2057)	45.8	0.08(0.07–0.09)	0.15(0.14–0.17)
Wage earners at basic level (n = 8507)	82.9	0.53(0.51–0.56)	0.68(0.60–0.71)
Wage earners at higher level (n = 3199)	91.5	1	
ACS diagnose			
Unstable angina (n = 2460)	75.1	1	1
AMI-STEMI (n = 4212)	80.1	1.42(1.36–1.51)	0.99(0.93–1.05)
NSTEMI (n = 2875)	81.7	1.64(1.54–1.74)	1.28(1.11–1.25)
AMI unspecified (n = 4231)	79.3	1.25(1.19–1.33)	0.98(0.92–1.04)
Year of diagnose			
2001–2003 (n = 4931)	80.8	1	1
2004–2006 (n = 4783)	78.5	1.19(1.15–1.25)	1.12(1.07–1.18)
2007–2009 (N = 4062)	77.1	1.80 (1.72–1.89)	1.51(1.44–1.59)
Procedures 30 days after admission			
No invasive procedure (n = 2724)	75.0	1	1
CAG, only (n = 5880)	79.6	1.56(1.49–1.64)	1.12(0.95–1.08)
PCI (n = 4363)	82.1	1.71(1.67–1-86	1.16 (1.11–1.22)
CABG (n = 708)	78.2	1.42(1.29–1.36)	0.89 (0.81–0.98)
Number of comorbidities			
None (n = 10,421)	83.7	1	1
1–2 (n = 2871)	67.9	0.48(0.45–-0.50)	0.50(0.48–0.53)
3 and more (n = 484)	51.4	0.28(0.25–0.32)	0.29(0.23–0.34)
Work status 30 days after diagnose			
Sick leave (n = 12029)	83.8	1	1
Unemployed (n = 1747)	48.1	0.16(0.15–0.18)	0.18(0.17–0.20)

*age underlying timescale.

the workforce without receiving economic compensation from the state. This is, however, very rare in Denmark and can be ignored in this study. We used invasive procedures during the first 30 days after diagnosis as covariates in our study. Thus, around 10% of those who only had a CAG actually had a PCI later. This information was not included in the analyses but might be a factor that could have an impact on return to work. Since some patients die during follow-up there might be a problem with competing risk

[23]. However, we did not use competing risk analysis, as the number of deaths was relatively small. Furthermore, such models do not provide simple relationships between variables [23].

The present study is conducted in a Nordic welfare system with high turnover rates in the labour market, high rates of participation and high degrees of social security. Expenditures for social protection in the Nordic countries including Denmark is relatively high compared to the rest of the European Union and countries such as the US and Canada, but these countries all have some degree of a social welfare system and universal health care. The size of economic compensation and duration of sick leave might have an impact on the consequence of a chronic disease but the risk factors and reasons for being on sick leave or returning to work is not only influenced by the political context but also by an individual's behaviour.

References

1. Schmidt M, Jacobsen JB, Lash TL, Botker HE, Sorensen HT (2012) 25-year trends in first time hospitalisation for acute myocardial infarction, subsequent short- and long-term mortality, and the prognostic impact of sex and co-morbidity: a Danish nationwide cohort study. BMJ 344:e356.
2. Rasmussen JN, Rasmussen S, Gislason GH, Buch P, Abildstrom SZ, et al. (2006) Mortality after acute myocardial infarction according to income and education. J Epidemiol Community Health 60:351–356.
3. Mital A, Desai A, Mital A (2004) Return to work after a coronary event. J Cardiopulm Rehabil 24:365–373.
4. Perk J, Alexanderson K (2004) Swedish Council on Technology Assessment in Health Care (SBU). Chapter 8. Sick leave due to coronary artery disease or stroke. Scand J Public Health Suppl 63:181–206.
5. Hallberg V, Palomaki A, Kataja M, Tarkka M, Hallberg V, et al. (2009) Return to work after coronary artery bypass surgery. A 10-year follow-up study. Scand Cardiovasc J 43:277–284.
6. Pinto N, Shah P, Haluska B, Griffin R, Holliday J, et al. (2012) Return to work after coronary artery bypass in patients aged under 50 years. Asian Cardiovasc Thorac Ann 20:387–391.
7. Voss M, Ivert T, Pehrsson K, Hammar N, Alexanderson K, et al. (2012) Sickness absence following coronary revascularisation. A national study of women and men of working age in Sweden 1994–2006. PLOS One 2012;7:e40952.
8. Hamalainen H, Maki J, Virta L, Keskimaki I, Mahonen M, et al. (2004) Return to work after first myocardial infarction in 1991–1996 in Finland. Eur J Public Health 14:350–353.
9. Thygesen LC, Daasnes C, Thaulow I, Brønnum-Hansen H (2011) Introduction to Danish (nationwide) registers on health and social issues: structure, access, legislation and archiving. Scand J Public Health 39 Suppl.:12–16.
10. (2006) IDA – an integrated database for labour market research. Main Report, 1991. Statistics Denmark, Copenhagen.
11. Hjollund NH, Larsen FB, Andersen JH (2007) Register-based follow-up of social benefits and other transfer payments: accuracy and degree of completeness in a Danish interdepartmental administrative database compared with a population-based survey. Scand J Public Health 35:497–502.
12. Joensen AM, Jensen MK, Overvad K, Dethlefsen C, Schmidt E, et al. (2009) Predictive values of acute coronary syndrome discharge diagnoses differed in the Danish National Patient Registry. J Clin Epidemio 62:188–94.
13. Pedersen J, Bjorner JB, Burr H, Christensen KB (2012) Transitions between sickness absence, work, unemployment, and disability in Denmark 2004–2008. Scand J Work Environ Health 38:516–526.
14. Vaccarino V, Krumholz HM, Yarzebski J, Gore JM, Goldberg RJ (2001) Sex differences in 2 years mortality after hospital discharge for myocardial infarction. Ann Int Med 134:173–181.
15. Radovanovic D, Erne O, Urban P, Bertel O, Rickli H, et al. (2007) Gender differences in management and outcomes in patients with acute coronary syndromes: results on 20,290 patients from the AMIS plus Registry. Heart 93:1369–1375.
16. Nielsen FE, Sorensen HT, Skagen K (2004) A prospective study found impaired left ventricular function predicted job retirement after acute myocardial infarction. J Clin Epidemiol 57:837–842.
17. Mittag O, Kolenda KD, Nordman KJ, Bernien J, Maurischat C (2001) Return to work after myocardial infarction/coronary artery bypass grafting: patients' and physicians' initial viewpoints and outcome 12 months later. Soc Sci Med 52:1441–1450.
18. Boudrez H, De BG (2000) Recent findings on return to work after an acute myocardial infarction or coronary artery bypass grafting. Acta Cardiol 55:341–349.
19. Mark DB, Lam LC, Lee KL, Clapp-Channing NE, Williams RB, et al. (1992) Identification of patients with coronary disease at high risk for loss of employment. A prospective validation study. Circulation 86:1485–1494.
20. Writing Group for the Bypass Angioplasty Revascularization Investigation (BARI. Investigators) (1997) Five-year clinical and functional outcome comparing bypass surgery and angioplasty in patients with multivessel coronary disease. A multicenter randomized trial. JAMA 277:715–721.
21. Pocock SJ, Henderson RA, Seed P, Treasure T, Hampton JR (1996) Quality of life, employment status, and anginal symptoms after coronary angioplasty or bypass surgery. 3-year follow-up in the Randomized Intervention Treatment of Angina (RITA). Trial. Circulation 942:135–142.
22. Thygesen SK, Christiansen CF, Christensen S, Lash TL, Sorensen HT (2011) The predictive value of ICD-10 diagnostic coding used to assess Charlson co-morbidity index conditions in the population-based Danish National Registry of Patients. BMC Med Res Methodol 11:83.
23. Andersen PK, Geskus RB, deWitte T, Putter H (2012) Competing risks in epidemiology: possibilities and pitfalls. Int J Epidemiol 41:861–70

Conclusion

In this study more than half of patients with first-time ACS stay in or return to work shortly after the event. Women, the socially disadvantaged, those with presumed more severe cardiac events and co-morbidity have lower rates of return when other clinical factors are accounted for. These factors should be considered during physical and social rehabilitation.

Author Contributions

Conceived and designed the experiments: MO. Performed the experiments: MO SM KC. Analyzed the data: MO. Contributed reagents/materials/analysis tools: MO SM KC. Wrote the paper: MO. Interpretation of data: MO SM EP KC. Revised the manuscript critically: MO.

11

The Value of a BP Determination Method Using a Novel Non-Invasive BP Device against the Invasive Catheter Measurement

Jinsong Xu[1,⁹], Yanqing Wu[1,⁹], Hai Su[1]*, Weitong Hu[1], Juxiang Li[1], Wenying Wang[1], Xin Liu[2], Xiaoshu Cheng[1]

1 Research Institute of Cardiovascular Diseases and Department of Cardiology, Second Affiliated Hospital of Nanchang University, Nanchang, Jiangxi, People' Republic of China, **2** Fuzhou Medical College of Nanchang University, Fuzhou, Jiangxi, People's Republic of China

Abstract

Objective: The aim of this study was to evaluate the accuracy of a new blood pressure (BP) measurement method (Pulse method).

Methods: This study enrolled 45 patients for selective percutaneous coronary intervention (PCI) via right radial artery. A BP device using either oscillometric (Microlife 3AC1-1) or Pulse method(RG-BP11)was used. At the beginning of each PCI, intra-radial BP was measured before Microlife BP or Pulse BP measurement as its own reference, respectively. At the end of PCI, BP was measured again with the measurement order of Microlife BP and Pulse BP reversed. The differences between intra-radial and Microlife (BPi-M) or Pulse BP (BPi-P) on SBP, DBP and mean artery pressure (MAP) were calculated. Meanwhile, in 48 patients the intra-brachial BP and intra-radial artery BP were measured to calculate the brachial -radial BP difference (BPr-b).

Results: The intra-radial SBP references used prior to both the Microlife and Pulse SBP that were similar (145.1 ± 27.7 vs 145.8 ± 24.2 mmHg), but the Microlife SBP was significantly lower than the Pulse SBP (127.7 ± 20.5 vs 130.3 ± 22.7 mmHg, $P<0.05$), thus the SBPi-M was higher than SBPi-P (18.1 ± 11.8 vs 14.8 ± 12.8 mmHg, $P<0.05$). As the mean SBPr-b was 12.4 mmHg, the Pulse SBP was closer to expected intra-brachial SBP by about 3.3 mmHg than was Microlife SBP to expected intra-brachial SBP. Meanwhile, Bland-Altman plots showed that the 95% limits of agreement for intra-radial SBP by Pulse SBP were narrower than those by Microlife SBP ($12.0\sim17.5$ vs $15.5\sim20.6$ mmHg). However, the 95% limits of agreement for Pulse DBP and MAP were similar to those for Microlife DBP and MAP.

Conclusion: Against the invasive BP measurement, the pulse method may provide more accurate SBP and comparable DBP and MAP as compared with the oscillometric method.

Editor: Xiongwen Chen, Temple University, United States of America

Funding: This work was supported by a grant from the National High Technology Research and Development Program of China (863 Program, No. 2012AA02A516). The funders had no role in study design, data collection and analysis, decision to publish, or preparation of the manuscript.

Competing Interests: The authors have declared that no competing interests exist.

* Email: suyihappy@sohu.com

⁹ These authors contributed equally to this work.

Introduction

Mercury sphygmomanometers will be replaced by new blood pressure (BP) devices in the near future because of their pollution problems. At present, most electronic automatic BP devices use the oscillometric method to determine systolic and diastolic BP (SBP and DBP). Although electronic automatic BP devices are widely used in clinical practice, controversy about their accuracy still exists [1–4].

Recently, some new non-invasive BP devices have been developed [5–7]. Among them, a novel automatic BP device (Pulse BP device) was developed and commercialized in China. This device uses a new "Pulse method" to determine SBP and DBP. Although this new BP device was patented in China and other countries [8,9], its accuracy against invasive catheter BP has

not been fully determined. The aim of this study is to compare the accuracy between the Pulse method and the oscillometric method against invasive catheter BP measurement.

Subjects and methods

The proposal and consent procedures of this study were approved by the Ethic Committee of the Second Affiliated Hospital of Nanchang University. For selective percutaneous coronary intervention (PCI) and BP measurement, all patients provided their written informed consent.

Subjects. From May to October of 2013, 45 patients undergoing PCI via the right radial artery were enrolled for this study. All of the patients enrolled were subjected to their first PCI via the right radial artery and had stable hemodynamics during the PCI.

We excluded any patients who experienced acute myocardial infarction, aortic coarctation, congenital heart disease, acute heart failure, hemiplegia, pulseless disease, previous trans-radial PCI or had arrhythmia at BP measurement. The information of the subjects was summarized in Table 1.

BP measurement and devices. Two types of automatic BP device were used in this study. One is by oscillometric method (Microlife BP 3AC1-1), and the other is by Pulse method (RG-BP11, the Ruiguang medical equipment co., LTD Shenzhen, China).

As a new device, the Pulse BP device has two features: First, it is equipped with two cuffs. The large cuff (14×27 cm) is placed on the middle of upper arm to compress brachial artery and to detect pressure, and the small cuff (7×23 cm) is placed on forearm near the fossa cubitalia to detect pulse wave of radial artery. The pressure curve in the large cuff and the pulse wave curve in the small cuff are simultaneously recorded. The second feature is the new determination method for SBP and DBP. When the pressure in the large cuff on upper arm decreases to the level that no longer blocks the brachial artery blood flow, pulse wave appears in the small forearm cuff. As the pressure decreases, the amplitudes of pulse waves in the small cuff gradually increase in a linear manner for the first several beats. The pressure in the large cuff that correlates with the cross point of the baseline line with the regression line in the small cuff is determined as SBP (Figure 1).

The determination of DBP is based on delay time, which is defined by the interval between the fluctuation signal in the large cuff and pulse wave in the small cuff. As the large cuff gradually deflates, the delay time gradually decreases. When the delay time becomes constant, the pressure in the large cuff is determined as DBP(Figure 1).

The BP measurement protocol

The examination was conducted in cardiac catheterization room. BP was taken when the patients lay on an operation table with right arm on a support pad. The large cuff of the Pulse BP device was also used for the Microlife BP device with a T-branch pipe in order to eliminate the effect of cuff size on BP measurement.

At first, the two cuffs of the Pulse BP device were properly placed according to the manufacturer's instructions. After sheathing (5Fr or 6Fr), a Judkins catheter was inserted into the lower edge of the small cuff at the position of the upper-middle part of the radial artery. When intra-radial BP curves became stable, the mean amplitude of ten pulse waves was recorded as intra-radial BP, and Pulse BP was taken subsequently. After 2 minutes, intra-radial BP curve was recorded again, followed by the reading of Microlife BP. At the end of PCI, the above-mentioned BP measurement procedure was repeated when the catheter was withdrawn back to the lower edge of the small cuff, while the order

Table 1. Summary of the information of the 45 patients.

Age(y)	69.4±20.1
HR(bpm)	72.7±12.8
SBP(mmHg)	127.6±20.5
DBP(mmHg)	95.1±15.2
Diabetes (%)	15(33.3)
Male (%)	34(75.6)
CHD (%)	33(73.3)

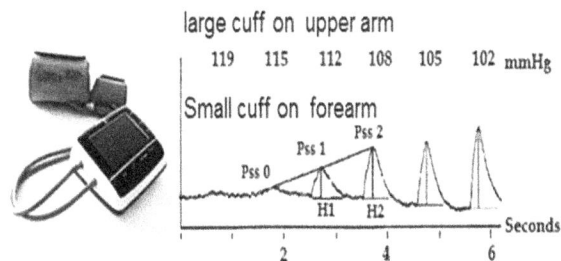

Figure 1. A Pulse BP device and the illustration for SBP determination. The numbers represent the pressure values (mmHg) in the large cuff. When the pressure decreases in the large cuff, the amplitudes of the first several pulse waves recorded from the small cuff gradually increases in a linear manner. Pss 0, Pss 1 and Pss 2 represent the first 3 pulse waves, respectively. H represents the vertical height of the pulse wave. The pressure in the large cuff at Pss0 is determined as SBP. Pss0 = (H2 X Pss1 -H1 X Pss2)/(H2— HI).

of two non-invasive BP devices was reversed. Therefore, both Microlife BP and Pulse BP had its own intra-radial artery BP as its gold standard.

The non-invasive mean arterial pressure (MAP) was calculated with the formula: MAP = (SBP+2×DBP)/3. The invasive MAP was read from the intra-artery pulse wave record (EP-Work Mate). The differences between intra-radial artery BP and Microlife BP (BPi-M) or Pulse BP (BPi-P) were calculated, respectively.

Meanwhile, in 48 patients (including the 20 patients received both Pulse and Microlife BP measurement) intra-brachial artery BP was recorded when the catheter was withdrawn to the middle of brachial artery in order to evaluate the difference between the intra-radial BP and the intra-brachial BP (BPr-b).

Statistical analysis

Data was entered in Excel 2003 and analyzed with SPSS10.0. Continuous variables were expressed as mean ± SD. The t-test, paired sample t-test and the analysis of variance (ANOVA) and the omnibus test were used for the statistical analysis. Linear regression analysis was performed to examine the correlation between BPs from invasive and noninvasive methods.

The inter-measurement agreement was evaluated by Bland-Altman plot method [10]. With this method, inter-measurement differences for SBP, DBP and MAP were plotted against their relative intra-radial artery parameters, respectively. The 95% limits of agreement (LoA) were determined (95% LoA = mean inter-measurement difference ±1.96 standard deviation). A p-value of less than 0.05 was considered statistically significant.

Results

As 4 patients had no complete paired Pulse and Microlife BP data, only 85 pairs of intra-radial and Microlife BPs and 85 pairs of intra-radial and Pulse BPs were finally used for analysis. The range (93–206 vs 88–226 mmHg) and the mean value of intra-radial SBP taken before Microlife BP were very similar to those taken before Pulse BP. However, the Microlife SBP was significantly lower than the Pulse SBP, so the SBPi-P was significantly lower than the SBPi-M. Significantly positive correlation was seen between intra-radial SBP and Pulse SBP (r = 0.89) or Microlife SBP (r = 0.87).

The range (49–102 vs 49–108 mmHg) and the mean value of intra-radial DBP taken before Microlife BP were also very similar to those taken before Pulse BP. Both Pulse DBP and Microlife

Table 2. The comparison between intra-radial and Microlife or Pulse BP.

	Microlife			Pulse		
	SBP	**DBP**	**MAP**	**SBP**	**DBP**	**MAP**
Intra-radial	145.8±24.2	69.9±10.2	95.2±12.8	145.1±27.7	70.5±11.6	95.4±14.9
Noninvasive	127.7±20.7*	74.6±10.9*	92.3±12.7*	130.3±22.7*	75.8±12.1*	94.0±13.9
BPi-n	18.1±11.8	−4.7±6.5	2.9±6.6	14.8±12.8$	−5.3±7.7	1.4±7.1
R	0.87#	0.81#	0.87#	0.89#	0.79#	0.88#

BPi-n: the difference between the intra-radial artery and noninvasive BP;
*: compared with intra-radial artery BP, P<0.05;
&: compared with Microlife SBP, P<0.05;
#: the coefficient, P<0.001;
(n=85,M±SD,mmHg).

DBP were significantly higher than their reference intra-radial DBPs, while the DBPi-P was similar to the DBPi-M. Meanwhile, the coefficient of the intra-radial DBP with Microlife DBP was similar to that with Pulse DBP (0.81 vs 0.79).

The reference intra-radial MAP for Pulse MAP was similar to that for Microlife MAP, although the MAPi-P was slightly lower than the MAPi-M. Nevertheless, the coefficients between the intra-radial MAP and Microlife MAP or Pulse MAP were nearly equal (Table 2).

In the 48 patients with both intra-radial and intra-brachial BP measurements in right arm, the intra-radial SBP and MAP were significantly higher than the intra-brachial SBP and MAP, while their intra-radial DBP was similar (Table 3).

Figure 2 shows the Bland-Altman plots for the intra-radial BP and the non-invasive BP. The 95% limits of agreement for Pulse SBP (12.0~17.5 vs 15.5~20.6 mmHg) and Pulse MAP (−0.2~2.9 vs 1.5~4.3 mmHg) were narrower than those for Microlife SBP and MAP.

However, the 95% limits of agreement for Pulse DBP (−7.0~−3.3 vs −6.9~−3.6 mmHg) were similar to those for Microlife DBP (Figure 2).

In the Bland-Altman plots, a positive linear correlation is observed between SBP and SBP difference for either Pulse (r=0.58, P<0.01) or Microlife (r=0.52, P<0.01) methods. Meanwhile, the coefficient is 0.27 for Pulse (P=0.012) and 0.21 for Microlife (P=0.049) between DBP and DBP difference, and the coefficient is 0.33 for Pulse (P=0.002) and 0.24 for Microlife (P=0.024) between MAP and MAP difference (Figure 2).

Table 3. The comparison between intra-radial and intra-brachial artery BPs.

	intra-radial	intra-brachial	BPr-b
SBP	146.0±25.4	133.5±22.8*	12.4±8.2
DBP	74.4±14.4	73.2±13.5	1.2±6.6
MAP	98.3±15.7	93.3±14.1*	5.0±6.0

BPr-b: the difference between intra-radial and intra-brachial artery BP.
*: compared with intra-radial, P<0.05.
(n=48, mmHg).

Discussion

The Pulse BP device used in this study has passed the validation process against sphygmomanometers according to the European Society of Hypertension International Protocol (by Doctor Wang W of Fuwai hospital, Beijing, China). This study aimed to evaluate the accuracy of Pulse BP method against intra-artery BP measurement.

The present study showed that at similar reference intra-radial SBP, the mean difference between intra-radial SBP and Pulse SBP was 14.8 mmHg, lower than the difference of 18.0 mmHg between intra-radial SBP and Microlife SBP. Meanwhile, this study confirmed SBP amplification phenomenon between intra-radial and intra-brachial artery [11,12], and this value was 12.4 mmHg in the 48 patients examined. When the SBP amplification phenomenon was taken in to consideration, the Pulse SBP was about 3 mmHg closer to the expected intra-brachial SBP as compared with Microlife SBP. Furthermore, the 95% limits of agreement of differences between intra-radial SBP and Pulse SBP were narrower than those between intra-radial SBP and Microlife SBP, and the coefficient of intra-artery SBP with Pulse SBP was slightly higher than that with Microlife SBP (0.89 vs 0.87). These results indicate that the Pulse method may provide more accurate brachial artery SBP as compared with the oscillometric method. For the oscillometric method, a state-of-the-art electronic measurement method, SBP is estimated by the average pressure and the empirical coefficient. Therefore, the reported BP may have relatively large individual differences, especially in some extreme clinical situations such as severe hypertension or hypotension.

This study showed that the two methods had comparable accuracy on MAP. After the correction for the MAP amplification phenomenon of 5.0 mm Hg, the Microlife MAP and the Pulse MAP were 2.1 and 3.6 mmHg higher than the expected intra-brachial MAP, respectively. Although the Microlife MAP was closer to the expected intra-brachial MAP by 1.5 mmHg, its 95% limits of agreement with intra-radial MAP were wider than those with Pulse MAP (1.5~4.3 vs −0.2~2.9 mmHg). Furthermore, their coefficients for intra-radial MAP were nearly equal; therefore, we suggest that these two methods have similar accuracy on MAP.

Although the Pulse BP device also uses a new delay time method, our study did not show that this method had advantage on DBP determination as compared with the oscillometric method, as similar coefficients and 95% limits of agreement were observed between intra-radial and Pulse or Microlife DBPs.

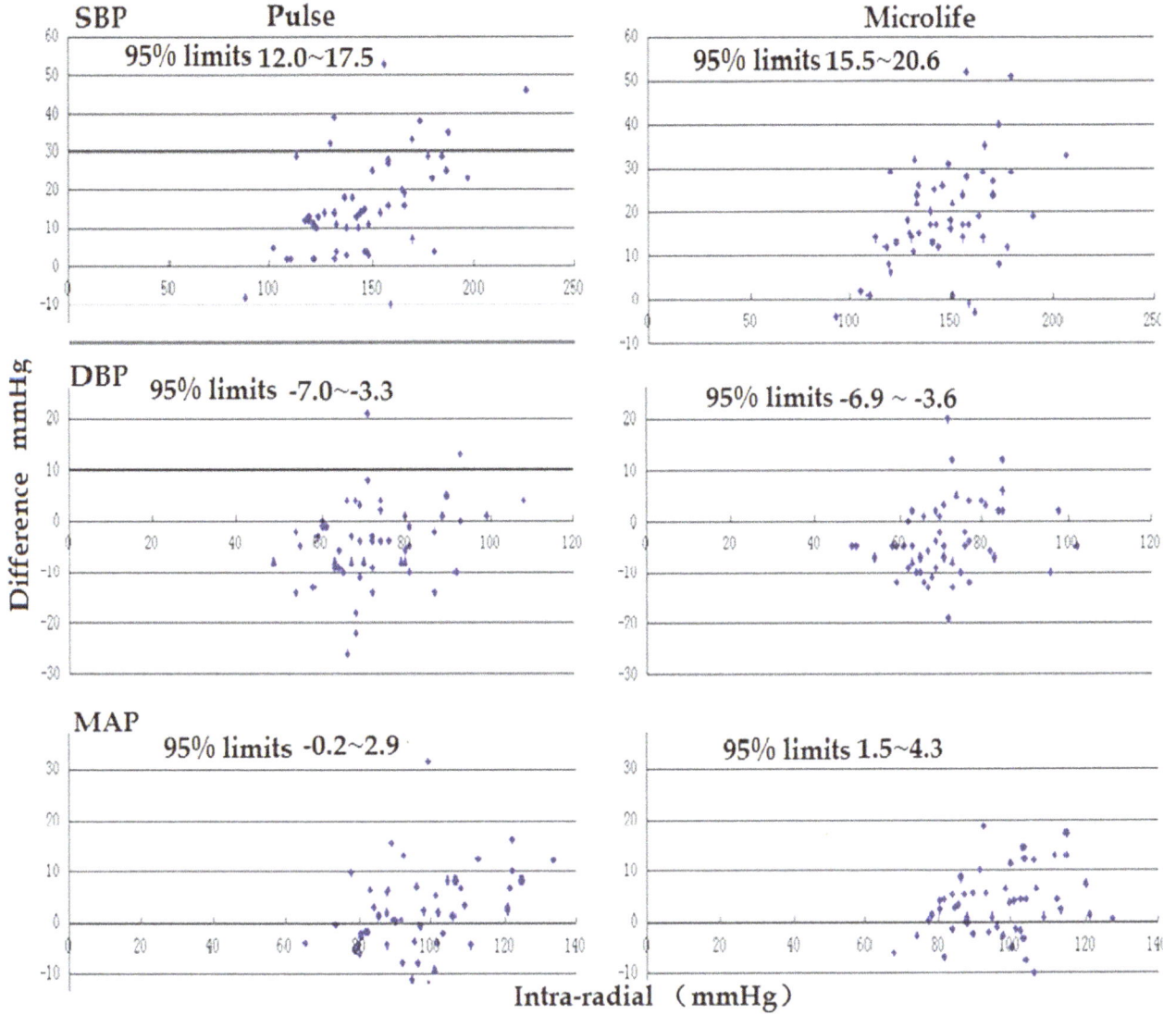

Figure 2. The Bland-Altman plots for the inter-measurement differences between intro-radial artery BP and Pulse BP or Microlife BP. Difference = intra-radial BP- non-invasive BP.

Meanwhile, this study showed no amplification phenomenon on DBP between brachial artery and radial artery.

In the Bland-Altman plots a positive linear correlation is observed between intra-radial SBP and SBP difference (intra-radial SBP- non-invasive SBP), between DBP and DBP difference, and between MAP and MAP difference for both methods. These results suggest that when the intra-radial BP is higher, the noninvasive brachial BP may be underestimated by both BP measurement methods, inducing higher intra-radial BP- non-invasive BP difference, especially for SBP. Meanwhile, the stronger correlation for Pulse method may indicate that the Pulse BP is more closely correlated with the intra-radial BP than with Microlife BP, especially for SBP.

Limitation

For ethical reasons, only some of the 45 patients who received both Pulse and Microlife BP measurement had intra-brachial artery BP values. The BP difference between intra-radial and intra-brachial artery used as the reference was partly obtained from other 48 patients, so the use of their data as the gold standard may result in some bias. However, the intra-radial SBP and DBP were very similar in the 2 groups of patients studied, suggesting this system error may not influence our conclusion.

Conclusion

Against the invasive BP measurement, the pulse method may provide more accurate SBP and comparable DBP and MAP as compared with the oscillometric method.

Author Contributions

Conceived and designed the experiments: HS JXL. Performed the experiments: JSX YQW. Analyzed the data: WTH WYW. Wrote the paper: XL HS XSC.

References

1. Babbs CF (2012) Ooscillometric measurement of systolic and diastolic blood pressures validated in a physiologic mathematical model. Biomed Eng Online 22: 11: 56.
2. Vos J, Vincent HH, Verhaar MC, Bos WJ (2013) Inaccuracy in determining mean arterial pressure with oscillometric blood pressure techniques. Am J Hypertens 26: 624–9.
3. Amoore JN (2012) Oscillometric sphygmomanometers: a critical appraisal of current technology. Blood Pressure Monitoring 17: 80–88
4. Raamat R, Talts J, Jagomägi K, Kivastik J (2013) Accuracy of some algorithms to determine the ooscillometric mean arterial pressure: a theoretical study. Blood Pressure Monitoring 18: 50–56.
5. Babbs CF (2012) Oscillometric measurement of systolic and diastolic blood pressures validated in a physiologic mathematical model. Biomed Eng Online. 11: 56.
6. Stergiou GS, Kollias A, Destounis A, Tzamouranis D (2012) Automated blood pressure measurement in atrial fibrillation: a systematic review and meta-analysis. J Hypertens 30: 2074–82.
7. Farsky S, Benova K, Krausova D, Sirotiaková J, Vysocanova P (2011) Clinical blood pressure measurement verification when comparing a Tensoval duo control device with a mercury sphygmomanometer in patients suffering from atrial fibrillation. Blood Pressure Monitoring 16: 252–257.
8. Xiaoguang Wu (2012) Inventors: Feb. 09. Non-invasive blood pressure measuring apparatus and measuring method thereof. CN2011/000866, International Classes: A61B5/0225
9. Xiaoguang Wu (2013) Inventor: May.30. Non-invasive blood pressure measuring apparatus and measuring method thereof. United States patent IPC8 Class: AA61B5022FI, USPC Class: 600493 Patent application number: 20130138001
10. Bland JM, Altman DG (1986). Statistical methods for assessing agreement between two methods of clinical measurement. The Lancet 327: 307–310.
11. Segers P, Mahieu D, Kips J, Rietzschel E, De Buyzere M, et al.(2009) Amplification of the Pressure Pulse in the Upper Limb in Healthy, Middle-Aged Men and Women. Hypertension 54: 414–420.
12. Ding FH, Li Y, Zhang RY, Zhang Q, Wang JG (2013) Comparison of the SphygmoCor and Omron devices in the estimation of pressure amplification against the invasive catheter measurement. J Hypertens 31: 86–93.

12

Shared Decision Making in Patients with Stable Coronary Artery Disease: PCI Choice

Megan Coylewright[1,2], Kathy Shepel[3], Annie LeBlanc[2], Laurie Pencille[2], Erik Hess[2,4], Nilay Shah[2,5], Victor M. Montori[2,5,6], Henry H. Ting[1,2]*

1 Division of Cardiovascular Diseases, Department of Medicine, Mayo Clinic, Rochester, Minnesota, United States of America, 2 Knowledge and Evaluation Research Unit, Mayo Clinic, Rochester, Minnesota, United States of America, 3 The Section of Creative Media at Mayo Clinic, Rochester, Minnesota, United States of America, 4 Division of Emergency Medicine Research, Department of Emergency Medicine, Mayo Clinic, Rochester, Minnesota, United States of America, 5 Division of Health Care Policy and Research, Department of Health Sciences Research, Mayo Clinic, Rochester, Minnesota, United States of America, 6 Division of Endocrinology, Diabetes, Metabolism, and Nutrition, Department of Medicine, Mayo Clinic, Rochester, Minnesota, United States of America

Abstract

Background: Percutaneous coronary intervention (PCI) and optimal medical therapy (OMT) are comparable, alternative therapies for many patients with stable angina; however, patients may have misconceptions regarding the impact of PCI on risk of death and myocardial infarction (MI) in stable coronary artery disease (CAD).

Methods and Results: We designed and developed a patient-centered decision aid (PCI Choice) to promote shared decision making for patients with stable CAD. The estimated benefits and risks of PCI+OMT as compared to OMT were displayed in a decision aid using pictographs with natural frequencies and text. We engaged patients, clinicians, health service researchers, and designers with over 20 successive iterations of the decision aid, which were field tested during real-world clinical encounters involving clinicians and patients. The decision aid is intended to facilitate knowledge transfer, deliberation based on patient values and preferences, and shared decision making.

Conclusions: We describe the methods and outcomes of the design and development of a decision aid (PCI Choice) to promote shared decision making between clinicians and patients regarding the choice of PCI+OMT vs. OMT for treatment of stable CAD. We will evaluate the impact of PCI Choice on patient knowledge, decisional conflict, participation in decision-making, and treatment choice in an upcoming randomized trial.

Editor: Giuseppe Biondi-Zoccai, Sapienza University of Rome, Italy

Funding: Dr. Ting was awarded a Program Development Grant from the Jeanne Sullivan Development fund to study shared decision making in coronary artery disease. This funding source had no role in study design, data collection and analysis, decision to publish or preparation of the manuscript.

Competing Interests: The authors have declared that no competing interests exist.

* E-mail: ting.henry@mayo.edu

Introduction

Percutaneous coronary intervention (PCI) does not lower the risk of death or myocardial infarction (MI) for patients with stable coronary artery disease (CAD) when added to optimal medical therapy (OMT) [1], although PCI is associated with more rapid improvement in symptoms [2,3].

Misconceptions exist among patients regarding the potential benefit of PCI+OMT for stable CAD as nearly 90% of patients in a recent study believed that PCI reduces the risk of MI [4]. The selection of PCI+OMT vs. OMT alone for stable CAD represents a preference-sensitive decision where comparable, alternative treatments exist. Shared decision making may improve patient knowledge and involvement in decision-making to promote an "informed, values-based choice among two or more medically reasonable alternatives." [5]

Clinicians want to "do the right thing" for patients with stable CAD, using professional society guidelines and appropriate use criteria to assist in decision making [6]. Often missing, however, are the skills and tools to best involve patients in a decision making

that reflects patient goals and preferences. In this paper, we describe the process of designing and testing a decision aid for the treatment of stable CAD to address these gaps for patients in whom a clinical choice exists between OMT or PCI+OMT. The decision aid is intended for use following stress testing and upstream from diagnostic angiography; if diagnostic angiography is performed, the minority of patients in whom a choice of surgery is then relevant would no longer utilize the decision aid, as this choice is not modeled. The process of decision aid creation included review of pertinent literature; design and development of the decision aid with input from patients, clinicians, designers and researchers; and the testing of successive iterations during real-world clinical encounters.

Methods

We used a practice-based, patient-centered, and participatory approach to design PCI Choice [7,8,9,10,11], requiring multidisciplinary input from clinicians (cardiologists, cardiology fellows, nurse practitioners, physician assistants, and nurses), health service researchers, design experts, statisticians, and patients. The process of decision aid design and development involves 1) review and synthesis of the available evidence and its endorsement by stakeholders; 2) analysis of usual practice; 3) development of an initial prototype; 4) field testing of the prototype in clinical settings under the study team's supervision; and 5) successive iterations and further testing of the prototype (Figure 1). The resulting decision aid is intended to be nondirective, encouraging clinicians to create a conversation with patients using their own communication styles, while simultaneously ensuring that key information is conveyed and that patient preferences are elicited [12]. We required sufficient evidence of ease of use and clarity of information from our study team, participating clinicians, and patients prior to selecting a final prototype. We tested the decision aid within the cardiovascular division at Mayo Clinic Rochester, which is comprised of 150 staff cardiologists (including 15 interventional cardiologists), 40 cardiovascular fellows, and approximately 700 allied health staff, including nurse practitioners, physician assistants, and specialized cardiac catheterization nurses. The outpatient cardiology practice is divided into 18 subspecialty clinics; prototypes of PCI Choice were tested in two clinics that see the highest volume of patients with stable CAD.

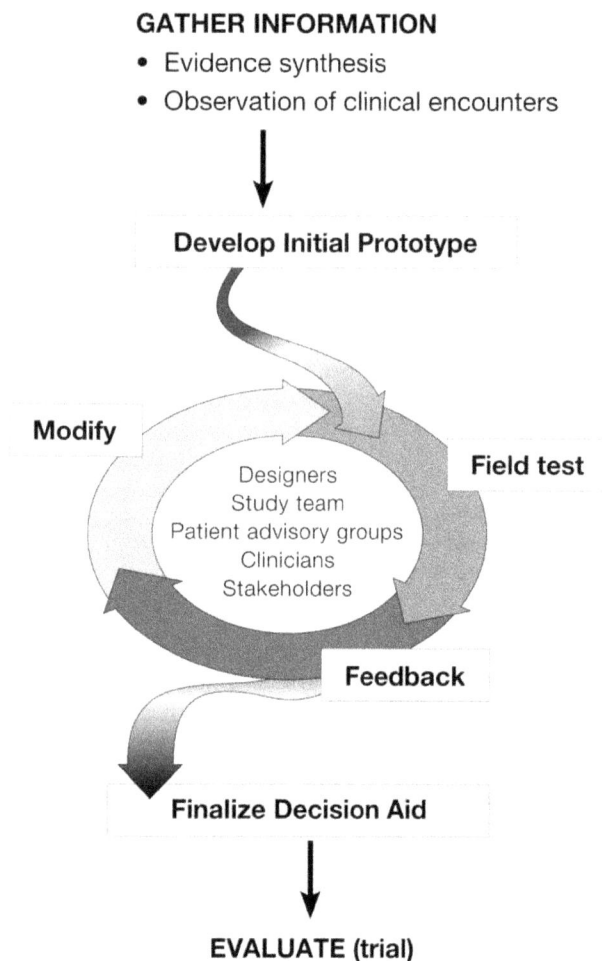

GATHER INFORMATION
- Evidence synthesis
- Observation of clinical encounters

Develop Initial Prototype

Modify

Field test

Designers
Study team
Patient advisory groups
Clinicians
Stakeholders

Feedback

Finalize Decision Aid

EVALUATE (trial)

Figure 1. Process for development and prototyping of decision aid.

Methods Step 1: Review and synthesis of the evidence

Synthesis of the evidence for the treatment of stable CAD was conducted by an interventional cardiologist (H.H.T.) and cardiology fellow (M.C.), up to date as of April 2012; we performed a detailed PubMed search, referenced American College of Cardiology/American Heart Association guidelines, and reviewed relevant bibliographies. The content of the decision aid was then vetted with cardiologists and cardiology fellows through a grand rounds presentation, focus groups, and individual interviews. Experts in the field of outcomes research in stable CAD at outside institutions were also included in reviewing the selected evidence base.

The study was approved by the Institutional Review Board (IRB) at Mayo Clinic-Rochester. All participants provided their verbal informed consent, as prespecified in our protocol submitted to, and approved by, the IRB. Documentation of the verbal script used to obtain consent was also submitted and approved by the IRB. Verbal consent was utilized given the minimal risk nature of the study in which a decision aid was being field tested and revised with feedback from patients involved. Verbal consent was obtained by trained study personnel involved in the testing of the decision aid, and receipt of verbal consent was documented within a spreadsheet that contained the name and medical record number of all patients considered for eligibility. This spreadsheet was distinct from the de-indentified database that included patient observations and feedback with use of the decision aid. Patients were not asked to submit written documents or complete surveys as part of this protocol.

Methods Step 2: Analysis of usual practice

Members of the study team undertook an in-depth evaluation of the usual flow of patient care at Mayo Clinic Rochester for patients with stable CAD. Outpatient clinical visits with both cardiovascular fellows and staff cardiologists were observed by study personnel to identify and document usual care patterns. Further observations were performed of specialized cardiac catheterization lab nurse interactions with patients in the outpatient setting in preparation for catheterization, and during the day of the procedure in the prep area of the catheterization lab. Lastly, observations were made in catheterization lab during the procedure and in the recovery room after the procedure. Multiple interactions in each area of care were observed to create a description of routine usual care patterns, in addition to direct observation of several patients from start to finish (starting with the initial cardiology consultation to the diagnostic catheterization and/or PCI procedure). Formal input was gathered from stakeholders regarding timing of the decision aid in relation to coronary angiography during a cardiovascular grand rounds presentation, as well as focus group sessions including cardiovascular fellows and staff, catheterization lab nurses, clinical assistants, nurse practitioners and physician assistants, and patients and their families.

Methods Step 3: Development of an initial prototype

Content experts (H.H.T, M.C.) and designers (K.S.) partnered to create the first iteration. Careful consideration of how to display numerical estimates of risk and benefit is integral to the process. The preferred method in risk communication is the use of pictographs, which specifically includes display of the proportion of patients who do not receive any benefit from the proposed treatment, as well as those that do benefit [13]. For example, we include language such as, "Out of 100 people, 60 will experience benefit, and 40 will not." The use of natural frequencies with a common denominator may be clearer to patients than communicating in relative risks [14]. We have found that using pictographs to display absolute risk improves communication of personalized benefit [15], and is effective across diverse socio-demographic groups [16].

Methods Step 4: Field testing

Field testing began with patient advisory groups with experience in decision aid development, which included the long-standing Diabetes Research Advisory Group (DAG), comprised of 15–20 community members with diabetes who meet with Mayo Clinic researchers on a monthly basis to provide feedback on research proposals and activities, as well as the Cardiovascular Patient and Family Advisory Council (comprised of over 25 patients and family members). The groups evaluated the decision aid early in the process with one-time focused meetings and reconvened to review our final prototype.

Methods Step 5: Successive iterations

A critical method in decision aid development is testing of successive iterations, with content and format adjustment based on clinical observations in real world clinical encounters. Study team members observed clinicians delivering the prototypes to patients with stable CAD. Clinical interactions were evaluated for ease of use and fit within flow of care; patient and clinician body language; and content of discussion. Our interest was in shifting the current technical dialogue (e.g., "Based on my experience, I recommend that you undergo PCI to treat a 70% blockage") to a conversation between the clinician and patient regarding the patient's health care goals ("Let's discuss what is important to you and alternative choices for treatment"). We have found that this shift in approach led to increased patient knowledge, decreased decisional conflict, and increased medication adherence [17]. After each clinical observation, the decision aid was revised by our development team over the course of 1–2 weeks. The process was repeated until there were consistent observations of knowledge transfer and elicitation of patient preferences.

Results

Results Step 1: Review and synthesis of the evidence

The 2011 revised ACC/AHA guidelines recommend PCI for stable CAD when symptoms persist while on OMT; [18] this is also reflected in the 2009 Appropriateness Criteria for Coronary Revascularization [19]. These recommendations are in part based upon COURAGE, a large, randomized trial demonstrating no difference in rates of MI or death for PCI+OMT over OMT in stable angina [20]. COURAGE was prefaced by years of data comparing PCI+OMT vs. OMT for stable CAD with similar results [21].

Quality of life data in the COURAGE trial [3], and other randomized trials of revascularization for stable angina such as BARI 2D [2], demonstrated an initial benefit of PCI+OMT early on for symptom relief which waned over time. We examined symptom-stratified quality of life data from COURAGE, creating two unique decision aids: one modeled Canadian Cardiovascular Class (CCS) Class I/II (mild) angina, and the second, CCS Class III (moderate) angina. The benefit of PCI+OMT is more dramatic in those patients with greater symptoms: for example, of patients with moderate angina (Class III) who chose PCI+OMT, 76% saw clinically significant improvement in their quality of life at one month as compared to 57% with mild symptoms (Class I/II) [3].

Large registries and clinical trials examining outcomes such as bleeding, death, and stent thrombosis provided data for risk estimates. A recent analysis of several trials of elective PCI demonstrated a 2% risk of periprocedural bleeding [22]. The risk of longer term bleeding (one year) was based on a registry of over 80,000 patients in which the risk of a major bleed with aspirin alone was 4% per patient-year, with the addition of clopidogrel raising the risk to 7% per patient-year [23]. We utilized data from COURAGE on need for revascularization with an initial strategy of OMT (14%) [20] and more recent data on restenosis risk in the drug-eluting stent era (7%) [24].

In PCI Choice, we specifically modeled population estimates for risk as opposed to personalized predictions for two reasons: 1) less clinician burden by eliminating the need to enter clinical variables or print a unique copy of the decision aid and 2) consistent observations that once patients understood there was no mortality benefit to PCI+OMT, risk estimates had little impact on decision making; instead, we observed that the severity of symptoms drove patient choice.

Results Step 2: Analysis of usual practice

Two clinicians (H.H.T. and M.C.) mapped the flow of care for patients with stable CAD at Mayo Clinic-Rochester, identifying potential points in time conducive to shared decision making regarding the choice of PCI vs. OMT. (Figure 2) Patients with chronic stable angina are typically first seen by a primary care provider, and are then referred to a cardiologist for consideration of PCI with or without a preceding stress test. Stress tests are often performed prior to PCI at some point in the flow of care. The majority of PCIs are performed ad hoc – that is, PCI is performed immediately following a diagnostic coronary angiogram on a sedated patient without a pause to discuss the benefits and risks of alternative treatment options. While the majority of PCI performed in our institution is ad hoc in the setting of unstable angina or myocardial infarction, PCI for stable CAD is also performed ad hoc (266/322; 83%). This trend is seen nationally; for example, in a recent publication from the comprehensive New York State database, when excluding patients with MI in the preceding 24 hours, more than 80% of PCI procedures were performed ad hoc [25].

After discussions with cardiologists, nurses, patients, and our development team, the consensus was that the optimal time for shared decision making in our practice is upstream from diagnostic catheterization during the clinical encounter between the cardiologist and the patient, accommodating the current practice of ad hoc PCI. We also recognize that some of the shared decision making may begin during the visit with the primary care provider, and that opportunities exist in the prep area of the catheterization lab as well as during a potential pause following diagnostic catheterization for shared decision making.

In a typical clinical encounter within the cardiology specialty clinics, prior to referral for coronary angiography, patients describe their symptoms and experience with medications to the clinician, undergo a physical examination, and then review pertinent testing, including stress testing, with their clinician. A computer may be used to display results of testing, with the clinician sitting at a desk and the patient sitting on an adjacent couch. If ischemia is detected on stress testing, or if anginal symptoms interfere with the patient's quality of life or are new, coronary angiography may be recommended. There is significant variability regarding type of information delivered and how it is communicated by clinicians; decision aids are not currently utilized during the clinical encounter, although patients may be given an educational pamphlet about coronary angiogram and PCI, and often watch a video with technical details of the procedure. Common language observed included, "If there is a severe blockage, we can go ahead and fix it at that time." We

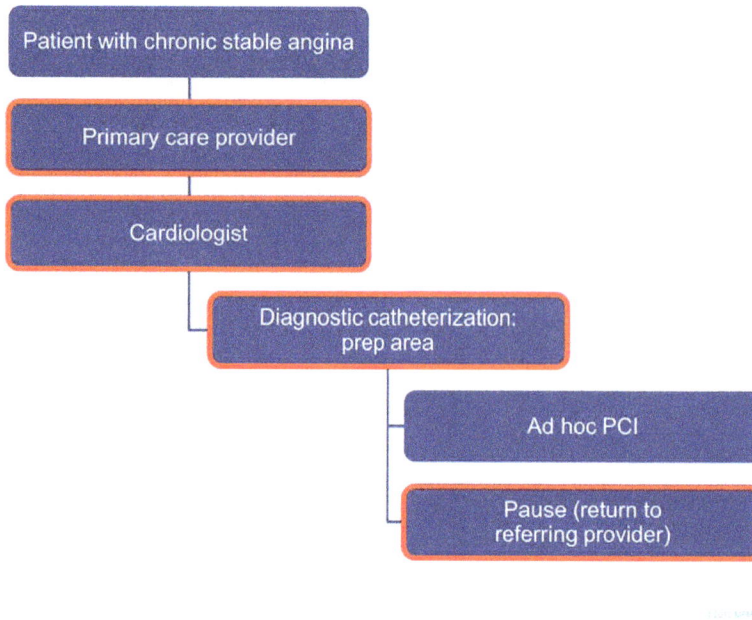

Figure 2. Flow of care for patients with chronic stable angina; red border indicates potential for shared decision making.

infrequently observed identification that there was a choice to be made or elicitation of patient values and preferences.

At our institution, patients who undergo coronary angiography typically do so on the day following consultation with a cardiologist, as many travel from a distance and request the convenience of next day scheduling. Informed consent is typically obtained by a cardiology fellow in the prep area of the catheterization lab and involves review of the risks, rather than potential benefits, of the procedure. There is not currently an opportunity to engage in shared decision making at this point for OMT vs. PCI+OMT, as the decision to proceed with coronary angiography with the possibility of PCI typically has already been made by the referring cardiologist with the patient; it is rare that patients expect to pause between diagnostic catheterization and intervention for shared decision making. Once the coronary anatomy is known, the interventional cardiologist will call the referring cardiologist on the phone while the sedated patient remains on the table. The interventional and referring cardiologist achieve consensus on whether to proceed with PCI, and the referring clinician follows the patient after procedure. For those patients in whom a choice of coronary artery bypass is relevant on the basis of diagnostic angiography, the decision aid is no longer applicable, as we have not modeled the choice of surgery at this time. Clinicians are encouraged at our institution to utilize a heart team approach and involve the cardiac surgeons, referring and interventional cardiologists, and the patient and their family, to select among PCI+OMT, PCI and coronary artery bypass surgery.

Results Step 3: Development of Initial Prototype

Two clinicians (H.H.T, and M.C.) partnered with a designer (K.S.) to create the first prototype. (Figure 3) Prominent in the initial design was modeling of benefit over time. Several delivery formats of the decision aid, PCI Choice, were considered, including desktop computer-based, handheld device-based, reusable plastic cards, and paper-based. We designed a one-page decision aid to confer portability, accessibility, scalability, and low cost features.

Results Step 4: Field testing of initial prototypes

The initial prototype was first tested with the Diabetes Research Advisory Group.

Most strikingly, the group stated the tool did not appear to be a true "decision aid" based on the benefits page alone, as they felt the decision was a "no-brainer" to choose medical therapy. Similar quotes were found among clinic patients who were asymptomatic; this was in stark contrast to those limited by angina, reinforcing the central nature of symptoms to this specific patient-centered decision making process. Based on this, we created two distinct decision aids that offered more personalized estimates of benefit for patients depending on the severity of their baseline angina.

The Cardiovascular Patient and Family Advisory group was comprised of many individuals with a history of PCI or coronary bypass surgery, and here we identified the challenge of communicating the lack of mortality benefit for patients who had already undergone PCI, as many members of the group believed in a mortality benefit of stents for stable CAD. Further modifications based on concerns raised by this group were made to emphasize the relevance of PCI Choice for stable, as compared to unstable, CAD.

Results Step 5: Successive iterations

In the real-word clinical encounters, over 20 patients with stable CAD were observed and interviewed while clinicians delivered iterative versions of the decision aid; 5 additional patients with a history of CAD were recruited from cardiac rehabilitation to provide feedback. We provided "just-in-time" training to the clinicians before the clinical encounter, reviewing the decision aid contents and recommending key concepts to reinforce.

Patients expressed an overwhelming preference for pictographs after we displayed benefit and risk in several ways, including shaded bars to depict relative differences between options, bar

Will having a stent placed in my heart prevent heart attacks or death?

NO. Stents will not lower the risk of heart attack or death when compared to using medicines alone.

How long will it take for me to feel better?

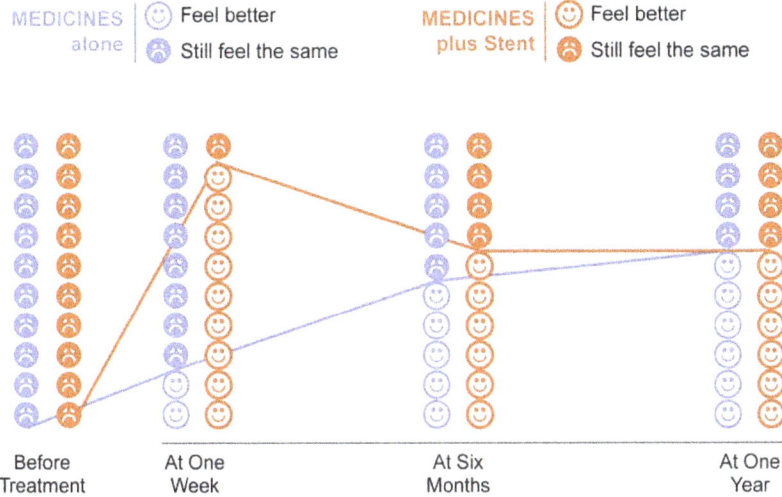

MEDICINES alone | 😊 Feel better | 😟 Still feel the same

MEDICINES plus Stent | 😊 Feel better | 😟 Still feel the same

Before Treatment   At One Week   At Six Months   At One Year

Figure 3. PCI Choice: early prototype of benefits page. Used with permission of Mayo Foundation for Medical Education and Research; Creative Commons License does not apply.

graphs in place of pictographs, and text-heavy descriptions. It became clear that the information central to the decision-making process was the benefit of PCI+OMT vs. OMT. This patient-based observation was striking, as risk was previously the focal point of discussions when considering PCI. Based on patient input, we added two sections: one on cross-over from medical therapy to PCI and another on risk of restenosis.

We found that excessive text limited the natural conversation between clinicians and patients, and thus focused on pictorial display. The number of graphs displaying risks was decreased due to a lack of patient interest in reviewing each individual risk. We inserted percentages next to the pictographs following observations of clinician difficulty with verbalizing graphical representation of data, which improved flow of the conversation. We placed a large-typed question at two points in the decision aid to lead both parties toward a discussion of patient goals and preferences.

The process of observing clinicians delivering the decision aid and directly interviewing patients regarding content and format of the decision aid was repeated over five months. Once the study team was satisfied, we met again with our patient advisory group, who approved the format and called the tool "enlightening." Finally, we were confident that the tool was likely to consistently create effective conversations around treatment choices for stable CAD and lead to decisions that reflected both the research evidence and the values and preferences of the informed patient. (Figure 4)

Discussion

Following the publication of comparative effectiveness research demonstrating no difference in death or MI with PCI+OMT for stable CAD compared to OMT, there has not been a substantial increase in the use of OMT [26]. Equally concerning is evidence of poor adherence with dual anti-platelet therapy following stent implantation, with the resulting risk in early to late stent thrombosis [27]. There is a growing literature base demonstrating overuse of coronary angiography and elective PCI [28,29], along with a call for a "pause" of ad hoc PCI to improve shared decision making [30]. With PCI being a common procedure (622 000 in 2007) [31] performed at a considerable cost (greater than $12 billion annually) [32], its appropriate use is a national health care priority [33]. Previous work clearly outlines misconceptions by patients regarding benefits of PCI, identifying an existing gap in the standard informed consent process [4,34]. We designed an individualized, patient-centered decision aid, PCI Choice, to assist clinicians and their patients considering PCI for stable CAD and to promote incorporation of patient values and preferences into decision making.

When examining the criteria for effective decision aids, PCI Choice addresses many of the key components of the International Patient Decision Aids Standards collaboration (IPDAS) including a systematic development process, presenting information on options and probabilities of outcomes, clarifying values, and using the scientific literature and patient stories on which to base the content, delivered in plain language [35].

Shared decision making tools can take many forms, including nurse-led group visits, personalized informed consent forms, videos, or decision coaches, among others [36,37,38]. For example, novel informed consent forms designed for use with patients undergoing angiography for stable angina successfully transfer knowledge about the mortality and bleeding risks associated with PCI and the benefit in target revascularization rates associated with drug-eluting vs. bare metal stents; these forms increase patient involvement in decision making across diverse sociodemographic groups [39]. However, decision aids, the type of tool used in this study, are distinct from traditional informed consent documents, with informed consent conventionally used once a treatment choice has been selected. Decision aids are

PCI Choice: Class I/II Stable Angina

This is a tool for you and your clinician to discuss treatment choices for stable angina. **In stable angina, stents are useful for symptom relief but do not reduce the risk of heart attack or death.** However, stents can reduce the risk of death in other heart diseases, such as unstable angina or heart attack.

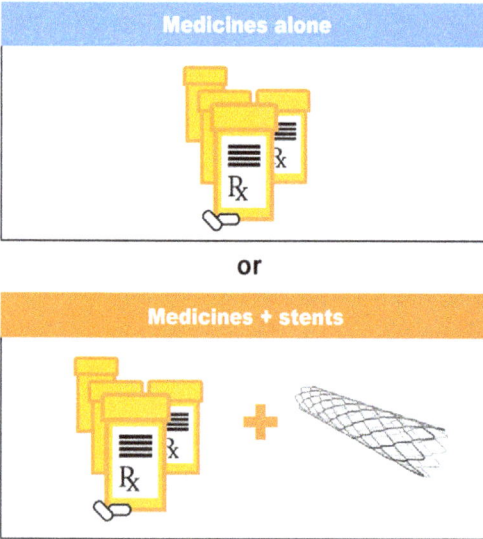

Medicines alone

or

Medicines + stents

Benefits

Prevention of heart attack or death in stable coronary artery disease with medicines + stents compared to medicines alone:

NO DIFFERENCE in heart attack or death.

How symptoms improve in 100 people with medicines + stents compared to medicines alone:

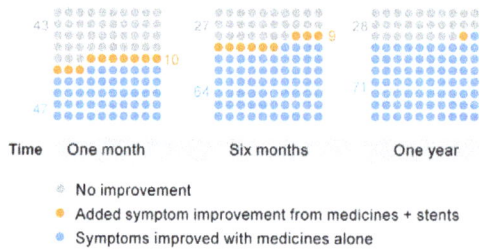

| Time | One month | Six months | One year |

43 / 10 / 47   27 / 9 / 64   28 / 1 / 71

◦ No improvement
● Added symptom improvement from medicines + stents
● Symptoms improved with medicines alone

Based upon the benefits, which choice do you prefer?

Risks

During the stent procedure:
Bleeding, heart attack, stroke or death

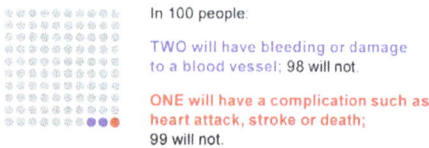

In 100 people:

TWO will have bleeding or damage to a blood vessel; 98 will not.

ONE will have a complication such as heart attack, stroke or death; 99 will not.

During the first year after stent:
Bleeding and heart attack

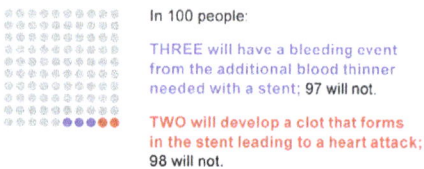

In 100 people:

THREE will have a bleeding event from the additional blood thinner needed with a stent; 97 will not.

TWO will develop a clot that forms in the stent leading to a heart attack; 98 will not.

Risks

During the first year after medicines alone or medicines + stents: Need for a procedure

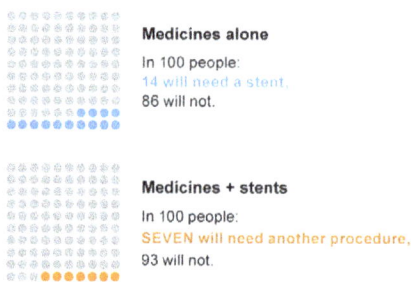

Medicines alone

In 100 people:
14 will need a stent; 86 will not.

Medicines + stents

In 100 people:
SEVEN will need another procedure, 93 will not.

Based upon the benefits and risks, which choice do you prefer?

Figure 4. PCI Choice: final prototype. Used with permission of Mayo Foundation for Medical Education and Research; Creative Commons License does not apply.

designed as an adjunct to a conversation that is already occurring between patient and clinician, helping to clarify and reinforce key issues specific to the individual patient as clinicians and patients select a treatment choice. Finally, decision aids differ from patient education materials, which are heavily text-based, designed to be read outside the clinical encounter, and are not tailored to the individual circumstances of the patient.

Conclusion

Significant misconceptions remain among patients with stable CAD regarding the benefits of PCI, a common, costly procedure that may be overused. In creating a patient-centered decision aid for stable CAD, we involved clinicians, health policy researchers, designers, patient focus groups and patients with stable angina to develop the best tool possible. We hypothesize that in an upcoming randomized trial, PCI Choice will lead to increased patient knowledge and patient involvement through effective translation of the best available comparative effectiveness evidence while incorporating patient values and preferences.

Acknowledgments

We are grateful for the generous contribution of members of the patient and family advisory groups, and of volunteer clinicians and patients who were willing to try the iterations of our prototype decision aids during their consultations while allowing our direct observation. We also appreciate the support of our colleagues from the Knowledge and Evaluation Research Unit and the Section of Creative Media at Mayo Clinic.

Author Contributions

Conceived and designed the experiments: MC VM HT. Performed the experiments: MC KS LP AL HT. Analyzed the data: MC KS LP AL HT. Contributed reagents/materials/analysis tools: KS AL EH NS VM HT. Wrote the paper: MC AL VM HT.

References

1. Stergiopoulos K, Brown DL (2012) Initial coronary stent implantation with medical therapy vs medical therapy alone for stable coronary artery disease: Meta-analysis of randomized controlled trials. Arch Intern Med 172: 312–319.
2. Brooks MM, Chung S-C, Helmy T, Hillegass WB, Escobedo J, et al. (2010) Health status after treatment for coronary artery disease and type 2 diabetes mellitus in the Bypass Angioplasty Revascularization Investigation 2 Diabetes Trial/Clinical perspective. Circulation 122: 1690–1699.
3. Weintraub WS, Spertus JA, Kolm P, Maron DJ, Zhang Z, et al. (2008) Effect of PCI on quality of life in patients with stable coronary disease. The New England Journal of Medicine 359: 677–687.
4. Rothberg MB, Sivalingam SK, Ashraf J, Visintainer P, Joelson J, et al. (2010) Patients' and cardiologists' perceptions of the benefits of percutaneous coronary intervention for stable coronary disease. Annals of Internal Medicine 153: 307–313.
5. O'Connor AM, Llewellyn-Thomas HA, Flood AB (2004) Modifying unwarranted variations in health care: Shared decision making using patient decision aids. Health Affairs.
6. Blankenship JC (2012) Progress toward doing the right thing. JACC: Cardiovascular Interventions 5: 236–238.
7. Breslin M, Mullan RJ, Montori VM (2008) The design of a decision aid about diabetes medications for use during the consultation with patients with type 2 diabetes. Patient Education and Counseling 73: 465–472.
8. Montori VM, Shah ND, Pencille LJ, Branda ME, Van Houten HK, et al. (2011) Use of a decision aid to improve treatment decisions in osteoporosis: The Osteoporosis Choice Randomized Trial. The American Journal of Medicine 124: 549–556.
9. Mullan RJ, Montori VM, Shah ND, Christianson TJ, Bryant SC, et al. (2009) The Diabetes Mellitus Medication Choice decision aid: A randomized trial. Archives of Internal Medicine 169: 1560–1568.
10. Pencille LJ, Campbell ME, Van Houten HK, Shah ND, Mullan RJ, et al. (2009) Protocol for the Osteoporosis Choice trial: A pilot randomized trial of a decision aid in primary care practice. Trials 10: 113.
11. Pierce M, Hess E, Kline J, Shah N, Breslin M, et al. (2010) The Chest Pain Choice trial: A pilot randomized trial of a decision aid for patients with chest pain in the emergency department. Trials 11: 57.
12. Montori VM, Breslin M, Maleska M, Weymiller AJ (2007) Creating a conversation: Insights from the development of a decision aid. PLoS Med 4: e233.
13. Hawley ST, Zikmund-Fisher B, Ubel P, Jancovic A, Lucas T, et al. (2008) The impact of the format of graphical presentation on health-related knowledge and treatment choices. Patient Education and Counseling 73: 448–455.
14. Kurz-Milcke E, Gigerenzer G, Martignon L (2008) Transparency in risk communication: Graphical and analog tools. Annals of the New York Academy of Sciences 1128: 18–28.
15. Kent DM, Shah ND (2011) Personalizing evidence-based primary prevention with aspirin: Individualized risks and patient preference. Circulation: Cardiovascular Quality and Outcomes 4: 260–262.
16. Coylewright M BM, Shah N, Hess E, LeBlanc A, Montori V, et al. (2012) Shared decision making increases patient knowledge across diverse patient subgroups: An encounter-level meta-analysis of six decision aid trials. American Heart Association Quality of Care and Outcomes Research Meeting. Atlanta, Georgia: Mayo Clinic.
17. Weymiller AJ, Montori VM, Jones LA, Gafni A, Guyatt GH, et al. (2007) Helping patients with type 2 diabetes mellitus make treatment decisions: Statin Choice randomized trial. Archives of internal medicine 167: 1076–1082.
18. Levine GN, Bates ER, Blankenship JC, Bailey SR, Bittl JA, et al. (2011) 2011 ACCF/AHA/SCAI guideline for percutaneous coronary intervention: A report of the American College of Cardiology Foundation/American Heart Association Task Force on Practice Guidelines and the Society for Cardiovascular Angiography and Interventions. Journal of the American College of Cardiology 58: e44–122.
19. Patel MR, Dehmer GJ, Hirshfeld JW, Smith PK, Spertus JA, et al. (2009) ACCF/SCAI/STS/AATS/AHA/ASNC 2009 Appropriateness criteria for coronary revascularization : A report of the American College of Cardiology Foundation Appropriateness Criteria Task Force, Society for Cardiovascular Angiography and Interventions, Society of Thoracic Surgeons, American Association for Thoracic Surgery, American Heart Association, and the American Society of Nuclear Cardiology. Endorsed by the American Society of Echocardiography, the Heart Failure Society of America, and the Society of Cardiovascular Computed Tomography. Catheterization and cardiovascular interventions : official journal of the Society for Cardiac Angiography & Interventions 73: E1–24.
20. Boden WE, O'Rourke RA, Teo KK, Hartigan PM, Maron DJ, et al. (2007) Optimal medical therapy with or without PCI for stable coronary disease. The New England Journal of Medicine 356: 1503–1516.
21. Coylewright M, Blumenthal RS, Post W (2008) Placing COURAGE in context: Review of the recent literature on managing stable coronary artery disease. Mayo Clinic Proceedings 83: 799–805.
22. Fleming LM, Novack V, Novack L, Cohen SA, Negoita M, et al. (2011) Frequency and impact of bleeding in elective coronary stent clinical trials: Utility of three commonly used definitions. Catheterization and Cardiovascular Interventions Nov 22.
23. Hansen ML, Sorensen R, Clausen MT, Fog-Petersen ML, Raunso J, et al. (2010) Risk of bleeding with single, dual, or triple therapy with warfarin, aspirin, and clopidogrel in patients with atrial fibrillation. Archives of Internal Medicine 170: 1433–1441.
24. Kandzari DE, Mauri L, Popma JJ, Turco MA, Gurbel PA, et al. (2011) Late-term clinical outcomes with zotarolimus- and sirolimus-eluting stents: 5-Year follow-up of the ENDEAVOR III (A randomized controlled trial of the Medtronic Endeavor drug [ABT-578] eluting coronary stent system versus the Cypher sirolimus-eluting coronary stent system in de novo native coronary artery lesions). JACC: Cardiovascular Interventions 4: 543–550.
25. Hannan EL, Samadashvili Z, Walford G, Holmes DR, Jacobs A, et al. (2009) Predictors and outcomes of ad hoc versus non-ad hoc percutaneous coronary interventions. JACC: Cardiovascular Interventions 2: 350–356.
26. Borden WB, Redberg RF, Mushlin AI, Dai D, Kaltenbach LA, et al. (2011) Patterns and intensity of medical therapy in patients undergoing percutaneous coronary intervention. JAMA : The Journal of the American Medical Association 305: 1882–1889.
27. Spertus JA, Kettelkamp R, Vance C, Decker C, Jones PG, et al. (2006) Prevalence, predictors, and outcomes of premature discontinuation of thienopyridine therapy after drug-eluting stent placement: Results from the PREMIER registry. Circulation 113: 2803–2809.
28. Korenstein D, Falk R, Howell EA, Bishop T, Keyhani S (2012) Overuse of health care services in the United States: An understudied problem. Archives of Internal Medicine 172: 171–178.
29. Chan PS, Patel MR, Klein LW, Krone RJ, Dehmer GJ, et al. (2011) Appropriateness of percutaneous coronary intervention. JAMA: The Journal of the American Medical Association 306: 53–61.
30. Nallamothu BK, Krumholz HM (2010) Putting ad hoc PCI on pause. JAMA : The Journal of the American Medical Association 304: 2059–2060.
31. Roger VL, Go AS, Lloyd-Jones DM, Adams RJ, Berry JD, et al. (2011) Heart disease and stroke statistics–2011 update: A report from the American Heart Association. Circulation 123: e18–e209.
32. Mahoney EM, Wang K, Arnold SV, Proskorovsky I, Wiviott S, et al. (2010) Cost-effectiveness of prasugrel versus clopidogrel in patients with acute coronary syndromes and planned percutaneous coronary intervention: Results from the trial to assess improvement in therapeutic outcomes by optimizing platelet inhibition with Prasugrel-Thrombolysis in Myocardial Infarction TRITON-TIMI 38. Circulation 121: 71–79.
33. Patel MR, Bailey SR, Bonow RO, Chambers CE, Chan PS, et al. (2012) ACCF/SCAI/AATS/AHA/ASE/ASNC/HFSA/HRS/SCCM/SCCT/SCMR/STS 2012 Appropriate use criteria for diagnostic catheterization: A report of the American College of Cardiology Foundation Appropriate Use Criteria Task Force, Society for Cardiovascular Angiography and Interventions, American Association for Thoracic Surgery, American Heart Association,

American Society of Echocardiography, American Society of Nuclear Cardiology, Heart Failure Society of America, Heart Rhythm Society, Society of Critical Care Medicine, Society of Cardiovascular Computed Tomography, Society for Cardiovascular Magnetic Resonance, and Society of Thoracic Surgeons. J Am Coll Cardiol 59: 1995–2027.

34. Chandrasekharan DP, Taggart DP (2011) Informed consent for interventions in stable coronary artery disease: Problems, etiologies, and solutions. European Journal of Cardio-Thoracic Surgery : Official Journal of the European Association for Cardio-Thoracic Surgery 39: 912–917.

35. O'Connor A, Llewellyn-Thomas H, Stacey D (2005) IPDAS Collaboration background document. In: Collaboration IPDAS, editor. pp. 54.

36. Arnold SV, Decker C, Ahmad H, Olabiyi O, Mundluru S, et al. (2008) Converting the informed consent from a perfunctory process to an evidence-based foundation for patient decision making/Clinical Perspective. Circulation: Cardiovascular Quality and Outcomes 1: 21–28.

37. Astley CM, Chew DP, Aylward PE, Molloy DA, De Pasquale CG (2008) A randomised study of three different informational aids prior to coronary angiography, measuring patient recall, satisfaction and anxiety. Heart, Lung and Circulation 17: 25–32.

38. Dontje K, Kelly-Blake K, Olomu A, Rothert M, Dwamena F, et al. (2012) Nurse-led group visits support shared decision making in stable coronary artery disease. The Journal of Cardiovascular Nursing.

39. Coylewright M GK, McNulty EJ, Spertus J, Ting HH (2012) Sociodemographic factors minimally impact patient experience with informed consent documents for percutaneous coronary intervention. Atlanta, Georgia: American Heart Association Quality Care and Outcomes Research Meeting.

13

Coronary Collateral Circulation in Patients of Coronary Ectasia with Significant Coronary Artery Disease

Po-Chao Hsu[1,2,6], Ho-Ming Su[1,6,7], Hsiang-Chun Lee[1,2], Suh-Hang Juo[3,4,5], Tsung-Hsien Lin[1,6*], Wen-Chol Voon[1,6], Wen-Ter Lai[1,6], Sheng-Hsiung Sheu[1,6]

1 Division of Cardiology, Department of Internal Medicine, Kaohsiung Medical University Hospital, Kaohsiung Medical University, Kaohsiung, Taiwan, 2 Graduate Institute of Medicine, College of Medicine, Kaohsiung Medical University, Kaohsiung, Taiwan, 3 Department of Medical Research, Kaohsiung Medical University Hospital, Kaohsiung Medical University, Kaohsiung, Taiwan, 4 Medical Genetics, Kaohsiung Medical University, Kaohsiung, Taiwan, 5 Center of Excellence for Environmental Medicine, Kaohsiung Medical University, Kaohsiung, Taiwan, 6 Faculty of Medicine, College of Medicine, Kaohsiung Medical University, Kaohsiung, Taiwan, 7 Department of Internal Medicine, Kaohsiung Municipal Hsiao-Kang Hospital, Kaohsiung, Taiwan

Abstract

Objectives: Patients with coronary ectasia (CE) usually have coexisting coronary stenosis resulting in myoischemia. Coronary collateral plays an important role in protecting myocardium from ischemia and reducing cardiovascular events. However, limited studies investigate the role of CE in coronary collaterals development.

Methods: We evaluated 1020 consecutive patients undergoing coronary angiography and 552 patients with significant coronary artery disease (SCAD), defined as diameter stenosis more than 70%, were finally analyzed. CE is defined as the ectatic diameter 1.5 times larger than adjacent reference segment. Rentrop collateral score was used to classify patients into poor (grades 0 and 1) or good (grades 2 and 3) collateral group.

Results: 73 patients (13.2%) had CE lesions which were most located in the right coronary artery (53.4%). Patients with CE had a lower incidence of diabetes (43.8% vs 30.1%, p = 0.03), higher body mass index (25.4±3.5 vs 26.7±4.6, p = 0.027) and poorer coronary collateral (58.2% vs 71.2%, p = 0.040). Patients with poor collateral (n = 331) had a higher incidence of CE (15.7% vs 9.5%, p = 0.040) and fewer diseased vessels numbers (1.96±0.84 vs 2.48±0.69, p<0.001). Multivariate analysis showed diabetes (odd ratio (OR) 0.630, p = 0.026), CE (OR = 0.544, p = 0.048), and number of diseased vessels (OR = 2.488, p<0.001) were significant predictors of coronary collaterals development.

Conclusion: The presence of CE was associated with poorer coronary collateral development in patients with SCAD.

Editor: Claudio Moretti, S.G.Battista Hospital, Italy

Funding: The authors have no support or funding to report.

Competing Interests: The authors have declared that no competing interests exist.

* E-mail: lth@kmu.edu.tw

Introduction

Coronary ectasia (CE) is an uncommon disease and its incidence has been reported as between 0.3 and 5% in different studies despite some exception [1–5]. It is defined as the diameter of the ectatic segment being more than 1.5 times larger compared with an adjacent healthy reference segment [2]. Most cases of CE are considered as a variant of coronary artery disease (CAD) [6]. The pathogenesis of CE is not completely illustrated. However, it is likely to involve the destruction of the arterial media, increased wall stress, thinning of the arterial wall, and progressive dilatation of the coronary artery segment [7].

The development of coronary collaterals is an adaptive response to chronic myoischemia and serves as a conduit bridging the significantly stenotic coronary vessels [8–10]. Collateral circulation can hence protect and preserve myocardium from episodes of ischemia, enhance residual myocardial contractility, and reduce angina symptoms and cardiovascular events [11–13]. However, there is inter-individual difference of coronary collateral formation and the mechanisms for the different individual ability to develop collateral circulation are still unclear.

Because CE are usually associated with atherosclerosis and even obstructive CAD resulting coronary ischemia, whether the presence of good coronary collateral or not is a very important issue for the CE population [2,6]. However, there were limited literatures discussing the coronary collateral formation in the CE population. Therefore we designed this study to investigate the role of CE in patients with obstructive CAD.

Patients and Methods

Study subjects

We evaluated 1020 patients scheduled for diagnostic coronary angiography from the Kaohsiung Medical University Hospital (KMUH) in Taiwan. Patients with coronary artery lumen diameter stenosis <70%, history of coronary artery bypass surgery (CABG), history of percutaneous coronary intervention (PCI), inadequate angiograms for CE evaluation were excluded. Finally

552 patients were recruited in our study. We collected patients' demographic and baseline information including sex, age, body mass index (BMI), duration of chest pain, history of diabetes, hypertension, hypercholesterolemia, and cigarette smoking.

Ethics Statement

The research protocol was approved and registered by the Institutional Review Board of the Kaohsiung Medical University Hospital (KMUH-IRB). Informed consents were obtained in written form from patients and all clinical investigation was conducted according to the principles expressed in the Declaration of Helsinki. The patients gave consent for the publication of the clinical details.

Coronary angiography

The coronary artery angiography films were reviewed by two experienced cardiologists blind to patients' clinical characteristics. A third reviewer blinded to the readings of the first two reviewers served as arbitrator of differences. Coronary angiography was performed by the femoral or radial approach with 6Fr diagnostic catheters. Images were recorded in multiple projections for left and right coronary arteries. Coronary artery stenosis was determined by quantitative coronary angiography. The presence of significant coronary artery disease (SCAD) is defined as coronary diameter stenosis more than 70%. CE is defined as the diameter of the ectatic segment being more than 1.5 times larger compared with an adjacent healthy reference segment [2]. The classification of CE developed by Markis et al. and based on the extent of ectatic involvement was used [14]. In decreasing order of severity, diffuse CE of two or three vessels was classified as Type I, diffuse disease in one vessel and localized disease in another vessel as Type II, diffuse CE of one vessel only as Type III and localized or segmental ectasia as Type IV. The recorded data also included the location, number of CAD and CE, percentage of stenosis of diseased vessels, the vessel to which the collaterals were connected, the grade of coronary collateral circulation, and the coronary artery disease severity scoring.

Collateral scoring and pathways evaluation by coronary angiography

In subjects with more than one SCAD vessel, the vessel with the highest collateral grade was chosen for analysis. The collateral scoring system developed by Rentrop and Cohen was used [15]. Grades of collateral filling from the contralateral vessel were: 0 = none; 1 = filling of side branches of the artery to be dilated via collateral channels without visualization of the epicardial segment; 2 = partial filling of the epicardial segment via collateral channels; 3 = complete filling of the epicardial segment of the artery being dilated via collateral channels. In subjects with more than one collateral vessel supplying the distal aspect of the diseased artery, the highest collateral grade was recorded. Patients were then classified according to their collateral grades as either poor (grade 0 or grade 1 collateral) or good (grade 2 or grade 3 collateral). In addition, the size of the collateral connection (CC) diameter was assessed by 3 grades: CC grade 0, no continuous connection between donor and recipient artery; CC grade 1, continuous, threadlike connection, and CC grade 2, continuous, small side branch-like size of the collateral throughout its course [16]. In the case of coexisting collateral connections, the prominent one was defined as the principal. The anatomic pathways were categorized according to Levin's pathways and summarized in 4 categories: septal, intra-arterial (bridging), epicardial with proximal takeoff (atrial branches), and epicardial with distal takeoff [10,17]. In the

case of coexisting collateral pathways, the principal pathway was defined as the one that was the first to opacify the stenotic epicardial segments.

Statistical analysis

All data were expressed as means ± standard deviation. Independent t test was used to compare continuous variables between the two groups. Chi-square test was used to compare categorical data. Subsequently, significantly correlated variables in the univariate analysis or relevant variables were further analyzed by binary logistic regression analysis to predict the collateral development (good vs. poor). All p values were two-sided with a significance level of $p<.05$. The Statistical Package for the Social Sciences 11.0 for Windows (SPSS Inc.,Chicago, IL) was used for statistical analysis.

Results

Clinical characteristics

Among the 1020 subjects initially evaluated, 468 patients were excluded for the following reasons: coronary artery lumen diameter stenosis <70%, history of CABG or PCI, or inadequate angiograms for collateral evaluation. The final study population was 552 subjects (443 male and 109 female; average age, 62.5 ± 12.5 years old). Regarding numbers of diseased vessels, 148 patients (26.8%) were 1 vessel disease (VD), 163 patients (29.5%) were 2VD, and 241 patients (43.7%) were 3VD.

Coronary ectasia and collaterals

There were 73 patients (13.2%) with CE with 24 patients (32.9%) 1VD, 26 (35.6%) 2VD, and 23 (31.5%) 3VD. Table 1 summarizes the angiographic characteristics of the patients with CE. 55 (75.3%) patients had CE involving one major vessel (right coronary artery: 39 patients, left anterior descending artery: 3 patient, left circumflex artery: 13 patients); 13 (17.8%) patients had CE involving two major vessel (right coronary artery and left anterior descending artery: 5 patients, right coronary artery and left circumflex artery: 7 patients, left anterior descending artery and left circumflex artery: 1 patients); 5 (6.8%) patients had CE involving all three vessels. For type of CE, 14 (19.2%) patients were type 1, 4 (5.5%) patients were type 2, 50 (68.5%) patients were type 3, and 5 (6.8%) patients were type 4. For coronary collateral grade and pathway evaluation, the 2 collaterals readers obtained a 96% agreement in the collateral classifications. Of the 73 patients with CE, the Rentrop coronary grade was distributed as follows: 40 (54.8%) patients with grade 0, 12 (16.4%) patients with grade 1, 13 (17.8%) patients with grade 2, and 8 (11%) patients with grade 3. The CC grade was distributed as follows: 49 (67.1%) patients with CC grade 0, 19 (26%) patients with CC grade 1, and 5 (6.8%) patients with CC grade 2. Furthermore, for the collateral pathways: the principal pathways was through septal connections in 57.6%, atrial-epicardial connections in 27.3%, bridging connections in 9.1%, and distal inter-arterial connections in 6.1%.

Baseline characteristics in patients with and without CE were shown in the Table 2. The patients with CE (n = 73) had a lower incidence of DM (30.1% vs 43.8%, p = 0.030), higher BMI (26.7 ± 4.6 vs 25.4 ± 3.5, p = 0.027), and poor coronary collateral (71.2% vs 58.2%, p = 0.040). The multivariate regression analysis of coronary collateral formation (good vs poor collateral) in CE population with SCAD and found that only number of diseased vessels (OR = 2.358, 95% CI = 1.148–4.843, p = 0.02) was a significant independent predictor of coronary collaterals development (Table 3).

Table 1. Angiographic Characteristics of the Patients With Coronary Ectasia.

Ectasia(s) location	N (%)
Right coronary artery	39 (53.4%)
Left anterior descending artery	3 (4.1%)
Left circumflex artery	13 (17.8%)
Right coronary artery + left anterior descending artery	5 (6.8%)
Right coronary artery + left circumflex artery	7 (9.6%)
Left anterior descending artery + left circumflex artery	1 (1.4%)
All three vessels	5 (6.8%)
Number of vessel(s) with coronary ectasia(s)	
1	55 (75.3%)
2	13 (17.8%)
3	5 (6.8%)
Type of coronary ectasia	
Type 1	14 (19.2%)
Type 2	4 (5.5%)
Type 3	50 (68.5%)
Type 4	5 (6.8%)
Rentrop collateral grade	
Grade 0	40 (54.8%)
Grade 1	12 (16.4%)
Grade 2	13 (17.8%)
Grade 3	8 (11%)
Collateral connection grades	
CC0	49 (67.1%)
CC1	19 (26%)
CC2	5 (6.8%)
Collateral pathway	
Septal	19 (57.6%)
Atrial-epicardial	9 (27.3%)
Bridging	3 (9.1%)
Distal inter-arterial	2 (6.1%)

CC, collateral connection

Table 2. Baseline Characteristics between Patients without and with Coronary Ectasia.

Parameters N (%)	Control (n = 479)	Ectasia (n = 73)	p Value
Sex (male)	379 (79.1)	64 (87.7)	0.113
Age (years)	62.8±12.1	60.3±14.8	0.174
DM	210 (43.8)	22 (30.1)	0.030
Hypertension	312 (65.1)	47 (64.4)	0.896
Smoking	280 (58.6)	50 (68.5)	0.124
Family history	16 (3.4)	2 (2.7)	1.000
Hypercholesterolemia (%)	264 (56.3)	36 (49.3)	0.311
CAD number			0.080
1-vessel disease	124 (25.9)	24 (32.9)	
2-vessel disease	137 (28.6)	26 (35.6)	
3-vessel disease	218 (45.5)	23 (31.5)	
BMI	25.4±3.5	26.7±4.6	0.027
Poor Collateral, n (%)	279 (58.2%)	52 (71.2%)	0.040

Data are presented as mean ± standard deviation or number (%); CAD, coronary artery disease; DM, diabetes mellitus; BMI, body mass index;

significant association between treatment strategies and presence of good or poor coronary collaterals (p = 0.284).

Discussion

There were three major findings in the present study. First, most CE lesion were located in the right coronary artery. Second, CE patients with significant coronary artery disease have poor coronary collateral development compared with non-CE patients. Third, CE is a significantly independent predictor of poor coronary collaterals in patients with SCAD.

The association between CE and coronary collaterals

CE is a variant of coronary artery abnormality [6]. It may be congenital or acquired. Acquired causes include atherosclerosis, Kawasaki disease, various inflammatory and infectious diseases, and so on [2–6]. However, most cases of CE are associated with atherosclerosis and had coexistence of obstructive CAD [2,6]. It

Coronary collaterals development in the whole population

Baseline characteristics in patients with poor and good collateral were shown in the Table 4, the patients with poor collateral (n = 331) had a higher incidence of CE (15.7% vs 9.5%, p = 0.040), and a fewer diseased vessels numbers (1.96±0.84 vs 2.48+0.69, p<0.001). Table 5 showed the multivariate analysis of coronary collateral formation (good vs poor collateral) in whole population with SCAD. We found diabetes (OR = 0.619, 95% CI = 0.410–0.934, p = 0.022), coronary ectasia (OR = 0.544, 95% CI = 0.297–0.996, p = 0.048), and number of diseased vessels (OR = 2.488, 95% CI = 1.917–3.228, p<0.001) were significant independent predictors of coronary collaterals development.

Treatment strategies in CE patients

Among the 73 patients with CE, 58 patients (79.5%) received PCI, 8 patients (11%) received CABG, and 7 patients (9.6%) only received medical treatment for the coronary lesions. There was no

Table 3. Multivariate logistic regression analysis of collateral circulation in CE population (poor collateral group as reference group).

	OR	95% CI	p Value
Sex (male vs female)	-	-	0.896
Age	-	-	0.110
Hypertension	-	-	0.881
DM	-	-	0.178
Smoking	-	-	0.330
Hypercholesterolemia	-	-	0.291
BMI	-	-	0.652
Number of diseased vessels	2.358	1.148–4.843	0.020

BMI, body mass index; CE, coronary ectasia; DM, diabetes mellitus

Table 4. Baseline Characteristics between good and poor collaterals.

Parameters N (%)	Poor (n = 331)	Good (n = 221)	p Value
Sex (male)	263 (79.5%)	180 (81.4%)	0.587
Age (years)	62.6±13.0	62.4±11.8	0.815
DM	143 (43.2%)	89 (40.3%)	0.538
Hypertension	214 (64.7%)	145 (65.6%)	0.856
Smoking	201 (60.7%)	129 (58.6%)	0.658
Family history	7 (2.1%)	11 (5.0%)	0.086
Hypercholesterolemia (%)	169 (52.3%)	131 (59.8%)	0.095
CAD number	1.96±0.84	2.48±0.69	<0.001
1-vessel disease	123 (37.2)	25 (11.3)	
2-vessel disease	97 (29.3)	66 (29.9)	
3-vessel disease	111 (33.5)	130 (58.8)	
BMI	25.5±3.74	25.7±3.6	0.553
Coronary ectasia, n (%)	52 (15.7%)	21 (9.5%)	0.040

Data are presented as mean ± standard deviation or number (%); CAD, coronary artery disease; DM, diabetes mellitus; BMI, body mass index

Table 5. Multivariate logistic regression analysis of collateral circulation in whole population (poor collateral group as reference group).

	OR	95% CI	p Value
Sex (male vs female)	-	-	0.395
Age	-	-	0.675
Hypertension	-	-	0.879
DM	0.619	0.410–0.934	0.022
Hypercholesterolemia	-	-	0.361
Smoking	-	-	0.270
BMI	-	-	0.318
Coronary ectasia	0.544	0.297–0.996	0.048
Number of diseased vessels	2.488	1.917–3.228	<0.001

BMI, body mass index; DM, diabetes mellitus

was considered to be a variant of CAD and is associated with the similar risk as the patients with CAD [2,14,18–19]. The clinical presentation and the long-term cardiac complications are associated with the severity of coexisting CAD [20]. Even in patients with isolated CE without coronary stenosis, there is still higher incidence of adverse events in this population compared to people with normal coronary arteries. The pathogenesis of CE is not completely understood, however, it is likely to involve the destruction of the arterial media, increased wall stress, thinning of the arterial wall, and progressive dilatation of the coronary artery segment[7]. The presence of ectatic segments produces sluggish blood flow, with exercise-induced angina and myocardial infarction, regardless of the severity of coexisting obstructive CAD [14. 18–19]. The possible causes of higher adverse events might be related to the repeated dissemination of microemboli to distal segments, or thrombotic occlusion of the dilated vessel. In addition, slow blood flow in the ectatic coronary arteries might be another cause which predisposes to the occurrence of AMI. Disturbances in blood flow filling and washout in the ectatic vessels were due to inappropriate coronary dilatation and were clearly associated with the severity of CE [21]. The turbulent and stagnant blood flow could induce endothelial damage, increase wall stress, and even cause extensive thrombosis. In past literature, all three coronary arteries can be affected by CE, but most patients had single-vessel involvement [22.23]. Furthermore, In CE patients with coexistent CAD, the right coronary artery is the most frequently involved. These findings were also similar with our current study.

The development of coronary collaterals can reduce angina and infarct size, preserve left ventricular ejection fraction, decrease aneurysmal dilatation, and provide a survival benefit in patients with SCAD [11–13]. However, there are limited studies discussing about the coronary collateral formation in the CE population and most of the studies were focused on the young patients with Kawasaki disease [24–25]. In children with Kawasaki disease, Onouchi Z et al. reported that coronary collaterals did not develop in the presence of localized stenosis regardless of the occurrence of

myocardial ischemia, but total occluded vessels had collateral development regardless of the presence of myocardial infarction [24]. Tatara K et al. also indicated that collateral circulation cannot be seen angiographically unless there is total occlusion and the presence of collateral circulation cannot provide protection against stress-induced myocardial ischemia [25]. These findings all suggest that relative poor collateral formation in the patients with etiology of Kawasaki disease. Despite of the etiologies different from previous studies, our study showed that CE is significantly associated with poor coronary collateral formation both in univariate and multivariate analysis. Although CE is reported to be associated with increased plasma levels of inflammatory markers, cytokines, and oxidative stress, the detailed mechanism of poor coronary collateral development is not well understood nowadays and may need further investigation in the future [26–28].

In addition, number of diseased vessels was not only a significant predictor of coronary collateral formation in the patients with SCAD, but also the only significant predictor in the CE population with SCAD. It is well known that coronary collateral formation is mainly dependent on the CAD severity [29–31]. Patients with good coronary collaterals appear to have a more extensive CAD. In previous studies, number of diseased vessels is a significant predictor of good collateral formation [32,33]. Hence, extent of coronary atherosclerosis significantly plays an important role in coronary collateral formation.

Limitations of the present study

First, the collateral formation was assessed by coronary angiography in this study. Measuring collateral flow index by intravascular Doppler guidewire may provide a more objective physiological measurement of collateral grade. However, the invasiveness of intravascular ultrasound limits its use in large-scale studies. Second, since this was only a clinical association study, potential mechanisms were not fully elucidated and long term follow-up of clinical outcome data will be needed to see whether CE patients with poorer coronary collaterals have higher incidence of cardiovascular adverse events in the future.

Conclusions

To our best, our study is the first study to show the poor coronary collateral development in the adult patients with CE and SCAD. Our data might partially explain why patients with CE have higher incidence of cardiovascular adverse events.

Author Contributions

Conceived and designed the experiments: PCH THL. Performed the experiments: PCH HMS THL SHS. Analyzed the data: HCL SHJ WCV WTL. Contributed reagents/materials/analysis tools: PCH HMS THL SHS. Wrote the paper: PCH THL.

References

1. Oliveros RA, Falsetti HL, Carroll RJ, Heinle RA, Ryan GF (1974) Atherosclerotic coronary artery aneurysm: report of five cases and a review of the literature. Arch Intern Med 134: 1072–1076.
2. Swaye PS, Fisher LD, Litwin P, Vignola PA, Judkins MP, et al. (1983) Aneurysmal coronary artery disease. Circulation 67: 134–138.
3. Hartnell GG, Parnell BM, Pridie RB (1985) Coronary artery ectasia. Its prevalence and clinical significance in 4993 patients. Br Heart J 54(4): 392–5.
4. Yilmaz H, Sayar N, Yilmaz M, Tangürek B, Cakmak N, et al. (2008) Coronary artery ectasia: clinical and angiographical evaluation. Turk Kardiyol Dern Ars 36: 530–535.
5. Sharma SN, Kaul U, Sharma S, Wasir HS, Manchanda SC, et al. (1990) Coronary arteriographic profile in young and old Indian patients with ischaemic heart disease: a comparative study. Indian Heart J 42(5): 365–9.
6. Swanton RH, Thomas ML, Coltart DJ, Jenkins BS, Webb-Peploe MM, et al. (1978) Coronary artery ectasia—a variant of occlusive coronary arteriosclerosis. Br Heart J 40(4): 393–400.
7. Rodbars S, Ikeda K, Montes M (1967) An analysis of mechanisms of poststenotic dilatation. Angiology 18: 349–353.
8. Fujita M, Sasayama S, Ohno A, Nakajima H, Asanoi H (1987) Importance of angina for development of collateral circulation. Br Heart J 57: 139.
9. Tayebjee MH, Lip GY, MacFadyen RJ (2004) Collateralization and the response to obstruction of epicardial coronary arteries. QJM 97: 259.
10. Levin DC (1974) Pathways and functional significance of the coronary collateral circulation. Circulation 50: 831–7.
11. Cohen M, Rentrop KP (1986) Limitation of myocardial ischemia by collateral circulation during sudden controlled coronary artery occlusion in human subjects: a prospective study. Circulation 74(3): 469–76.
12. Meier P, Gloekler S, Zbinden R, Beckh S, de Marchi SF, et al. (2007) Beneficial effect of recruitable collaterals: a 10-year follow-up study in patients with stable coronary artery disease undergoing quantitative collateral measurements. Circulation 116(9): 975–83.
13. Regieli JJ, Jukema JW, Nathoe HM, Zwinderman AH, Ng S, et al. (2009) Coronary collaterals improve prognosis in patients with ischemic heart disease. Int J Cardiol 132(2): 257–62.
14. Markis JE, Joffe CD, Cohn PF, Fen DJ, Herman MV, et al. (1976) Clinical significance of coronary artery ectasia. Am J Cardiol 37: 217–222.
15. Rentrop KP, Cohen M, Blanke H, Phillips RA (1985) Changes in collateral channel filling immediately after controlled coronary artery occlusion by an angioplasty balloon in human subjects. J Am Coll Cardiol 5(3): 587–92.
16. Werner GS, Ferrari M, Heinke S, Kuethe F, Surber R, et al. (2003) Angiographic assessment of collateral connections in comparison with invasively determined collateral function in chronic coronary occlusions. Circulation 107: 1972–7.
17. Brown G, Rockstroh J (2002) Coronary collateral size, flow capacity, and growth estimates from the angiogram in patients with obstructive coronary disease. Circulation 105: 168–73.
18. Befeler B, Aranda JM, Embi A, Mullin F, Ei-Sherif N, et al. (1977) Coronary artery aneurysms: Study of their etiology, clinical course and effect on left ventricular function and prognosis. Am J Cardiol 62: 597–607.
19. Demopoulos VP, Olympios CD, Fakiolas CN, Pissimissis EG, Economides NM, et al. (1997) The natural history of aneurysmal coronary artery disease. Heart 78: 136–141.
20. Manginas A, Cokkinos DV (2006) Coronary artery ectasias: imaging, functional assessment and clinical implications. Eur Heart J 27(9): 1026–31.
21. Mavrogeni S (2010) Coronary artery ectasia: from diagnosis to treatment. Hellenic J Cardiol 51(2): 158–63.
22. Daoud AS, Pankin D, Tulgan H, Florentin RA (1963) Aneurysms of the coronary artery. Report of ten cases and review of literature. Am J Cardiol 11: 228–237.
23. al-Harthi SS, Nouh MS, Arafa M, al-Nozha M (1991) Aneurysmal dilatation of the coronary arteries: diagnostic patterns and clinical significance. Int J Cardiol 30: 191–194.
24. Onouchi Z, Hamaoka K, Kamiya Y, Hayashi S, Ohmochi Y, et al. (1993) Transformation of coronary artery aneurysm to obstructive lesion and the role of collateral vessels in myocardial perfusion in patients with Kawasaki disease. J Am Coll Cardiol 21(1): 158–62.
25. Tatara K, Kusakawa S, Itoh K, Honma S, Hashimoto K, et al. (1991) Collateral circulation in Kawasaki disease with coronary occlusion or severe stenosis. Am Heart J 121: 797–802.
26. Ozbay Y, Akbulut M, Balin M, Kayancicek H, Baydas A, et al. (2007) The level of hs-CRP in coronary artery ectasia and its response to statin and angiotensin-converting enzyme inhibitor treatment. Mediators Inflamm 89649.
27. Li JJ, Nie SP, Qian XW, Zeng HS, Zhang CY (2009) Chronic inflammatory status in patients with coronary artery ectasia. Cytokine 46(1): 61–4.
28. Sezen Y, Bas M, Polat M, Yildiz A, Buyukhatipoglu H, et al. (2010) The relationship between oxidative stress and coronary artery ectasia. Cardiol J 17(5): 488–94.
29. Abaci A, Oğuzhan A, Kahraman S, Eryol NK, Unal S, et al. (1999) Effect of diabetes mellitus on formation of coronary collateral vessels. Circulation 99(17): 2239–2242.
30. Helfant RH, Kemp HG, Gorlin R (1970) Coronary atherosclerosis, coronary collaterals, and their relation to cardiac function. Ann Intern Med 73: 189–193.
31. Sezer M, Ozcan M, Okular I, Elitok A, Umman S, et al. (2007) A potential evidence to explain the reason behind the devastating prognosis of coronary artery disease in uraemic patients: renal insufficiency is associated with poor coronary collateral vessel development. Int J Cardiol 115(3): 366–372.
32. Gulec S, Ozdemir AO, Maradit-Kremers H, Dincer I, Atmaca Y, et al. (2006) Elevated levels of C-reactive protein are associated with impaired coronary collateral development. Eur J Clin Invest 36(6): 369–75.
33. Resar JR, Roguin A, Voner J, Nasir K, Hennebry TA, et al. (2005) Hypoxia-inducible factor 1alpha polymorphism and coronary collaterals in patients with ischemic heart disease. Chest 128(2): 787–91.

14

Viral Cross-Class Serpin Inhibits Vascular Inflammation and T Lymphocyte Fratricide; A Study in Rodent Models In Vivo and Human Cell Lines In Vitro

Kasinath Viswanathan[1,9], Ilze Bot[2,3,9], Liying Liu[1,4], Erbin Dai[1,4], Peter C. Turner[5], Babajide Togonu-Bickersteth[1,4], Jakob Richardson[1], Jennifer A. Davids[5], Jennifer M. Williams[4], Mee Y. Bartee[4,5], Hao Chen[4], Theo J. C. van Berkel[2,3], Erik A. L. Biessen[2,3], Richard W. Moyer[5], Alexandra R. Lucas[1,4,5*]

1 Vascular Biology Research Group, Robarts' Research Institute, London, Canada, 2 Division of Biopharmaceutics, Leiden/Amsterdam Center for Drug Research, Leiden, The Netherlands, 3 University of Maastracht, Maastracht, The Netherlands, 4 Department of Medicine, Divisions of Cardiovascular Medicine and Rheumatology, University of Florida, Gainesville, Florida, United States of America, 5 Department of Molecular Genetics and Microbiology, University of Florida, Gainesville, Florida, United States of America

Abstract

Poxviruses express highly active inhibitors, including *serine proteinase inhibitors* (*serpins*), designed to target host immune defense pathways. Recent work has demonstrated clinical efficacy for a secreted, myxomaviral serpin, Serp-1, which targets the thrombotic and thrombolytic proteases, suggesting that other viral serpins may have therapeutic application. Serp-2 and CrmA are intracellular cross-class poxviral serpins, with entirely distinct functions from the Serp-1 protein. Serp-2 and CrmA block the serine protease granzyme B (GzmB) and cysteine proteases, caspases 1 and 8, in apoptotic pathways, but have not been examined for extracellular anti-inflammatory activity. We examined the ability of these cross-class serpins to inhibit plaque growth after arterial damage or transplant and to reduce leukocyte apoptosis. We observed that purified Serp-2, but not CrmA, given as a systemic infusion after angioplasty, transplant, or cuff-compression injury markedly reduced plaque growth in mouse and rat models *in vivo*. Plaque growth was inhibited both locally at sites of surgical trauma, angioplasty or transplant, and systemically at non-injured sites in ApoE-deficient hyperlipidemic mice. With analysis *in vitro* of human cells in culture, Serp-2 selectively inhibited T cell caspase activity and blocked cytotoxic T cell (CTL) mediated killing of T lymphocytes (termed fratricide). Conversely, both Serp-2 and CrmA inhibited monocyte apoptosis. Serp-2 inhibitory activity was significantly compromised either *in vitro* with GzmB antibody or *in vivo* in ApoE/GzmB double knockout mice. ***Conclusions*** The viral cross-class serpin, Serp-2, that targets both apoptotic and inflammatory pathways, reduces vascular inflammation in a GzmB-dependent fashion *in vivo*, and inhibits human T cell apoptosis *in vitro*. These findings indicate that therapies targeting Granzyme B and/or T cell apoptosis may be used to inhibit T lymphocyte apoptosis and inflammation in response to arterial injury.

Editor: Santanu Bose, The University of Texas Health Science Center at San Antonio, United States of America

Funding: This work was funded by research grants from the Canadian Institutes of Health research (CIHR), the Heart and Stroke foundation of Ontario (HSFO), the National Institutes of Health (NIH) ARRA grant 1RC1HL100202–01, and the American Heart Association (AHA) grant 0855421 E. The funders had no role in study design, data collection and analysis, decision to publish, or preparation of the manuscript.

Competing Interests: ARL is the chief clinical officer and holds shares in a small Biotechnology company, Viron Therapeutics, Inc in London, Canada, which is developing another viral serpin for clinical use. The cross-class serpins in this paper have different molecular targets and are not in any way connected to, nor under development by, this biotech company.

* E-mail: alexandra.lucas@medicine.ufl

9 These authors contributed equally to this work.

Introduction

Serine protease inhibitors or *serpins* have extensive regulatory actions, moderating thrombotic and immune responses [1,2]. Poxviruses encode highly active serpins, including a secreted serpin Serp-1, which inhibits extracellular thrombolytic and thrombotic proteases and markedly reduces arterial inflammation and plaque growth in animal models [2–4]. This serpin, when injected as a purified protein, also significantly reduces markers of myocardial damage after stent implant in patients with unstable coronary syndromes [5]. These studies suggest that other viral serpins may have therapeutic potential. With the studies reported

herein we explore a second class of viral cross-class serpins with different protease targets that block apoptosis and inflammation.

Serp-2, encoded by myxoma [6,7], and CrmA (cytokine response modifier-A) encoded by cowpox [8,9] are poxviral cross-class serpins that inhibit the serine protease, granzyme B, and cysteine proteases, caspases 1 and 8. These serpins are purportedly intracellular defense proteins; however, both serpins inhibit pathways with potential extracellular activity. CrmA is a more potent inhibitor *in vitro*, binding caspase 1, caspase 8, and granzyme B (GzmB), with greater inhibition in chicken chorioallantoic membranes [8-11]. In contrast, Serp-2 binds caspases 1 and GzmB with lower affinity *in vitro* [6,7,10,11], but has greater effects on viral virulence *in vivo* in rabbits infected with Serp-2 deficient myxomavirus [6–8,11].

Key pathways to cellular apoptosis, also termed programmed cell death, are mediated by serine and cysteine proteases [10,12–18]. Caspases are cysteine proteases, some of which drive intracellular apoptotic pathways, whereas the serine protease GzmB is released by activated T cells into the surrounding medium and inserted into target cells. GzmB initiates apoptosis, either via interaction with perforin or through less defined pathways [13,16–22]. Granzyme B thus has both intracellular and extracellular activities, initiating two-tiered caspase activation in which caspases 3, 7, 8, and Bid (BH3-interacting domain death agonist) play central roles [10,12,14,15]. Granzyme B also cleaves proteases and inhibitors that protect against DNA degradation, specifically topoisomerase, poly (ADP ribose) polymerase (PARP), and inhibitor of caspase-activated deoxyribonuclease (iCAD) [15]. Topoisomerase is part of the DNA repair machinery, PARP releases topoisomerase stalled in the repair process, and iCAD blocks caspase activation of deoxyribonuclease (DNAse).

Apoptosis of endothelial cells, monocytes, and T cells leads to release of pro-inflammatory mediators, creating a cycle of inflammation and cell death. Caspase 1 directly activates interleukin-1beta (IL-1β) and the inflammasome, involved in the macrophage cell death pathway called pyroptosis [23,24]. In atherosclerotic plaques, increased numbers of apoptotic cells, including T cells, are found at sites of plaque rupture. Monocyte and T lymphocyte invasion, together with endothelial cell dysfunction, are closely linked to atherosclerotic plaque growth and vessel occlusion [16,25]. Apoptosis induces a pro-thrombotic and pro-inflammatory state in endothelium [13,16–18,25], while in macrophages and smooth muscle cells [13,16–18] apoptosis is implicated in plaque rupture, the underlying cause for sudden arterial thrombotic occlusion in heart attacks and strokes [16,17].

While environmental factors such as smoking, high fat or high cholesterol diets, lack of exercise or diabetes can cause initial injury to the arteries, plaques can be found in otherwise healthy individuals at the branching points of arteries, as they have low shear stress and unpredictable blood flow and thus recruit additional inflammatory cells [5,16–18]. Increased numbers of cytotoxic, perforin-positive T lymphocytes are present in inflammatory vascular disease, unstable coronary syndromes, and accelerated transplant vasculopathy [19–21], potentially driving cell death. Additionally, activated T cells express CD154 which binds to CD40L present on macrophages and allows for cross-talk and cross-activation of the innate and humoral immune systems. Monocytes secrete cytokines such as interleukin-2 (IL-2) and interferon γ (IFN γ) to alert other lymphocytes to the injury and stimulate them to mature into macrophages and effector T cells [22]. Interference with T cell apoptosis in rats [13] leads to a transplant tolerant state whereas GzmB deficiency in mice reduces transplant vasculopathy in some models [20]. Fas Ligand (FasL) has been reported to either block [26] or to accelerate [27] atheroma development in ApoE-deficient mice. FasL and GzmB are also associated with T cell death induced by other cytotoxic T cells (CTL) changing the balance of T cell subsets {e.g. CD8 T cells, CD4 T helper cells (TH1, TH2, TH17), and CTL} and altering immune responses [28–30]. T cell apoptosis may thus contribute toward plaque progression [12,13,16,17,19–22,26,27] but the precise role and effects on the balance of different T cell subsets remains only partially defined.

We present here a series of studies examining potential extracellular effects of intracellular cross-class serpins, Serp-2 and CrmA on inflammatory vascular disease in animal models [2–4,31–33], with selective analysis of GzmB mediated cellular apoptosis and T cell fratricide.

Results

Serp-2 reduces plaque growth in arterial surgical injury models, in vivo

To assess potential extracellular effects of Serp-2 and CrmA on arterial plaque growth, we infused a single dose of individual purified proteins immediately after arterial surgery (**Table 1**) Two animal models were initially examined; 1) a balloon angioplasty injury model [2,31,33] and 2) an aortic transplant model [3,4]. Saline, Serp-2, CrmA and two Serp-2 mutants were individually assessed after balloon angioplasty (N = 126, **Table 1, Fig. 1A–C**). Serp-2 treatment (6 rats/dose; total N = 24) significantly reduced plaque growth at doses of 30 ng (0.10 ng/g) or higher (**Fig. 1A**: 3 ng/ p = 0.400; 30 ng/p<0.006; 300 ng/p<0.006; 3000 ng/ p<0.004) after mechanical angioplasty injury when compared to saline (N = 6). Treatment with CrmA (12 rats/dose; total N = 60; **Table 1, Fig. 1B**: 0.03 ng/p = 0.466; 0.3 ng/p = 0.121; 3 ng/ p = 0.148; 30 ng/0.094; 300 ng/p = 0.279 and 3000 ng/ p = 0.612) or either of the two active site mutations of Serp-2, D294E (6 rats/dose; N = 18; **Fig. 1C**: 0.3 ng/p = 0.377; 30 ng/ p = 0.138 and 3000 ng/p = 0.567) or D294A (6 rats/dose; N = 18; 0.3 ng/p = 0.821; 30 ng/p = 0.076 and 3000 ng/p = 0.623, not shown) showed a trend toward reduced plaque at the 30 ng dose, but failed to inhibit plaque growth at higher concentrations. These results demonstrate that Serp-2 consistently reduced plaque growth in a rat iliofemoral angioplasty model when compared to CrmA, and Serp-2 RCL mutants.

Balloon angioplasty injury predominately induces endothelial denudation with smooth muscle cell proliferation and connective tissue scarring, but with less pronounced inflammation. Therefore, treatment with each serpin was assessed after aortic allograft transplant where greater inflammatory cells responses are detected [2,3,4,31,33]. Plasminogen activator inhibitor-1 (PAI-1) is a mammalian serpin that regulates thrombolytic proteases and PAI-1$^{-/-}$ aortic allografts have increased inflammatory cell invasion and plaque growth [2,3,4,34]. We therefore examined plaque growth in PAI-1$^{-/-}$ donor to Balb/C recipient mouse aortic allografts (N = 33 total transplants). Serp-2 (N = 6) again reduced plaque growth in transplanted aortic segments [p<0.05 compared to saline (N = 6); p<0.026 compared to CrmA (N = 9)], while CrmA and the two Serp-2 mutants, D294A (N = 5) and D294E (N = 7), did not reduce plaque (**Fig. 1D**). Mutant D294E was predicted to increase inhibitory activity due to preserved negative charge, however, no significant anti-plaque activity was detected with D294E or D294A ; conversely, D294A increased plaque (**Fig. 1D**) when compared to CrmA (p<0.047), D294E (p<0.025), or Serp-2 (P p<0.0005) treatments.

Histological cross sections from aortic allograft transplant (B6.129S2-*Serpine1*^{tm1Mlg} PAI-1$^{-/-}$ to Balb/C recipient) with saline treatment (**Fig. 1D, 1E**) or CrmA treatment (**Fig. 1D, 1F**) displayed rapid plaque growth at 4 weeks with mononuclear cell invasion (**Fig. 1F**, indicated by arrow heads). Serp-2 significantly reduced plaque growth at doses of 1.5 μg (50 ng/g), with reduced inflammatory cell invasion (**Fig. 1D, 1G**; plaque thickness demarcated by arrows; p<0.044), whereas Serp-2 mutants D294A and E (**Fig. 1D, 1H**) did not reduce plaque growth.

Serp-2 reduced inflammatory cell invasion in the adventitia (N = 10, 39.53+4.51 cell counts per high power field) when compared to saline (N = 10, 71.43+6.48 cells, p<0.019) and CrmA (N = 10, 77.27+9.59 cells, p<0.007). Conversely, D294A increased inflammatory cell invasion in the intima (N = 6, mean: 25.18

Table 1. Animal models.

Strain	Total No.	No. Survival	(%) Survival	Treatment
STUDY 1A – Rat Iliofemoral Angioplasty: 4wks				
SD	6	6	100%	Saline
SD	6	6	100%	Serp-2 3ng
SD	6	6	100%	Serp-2 30ng
SD	6	6	100%	Serp-2 300ng
SD	6	6	100%	Serp-2 3000ng
SD	6	6	100%	CrmA 0.03ng
SD	6	6	100%	CrmA 0.03ng
SD	12	12	100%	CrmA 3ng
SD	12	12	100%	CrmA 30ng
SD	12	12	100%	CrmA 300ng
SD	12	12	100%	CrmA 3000ng
SD	6	6	100%	D294A 0.3ng
SD	6	6	100%	D294A 30ng
SD	6	6	100%	D294A 300ng
SD	6	6	100%	D294A 3000ng
SD	6	6	100%	D294E 0.3ng
SD	6	6	100%	D294E 30ng
SD	6	6	100%	D294E 300ng
SD	6	6	100%	D294E 3000ng
Total	126	126	100%	
STUDY 3 – Mouse Carotid Cuff Injury				
$ApoE^{-/-}$	11	11	100%	Saline
$ApoE^{-/-}$	11	11	100%	Serp-2 1.8µg/d
$ApoE^{-/-}$	11	11	100%	CrmA 240 ng/d
Total	33	33	100%	

Strain	Total No.	No. Survival	(%) Survival	Treatment
STUDY 1B – Rat Angioplasty: 0– 72 hrs				
SD	20	20	100%	Saline
SD	20	20	100%	Serp-2 300ng
SD	20	20	100%	CrmA 300ng
SD	20	20	100%	D294A 300ng
SD	20	20	100%	D294E 300ng
Total	100	100	100%	
STUDY 2 – Mouse Aortic Allograft				
$PAI\text{-}1^{-/-}$	6	5	83.30%	Saline
$PAI\text{-}1^{-/-}$	6	5	83.30%	Serp-2 15µg
$PAI\text{-}1^{-/-}$	9	6	66.70%	CrmA 15µg
$PAI\text{-}1^{-/-}$	5	5	100%	D294A 15µg
$PAI\text{-}1^{-/-}$	7	5	71.40%	D294E 15µg
$ApoE^{-/-}$	5	5	100%	Saline
$ApoE^{-/-}$	5	5	100%	Serp-2 15µg
$ApoE^{-/-}$	6	5	83.30%	CrmA 15µg
$GzmB^{-/-}$	6	6	100%	Saline
$GzmB^{-/-}$	5	5	100%	Serp-2 15µg
$GzmB^{-/-}$	6	5	83.30%	CrmA 15µg
$GzmB^{-/-}$	7	5	71.40%	D294A 15µg
$GzmB^{-/-}$	5	5	100%	D294E 15µg
$ApoE^{-/-}$, $GzmB^{-/-}$	6	5	83.30%	Saline
$ApoE^{-/-}$, $GzmB^{-/-}$	6	5	83.30%	Serp-2 15µg
$ApoE^{-/-}$, $GzmB^{-/-}$	6	5	83.30%	CrmA 15µg
Total	96	82	85.40%	

SD – Sprague Dawley; $ApoE^{-/-}$ – Apolipoprotein E; $GzmB^{-/-}$ – Granzyme B (B6.129S2-*Gzmbtm1Ley*/J); $PAI\text{-}1^{-/-}$ – Plasminogen Activator Inhibitor-1 (B6.129S2-*Serpine1^{tm1Mlg}*).

+2.21, $p<0.034$, saline $N = 10$, 23.7 +1.90) and decreased it in the adventitia ($N = 6$, 46.06 +12.99, $p<0.0341$, saline $N = 10$, 71.43+6.48), whereas D294E had no significant effects compared to saline.

Serp-2 treatment also reduced plaque in rat aortic transplant models (ACI donor to Lewis recipient, $p<0.05$, data not shown) and reduced mononuclear cell invasion, when compared to CrmA, in both intimal ($p<0.0001$, data not shown) and adventitial layers.

These initial studies demonstrate an arterial anti-inflammatory effect for an intracellular viral serpin, Serp-2, in both angioplasty injury as well as aortic allograft transplant models in rodents, when infused into the circulating blood immediately after injury. This effect was specific to Serp-2 and was neither reproduced by another intracellular serpin, CrmA nor by two active site mutants of Serp-2.

Serp-2 reduces plaque growth in Apolipoprotein E deficient ($ApoE^{-/-}$) mice

Serpin treatment in hyperlipidemic $ApoE^{-/-}$ mice after carotid cuff compression injury was examined, both at the site of cuff injury and at the aortic root where no surgical injury occurs (**Fig. 2**) [32]. This model provides a means to assess both effects of serpin treatment after arterial surgical injury and also at a site of de novo growth of plaque induced by genetic hyperlipidemia with no arterial surgical injury (e.g. apolipoprotein E deficiency). Serp-2 significantly reduced plaque area in the aortic root ($N = 11$, $p<0.001$, **Fig. 2B, 2D**) where there was no surgical injury, but with borderline significance at sites of carotid cuff compression injury ($N = 11$, $p = 0.06$, **Fig. 2E**), when compared to saline (**Fig. 2A, 2D**). Plaque reductions with Serp-2 treatment were comparable at both sites, 42% for aortic root versus 44% for the carotid (**Fig. 2D, 2E**), while CrmA treatment ($N = 11$) had no effect (**Fig. 2C, 2D, 2E**). Compared to saline, plaque lipid content was also significantly reduced on Oil-red O stained sections with Serp-2 treatment, but not with CrmA (**Fig. 2F**). This reduction in lipid-laden cells is similar to the reduction in inflammatory cell invasion seen with Serp-2 treatment in the aortic angioplasty and allograft models.

Cross-class serpin treatments modify apoptotic responses in vitro

Effects of serpin treatments on cellular apoptotic responses were assessed both at early times after angioplasty injury *in vivo* and *in*

A. Serp-2: Rat balloon angioplasty

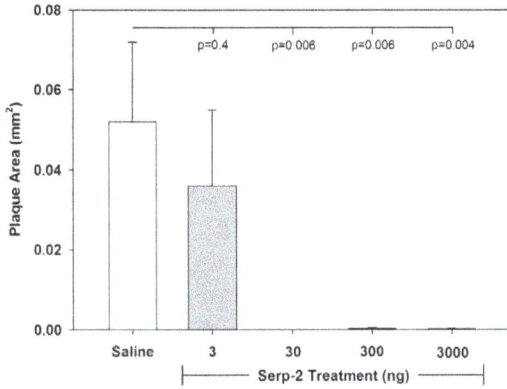

B. CrmA: Rat balloon angioplasty

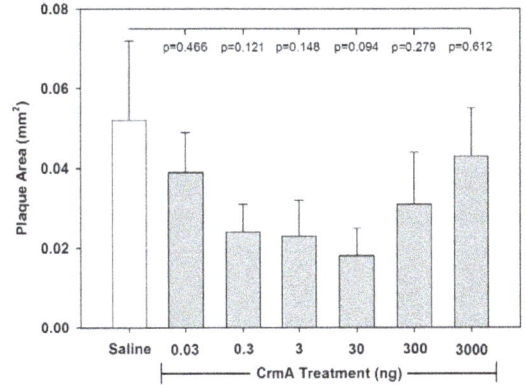

C. D294E: Rat balloon angioplasty

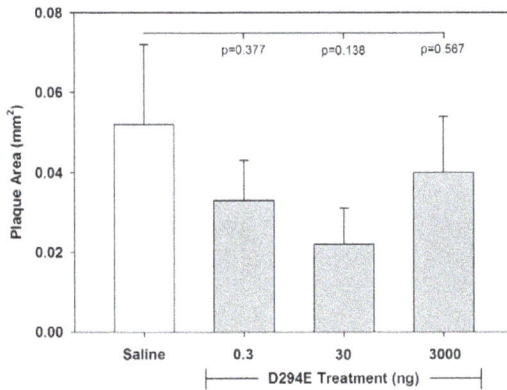

D. Mouse aortic allograft

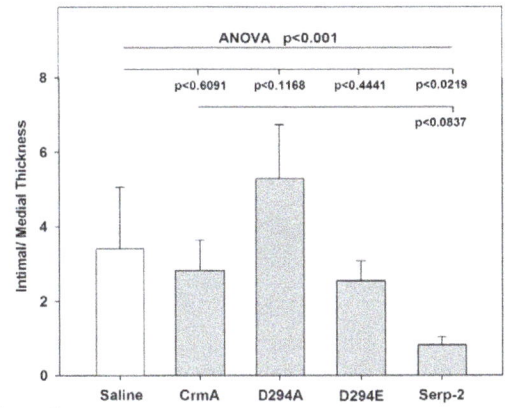

E. Saline

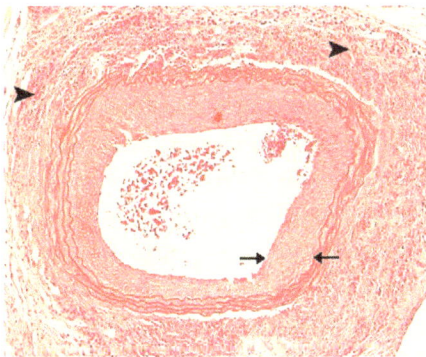

F. CrmA

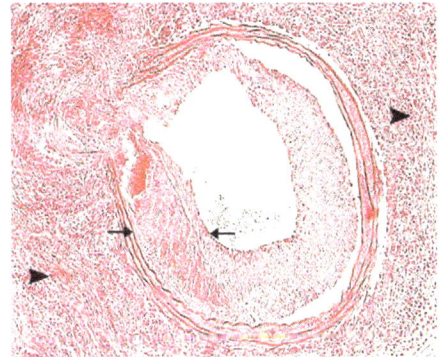

G. Serp-2

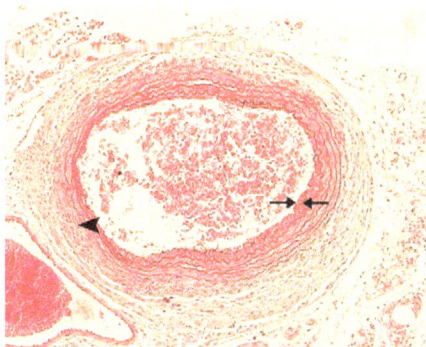

H. D294A

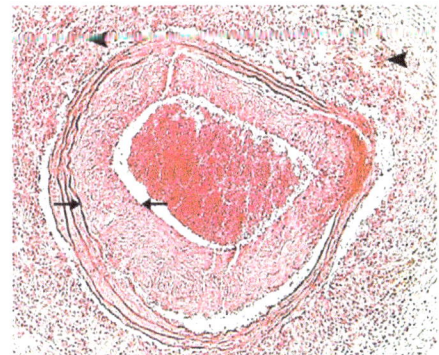

Figure 1. Serp-2 reduces plaque growth in arterial surgery models. Treatment of rat models of arterial injury with viral cross-class serpins demonstrates reduced vasculopathy. Haematoxylin and eosin stained sections of rat iliofemoral arterial sections harvested at 4 weeks and the mean plaque area were measured and presented as mean ± SE. The results demonstrated reduced plaque growth with Serp-2 (6 rats/dose; 3–3000 ng total N = 24) treatment at doses >30 ng (**A**). CrmA (6–12 rats/dose, 0.03–3000 ng; total N = 60) (**B**) and the Serp-2 reactive center loop mutant D294E (6 rats/dose, 0.3–3000 ng; total N = 18) treatments (**C**) demonstrated a non-significant trend toward reduced plaque at 30 ng, with no significant inhibition of plaque growth at higher concentrations. (**D**) In the mouse aortic allograft transplant model (PAI-1$^{-/-}$, B6.129S2-*Serpine1*^{tm1Mlg} donor to Balb/C recipient) Serp-2 again significantly reduced plaque (p<0.026), whereas CrmA and the D294A and D294E Serp-2 RCL mutants did not reduce plaque (total mice 33). (**E–H**) Five micron thick cross sections of mouse aortic allograft transplants taken from within the transplanted donor aortic section, demonstrate the marked intimal hyperplasia and associated mononuclear cell invasion in the adventitial layers in saline (**E**) or CrmA (**F**) treated mice. Treatment with Serp-2 (**G**) but not Serp-2 D294E mutants (**H**), displayed reduced plaque and inflammation. Arrows bracket intimal plaque limits. Arrowheads point to areas of mononuclear cell invasion. Magnification 100X.

vitro in human cell lines. Changes in individual cells in the arterial wall may be masked by analysis of arterial extracts, therefore effects of serpins on apoptosis were examined in individual cell lines in addition to assessing changes in the arterial wall.

At early times post aortic angioplasty injury (12h) in rat arteries, increased fragmented nucleosomes and higher levels of caspase 3, 7, 8, and granzyme B were detected when compared to saline control treatment (p<0.0001). Treatment with individual serpins demonstrated a trend towards reduced caspase and GzmB activity, but no significant reduction was detectable. For instance when DEVDase (caspase 3 and 7) activity was tested, Serp-2 (1.52±0.18; p<0.017), CrmA (1.56±0.18; p<0.0001), D294A (1.8±0.31; p<0.037), or D294E (1.67±0.25; p<0.008) treatment produced significant differences when compared to saline (2.3±0.4), but did not show any difference in activity between Serp-2, Serp-2 mutants, and CrmA treatments.

To test for potential effects on individual cell types associated with arterial inflammation and plaque growth, inhibition of apoptotic responses were measured in HUVEC (human umbilical vein endothelial cells), THP-1 monocytes, and Jurkat T lymphocytes *in vitro*, with and without serpin treatment. Apoptotic responses were induced through three pathways using staurosporine (STS; intrinsic pathway), and camptothecin (CPT; double strand break initiation).

In T cells, caspase 3 and 7 activity (as measured by DEVDase assay) were significantly increased after camptothecin (**Fig. 3A**, P<0.001) and staurosporine (**Fig. 3B**, P<0.0001) treatment [48]. Granzyme B and caspase 8 (as measured by IEPDase assay) [35] were significantly increased by STS (P<0.0001, **Fig. S1**). Serp-2 reduced caspase 3 and 7 in T cells after camptothecin (**Fig. 3A**, P<0.001) and after staurosporine (**Fig. 3B**, P<0.033) treatment, while CrmA did not alter T cell responses after CPT or STS (**Fig. 3A**). Serp-2 inhibition was more pronounced with CPT treatment (**Fig. 3A**) than after STS (**Fig. 3B**) in T cells. Serp-2 also significantly reduced apoptosis measured by cell death ELISA in T cells after CPT treatment (**Fig. 3C**, p<0.012), while CrmA did not.

In THP-1 monocytes, camptothecin (**Fig. 3D**, p<0.001) and staurosporine (p<0.0009, not shown), both significantly increased caspase 3 and 7 activity, but had little effect on caspase 8 and GzmB (**Fig. S1B**). In monocytes, caspase 3 and 7 were significantly reduced by both Serp-2 (p<0.032) and CrmA (p<0.001) after CPT treatment (**Fig. 3D**), with CrmA producing greater inhibition. Conversely, neither Serp-2 nor CrmA significantly altered GzmB and caspase 8 in THP-1 cells treated with STS (**Fig. S1**).

The Serp-2 mutants, D294A and D294E, did not alter caspase activity in T cells after camptothecin treatment (**Fig. 3A**, p = 0.11), but D294E (although not D294A) did reduce caspase 3, 7, 8 and GzmB with staurosporine (**Fig. 3B**, p<0.016), indicating that the D294E RCL mutant retains some anti-apoptotic activity that

differs from endogenous Serp-2. D294A and D294E had no inhibitory activity when tested in THP-1 monocytes after camptothecin or staurosporine treatment (**Fig. 3D**, p = 0.104).

In HUVEC cultures treated with serum deprivation, staurosporine, or camptothecin caspase 3, 7, 8 and GzmB were increased (p<0.001, not shown). Serp-2 and CrmA both significantly reduced caspase 8 after CPT treatment (p<0.0001) in HUVEC, but had no effect on caspase 3 and 7 (not shown). STS-induced apoptosis was not altered by Serp-2, CrmA, D294A, or D294E in HUVEC (not shown). In all cell lines tested after FasL treatment Serp-2, CrmA, and D294A had no inhibitory activity (not shown). The Serp-2 RCL mutant, D294E did, however, reduce caspase 3, 7, 8 and GzmB activity after FasL treatment of T cells (p<0.0005, not shown). Cathepsin K, S, L, V activity in T cells was not affected by serpin treatment (p = 0.386, not shown).

In summary, Serp-2, but not CrmA, inhibited camptothecin- and staurosporine-induced caspase activity in T cells *in vitro*. Both Serp-2 and CrmA inhibited camptothecin-induced caspase activity in monocytes with CrmA displaying greater inhibitory activity in monocytes, suggesting T lymphocytes as a primary target for Serp-2. No differential effects were produced by Serp-2 and CrmA *in vivo* in arterial sections isolated early after angioplasty injury, which may be due to the fact that multiple cell types are assessed in arterial sections.

Serp-2 reduces T cell apoptotic responses to cytotoxic T lymphocyte (CTL) granzyme B

Activated T cells (TH1) and cytotoxic T lymphocytes/ natural killer (CTL/NK) cells release GzmB into the surrounding medium, initiating death responses in other cells, and also in T lymphocytes [12,14,15]. The role of GzmB in Serp-2 mediated anti-apoptotic activity was assessed using medium from T cells activated to a CTL-like state with phorbol myristic acid (PMA) and ionophore [12,14]. These activated CTL-like cells express and secrete increased GzmB. Naive HUVEC, THP-1, and Jurkat cells were then treated with medium from the CTL-like T cells (CTLm) with and without serpin treatments (**Fig. 4, Fig. S1**).

Increased secreted extra-cellular GzmB was detected in PMA and ionophore treated Jurkat cultures (**Fig. 4A**). Both anti-GzmB antibodies and the tetrapeptide ZAAD – Chloromethylketone (ZAAD-CMK), a chemical intracellular inhibitor of GzmB, reduced granzyme B and caspase 8 activity (IEPDase) in these CTL cultures (**Fig. 4A**, P<0.001).

IEPDase (GzmB and caspase 8 p<0.0001) activity and DEVDase (caspase 3 and 7 p<0.0001) activity were increased significantly in T cells treated with CTL medium (**Fig. 4C, 4D**), but not significantly in CTLm treated HUVECs (**Fig. 4B**, p = 0.836) nor monocytes (not shown) [35,36]. Serp-2, reduced caspase 3 and 7 (**Fig. 4B**, p<0.01) and caspase 8 (not shown, p<0.01) in HUVEC cultures, but not in THP-1 (not shown).

A. Saline

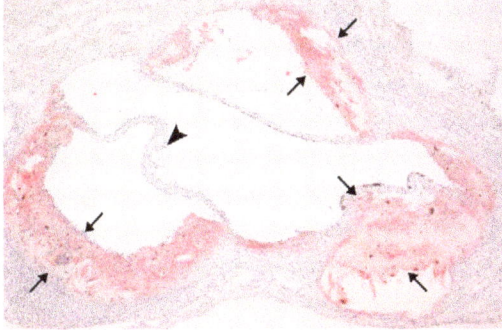

B. Serp-2

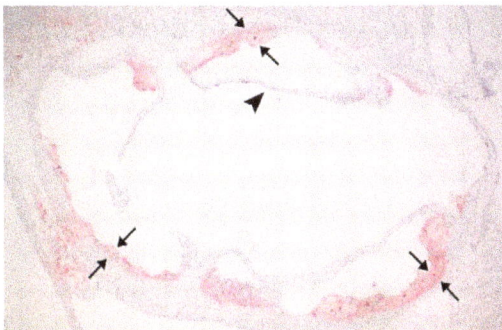

C. CrmA

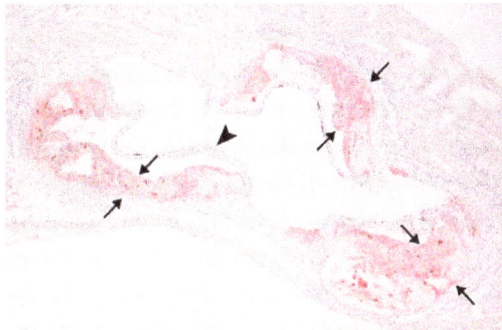

D. Aortic root

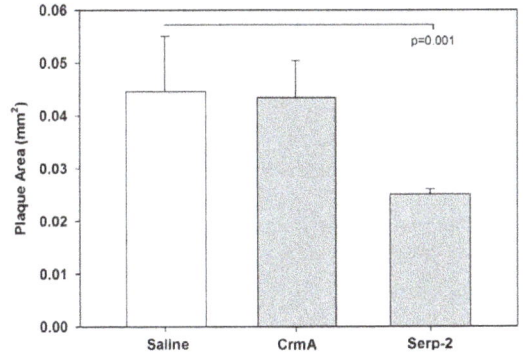

E. Carotid cuff compression

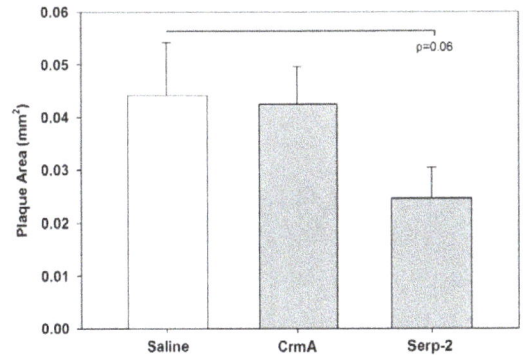

F. Aortic root: Oil red O stain

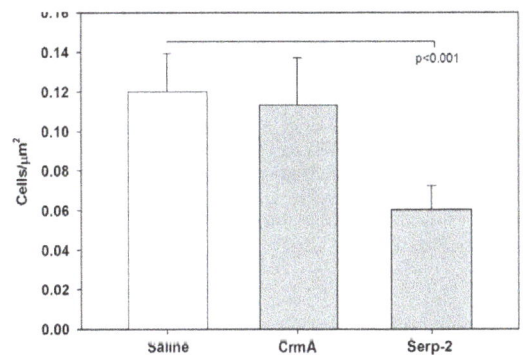

Figure 2. Serp-2 reduces plaque growth in Apolipoprotein E deficient (ApoE$^{-/-}$) mice. Hyperlipidemic ApoE$^{-/-}$ mice were infused with a bolus of Serp-2, CrmA or control saline after carotid cuff compression injury. Histological sections taken at the aortic root, where no surgical injury occurs, and distally at the site of cuff injury were examined. Cross sections taken at the aortic valve level (Oil red O staining) demonstrate plaque growth in saline treated control mice (A) (N = 11). A significant reduction in plaque area is detectable with Serp-2 (**B**, N = 11), but not with CrmA (**C**, N – 11) treatment compared to saline treated controls. Morphometric analysis of plaque area at the aortic root in ApoE$^{-/-}$ mice, where no surgery has been performed, demonstrated that Serp-2 inhibited aortic plaque and macrophage/foam cell invasion (**D**, p<0.001) to a greater extent than at sites of vascular carotid compression surgery in the same model (**E**, P = 0.06). Oil red O staining confirmed a reduction in fatty plaque in the ApoE$^{-/-}$ aortic root (**F**), indicating decreased foam cell/macrophage invasion (p<0.001). Thin arrows bracket intimal plaque limits, larger arrows identify an aortic leaflets, large arrow with open base points to area of fatty, foam cell (macrophage) invasion; Magnification – 100X.

CrmA did not decrease caspase activity in HUVEC cultures treated with CTLm (p = 0.249, **Fig. 4B**).

In T cells treated with CTLm, Serp-2 produced a significant reduction in CTLm-mediated increases in caspase 8/GzmB (p<0.01, **Fig. 4C**) and in caspase 3/7 (p<0.0009, **Fig. 4D**). Concomitant treatment with antibody to GzmB or perforin blocked Serp-2 inhibition of caspase 8/GzmB (**Fig. 4D**, p<0.0004 compared to Serp-2 and CTLm treatment for GzmB antibody, p = 0.412 for perforin antibody compared to CTLm alone) and caspase 3/7 activity (**Fig. 4D**, p = 0.149 compared to CTLm treatment alone, p<0.0193 for perforin antibody compared to CTLm treatment alone).

A. T cells-Camptothecin treatment

B. T cells-Staurosporin treatment

C. T cells-Camptothecin treatment

D. Monocytes-Camptothecin treatment

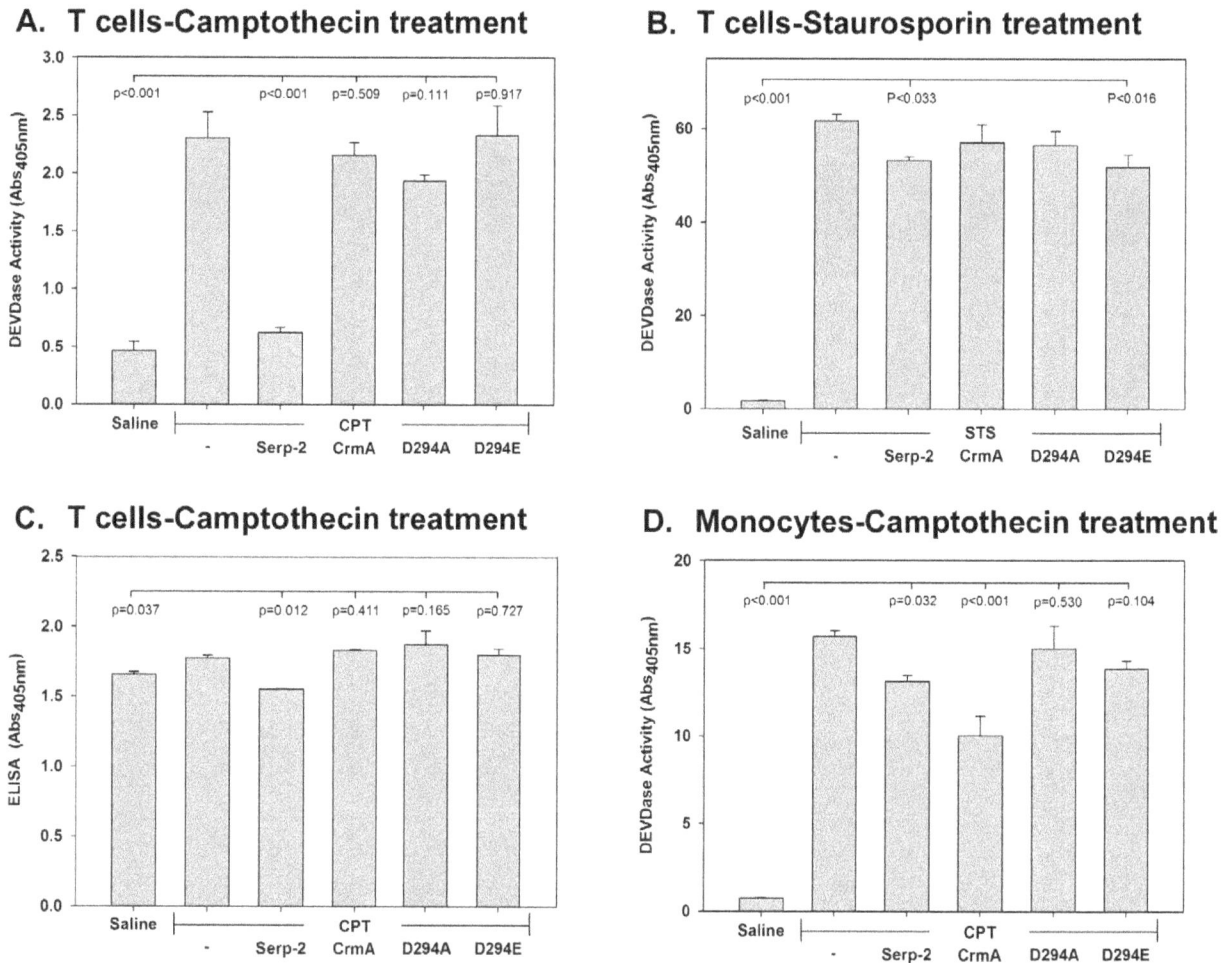

Figure 3. Viral cross-class serpins alter apoptotic responses in T cells and monocytes, *in vitro*. Apoptotic responses were induced in T cells and monocytes using camptothecin or staurosporine. Inhibition of caspase 3 and 7 activity was measured after treatment with Serp-2, CrmA, or the two Serp-2 mutants by analysis of changes in DEVDase activity, with comparison to untreated controls. Serp-2, but not CrmA nor D294A and D294E treatment of Jurkat T cells reduced caspase 3 activity (DEVDase) after camptothecin (CPT) (**A**, $p \leq 0.001$) or staurosporine (STS) (**B**, $p \leq 0.033$) apoptosis actuator treatment. Cell death in T cells measured as fragmented DNA by ELISA was also blocked in CPT treated T cells (**C**, $p \leq 0.012$). Serp-2 ($p \leq 0.032$) and CrmA ($p \leq 0.001$) both significantly reduced CPT-induced elevations in caspase 3 and 7 activity in monocytes (**D**). The results shown here represent mean ± SE from 3 to 5 replicates for each experiment. Significance was assessed by analysis of variance (ANOVA) with secondary Fishers least significant difference and Mann Whitney analysis.

Serp-2 binding to T cells is reduced with granzyme B inhibition

To determine whether Serp-2 or CrmA binds to T cells, FITC-labeled Serp-2 and CrmA binding was measured by flow cytometry (**Fig. 5A**) and fluorescence microscopy (**Fig. 5B**). In these studies Serp-2 displayed a greater binding affinity than CrmA (**Fig. 5A, 5B**) for T cells *in vitro* and mouse peripheral circulating lymphocytes *in vivo* (not shown). Serp-2 significantly reduced caspases 3/7 activity in CTLm treated T cells (**Fig. 5C**, $p < 0.001$) and treatment with the GzmB inhibitor ZAAD-CMK, which predominately inhibits intracellular granzyme B, further increased Serp-2-mediated inhibition of caspases, indicating that Serp-2 actions may be predominately extra-cellular (**Fig. 5C**, $p < 0.005$). The uptake of FITC-labeled Serp-2 into Jurkat T cells, as measured by soluble lysate content, was also reduced after treatment with antibody to GzmB (**Fig. 5D**, $p < 0.003$) or perforin (**Fig. 5D**, $p < 0.012$), further supporting a role for Serp-2 binding to GzmB and inhibiting of T cell responses.

Serp-2 inhibition of aortic plaque is reduced in granzyme B knockout aortic allografts

We postulated that Serp-2 mediates extracellular anti-inflammatory and anti-atherogenic activity via selective targeting of granzyme B (GzmB). Plaque growth in GzmB$^{-/-}$ single and ApoE$^{-/-}$, GzmB$^{-/-}$ double knockout (ApoE$^{-/-}$, GzmB$^{-/-}$ DKO) aortic allografts was assessed with and without Serp-2 or CrmA treatment. Donor ApoE$^{-/-}$GzmB$^{-/-}$ DKO aortic allografts (N = 18) were compared with ApoE$^{-/-}$ (N = 16) and GzmB$^{-/-}$ (N = 29) allografts (B6 into C57Bl/6 background). ApoE$^{-/-}$ hyperlipidemic mice are expected to have greater *de novo* plaque buildup and thus are predicted to enhance the capacity to detect changes / reductions in plaque growth in GzmB deficient mice. GzmB deficiency has the potential to reduce baseline plaque and thus prevent detection of a further reduction in plaque size after serpin treatment. ApoE$^{-/-}$GzmB$^{-/-}$ DKO and single GzmB$^{-/-}$ or single ApoE$^{-/-}$ knockout allografts were therefore assessed for differences in plaque production. In our model, 4 weeks post-transplantation, saline treated ApoE$^{-/-}$GzmB$^{-/-}$

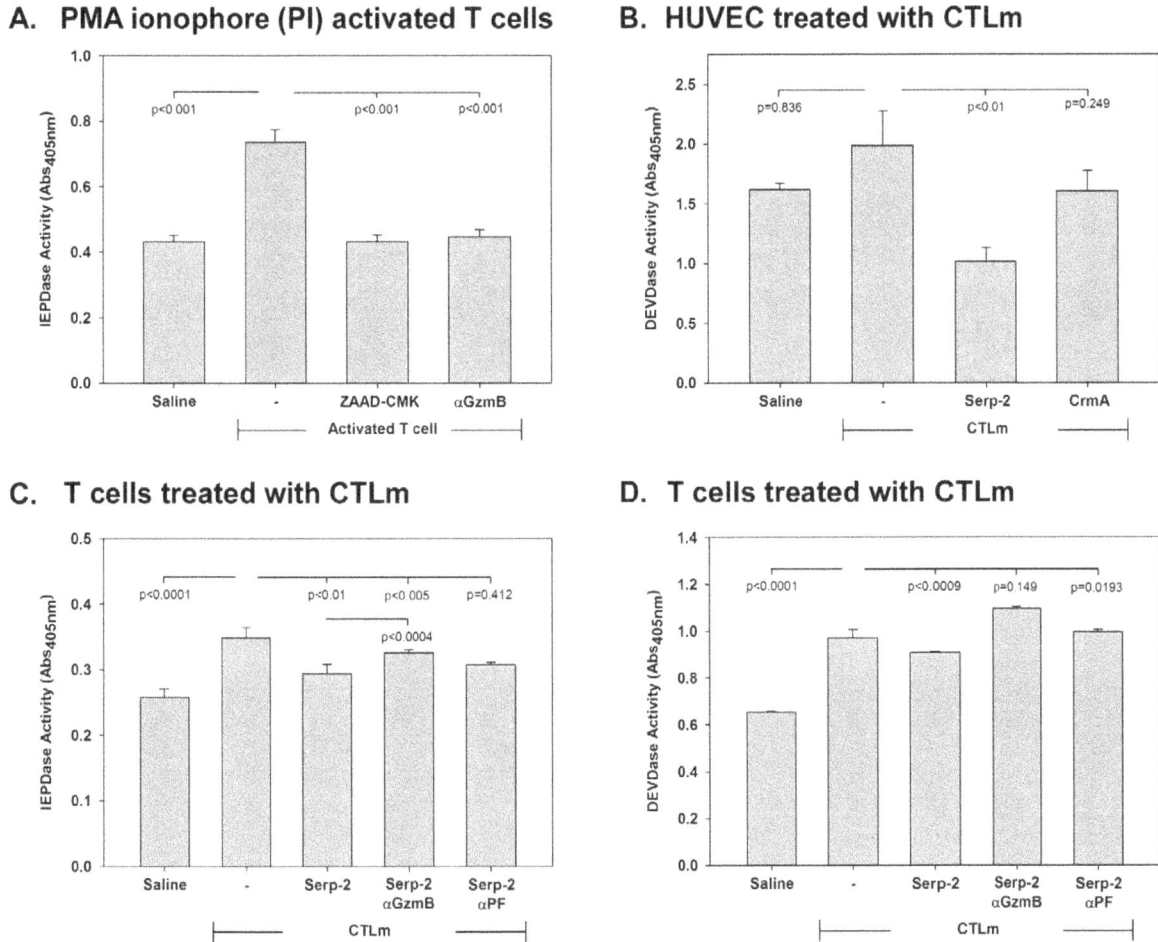

Figure 4. Blockade of granzyme B reduces viral cross-class serpin inhibition of T cell induced T cell apoptosis. Jurkat T cells were treated with PMA and ionophore (PI) and the level of granzyme B expressed was measured by IEPDase assay and caspase 3 and 7 activity by DEVDase assay (**A**). Increased granzyme B (GzmB, $p < 0.001$) secreted by these cells and was inhibited by treating the cells with an intracellular inhibitor of granzyme B, ZAAD-CMK ($p < 0.001$) or anti-granzyme B antibody ($p < 0.001$) (**A**). The medium containing granzyme B from PI treated T cells (CTLm) was applied to naive HUVECs to induce apoptosis (**B**). Treatment with Serp-2, but not CrmA, reduced caspase activity in CTLm treated HUVECs (**B**). The CTLm was also applied to naive T cells in culture to induce apoptosis and increased levels of caspase 3 and granzyme B were observed as IEPDase activity (**C**, $p < 0.0001$) and DEVDase activity (**D**, $p < 0.0001$) respectively. Treatment with Serp-2 reduced both granzyme B (**C**, $p < 0.01$) and caspase 3 (**D**, $p < 0.0009$) activities significantly. Antibody to granzyme B (GzmB) blocked Serp-2 mediated reductions in CTLm induced granzyme B (**C**) when compared to Serp-2 treatment alone ($p < 0.0004$), but with a still significant decrease ($p < 0.005$) when compared to CTLm treatment alone. Antibody to granzyme B also blocked the Serp-2 mediated decrease in caspase 3 (**D**, $p < 0.149$) when compared to CTLm activation. This Serp-2 mediated inhibition of CTLm induced granzyme B activity was also blocked by incubation of cells with antibody to perforin (**C**, $p = 0.412$) but not the caspase 3 activity (**D**, $p < 0.0193$). The results shown here represent mean ± SE from 3 to 5 replicates for each experiment. Significance was assessed by analysis of variance (ANOVA) with secondary Fishers least significant difference and Mann Whitney analysis.

DKO allografts had a significant trend toward reduced plaque area (**Fig. 6A**) and IMT (**Fig. 6B**) when compared to saline treated ApoE$^{-/-}$ allografts (**Fig. 6A**), suggesting that GzmB deficiency in donors has variable effects on plaque growth. At 4 weeks follow up Serp-2 significantly reduced plaque area (**Fig. 6A**, $p < 0.036$) and intimal to medial thickness (IMT) ratios (**Fig. 6B**, $p < 0.045$) in the ApoE$^{-/-}$ allografts. Serp-2 no longer significantly reduced plaque area (**Fig. 6A**) or IMT ratios (**Fig. 6B**) in GzmB$^{-/-}$ ($p = 0.995$ for plaque area and $p = 0.992$ for IMT) or in ApoE$^{-/-}$GzmB$^{-/-}$ DKO allografts ($p = 0.704$ for plaque area, $p = 0.353$ for IMT). Conversely, CrmA significantly increased plaque area in ApoE$^{-/-}$ donor allografts (**Fig. 6A**, $P < 0.026$). CrmA increased plaque area in GzmB$^{-/-}$ ($p < 0.041$), but not in ApoE$^{-/-}$GzmB$^{-/-}$ DKO ($p = 0.973$) allografts (**Fig. 6A**) and had

no significant effect on IMT (**Fig. 6B**). The increase in plaque area detected with CrmA treatment in ApoE$^{-/-}$ donor allografts (**Fig. 6A**, $p < 0.026$) was significantly reduced in CrmA treated ApoE$^{-/-}$GzmB$^{-/-}$ DKO allografts (**Fig. 6A, 6B**, $p < 0.021$ for plaque area and $p < 0.006$ for IMT). Serp-2, but not the mutant D294E protein, was able to reduce the amount of active Caspase 3 staining in cross sections of mouse aorta 4 weeks after transplant injury (**Fig. 6C**). Reduced staining was visible in mononuclear cells in the adventitia ($p < 0.024$) for Serp-2 treatment when compared to the less active D294E mutant (**Fig. 6D**).

These studies support GzmB as one of the central targets for Serp-2 mediated anti-inflammatory and anti-atherogenic activity.

A. Flow Cytometry

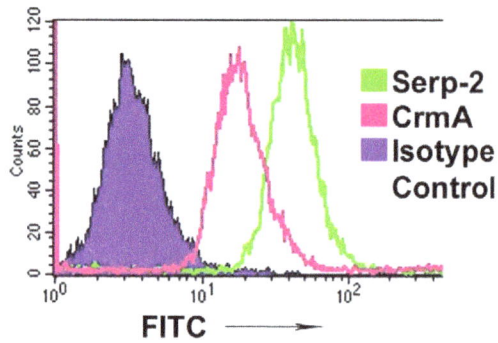

B. Fluorescence Microscopy

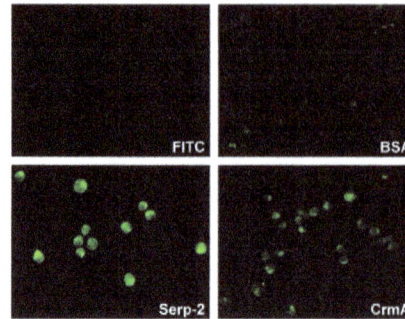

C. Caspase 3/7 Assay

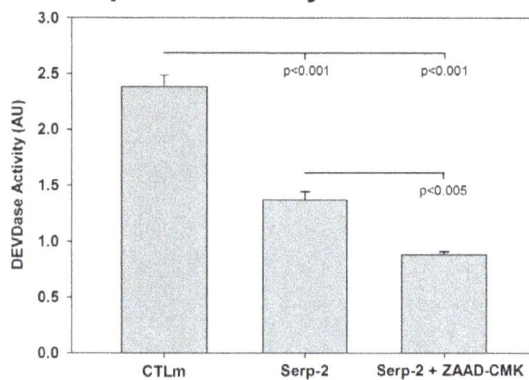

D. FITC-Serp-2 Binding Assay

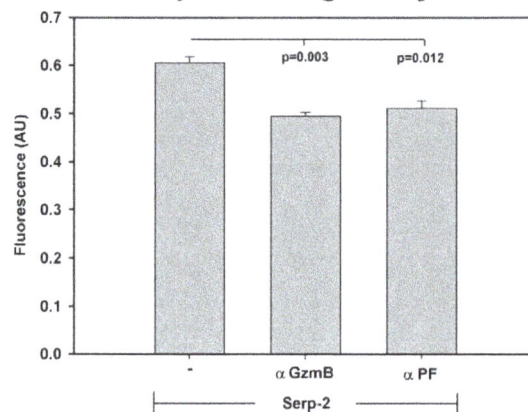

Figure 5. Serp-2 binds T cells *in vitro* with greater affinity than CrmA. Jurkat T cells were treated with FITC labeled Serp-2 or CrmA and binding/ association of these viral proteins with T cells was analyzed using Flow cytometry (FACS) analysis (**A**) and fluorescence microscopy (**B**, Magnification 10X). Extracellular, surface FACS analysis shows both Serp-2 and CrmA bind to the T cell surface (**A**). This observation was also supported by the fluorescent microscopic analysis (**B**). Intracellular ZAAD-CMK granzyme B inhibitor decreased Serp-2 mediated inhibition of caspase 3 activity in response to treatment with CTLm (cytotoxic-like T cell medium) (**C**, $p<0.005$). Treatment with antibody to granzyme B (α GzmB) or perforin (α PF) partially blocked Serp-2 binding (**D**, $p<0.003$ and $p<0.012$, respectively). The results represent mean $\pm$ SE from 3 to 5 replicates for each experiment. Significance was assessed by analysis of variance (ANOVA) with secondary Fishers least significant difference and Mann Whitney analysis.

Serp-2 reduces early apoptosis in invading inflammatory cells after aortic allograft transplant

Early changes in T cell and macrophage responses can initiate inflammatory responses that drive plaque development and plaque growth at later times in arterial plaque growth and disease. To assess effects of Serp-2 and CrmA on inflammatory T cell responses *in vivo* in a mouse model, we examined markers for T cell invasion and apoptosis in aortic allograft transplants in mice at early 72 hour follow up (**Fig. 7**). Serp-2 treatment (**Fig. 7**) induced no significant T lymphocyte responses at 72 hrs follow up, although there is a minor trend toward an increase in CD3 positive T cells. On immunohistochemical staining, however, Serp-2 but not CrmA, markedly reduced inflammatory cell apoptosis (**Fig. 7G,** $p<0.0002$).

Discussion

Many cell types are associated with atherosclerotic plaque growth. Injury to the arterial wall is believed to cause endothelial cell dysfunction and activation of inflammatory cells, specifically monocytes that transform into macrophages, T lymphocytes as well as smooth muscle cells, and other cells types such as mast cells, neutrophils and even B lymphocytes. Damage to the arterial wall and loss of supporting connective tissue can additionally cause programmed cell death or apoptosis, which can lead to release of increased levels of inflammatory cytokines. Activated or dysfunctional T cells can also induce transformation of other cells to a suicidal or apoptotic state. These initial changes in inflammatory cell responses are believed to then drive further damage to the arterial wall and cause intimal plaque growth and arterial narrowing.

It is evident that there are multiple factors that drive plaque growth with some known shared or common pathways. We elected to assess the effect of an anti-apoptotic serpin, as the apoptotic pathways are becoming recognized as a driving force in arterial injury responses and inflammation. Apoptosis in endothelial and in macrophage cells has been reported, as has apoptosis in SMC and T cells in plaque development. However, apoptosis altering the many T cell sub-populations remains poorly defined. It is not known whether interruption of apoptotic responses will alter plaque development and whether this applies to the wide range of arterial injury states that can cause plaque formation.

It is for this reason we have elected to assess plaque growth and responses to the viral anti-inflammatory serpin, Serp-2, in a range

A. Plaque Area

B. Intimal / Medial Thickness

C. Active Caspase 3 Localization

D. Active Caspase 3 Histology

D294E   Serp-2

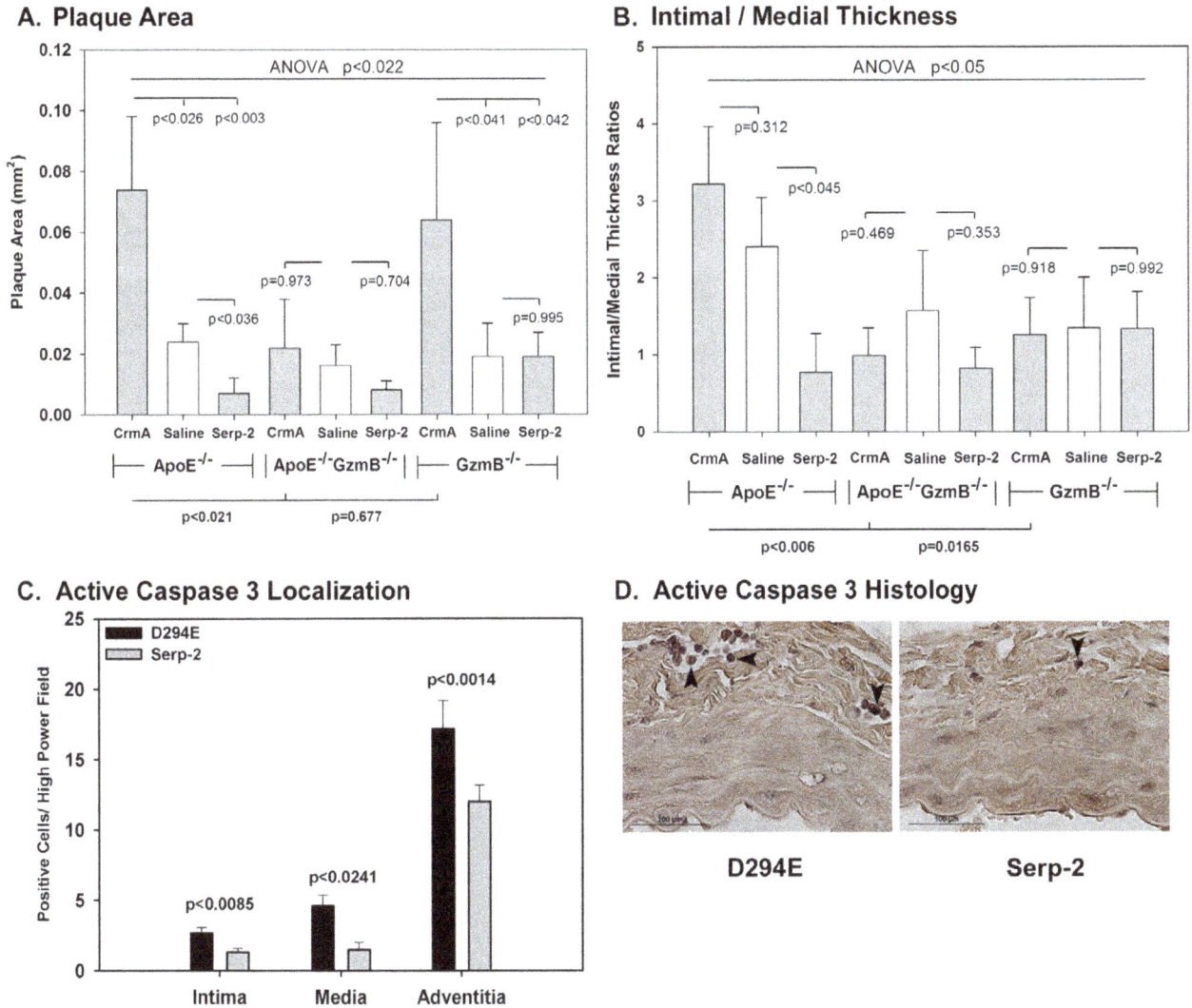

Figure 6. Granzyme B deficiency (GzmB$^{-/-}$) in donor aorta interferes with Serp-2 inhibition of plaque growth after aortic allograft transplant. ApoE$^{-/-}$ (C57Bl/6) donor aortic allograft transplant into Balb/C recipient mice (N = 16) induced plaque growth at 4 weeks follow up as measured by plaque area (**A**) and intimal to medial thickness (IMT) ratios (**B**). Serp-2 treatment significantly reduced plaque area (**A**, $p<0.036$) and IMT ratios (**B**, $p<0.045$) when compared to saline treatment. CrmA treatment markedly increased plaque area (**A**, $p<0.026$) and non-significantly increased IMT ratios (**B**, $p = 0.312$). Saline treated ApoE$^{-/-}$ GzmB$^{-/-}$ DKO allografts (N = 18) had non-significant reductions in plaque area and IMT when compared to ApoE$^{-/-}$ donor allografts (**A, B**). CrmA treated ApoE$^{-/-}$ GzmB$^{-/-}$ DKO allografts had significantly reduced plaque area (A, $p<0.021$) and IMT (**B**, $p<0.006$) when compared to CrmA treated ApoE$^{-/-}$ donor allografts. Serp-2 no longer reduced plaque area (**A**) or IMT (**B**) in either GzmB$^{-/-}$ allografts ($p = 0.995$ for plaque area and $p = 0.992$ for IMT) or ApoE$^{-/-}$ GzmB$^{-/-}$ DKO ($p = 0.704$ for plaque area and $p = 0.353$ for IMT). Serp-2 but not Serp-2 mutant D294E significantly reduced caspase 3 staining in all three arterial layers (Fig 6C, $p<0.024$) in PAI-1$^{-/-}$ mice 4 weeks post-aortic transplant. Immunostained sections for caspase 3 illustrate reduced staining in mononuclear cells in Serp-2 treated PAI-1$^{-/-}$ aortic transplants when compared toD294E treatment (Fig 6D, Mag 400X).

of models to determine whether the effects of this protein will be evident in different animal models of arterial disease in order to assess whether this will be of more widespread potential interest. Furthermore, in order to better isolate the contributions of individual cellular subpopulations, individual serpins were tested on human cell lines. Activated or dysfunctional T cells can also induce apoptosis of endothelial cells and monocytes/ macrophages, among other cell types; in the plaque, this leads to an increased release of cytokines and activate thrombolytic serine proteases tissue- and urokinase-type plasminogen activators (tPA and uPA, respectively) and the matrix metalloproteases (MMPs), which breakdown collagen and elastin, weakening the plaque's fibrotic cap [45–47]. In addition to these activated and apoptotic cells, the

newly exposed necrotic core and eroded cap structure also activate leukocytes and may initiate plaque rupture, subsequent thrombus formation, leading to heart attacks and strokes. Through a series of complex cross-talk and feedback mechanisms, the serine proteases in the coagulation and fibrinolytic pathways interact on many levels with the inflammatory and apoptotic responses and vice versa.

It is evident that there are multiple factors that drive plaque growth with some known shared or common pathways. We elected to assess the effect of an anti-apoptotic serpin, as the apoptotic pathways are now becoming recognized as a driving force in arterial injury responses and inflammation [48]. Apoptosis in endothelial cells and in macrophage has been reported as has

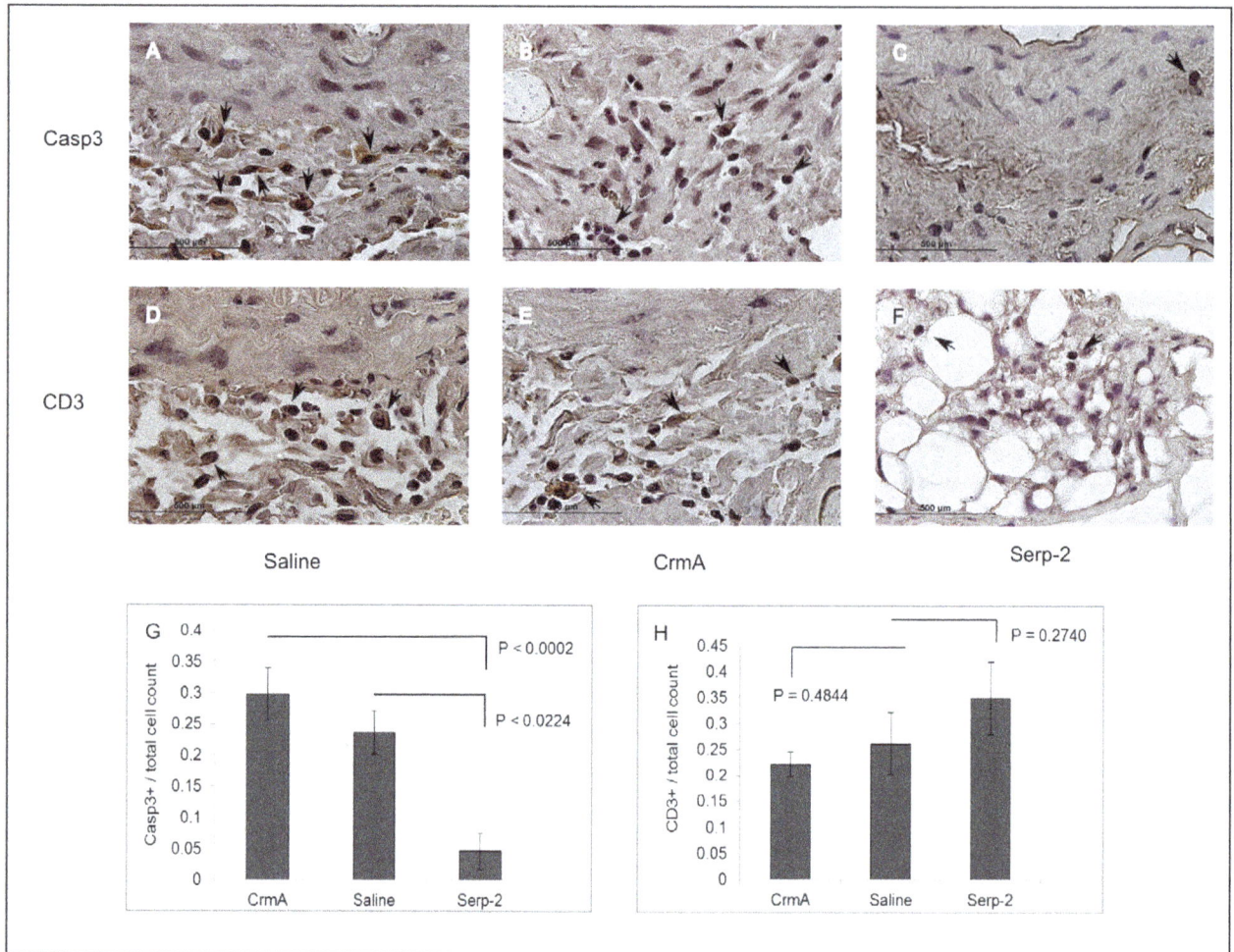

Figure 7. CD3 and active Caspase 3 populations 72 hrs after mouse aortic allograft. C57Bl/6 donor aortic allografts were transplanted into Balb/C recipient mice (N = 3 per treatment) and followed up at 72 hrs. Compared to saline, Serp-2 but not CrmA treatment reduced caspase 3 activity (panels A-C,G; p<0.0224). Neither protein treatment significantly reduced CD3+ T cells (panels D-F,H).

apoptosis in SMC and T cells in plaque development. However, apoptosis altering the many T cell sub-populations remains poorly defined. It is not known whether interruption of apoptotic responses will alter plaque development and whether this applies to the wide range of arterial injury states that can cause plaque formation. For this reason, we have elected to assess plaque growth and responses to the viral anti-inflammatory serpin, Serp-2, in a range of models to determine whether the effects of this protein will be evident in different animal models of arterial disease. Furthermore, in order to better tease apart the contributions of individual cellular subpopulations, individual serpins were tested on human cell lines.

Intravenous infusion of Serp-2, a reputed intracellular myxomaviral cross-class serpin, effectively inhibited plaque growth in a series of animal models of vascular disease (**Figs. 1, 2**) irrespective of the model being vascular surgery based or hyperlipidemic mice. These studies demonstrate marked extracellular, GzmB-dependent inhibitory actions for Serp-2, previously thought to function in a predominantly intracellular capacity. This inhibitory activity was unique to Serp-2; the cowpox viral serpin, CrmA and two Serp-2 active site mutants were inactive in these models.

Serp-2 blockade of plaque growth in donor aortic allografts was absent when the transplanted tissue was from $GzmB^{-/-}$ donors.

Local deficiency of GzmB was not sufficient to reduce plaque growth in donor allografts treated with saline, but did block increased plaque in $ApoE^{-/-}$ mice treated with CrmA. Thus, granzyme B may have greater effects on vascular disease when active locally rather than systemically during inflammatory cell responses. Although Serp-2 was infused systemically, the loss of activity in donor allografts from knockout mice suggests that Serp-2 acts locally on donor aorta after infusion (**Fig. 6**). *In vitro* studies suggest that Serp-2 specifically inhibits T cell apoptosis. Further work using isografts, $GzmB^{-/-}$ transplant recipients, and caspase 1 deficient transplants is needed to assess and contrast the roles of systemic GzmB and caspase 1 in allograft vasculopathy and as a target for Serp-2.

To try to separate out the effects of different cell lineages found in plaques, the effects of the serpins on apoptosis-induced cell lines were examined. Serp-2 bound to T cells *in vitro* in culture and selectively inhibited caspase 3/7 in camptothecin (CPT)-treated Jurkat T cells (**Figs. 3 and 4**) and was dependent upon GzmB and perforin (**Figs. 5 and 6**). Additionally, Serp-2 but not Serp-2 D294E was able to reduce levels of active caspase 3 in ApoE and ApoE/GzmB knockout mouse aortic cross-sections after transplant (**Fig. 6**). This Serp-2 mediated reduction for apoptosis was substantiated when comparing Serp-2 to CrmA and saline 72hrs after C57Bl/6 aortic transplant into Balb/C mice (**Fig. 7A–C, 7H**). Based upon these studies we postulate that Serp-2 decreases T cell mediated apoptosis, inducing a generalized reduction in vascular inflammation.

The extracellular activity for this viral serpin is predicted to begin with binding to GzmB. GzmB mediates apoptosis upon release from T cells and can also induce apoptosis in other T cells. Many viral proteins have multiple functions [2,8,31] and expanded actions of these cross-class serpins upon release from infected cells is predicted [2–9,31–33]. This inhibitory activity is present either with camptothecin treatment of T cells or after treatment with CTL medium from PMA and ionophore treated T cells, containing granzyme B. Serp-2 may thus either bind GzmB outside the cell or may be internalized via perforin pathways. The GzmB inhibitor ZAAD-CMK, which is cell membrane permeable and inhibits GzmB inside the cell, further increased Serp-2 inhibition of caspase activity indicating that Serp-2 actions are extra-cellular. Serp-2 inhibition of camptothecin-mediated apoptosis is consistent with GzmB inhibition.

Many viral proteins are also reported to derive functions through mimicking mammalian genes, as well as the converse. Two mammalian serpins, murine serine protease inhibitor 6 (SPI-6) [36] and human protease inhibitor 9 (PI-9) [37] target GzmB and protect cells from CTL-induced apoptosis. Serp-2 protein may thus mimic this mammalian serpin pathway, hindering T cell apoptosis and inflammation, e.g. T cell fratricide. We have not yet, however, determined whether selected T cell subsets are targeted by Serp-2 protection. It is undeniable that Serp-2 is protecting both T cells and other lineages from GzmB mediated apoptosis (**Fig. 4**) *in vitro*.

GzmB mediates DNA degradation, interfering with DNA repair responses. Topoisomerase, iCAD, and PARP are involved in DNA damage repair and are GzmB substrates. Camptothecin binds topoisomerase I, an enzyme class that alters DNA topography, interfering with DNA re-ligation [38] and creating persistent DNA breaks. Inhibition of topoisomerase also leads to caspase activation [37]. Poly (ADP ribosylation, PAR) is a post-translational modification driven by the PAR polymerase-1 (PARP-1) that reactivates topoisomerase complexes, preventing further damage [39] and is also a transcription initiation factor for NFκB [40]. Once cleaved, iCAD no longer inhibits caspase activated DNAse permitting DNA degradation [41]. Serp-2 mediated inhibition of GzmB or inhibition of secondary induction of caspase 3 may alter the balance between DNA repair and damage in T cells [42–44].

We conclude that Serp-2, a viral anti-apoptotic cross class serpin, has the potential to inhibit arterial vascular disease progression in animal models through inhibition of GzmB-dependent T cell apoptosis. Granzyme B-inhibition of T cell fratricide may represent a potential new target for intervention in inflammation-based disease. Serp-2 inhibition is generalized, with expanded inhibitory function for plaque growth in hyperlipidemic ApoE$^{-/-}$ mice and after arterial surgery, indicative of blockade of central regulatory pathways.

Materials and Methods

Animal Models

All research protocols and general animal care were approved by the Robarts' Research Institute, University of Western Ontario, London, Canada, laboratory animal ethics committee and the University of Florida, Gainesville, USA, Institutional Animal Care Committee, (IACUC, Protocol number – 102004234) and conformed to national guidelines. Effects of each serpin on plaque growth were assessed in three animal models; 1} angioplasty injury

in 250–300 g male Sprague Dawley rats (SD, Charles River Laboratories, Wilmington, Mass USA; N = 126) [2,31,33], 2} aortic allograft transplant from inbred 250–300 g ACI to Lewis rats (N = 60) [2,31], as well as C57Bl/6 to Balb/C mice (N = 96) [2,3,4,31] (Charles River Laboratories), and 3} carotid cuff compression injury in 12–14 week old C57Bl/6 ApoE$^{-/-}$ mice (N = 33) [32] (TNPO-PG, Leiden, the Netherlands) with all surgeries performed as previously described (**Table 1**). In a second study, ApoE$^{-/-}$ (N = 15), GzmB$^{-/-}$ (B6.129S2-Gzmbtm1Ley/J; N = 15), PAI-1$^{-/-}$ (B6.129S2-Serpine1^{tm1Mlg}; N = 14) (The Jackson Laboratory, Bar Harbor, Maine) as well as GzmB$^{-/-}$/ApoE$^{-/-}$ DKO mice (C57Bl/6 background, N = 15) used in aortic allograft transplant studies [2–4]. GzmB$^{-/-}$/ApoE$^{-/-}$ DKO mice (C57Bl/6 background) were generated at the Breeding Facility at the University of Florida from ApoE and GzmB single knockout mice purchased from Jackson Laboratories and tested for homozygous double knockout status before being used in experiments. All research protocols and general animal care were approved by University laboratory animal ethics and conformed to national guidelines. All surgeries were performed under general anesthetic, 6.5 mg per 100 g body weight Somnotrol (MTC Pharmaceuticals, Cambridge, Canada) intra-muscular injection for rats [2–4,31,33] and subcutaneous 60 mg/kg ketamine (Eurovet Animal Health), 1.26 mg/kg Fentanyl, and 2.0 mg/kg fluanisone (Janssen Animal Health) for carotid cuff placement in ApoE$^{-/-}$ mice [32].

Viral serpins were infused intravenously (i.v.) immediately after surgery in rats at doses of 0.3 ng – 3000 ng/rat (0.001–10 ng/g), with follow up at 4 weeks (Table 1). Daily subcutaneous injections of saline, CrmA (240 ng/mouse/day, 12 ng/g/day) and Serp2 (1800 ng/mouse/day, 90 ng/g/day) were started two weeks after collar placement in ApoE$^{-/-}$ mice and continued for 4 weeks until sacrifice. ^{125}I labeled CrmA and Serp-2 were injected on the first day and the last two days in two ApoE$^{-/-}$ mice detecting serum concentrations of 0.16 nM for CrmA and 1.72 nM for Serp-2. For the mouse aortic transplant studies a single i.v. injection (15 μg/ mouse; 500 ng/g) of Serp-2, CrmA, or D294A or D294E mutants was administered immediately after allograft surgery. A separate group of 100 rats had angioplasty injury with 300 ng of each serpin by i.v. injection for early follow up at 0, 12, or 72 hours to assess early apoptotic pathway enzyme activity (6 animals/treatment group; Table 1). There were no deaths after angioplasty or aortic transplant in the rats, 14 mice died after aortic transplant, and one mouse died during placement of the carotid cuff. In the mouse aortic transplant model two mice died after treatment with Serp-2, 5 after CrmA, 2 after D294A, 2 after D294E, and 2 after saline treatment with overall survival of 85.4% (p = NS). Body weight was measured weekly and mice were checked daily for signs of distress and necessity for analgesic.

Histological, Morphometric, and Fluorescence Analysis

At the designated study end (4 weeks for plaque analysis and 0–72 hours for protease activity or apoptosis) rats and mice were sacrificed with Euthanyl (Bimenda MTC Animal Health Company, Cambridge, Ontario, Canada). For mouse and rat angioplasty and allograft transplant models, arterial sections were fixed, processed, paraffin embedded, and cut into 5 μm sections (2–3 sections per site) for histological analysis, as previously described [2–4,31–34]. For the ApoE$^{-/-}$ mice with carotid cuff compression, the aortic valve area (10 μm sections throughout the valve area) and the carotid artery from the bifurcation through the site of cuff compression (5 μm sections at 25 μm intervals) were assessed. Sections were stained with Haematoxylin/ Eosin, Trichrome and Oil Red O for analysis of plaque area, thickness, and invading mononuclear cells, as previously described [2–4,31–33]. Plaque area as well as intimal thickness and medial thickness were measured by morphometric analysis via the Empix Northern Eclipse trace application program (Mississauga, ON, Canada) on images captured by a video camera (Olympus, Orangeburg, NY, USA) attached to and calibrated to the Olympus microscope objective. The mean total cross-sectional area of the intima as well as diameter of the intima and media were calculated for each arterial section. For immunohistochemistry, T cells were labeled with rabbit anti-mouse CD3 antibody, both then labeled with secondary goat anti-rabbit antibody (CD3; Cat # AB5690, Secondary anti-rabbit; Cat# AB80437. Abcam, Cambridge, MA, USA). For Caspase 3 staining, sections were incubated with anti-caspase 3 polyclonal antibody (Cat# AB3623 1:20) as primary antibody with secondary rabbit specific-HRP conjugated antibody (Cat # AB80437). Either numbers of positively stained cells in three high power fields in the intimal, medial, and adventitial layers were counted and the mean calculated for each specimen or, when fewer cells were detected, (displayed in earlier follow up times) cell counts for positive staining in all three layers were averaged.

For spectroscopic analysis of Serp-2 and CrmA binding, 1×10^6 cells/mL were treated with 1ug/mL of FITC-labeled protein for two hours, lysed with cell lysis buffer, and fluorescence emission at 525 nm quantified during excitation at 485 nm. For fluorescence microscopy, cells treated with Serp-2 FITC for 2 hrs at 4°C, then fixed with 2% formaldehyde, mounted with 10% glycerol mounting solution and viewed with a Zeiss fluorescent microscope as previously described [4]. For FACS analysis, 1×10^6 cells/mL were treated with 1 µg/mL of FITC labeled Serp-2 or CrmA for two hours and run on FACS (FACS Calibur, BD Falcon) acquiring data for 20,000 events with three replicates (Cell Quest data analysis program). To measure uptake of Serp-2, Jurkat T cells were treated with PMA and ionophore to stimulate granzyme B production, then FITC-labeled Serp-2 was added to the activated cells and incubated. Cells were lysed and the membrane and insoluble fractions were separated by centrifugation. FITC-Serp-2 presence was quantitated by absorbance at 525 nm (Fluorscan) measurements for both fractions.

Cell culture

Human umbilical vein endothelial cells (HUVEC, CC-2519 Clonetics, Walkersville, MD, passages 2–5), THP-1 cells (American Type Culture Collection, Rockville, MD, USA, ATCC TIB-202), or Jurkat cells (E6.1 clone, ATCC TIB-152) ($0.5 – 1.0 \times 10^6$ cells/ml) were incubated with saline control, one of the apoptosis inducing agents (3 ng/ml membrane bound FasL, 0.5 µM STS, or 2 –10 µM CPT) together with individual serpins (500 ng/10^6 cells/ml) [4]. Media was supplemented with 10% Fetal Bovine Serum (Invitrogen Canada Inc., Burlington, ON), Penicillin (100 units/ml), and Streptomycin (100 µg/ml, Gibco BRL).

Source and Purification of Serp-2, CrmA, D294A, and D294E

All serpins were His-tagged at the amino-terminus, expressed in vaccinia/T7 vector in HeLa cells (Dr Richard Moyer, University of Florida, Gainesville, USA) [6], and purified by immobilized metal affinity using His-Bind resin (Novagen) [2–8,31,33]. The D294A protein is a site-directed mutant of Serp-2 with P1 Aspartate 294 changed to Alanine to inactivate the serpin, while the D294E protein has P1 Aspartate 294 replaced by Glutamic acid to alter the inhibition spectrum [6–8]. Eluted proteins were judged >90% pure by SDS-12% PAGE, silver staining and immunoblotting. Serp-2 and CrmA were tested for Casp 1 and

GzmB inhibitory activity, CrmA displaying greater (>5–6 fold) Casp 1 inhibition than Serp-2 (data not shown), as previously reported [6–9].

Serp-2 and CrmA were labeled with Fluorescein Isothionate (Fluorotag FITC conjugation kit, Sigma-Aldrich Canada Ltd., Mississauga, Ontario) and passed through G-25M gel filtration column to separate unbound FITC. The F/P (FITC/protein) ratio was 2.2 and 2.1, for Serp-2 and CrmA respectively. The caspase 1 inhibitory activity of FITC labeled proteins was assayed, displaying normal activity. BSA was labeled in parallel with FITC and used as control in entry assays.

Enzyme activity analyses

For whole arterial lysates Serp-2, CrmA, 294A, or 294E treated rat femoral arteries (2–3 cm length) were excised at 0, 12, and 72 hours after angioplasty injury. The tissues were homogenized, lysed and extracted in 1mM EDTA buffer, centrifuged at 10,000 rpm, 8°C for 10 min to remove un-dissolved solids and supernatant stored at 80°C. For cell lysates, $1 \times 10^7/1$ ml volume (HUVEC, THP-1, or T-cells) were treated with saline or apoptosis actuators (CPT, 2 µM for THP-1 and 10 µM for T cells; STS 0.5 µM from Sigma, Oakville, ON, Canada; or FasL, 3 ng/mL from Upstate solutions, Charlottesville, VA, U.S.A.), and each actuator given in combination with either Serp-2, CrmA, 294A, or 294E (500 ng/ml). Cells were collected at 6 hours, washed with cold saline and treated with 60 µl lysis buffer (150 mM NaCl, 20 mM Tris base, 1% (v/v) Triton-X 100 at pH 7.2, for 10 min, 4°C) followed by centrifugation at 10,000 rpm for 10 min, 8°C. Supernatant was collected and stored at -80°C until use. Protein concentration was measured (Bio-Rad Protein assay, Bio-Rad Laboratories, Hercules, CA, U.S.A.).

A subset of T cell cultures were treated with phorbol myristic acid (PMA, 1 ug/mL) and Ionophore A23187 (1 µg/mL) to induce a CTL-like (cytotoxic T lymphocyte) state. Medium from treated T cell cultures containing GzmB and perforin was removed after 2 hours incubation and applied to fresh, untreated T cell cultures together with Serp-2, CrmA, or D294A or E, with and without antibody to GzmB or perforin (Sigma) or the cell permeable small molecule inhibitor, ZAAD-CMK (ZAAD-chloromethylketone, Calbiochem, CedarLane, Hornby, ON), incubation for 12 or 24 hours [44].

To analyze cell death ELISA assay, fragmented nucleosomes were detected using quantitative sandwich-enzyme immunoassay as per the manufacturer's directions (Cell Death ELISA kit, Roche Diagnostics, Germany) with conjugated peroxidase measured photometrically at 405 nm with ABTS (2,2Ã-azino-di [3]-ethylbenzthiazoline sulfonate) as substrate using a Multiscan Ascent Spectrophotometer (Thermo LabSystems Inc., Beverly, MA, US).

For the DEVDase (Casp 3 and 7), 10 µl of the cell/tissue lysate was incubated at 37°C for one hour in 90 µl of reaction buffer (100 mM Acetyl-DEVD(Asp-Glu-Val-Asp)-AFC(7-amino-4-trifluoromethylcoumarin) (Bachem, Torrance, CA, U.S.A.), 100 mM HEPES, 0.5 mM EDTA, 20% (v/v) Glycerol and 5 mM DTT, pH 7.5). For IEPDase, 10 µl of the cell /tissue lysate was incubated at 37°C for one hour in 90 µl of reaction buffer (100 mM Acetyl-IEPD(Ile-Glu-Pro-Asp)-AFC(7-amino-4-trifluoromethylcoumarin) (Kamiya Biomedical Company, Seattle, WA, 50 mM HEPES, 0.05% (w/v) CHAPS, 10% (w/v) Sucrose and 5 mM DTT, pH 7.5) [35,41,42]. For the Cathepsin K, S, L, and V assays, 10 µl of the cell /tissue lysate was incubated in 90 µl of reaction buffer (5 mM Rhodamine 110, bisCBZ-L-Phenylalanyl-L-arginine amide, 50 mM Sodium acetate, 1 mM EDTA and 4 mM DTT, pH5.5) (Bachem, Torrance, CA, U.S.A.) [39]. For

DEVDase and IEPDase hydrolyzed fluorochrome, 7-amino-4-trifluoromethyl coumarin was measured using a Spectrofluorometer (Fluoroskan; with excitation 405 nm, emission 527 nm) (Thermo LabSystems Inc., Beverly, MA, US) [39]. For the Cathepsin assay hydrolyzed fluorochrome, Rhodamine110 was measured using excitation 485 nm, emission at 527 nm. Final values are corrected for protein concentration. All these experiments were performed in triplicate, with three separate experiments performed for each condition, and the arbitrary fluorescent units from each reading used to derive the mean ± standard error for individual treatments and presented in the figures as bar graph with error bars indicating standard error.

Statistical Analysis

The apoptotic enzyme activity measurement results unless otherwise mentioned represents mean ± SE from 3 to 5 replicates for each experiment. Significance was assessed by analysis of variance (ANOVA) with secondary Fishers least significant difference and Mann Whitney; p values <0.05 considered significant.

Supporting Information

Figure S1 Viral cross-class serpins alter Staurosporine-induced apoptotic responses in T cells and monocytes, *in vitro*. Apoptotic responses were induced in T cells and monocytes using staurosporine. The ability of Serp-2, CrmA, or

Serp-2 mutants to counteract this induction was measured by granzyme B and caspase 8 activity by IEPDase activity. Serp-2, but not CrmA nor D294A and D294E treatment of Jurkat T cells reduced caspase 8 and Granzyme B activity after staurosporine (STS) (**A**, p≤0.001) apoptosis actuator treatment. In THP-1 human monocytes, no cross-class serpins significantly reduced granzyme B or caspase 8 activity (**B**). The results shown here represent mean ± SE from 3 to 5 replicates for each experiment. Significance was assessed by analysis of variance (ANOVA) with secondary Fishers least significant difference and Mann Whitney analysis.

Acknowledgments

We would like to thank Dr. Grant McFadden for many thoughtful discussions.

Author Contributions

Conceived and designed the experiments: KV IB PCT LYL ED RWM EALB TJCvB ARL. Performed the experiments: KV IB LYL ED EALB PCT RM JMW JAD HC JR BTB ARL. Analyzed the data: KV IB LYL ED EB RWM JMW JAD BTB JR MYB ARL. Contributed reagents/materials/analysis tools: KV IB LYL ED EB PCT RM JMW JAD BTB JR MYB TJCvB ARL. Wrote the paper: KV IB LYL ED EB PCT RM JMW JAD BTB JR MYB TJCvB ARL.

References

1. Silverman GA, Whisstock JC, Bollomley SP, Huntington JA, Kaiserman D, et al (2010) Serpins flex their muscle I. Putting the clamps on proteolysis in diverse biological systems. J Biol Chem. 285: 24299–24305.
2. Lucas A, Liu L, Dai E, Bot I, Viswanathan K, et al. (2008) The serpin saga; Development of a new class of virus derived anti-inflammatory protein immunotherapeutics. In Pathogen-Derived Immunomodulatory Molecules. Adv Exp Med Biol. 666:132–156.
3. Dai E, Viswanathan K, Sun YM, Li X, Liu L, et al. (2006) Identification of myxomaviral serpin reactive site loop sequences that regulate innate immune responses. J Biol Chem. 281: 8041–8050.
4. Viswanathan K, Richardson J, Bickersteth B, Dai E, Liu L, et al. (2009) Myxoma viral serpin, Serp-1, inhibits human monocyte activation through regulation of actin binding protein filamin B. J Leukocyte Biol. 85: 418–426.
5. Tardif J-C, L'Allier P, Grégoire J, Ibrahim R, McFadden G, et al. (2010) A phase 2, double-blind, placebo-controlled trial of a viral Serpin (Serine Protease Inhibitor), VT-111, in patients with acute coronary syndrome and stent implant. Circ Cardiovasc Intervent. 3(6):543–548.
6. Turner PC, Sancho MC, Thoennes SR, Caputo A, Bleackley RC, et al. (1999) Myxoma virus Serp2 is a weak inhibitor of GzmB and interleukin-1-converting enzyme in vitro and unlike CrmA cannot block apoptosis in cowpox virus-infected cells. J Virol. 73: 6394–6404.
7. Messud-Petit F, Geifi J, Delverdier M, Amardeilh MF, Py R, et al. (1998) Serp2, an inhibitor of the interleukin-1beta-converting enzyme, is critical in the pathobiology of myxomavirus. J Virol.72: 7830–7839.
8. Turner PC, Moyer RW (2001) Serpins enable poxviruses to evade immune defenses. Am Soc Microbiol News.67: 201–209.
9. Komiyama T, Ray CA, Pickup DJ, Howard AD, Thornberry NA, et al. (1994) Inhibition of interleukin-1-beta converting enzyme by the cowpox virus serpin CrmA. An example of cross-class inhibition. J Biol Chem.269: 19331–19337.
10. Barry M, Bleackley C (2002) Cytotoxic T lymphocytes: all roads lead to death. Nature Rev.2: 401–409.
11. Nathaniel R, MacNeill AL, Wang YX, Turner PC, Moyer RW (2004) Cowpox virus CrmA, Myxoma virus SERP2 and baculovirus P35 are not functionally interchangeable caspase inhibitors in poxvirus infections. J Gen Virol.85: 1267–1278.
12. Adrain C, Murphy BM, Martin SJ (2005) Molecular ordering of the caspase activation cascade initiated by the cytotoxic T lymphocyte/ natural killer (CTL/NK) protease granzyme. Br J Biol Chem. 280: 4668–4679.
13. Akyurek LM, Johnson C, Lange D, Georgii-Hemming P, Larsson E, et al. (1998) Tolerance induction ameliorates allograft vasculopathy in rat aortic transplants. Influence of Fas-mediated apoptosis. J Clin Invest. 101: 2889–2899.
14. Gorak-Stolinska P, Truman J-P, Kemeny DM, Noble A (2001) Activation-induced cell death of human T-cell subsets is mediated by Fas and granzyme B but is independent of TNFa. J Leukocyte Biol.70: 756–766.
15. Lieberman J (2003) The ABC of Granule mediated cytotoxicity: New weapons in the arsenal. Nature Rev Immunol.3: 361–370.
16. Littlewood TD, Bennett MR (2003) Apoptotic cell death in atherosclerosis. Curr Opin Lipidol. 14: 469–475.
17. Rossig L, Dimmeler S, Zeiher AM (2001) Apoptosis in the vascular wall and atherosclerosis. Bas Res Cardiol.96: 11–22.
18. Stoneman VEA, Bennett MR (2004) Role of apoptosis in atherosclerosis and its therapeutic implications. Clin Sci.107: 343–354.
19. Alcouffe J, Therville N, Segui B, Nazzal D, Blaes N, et al. (2004) Expression of membrane-bound and soluble FasL in Fas- and FADD-dependent T lymphocyte apoptosis induced by mildly oxidized LDL. FASEB. J.18: 122–124.
20. Choy JC, Cruz RP, Kerjner A, Geisbrecht J, Sawchuk T, et al. (2005) Granzyme B induces endothelial cell apoptosis and contributes to the development of transplant vascular disease. Am J Transplant.5: 494–499.
21. Fox WM, Hameed A, Hutchins GM, Reitz BA, Baumgartner WA, et al. (1993) Perforin expression localizing cytotoxic lymphocytes in the intimas of coronary arteries with transplant – related accelerated arteriosclerosis. Hum Pathol.24: 477–482.
22. Ross R (1999) Atherosclerosis - An Inflammatory Disease. 2, NEJM, 340: 115–126.
23. Duewell P, Kono H, Rayner KJ, Sirois CM, Vladimer G, et al. (2010) NLRP3 inflammasomes are required for atherogenesis and activated by cholesterol crystals. Nature. 464:1357–1361.
24. Seto T, Kamijo S, Wada Y, Yamaura K, Takahashi K, et al. (2010) Upregulation of the apoptosis-related inflammasome in cardiac allograft rejection. J. Heart Lung Transplant.29: 352–359.
25. Hansson GK (2005) Inflammation, atherosclerosis, and coronary artery disease. N Engl J Med. 352: 1685–1695.
26. Yang J, Sato K, Aprahamian T, Brown NJ, Hutcheson J, et al. (2004) Endothelial overexpression of FasL decreases atherosclerosis in apolipoprotein E-deficient mice. Arterioscler Thromb Vasc Biol. 24: 1466–1473.
27. Zadelaar ASM, von der Thusen JH, Boesten LSM, Hoeben RC, Kockx MM, et al. (2005) Increased vulnerability of pre-existing atherosclerosis in ApoE-deficient mice following adenovirus-mediate FasL gene transfer. Atherosclerosis.183: 244–250.
28. Callard RE, Stark J, Yates AJ (2003) Fratricide: A mechanism for T memory cell homeostasis. Trends Immunol. 24: 370–375.
29. Liu Z-X, Govindarajan S, Okamoto S, Dennert G (2001) Fas-mediated apoptosis causes elimination of virus-specific cytotoxic T cells in the virus-infected liver. J Immunol.166: 3035–3041.
30. Waggoner SN, Taniguchi RT, Mathew PA, Kumar V, Welsh RM (2010) Absence of mouse 2B4 promotes NK cell-mediated killing of activated CD8+ T cell, leading to prolonged viral persistence and altered pathogenesis J Clin Invest.120: 1925– 1938.

31. Liu LY, Lalani A, Dai E, Seet B, Macauley C, et al. (2000) A viral anti-inflammatory chemokine binding protein, M-T7, reduces intimal hyperplasia after vascular injury. J Clin Invest.105: 1613–1621.

32. Bot I, von der Thusen JH, Donners MM, Lucas A, van Berkel TJC, et al. (2003) The Serine Protease Inhibitor Serp-1 Strongly Impairs Atherosclerotic Lesion Formation and Induces a Stable Plaque Phenotype in ApoE$^{-/-}$ Mice. Circ Res. 93: 464–471.

33. Lucas AR, Liu LY, Macen J, Nash P, Dai E, et al. (1996) Virus-encoded serine proteinase inhibitor, SERP-1, inhibits atherosclerotic plaque development after balloon angioplasty. Circ. 94: 2890–2900.

34. Gramling MW, Church FC (2010) Plasminogen activator inhibitor-1 is an aggregate response factor with pleiotropic effects on cell signaling in vascular disease and the tumor microenvironment. Thromb Res. 125: 377–381.

35. Korkmaz B, Attucci S, Hazouard E, Ferrandiere M, Jourdan ML, et al. (2002) Discriminating between the activities of human neutrophil elastase and proteinase 3 using Serpin-derived fluorogenic substrates. J Biol Chem. 277: 39074–39081.

36. Medema JP, Schuurhuis DH, Rea D, van Tongeren J, de Jong J, et al. (2001) Expression of the serpin serine protease inhibitor 6 protects dendritic cells from cytotoxic T lymphocyte-induced apoptosis: Differential modulation by T helper " type 1 and type 2 cells. J Exp Med. 194: 657–667.

37. Trapani JA, Sutton VR (2001) Granzyme B: pro-apoptotic, anti-viral and anti-tumor functions Curr Opin Immunol.2003; 15: 533–543.

38. Rasheed ZA, Rubin EH (2003) Mechanism of resistance to topoisomerase I - targeting drugs. Oncogene. 22: 7296–7304.

39. Managa M, Althaus FR (2004) Poly(ADP-ribose) reactivates stalled DNA topoisomerase I and induces DNA strand break resealing. J Biol Chem.279: 5244–5248.

40. Hassa PO, Buerki C, Lombardi C, Imhof R, Hottiger MO (2002) Transcriptional coactivation of nuclear factor-B-dependent gene expression by p300 is regulated by poly(ADP)ribose polymerase-1. J Biol Chem.278: 48145–45149.

41. Solovyan VT, Bezvenyuk ZA, Salminen A, Austin CA, Courtney CA (2002) The role of topoisomerase II in the excision of DNA loop domains during apoptosis. J Biol Chem. 277: 21458–21467.

42. Alam A, Cohen LY, Aouad S, Sekaly R-P (1999) Early activation of caspases during T lymphocyte stimulation results in selective substrate cleavage in nonapoptotic cells. J Exp Med. 190: 1879–1890.

43. Kennedy NJ, Kataoka T, Tschopp J, Budd RC (1999) Caspase activation is required for T cell proliferation. J Exp Med. 190, 1891–1895.

44. Rogge L, Bianchi E, Biffi M, Bono E, Chang SY, et al. (2000) Transcript imaging of the development of human T-helper cells using oligonucleotide arrays. Nat. Genetics. 25: 96–101.

45. Schneider DF, Glenn CH, Faunce DD (2007) Innate lymphocyte subsets and their immunoregulatory roles in burn injury and sepsis. J Burn Care and Res, 28, 365–379.

46. Opal SM, Esmon CT (2003) Bench-to-bedside review: Functional relationships between coagulation and the innate immune response and their respective roles in the pathogenesis of sepsis. Critical Care, 7, 23–38.

47. Jancaiuskiene S (2001) Conformational properties of serine proteinase inhibitors (serpins) confer multiple pathophysiological roles. Biochem Biophys Acta, 1535, 221–235.

48. Gerner C, Frohwein U, Gotzmann J, Bayer E, Gelbmann D, et al. (2001) The Fas-induced apoptosis analyzed by high throughput proteome analysis. J Biol Chem. 275, 39018–39026.

Lesion Length Impacts Long Term Outcomes of Drug-Eluting Stents and Bare Metal Stents Differently

Shang-Hung Chang, Chun-Chi Chen, Ming-Jer Hsieh, Chao-Yung Wang, Cheng-Hung Lee, I-Chang Hsieh*

Second Section of Cardiology and Percutaneous Coronary Intervention Center Department of Medicine, Chang Gung Memorial Hospital and Chang Gung University, Taipei, Taiwan

Abstract

Background: Long lesions have been associated with adverse outcomes in percutaneous coronary interventions with bare metal stents (BMS). However, the exact impact of lesion length on the short- and long-term outcomes of drug-eluting stent (DES) implantations is not as clear.

Methods and Results: This study compared the impact of lesion length on angiographic and clinical outcomes of BMS and DES in a single-center prospective registry. Lesion length was divided into tertiles. The primary endpoints were angiographically defined binary in-stent restenosis (ISR) rate and major adverse cardiac event (MACE). Of the 4,312 de novo lesions in 3,447 consecutive patients in the CAPTAIN registry, 2,791 lesions (of 2,246 patients) received BMS, and the remaining 1,521 lesions (of 1,201 patients) received DES. The mean follow-up duration was 4.5 years. The longer the lesion, the higher the ISR rate (14%, 18%, and 29%, p<0.001) and the lower the MACE-free survivals (p = 0.007) in the BMS group. However, lesion length showed no such correlation with ISR rates (4.7%, 3.3%, and 7.8%, p = 0.67) or MACE-free survivals (p = 0.19) in the DES group.

Conclusions: In our single-center prospective registry, lesion length defined in tertiles has no impact on the short-term (ISR) or long-term (MACE) outcomes of patients implanted with DES. In contrast, longer lesion correlates with higher ISR and MACE rates in BMS group.

Editor: Giuseppe Biondi-Zoccai, Sapienza University of Rome, Italy

Funding: Shang-Hung Chang was supported by a grant from Chang Gung Memorial Hospital (CMRPG350214). I-Chang Hsieh was supported by a grant from the Taiwan National Science Council (98-2314-B-182-060). The funders had no role in study design, data collection and analysis, decision to publish, or preparation of the manuscript.

Competing Interests: The authors have declared that no competing interests exist.

* E-mail: hsiehic@ms28.hinet.net

Introduction

The management of long coronary lesions has become increasingly important in clinical practice because of the rising incidence of long or complex lesions in aging populations and their increasing comorbidity [1]. In-stent restenosis (ISR) is one of the main challenges in treating long lesions with stents while major adverse cardiac events (MACE) free survival is the gold standard for stents comparisons. Generally speaking, drug-eluting stents (DES) have been shown to be more efficacious than bare metal stents (BMS) in reducing ISR and MACE [2–5]. Stent length and lesion length have both been reported as very important predictors of ISR in the BMS era [6–9]. These two factors are thought to be less important in the DES era because DES reduce ISR dramatically in almost every type of lesion [10–11]. On the other hand, the effect of lesion length on the long term outcomes in the DES era has been ignored. A very recent study suggested that longer stents are associated with increased MACE rates at 1 year [12]. The exact difference in impact of lesion length on the long term outcomes for BMS and DES, however, is not clear. To bridge this gap, this study was conducted with the aim of comparing the real impact of lesion length on BMS and DES in terms of ISR and MACE-free survival. Data were collected from a prospectively created database, and angiographic follow-up was decided upon prior to data interpretation.

Methods

Subjects

The CAPTAIN (Cardiovascular Atherosclerosis and Percutaneous TrAnsluminal INterventions) registry is a physician-initiated prospective single-center observational study in a tertiary medical center, which enrolls consecutive patients undergoing stent implantation.

Both short and long term outcomes of stent implantations are examined in this paper. For short-term outcomes, a total of 4,745 consecutive patients with de novo native coronary artery lesions who had undergone successful emergency or elective percutaneous coronary intervention (PCI) at this hospital between November 1996 and December 2010 were registered. Patients were referred for coronary angiography based on angina, an abnormal stress test, or elevated markers of myocardial damage. Because of different timelines of restenosis between BMS and DES, follow-up angiographies were performed for 4,312 target lesions in 3,447 patients at either 6 months (in the BMS group) or 9 months (in the DES group) after the index procedure [13–18]. For long term outcomes, patients were scheduled to undergo clinical follow-up at 30 days, 6, 9, 12 months, and thereafter annually. The stents used in this study were either BMS (Palmaz-Schatz, Crown, Bx, Multilink, Duet, Tristar, Penta, Pixel, Express, Liberte, S7, Driver, and Vision), or DES (Cypher, Taxus, Endeavor, Xience V). The BMS used in this study measured between 2.5 mm and 5 mm in diameter and between 7 mm and 38 mm in length. The DES used were between 2.25 and 4 mm in diameter and between 12 and 38 mm in length. After stent implantation, dual antiplatelet treatment of aspirin and a thienopyridine derivative (ticlopidine, 200 mg/day or clopidogrel, 75 mg/day) was to be maintained for 3–12 months. Thereafter, the decision regarding the duration of dual antiplatelet therapy was left to the discretion of each attending physician. Lifelong use of aspirin was suggested after the procedure except when a contraindication existed.

Lesions were classified into tertiles, and cut points were 14 and 21 mm for the BMS group and 16 and 24 mm for the DES group. If a patient had multiple stent implantations, the longest lesion was used in analysis.

Definition of endpoints

The primary endpoints are binary ISR and MACE. Binary ISR at follow-up was defined as a stenosis occupying ≥50% of vessel diameter and occurring in the segment inside the stent or within a 5 mm segment proximal or distal to the stent. MACE was defined as a composite of cardiac death, ST-elevation and non–ST-elevation myocardial infarction (MI), coronary artery bypass grafting (CABG), or target lesion revascularization (TLR). An independent researcher unaware of the patient's treatment reviewed all clinical end points during follow-up. Lesion length was measured as the length of contiguous coronary narrowing (defined as percent diameter stenosis >50%) [19]. Angiographic variables derived from the index procedure and restudy, including absolute lesion length, stent length, reference vessel diameter, minimal luminal diameter, percent diameter stenosis, and late loss, were measured by automated edge detection or a digital caliber before and after stent deployment at baseline and follow-up coronary angiography, using the contrast-filled guiding catheter as a calibration reference [20]. A small vessel was defined as one having a pre-procedural reference diameter of less than 2.5 mm. Baseline clinical characteristics were collected during the index procedure. Lesions were qualitatively classified using the modified American College of Cardiology/American Heart Association grading system.

Statistics

Categorical data were shown as percentages and compared between groups using chi-square. Continuous variables are presented as the mean ± standard deviation, and comparisons were made by analysis of variance (ANOVA). Spearman rank correlation was applied for association between ordinal variables. Cumulative curves for MACE were obtained using the Kaplan-Meier method and the groups were compared in terms of survival on log-rank tests. Data analysis was performed using STATA version 10 (StataCorp LP. College Station, TX, USA). A p value <0.05 was considered significant.

Results

In a 14-year period, 3,447 patients were entered into a prospectively collated database. Angiographic follow-ups were 80% and 79% in the BMS and DES groups, respectively. ISR and late loss were assessed angiographically in 4,312 lesions (2,791 implanted with BMS and 1,521 with DES). MACE was followed in 3,447 patients (2,246 patients with BMS and 1,201 with DES). In both the BMS and DES groups, the patients had generally similar demographic and baseline clinical characteristics irrespective of lesion length, with the following exceptions: In the DES group, the middle subgroup had the lowest incidence of hypertension (Table 1). Lesion characteristics distribute similarly in the BMS and DES groups. The reference diameter of the target lesions in all subgroups for either BMS or DES was about 3.2 mm. In both BMS and DES groups, longer lesions were more calcified, more complex, and had been treated by multiple stents. The incidence of small vessels was generally very low in all subgroups (Table 2).

The overall angiographic ISR rate was much higher for the BMS group than for the DES group (20.3% vs. 5.3%, p<0.001). In the BMS group, the ISR rate correlated perfectly with lesion length (14%, 18%, and 29%, Spearman's rho = 1, p<0.001) (Figure 1). However, ISR rates showed no such correlation with lesion length in the DES group (4.7%, 3.3%, and 7.8%, Spearman's rho = 0.5, p = 0.67).

On chronic results, BMS and DES patients were both divided into tertiles based on lesion length. The BMS patients were followed up for ten years, and the DES patients were followed up for eight years. The survival curve for the BMS group shows that lesion length affected survival rates (p = 0.007). On the other hand, the survival rates of DES patients did not differ among the lesion length tertiles (p = 0.19) (Figure 2).

Discussion

This study presents three major findings. First, the DES group had much lower ISR and better MACE-free survival than the BMS group at any lesion length. Second, ISR rates correlated perfectly and positively with lesion lengths in the BMS group. However, lesion length had no such correlation to ISR in the DES group. Finally, longest lesions had the worst long-term MACE-free survival in the BMS group while such results were not as pronounced in the DES group.

Lesion length and stent length have been reported as important predictors of ISR for various types of BMS and DES [19]. From a very early stage of coronary intervention, studies have shown that shorter BMSs were associated with fewer clinical events and lower ISR rates [21]. Stented segment length was also found to be an important and independent predictor of restenosis when using various types of BMS in more than 1000 lesions [6]. Kereiakes et al, in their meta-analysis of 4 multi-link stent trials, described a fairly linear correlation between stent lengths and IRS rates for stents in 6 length groups [22]. That assertion is supported by the present study, in which we also observed that in the BMS group, the longer the lesion length, the higher the ISR rates. Similarly, stent length and lesion length have been reported as independent predictors of IRS in various DES such as sirolimus-eluting stents [23–25]. However, in the present study we did not see the same result. According to our data, lesion length has no significant effect on ISR rate for DES until lesions are longer than 24 mm.

Several studies have suggested that longer lesions were associated with higher MACE rates in the BMS and DES eras [12,26,27]. Our results showed similar results in the BMS group, but not in the DES group. Although different populations, follow-up protocols, and definitions of endpoints prevented direct comparisons between this and these observational studies, our study is distinctive in its very long follow-up time frame. In both BMS and DES groups, most of the MACEs were contributed mainly by TLR performed in scheduled angiography. The impact of lesion length on MACE in BMS would have been much smaller

Table 1. Clinical characteristics.

Tertile (mm)	BMS (r = 2,246)				DES (n = 1,201)				BMS vs. DES (p)
	Shortest (<14) (n = 812)	Middle (14–21) (n = 825)	Longest (>21) (n = 609)	p	Shortest (<16) (n = 401)	Middle (16–24) (n = 411)	Longest (>24) (n = 389)	p	
Age (years)	61±10	61±11	60±11	NS	62±12	61±12	60±11	NS	60.8±0.2 vs. 60.9±0.3 (NS)
Male (%)	82	83	83	NS	81	84	81	NS	82.3 vs. 82 (NS)
Hypertension (%)	51	48	49	NS	60	52	59	0.04	50.7 vs. 57 (<0.001)
Diabetes (%)	23	22	22	NS	26	26	28	NS	23 vs. 27.3 (0.003)
Smoking (%)	50	49	50	NS	38	42	41	NS	49.6 vs. 40.7 (<0.001)
Dyslipidemia (%)	58	60	62	NS	53	55	54	NS	59.5 vs. 53.8 (0.001)
% of diseased coronary arteries				0.02				0.02	(NS)
1-vessel	37	43	43		40	46	39		40.7 vs. 41.6
2-vessel	34	33	32		33	31	35		33.1 vs. 33
3-vessel	26	23	24		24	22	25		24.5 vs. 23.77
Left main	3	1	1		3	1	1		1.6 vs. 1.6

Values are mean ± SD where appropriate. BMS, bare metal stent; DES, drug-eluting stent NS, not significant.

Table 2. Lesions and Procedural Characteristics.

Tertile (mm)	BMS (n=2,791) Shortest (<14) (n=906)	Middle (14–21) (n=1,012)	Longest (>21) (n=873)	p	DES (n=1,521) Shortest (<16) (n=447)	Middle (16–24) (n=519)	Longest (>24) (n=555)	p	BMS vs. DES (p)
Lesion length (mm)	12.1±2.2	16.9±2.2	29.4±8.8	<0.0001	12.6±2.2	19.1±1.9	33.8±13	<0.0001	18.3±0.2 vs. 22.6±0.3 (<0.001)
Reference (mm)	3.2±0.5	3.2±0.5	3.1±0.5	NS	3.2±.05	3.2±0.4	3.2±0.4	NS	3.18±0.01 vs. 3.19±0.01 (NS)
Multiple stents (%)	0	2	23	<0.0001	0	1	34	<0.0001	8 vs. 12.9 (<0.001)
AHA type B2+C (%)	60	74	97	<0.0001	71	82	98	<0.0001	76.9 vs. 84.6 (<0.001)
Lesion site (%)				<0.0001				<0.0001	NS
Left Main	4	1	1		4	1	2		2.2 vs. 2.2
LAD	44	45	51		44	50	51		47.7 vs. 50.8
LCX	18	19	12		22	19	12		17.1 vs. 17.8
RCA	29	33	34		23	26	34		33 vs. 29.3
Calcification (%)	13	13	25	<0.0001	12	11	16	0.04	16.7 vs. 12.9 (0.001)
Angulated >45° (%)	7	6	7	NS	3	2	2	NS	6.7 vs. 2.1 (<0.001)
Eccentric (%)	58	49	36	<0.0001	46	43	31	<0.0001	48 vs. 39.6 (<0.001)
Small vessel (%)	8	4	5	0.005	3	4	1	0.003	5.8 vs. 2.7 (0.001)
Bifurcation lesion (%)	11	10	10	NS	11	11	10	NS	10 vs. 10.1 (NS)
Ostial lesion (%)	9	4	6	0.001	14	7	8	<0.0001	6.1 vs. 9.6 (<0.001)
Chronic total occlusion (%)	5	12	22	<0.0001	10	24	24	<0.0001	13 vs. 20 (<0.001)
Angiographic follow up									
Late loss (mm)	0.9±0.6	1±0.66	1.2±0.7	<0.0001	0.38±0.58	0.35±0.56	0.51±0.7	<0.0001	1.05±0.01 vs. 0.42±0.02 (<0.001)
Restenosis (%)	14	18	29	<0.0001	4.7	3.3	7.8	0.004	20.3 vs. 5.3 (<0.001)

BMS, bare metal stent; DES, drug-eluting stent; LAD, left anterior descending; LCX, left circumflex; RCA, right coronary artery.

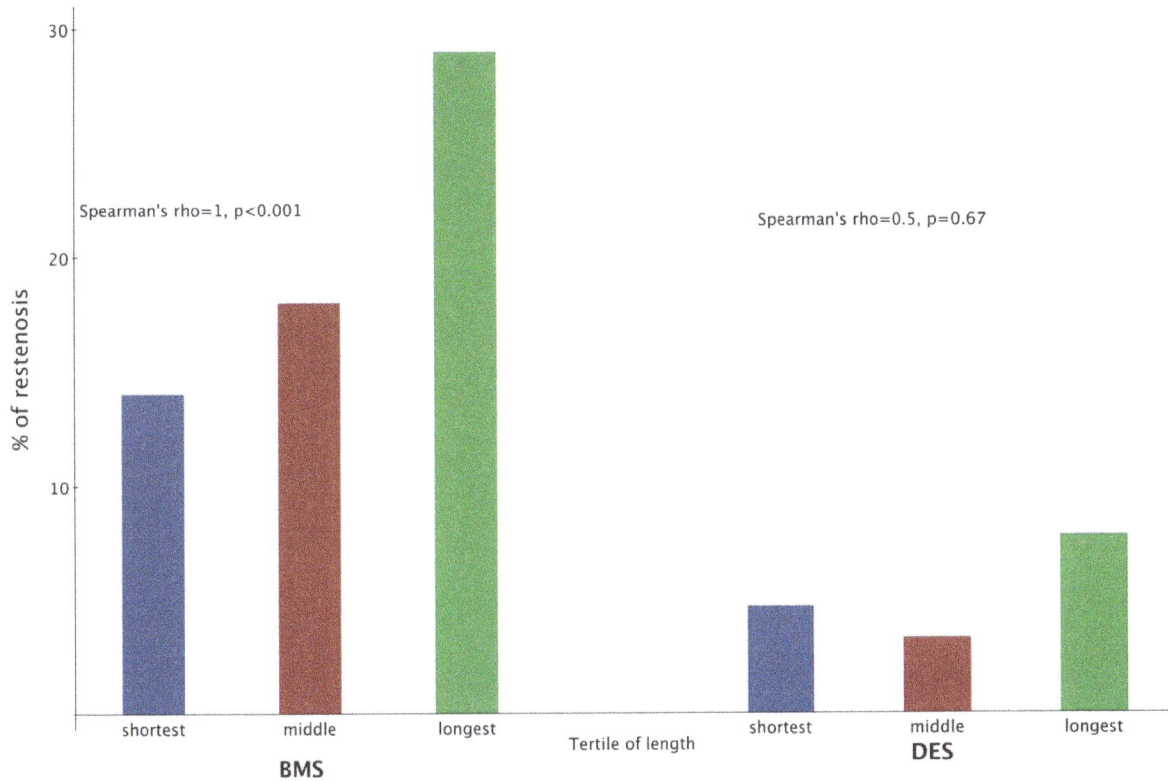

Figure 1. Intra-stent restenosis rate defined by scheduled angiographic follow-up of various lesion length. BMS: bare metal stent. DES: drug-eluting stents.

if only "hard" endpoints such as cardiac deaths and myocardial infractions had been considered as endpoints.

To our knowledge, this report is the first one that has directly compared IRS or very long term MACE-free survival between BMS and DES for every lesion length subgroups of a single registry. DES decreases IRS more dramatically than does BMS [23,28]. For example, Dawkins reported 12% vs. 36% ISR rates of DES vs. BMS in a TAXUS VI trial [29]. The present study supports these findings. Most data from numerous trials regarding lesion length and ISR in the DES era showed that DES resolved the issue of restenosis in lesions of various lengths [30,31]. Again, this paper supports that conclusion, but only for lesions that are shorter than 24 mm. DES is still superior to BMS in lesions longer than 24 mm, but the advantage is not as great as in shorter lesions.

The results of this study may have some clinical implications for the daily practice of interventional cardiologists. DES has lessened the impact of lesion length on ISR rate and MACE-free survival to some degree; therefore operators might feel comfortable in deploying DES for long lesions. One should be aware that some long lesions in this study (23% in BMS and 34% in DES) were covered by multiple overlapping stents, implying that DES were more effective in treating long lesions even when multiple stenting was involved. For example, Räber et al. reported a relatively high (18%) target lesion revascularization rate in 333 patients who had received multiple and overlapping DES [32]. However, before further evidence becomes available, one may argue that lesion length per se—instead of being a true underlying reason for higher ISR rate in the DES group—might merely be a surrogate for many other factors such as severity of disease, flow reserve, local inflammation, or lesion complexity. For example, the extent of intimal hyperplasia is significantly greater in lesions treated with

longer stents [33]. Therefore, more studies regarding the pathological effects of lesion length are needed. Nevertheless, lesion length is still a convenient parameter for making clinical decisions and predicting outcomes.

The present study has several limitations that should be mentioned. First, this is a registry observation from a single center, so the choice of stents and follow-up angiography might be biased considerably by operators, patients, or the availability of devices. Second, optimal medication choices, especially antiplatelet therapy, the technique and concept of percutaneous coronary intervention, and the design of devices, were evolving greatly during the long period of this study, the effect of which this analysis did not take into account. The difference of ticlopidine and clopidogrel, however, were examined, and it showed no effects on MACE. (Figure S1 of supplement data) Third, a major consideration that should be emphasized is the heterogeneity of DES. Recent randomized trials have shown that second-generation DES are superior to first-generation DES (especially palitaxel-eluting stents) in their ability to lower incidence of restenosis [34]. However, the very long term follow-up frame might have partially compensated for these limitations. The 'all comers' design of this study, which included a variety of stents, lesions, and patients, should be able to reflect the true impact of lesion length in the real world.

In conclusion, lesion length has different effects on ISR rates and MACE-free survival in BMS and DES in the real world. Lesion length positively associates with ISR rate for BMS,and longest lesions have the worst MACE-free survival. DES considerably lowers the effects of lesion length on ISR rates and MACE-free survival.

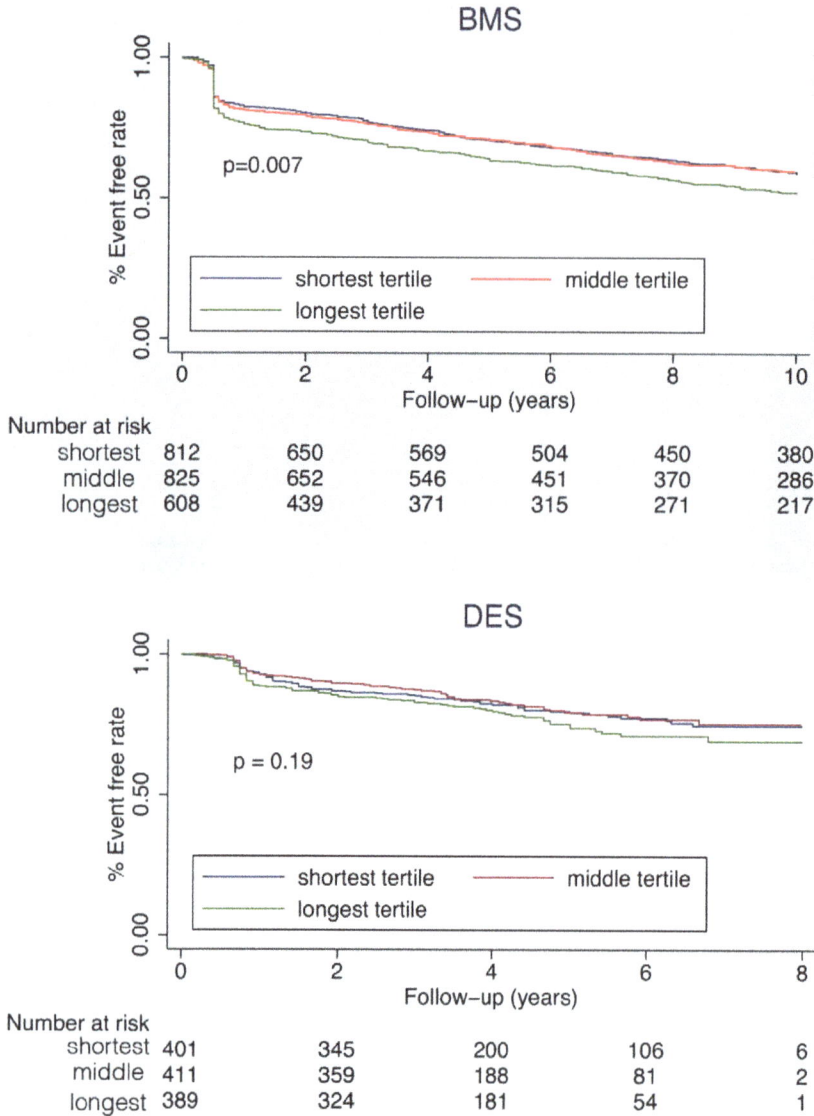

BMS

p=0.007

shortest tertile — middle tertile
longest tertile

Number at risk

shortest	812	650	569	504	450	380
middle	825	652	546	451	370	286
longest	608	439	371	315	271	217

DES

p = 0.19

shortest tertile — middle tertile
longest tertile

Number at risk

shortest	401	345	200	106	6
middle	411	359	188	81	2
longest	389	324	181	54	1

Figure 2. Kaplan-Meier estimates: major adverse cardiac events (MACE) free survival of patients with various lesion length. BMS: bare metal stent. DES: drug-eluting stents.

Supporting Information

Figure S1 MACE free survival of BMS group before and after clopidogrel era were similar. (Logrank p = 0.5). Blue line indicates the survival curve of patients treated with ticlopidine while red line indicates the curve of patients treated with clopidogrel.

Author Contributions

Conceived and designed the experiments: SHC ICH. Performed the experiments: CCC MJH CYW CHL. Analyzed the data: SHC. Contributed reagents/materials/analysis tools: CCC MJH CYW CHL. Wrote the paper: SHC ICH.

References

1. Boden WE, O'rourke RA, Teo KK, Hartigan PM, Maron DJ, et al. (2007) The evolving pattern of symptomatic coronary artery disease in the United States and Canada: baseline characteristics of the Clinical Outcomes Utilizing Revascularization and Aggressive DruG Evaluation (COURAGE) trial. Am J Cardiol 99: 208–212.
2. Liistro F, Stankovic G, Di Mario C, Takagi T, Chieffo A, et al. (2002) First clinical experience with a paclitaxel derivate-eluting polymer stent system implantation for in-stent restenosis: immediate and long-term clinical and angiographic outcome. Circulation 105: 1883–1886.
3. Koh AS, Chia S, Choi LM, Sim LL, Chua TSJ, et al. (2011) Long-term outcomes after coronary bare-metal-stent and drug-eluting-stent implantations:

a 'real-world' comparison among patients with diabetes with diffuse small vessel coronary artery disease. Coronary Artery Disease 22: 96–99.
4. Violini R, Musto C, De Felice F, Nazzaro MS, Cifarelli A, et al. (2010) Maintenance of long-term clinical benefit with sirolimus-eluting stents in patients with ST-segment elevation myocardial infarction 3-year results of the SESAMI (sirolimus-eluting stent versus bare-metal stent in acute myocardial infarction) trial. J Am Coll Cardiol 55: 810–814.
5. Menichelli M, Parma A, Pucci E, Fiorilli R, De Felice F, et al. (2007) Randomized trial of Sirolimus-Eluting Stent Versus Bare-Metal Stent in Acute Myocardial Infarction (SESAMI). J Am Coll Cardiol 49: 1924–1930.

6. Kobayashi Y, De Gregorio J, Kobayashi N, Akiyama T, Reimers B, et al. (1999) Stented segment length as an independent predictor of restenosis. J Am Coll Cardiol 34: 651–659.

7. Kastrati A, Elezi S, Dirschinger J, Hadamitzky M, Neumann FJ, et al. (1999) Influence of lesion length on restenosis after coronary stent placement. Am J Cardiol 83: 1617–1622.

8. Mehran R, Dangas G, Abizaid AS, Mintz GS, Lansky AJ, et al. (1999) Angiographic patterns of in-stent restenosis: classification and implications for long-term outcome. Circulation 100: 1872–1878.

9. de Feyter PJ, Kay P, Disco C, Serruys PW (1999) Reference chart derived from post-stent-implantation intravascular ultrasound predictors of 6-month expected restenosis on quantitative coronary angiography. Circ 100: 1777–1783.

10. Rozenman Y, Witzling V, Tamari I, Turkisher V, Kriviski M, et al. (2009) Impact of stent length on restenosis in patients with acute myocardial infarction treated with primary percutaneous coronary intervention: analysis based on data from the Trial to Assess the Use of the Cypher Stent in Acute Myocardial Infarction Treated with Balloon Angioplasty (TYPHOON). EuroIntervention 5: 219–223.

11. Rathore S, Terashima M, Katoh O, Matsuo H, Tanaka N, et al. (2009) Predictors of angiographic restenosis after drug eluting stents in the coronary arteries: contemporary practice in real world patients. EuroIntervention 5: 349–354.

12. Caputo RP, Goel A, Pencina M, Cohen DJ, Kleiman NS, et al. (2012) Impact of Drug Eluting Stent Length on Outcomes of Percutaneous Coronary Intervention (from the EVENT Registry). The American journal of cardiology 110: 350–355.

13. Cutlip DE, Chauhan MS, Baim DS, Ho KKL, Popma JJ, et al. (2002) Clinical restenosis after coronary stenting: perspectives from multicenter clinical trials. J Am Coll Cardiol 40: 2082–2089.

14. Kimura T, Abe K, Shizuta S, Odashiro K, Yoshida Y, et al. (2002) Long-term clinical and angiographic follow-up after coronary stent placement in native coronary arteries. Circ 105: 2986–2991.

15. Hsieh I-C, Huang H-L, See L-C, Chang S-H, Chang H-J, et al. (2006) Improvement in left ventricular function following coronary stenting in patients with acute myocardial infarction: 6-month and 3-year follow-up. International journal of cardiology 111: 209–216.

16. Kimura T, Yokoi H, Nakagawa Y, Tamura T, Kaburagi S, et al. (1996) Three-year follow-up after implantation of metallic coronary-artery stents. N Engl J Med 334: 561–566.

17. Teirstein PS (2010) Drug-eluting stent restenosis: an uncommon yet pervasive problem. Circ 122: 5–7.

18. Park KW, Kim C-H, Lee H-Y, Kang H-J, Koo B-K, et al. (2010) Does "late catch-up" exist in drug-eluting stents: insights from a serial quantitative coronary angiography analysis of sirolimus versus paclitaxel-eluting stents. Am Heart J 159: 446–453.e443.

19. Mauri L, O'Malley AJ, Cutlip DE, Ho KKL, Popma JJ, et al. (2004) Effects of stent length and lesion length on coronary restenosis. Am J Cardiol 93: 1340–1346, A1345.

20. Hsieh I-C, Chang H-J, Huang H-L, See L-C, Chern M-S, et al. (2004) Acute and long-term clinical and angiographic outcomes of coronary stenting using

Palmaz-Schatz stent and ACS Multi-Link stent. Catheter Cardiovasc Interv 62: 453–460.

21. Foley DP, Pieper M, Wijns W, Suryapranata H, Grollier G, et al. (2001) The influence of stent length on clinical and angiographic outcome in patients undergoing elective stenting for native coronary artery lesions; final results of the Magic 5L Study. Eur Heart J 22: 1585–1593.

22. Kereiakes D, Linnemeier TJ, Baim DS, Kuntz R, O'Shaughnessy C, et al. (2000) Usefulness of stent length in predicting in-stent restenosis (the MULTI-LINK stent trials). Am J Cardiol 86: 336–341.

23. Moses JW, Leon MB, Popma JJ, Fitzgerald PJ, Holmes DR, et al. (2003) Sirolimus-eluting stents versus standard stents in patients with stenosis in a native coronary artery. N Engl J Med 349: 1315–1323.

24. Holmes DR, Leon MB, Moses JW, Popma JJ, Cutlip D, et al. (2004) Analysis of 1-year clinical outcomes in the SIRIUS trial: a randomized trial of a sirolimus-eluting stent versus a standard stent in patients at high risk for coronary restenosis. Circulation 109: 634–640.

25. Mauri L, O'Malley AJ, Popma JJ, Moses JW, Leon MB, et al. (2005) Comparison of thrombosis and restenosis risk from stent length of sirolimus-eluting stents versus bare metal stents. Am J Cardiol 95: 1140–1145.

26. Tcheng JE, Lim IH, Srinivasan S, Jozic J, Gibson CM, et al. (2009) Stent parameters predict major adverse clinical events and the response to platelet glycoprotein IIb/IIIa blockade: findings of the ESPRIT trial. Circ Cardiovasc Interv 2: 43–51.

27. Shirai S, Kimura T, Nobuyoshi M, Morimoto T, Ando K, et al. (2010) Impact of multiple and long sirolimus-eluting stent implantation on 3-year clinical outcomes in the j-Cypher Registry. JACC Cardiovasc Interv 3: 180–188.

28. Dibra A, Kastrati A, Alfonso F, Seyfarth M, Pérez-Vizcayno M-J, et al. (2007) Effectiveness of drug-eluting stents in patients with bare-metal in-stent restenosis: meta-analysis of randomized trials. J Am Coll Cardiol 49: 616–623.

29. Dawkins KD, Grube E, Guagliumi G, Banning AP, Zmudka K, et al. (2005) Clinical efficacy of polymer-based paclitaxel-eluting stents in the treatment of complex, long coronary artery lesions from a multicenter, randomized trial: support for the use of drug-eluting stents in contemporary clinical practice. Circulation 112: 3306–3313.

30. Kim Y-H, Park S-W, Lee S-W, Park D-W, Yun S-C, et al. (2006) Sirolimus-eluting stent versus paclitaxel-eluting stent for patients with long coronary artery disease. Circulation 114: 2148–2153.

31. Grube E, Dawkins K, Guagliumi G, Banning A, Zmudka K, et al. (2009) TAXUS VI final 5-year results: a multicentre, randomised trial comparing polymer-based moderate-release paclitaxel-eluting stent with a bare metal stent for treatment of long, complex coronary artery lesions. EuroIntervention 4: 572–577.

32. Räber L, Jüni P, Löffel L, Wandel S, Cook S, et al. (2010) Impact of stent overlap on angiographic and long-term clinical outcome in patients undergoing drug-eluting stent implantation. J Am Coll Cardiol 55: 1178–1188.

33. Kang S-J, Mintz GS, Park D-W, Lee S-W, Kim Y-H, et al. (2011) Mechanisms of in-stent restenosis after drug-eluting stent implantation: intravascular ultrasound analysis. Circ Cardiovasc Interv 4: 9–14.

34. Dangas GD, Claessen BE, Caixeta A, Sanidas EA, Mintz GS, et al. (2010) In-stent restenosis in the drug-eluting stent era. J Am Coll Cardiol 56: 1897–1907.

16

National Trends over One Decade in Hospitalization for Acute Myocardial Infarction among Spanish Adults with Type 2 Diabetes: Cumulative Incidence, Outcomes and Use of Percutaneous Coronary Intervention

Ana Lopez-de-Andres*, Rodrigo Jimenez-Garcia, Valentin Hernandez-Barrera, Isabel Jimenez-Trujillo, Carmen Gallardo-Pino, Angel Gil de Miguel, Pilar Carrasco-Garrido

Preventive Medicine and Public Health Department. Rey Juan Carlos University. Alcorcón, Madrid, Spain

Abstract

Background: This study aims to describe trends in the rate of acute myocardial infarction (AMI) and use of percutaneous coronary interventions (PCI) in patients with and without type 2 diabetes in Spain, 2001–2010.

Methods: We selected all patients with a discharge of AMI using national hospital discharge data. Discharges were grouped by diabetes status: type 2 diabetes and no diabetes. In both groups PCIs were identified. The cumulative incidence of discharges attributed to AMI were calculated overall and stratified by diabetes status and year. We calculated length of stay and in-hospital mortality (IHM). Use of PCI was calculated stratified by diabetes status. Multivariate analysis was adjusted by age, sex, year and comorbidity. Results: From 2001 to 2010, 513,517 discharges with AMI were identified (30.3% with type 2 diabetes). The cumulative incidence of discharges due to AMI in diabetics patients increased (56.3 in 2001 to 71 cases per 100,000 in 2004), then decreased to 61.9 in 2010. Diabetic patients had significantly higher IHM (OR, 1.14; 95%CI, 1.05–1.17). The proportion of diabetic patients that underwent PCI increased from 11.9% in 2001 to 41.6% in 2010. Adjusted incidence of discharge in patients with diabetes who underwent PCI increased significantly (IRR, 3.49; 95%CI, 3.30–3.69). The IHM among diabetics patients who underwent a PCI did not change significantly over time.

Conclusions: AMI hospitalization rates increased initially but declining slowly. From 2001 to 2010 the proportion of diabetic patients who undergo a PCI increased almost four-fold. Older age and more comorbidity may explain why IHM did not improve after a PCI.

Editor: Giovanni Targher, University of Verona, Ospedale Civile Maggiore, Italy

Funding: This study forms part of research funded by the FIS (Fondo de Investigaciones Sanitarias—Health Research Fund, grant no. PI10/00360, Instituto de Salud Carlos III). The funders had no role in study design, data collection and analysis, decision to publish, or preparation of the manuscript.

Competing Interests: The authors have declared that no competing interests exist.

* E-mail: ana.lopez@urjc.es

Introduction

Diabetes is a major risk factor for atherosclerosis, which predisposes patients to occlusive coronary artery disease (CAD), acute myocardial infarction (AMI), and death [1]. It is well established that the long-term prognosis of AMI is worse in patients with diabetes than in those without diabetes [2,3]. In fact, the mortality rate for AMI is approximately double in patients with diabetes [3].

Patients with diabetes are prone to a diffuse and rapidly progressive form of CAD, which increases their likelihood of undergoing revascularization procedures [4]. Approximately one-third of all percutaneous coronary interventions (PCI) performed each year in the US are in patients with diabetes [5]. As the prevalence of diabetes increases, the number of patients with diabetes requiring revascularization for advanced CAD will escalate [6]. Although management of patients with CAD has improved considerably, coronary event rates remain very frequent, and mortality is greater among patients with diabetes [7].

Secular trends in the use of PCI in patients with diabetes have been examined [8,9]. In the UK, Vamos *et al.* [9] found that PCI rates increased significantly (IRR, 1.01, 95%CI, 1.005–1.03) in people with diabetes during 2004–2009. However, no studies have investigated national trends in the use and outcomes of PCI after AMI in diabetic patients in Spain.

In this study, we used national hospital discharge data to describe trends in the rate of AMI and use of PCI in patients with and without type 2 diabetes between 2001 and 2010 in Spain. In particular, we analyzed patient comorbidities and in-hospital outcomes such as length of stay and in-hospital mortality (IHM). Finally we analyzed the association between the use of PCI and IHM.

Materials and Methods

Ethics Statement

The Spanish National Hospital Database (CMBD) is hosted by the Ministry of Health Social Services and Equality (MSSSI). Researchers working in public and private institutions can request the databases by filling, signing and sending the questionnaire available the MSSSI web [10]. In the questionnaire the following information is required: 1. Researchers information. 2. Variables (years, diagnosis, procedures, outcomes and socio-demographic variables). 3. Objectives. 4. Analysis of patient records. 5. Proposed results dissemination. 6. Confidentiality Commitment.

All data used in this investigation was anonymized and de-identified by the MSSSI before it was provided to us.

Our investigation was presented and approved by the Institutional Review Board of the Rey Juan Carlos University.

According to the Confidentiality Commitment signed with the MSSSI we cannot provide anonymized or de-identified data to other researchers upon request. These researchers must request the data directly to the MSSSI.

Design

We performed a retrospective, descriptive, epidemiology study using the CMBD, which compiles all public and private hospital data and therefore covers more than 95% of hospital discharges [11]. The CMBD is managed by the MSSSI and includes patient variables (sex, date of birth), date of admission, date of discharge, up to 14 discharge diagnoses, and up to 20 procedures performed during the admission. The MSSSI sets standards for registration and performs periodic audits [11].

We selected discharges for AMI in patients whose main medical diagnosis was classified according to the International Classification of Diseases-Ninth Revision, Clinical Modification (ICD-9-CM), codes 410.0–419.0. Discharge grouped by diabetes status as follows: no diabetes and type 2 diabetes (ICD-9-CM codes 250.x0 and 250.x2). Patients with type 1 diabetes were excluded (ICD-9-CM codes: 250.x1; 250.x3). PCIs were identified using the ICD-9-CM codes 00.66, 36.06, and 36.07.

We calculated the cumulative incidence of discharge rates after AMI for patients with type 2 diabetic and non-diabetes patients per 100,000 inhabitants. We also calculated the yearly age- and sex-specific cumulative incidence rates for diabetic and non-diabetic patients by dividing the number of cases by year, sex, and age group by the corresponding number of people in that population group according to data from the Spanish National Institute of Statistics, as reported at December 31 of each year [12].

The outcomes of interest included the proportion of patients who died during admission (IHM) and the mean length of hospital stay (LOS).

Clinical characteristics included information on overall comorbidity at the time of surgery, which was assessed by computing the Charlson comorbidity index (CCI). The index applies to 17 disease categories whose scores are totaled to obtain an overall score for each patient [13]. The index is subsequently categorized into three levels: 0, no disease; 1, one or two diseases; and 3, more than three diseases. To calculate the CCI we used 15 disease categories, excluding diabetes and AMI, as described by Thomsen RW *et al.* [14].

The percentage of use of PCI was calculated during the study period in patients with and without type 2 diabetes. We calculated LOS and IHM after PCI by diabetes status.

Statistical Analysis

A descriptive statistical analysis was performed. Statistical significance was set at $p<0.05$ (2-tailed). In order to test the time trend in the use of PCI, we fitted separate Poisson regression models for patients with and without type 2 diabetes, using year of discharge, sex, age, and CCI as independent variables. For IHM, logistic regression analyses were performed with mortality as a binary outcome using the same variables for the group with and without diabetes and for the entire population. Statistical analyses were performed using Stata version 10.1 (Stata, College Station, Texas, USA).

Results

During the 10-year study period, 513,517 discharges with AMI were identified. Patients with type 2 diabetes accounted for 30.3% of the total (155,676). Mean age was 67.26 ± 13.95 years, and 60.5% were men. In patients without diabetes, the mean age was 71.38 ± 11.18 years, and 73.2% were men ($p<0.05$).

Table 1 shows the annual hospital discharges rates for patients with and without type 2 diabetes. The cumulative incidence of discharges due to AMI in patients with diabetes increased from 56.3 cases per 100,000 inhabitants in 2001 to 71 cases per 100,000 inhabitants in 2004 and then decreased to 61.9 cases per 100,000 inhabitants in 2010. Cumulative incidence was significantly higher for men in both groups and in all the years studied.

The mean length of stay fell from 10.4 days in 2001 to 8.6 days in 2010 for patients with type 2 diabetes ($p<0.05$) and from 9.9 days in 2001 to 7.7 days in 2010 for patients without diabetes ($p<0.05$). LOS was significantly higher among men and women with than without diabetes in all the years analyzed ($p<0.05$).

Patients with type 2 diabetes had significantly higher IHM than patients without diabetes (11.5% vs. 9.2%). IHM decreased significantly from 13.2% in 2001 to 9.8% in 2010 among diabetic adults and from 11.2% to 7.7% among non-diabetic adults.

IHM decreased for both sexes, although it was always greater in women with type 2 diabetes than in men with type 2 diabetes (Figure 1).

Table 2 presents the results of a multivariate analysis of the factors associated with cumulative incidence and IHM after AMI. When the year 2004 was used as the reference and after controlling for possible confounders, we observed that the cumulative incidence of discharges in patients with type 2 diabetes did not change significantly after this year (IRR, 0.98; 95%CI, 0.96–1.01).

IHM was significantly greater in women with diabetes than in men with diabetes (OR, 1.28; 95%CI, 1.24–1.32) and in those with more diabetes-associated comorbidities (OR, 1.88; 95%CI, 1.82–1.95 [for those with 1 or 2 comorbidities] and OR, 2.64; 95%CI, 2.52–2.78 [for those with 3 or more comorbidities]). Those diabetic patients who did not receive a PCI had a 2.41 fold (95%CI, 2.32–256) higher probability of dying during their stay than those who underwent this procedure.

When we analyzed the entire database, patients with type 2 diabetes had significantly higher mortality than patients without diabetes after adjusting for age, gender, CCI, and year (OR, 1.14; 95%CI, 1.05–1.17).

Coronary revascularization

Between 2001 and 2010, the overall number of PCIs in Spain was 168,537 (44,331 among patients with type 2 diabetes [26.3%]). There was a considerable male predominance in both patients with and patients without diabetes (70.0% and 81.2%, respectively). The mean age at the time of the PCI was

Table 1. Hospital discharges due to acute myocardial infarction among patients with and without type 2 diabetes in Spain, 2001–2010.

Year	With Type 2 Diabetes				Without Diabetes			
	Total	Incidence	LOS (SD)	%IHM	Total	Incidence	LOS (SD)	% IHM
2001	12235	56.3	10.4(8.5)	13.2	34131	156.9	9.9(9.4)	11.2
2002	13864	62.9	10.6(9.1)	13.8	36904	167.5	9.8(9.6)	10.5
2003	15955	70.7	10.4(9.1)	12.9	36870	163.5	9.3(8.6)	10.3
2004	16396	71	10(8.3)	11.8	36550	158.3	9.1(10.3)	9.7
2005	16608	70.4	9.8(8.4)	12.1	36187	153.4	8.8(8.8)	9.2
2006	15754	65.4	9.6(8.7)	11.2	35566	147.5	8.5(8.4)	8.5
2007	16082	65.3	9.2(8.6)	11.0	35537	144.4	8.3(8.9)	8.5
2008	16221	64.6	9.2(8.3)	10.6	35799	142.5	8.1(8.7)	8.3
2009	16390	63.9	8.9(9.6)	9.8	35309	137.7	7.8(8.3)	7.9
2010	16171	61.9	8.6(9)	9.8	34988	133.8	7.7(9.5)	7.7
Total Men	94199	83.1	9.5(8.9)	9.4	262013	231.1	8.6(9.1)	7.4
Total Female	61477	50.1	9.9(8.6)	14.9	95828	78.1	9(9.1)	14.1
Total	155676	65.2	9.6(8.8)	11.5	357841	149.9	8.7(9.1)	9.2

Cumulative Incidence per100,000. Cumulative Incidence was calculated using the Spanish National Statistics Institute census projections [11]. LOS (SD): Mean length of stay (standard deviation). %IHM: In-Hospital Mortality.

significantly higher in patients with type 2 diabetes (67.2±0.05 years vs. 62.5±0.04 years).

Among those who underwent PCI, the mean LOS was significantly higher in patients with diabetes than in those without diabetes (9.31±0.04 days vs. 8.23±0.02 days). In addition, IHM was significantly higher in patients with diabetes (4.4% vs. 3.1%).

Patients with type 2 diabetes undergoing PCIs had a higher CCI than those without diabetes (39.2% vs. 28.5% with ≥1, respectively).

Table 3 shows the time trend for annual PCIs in patients with and without type 2 diabetes in Spain during 2001–2010. We found that use of PCI increased significantly in patients with and without diabetes. In 2001, 11.9% of patients with type 2 diabetes and 16.7% of patients without type 2 diabetes underwent PCI; in 2010,

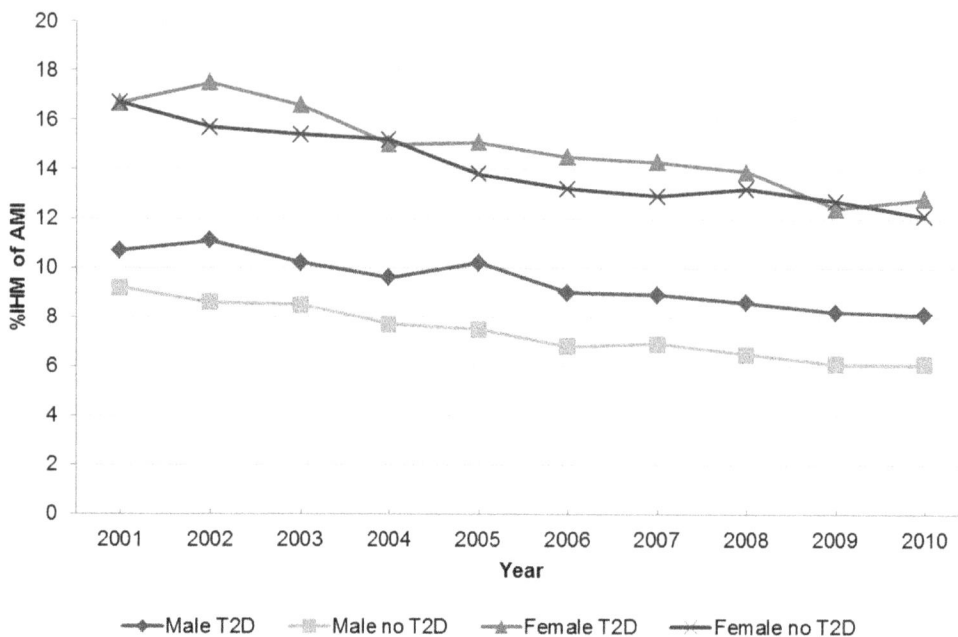

Figure 1. In-hospital mortality after AMI in patients with and without type 2 diabetes according to sex. IHM of AMI: In-hospital mortality after acute myocardial infarction. Male T2D: Men with type 2 diabetes. Male no T2D: Men without type 2 diabetes. Female T2D: Women with type 2 diabetes. Female without T2D: Women without type 2 diabetes.

Table 2. Multivariate analysis of the factors associated with cumulative incidence and in-hospital mortality after acute myocardial infarction in patients with and without type 2 diabetes in Spain, 2001–2010.

		With Type 2 Diabetes		Without Diabetes	
		Incidence (IRR)*	IHM (OR)†	Incidence (IRR)*	IHM (OR)†
Age (years)	35–60 years	1	1	1	1
	61–70 years	1.32 (1.30–1.34)	1.97 (1.82–2.13)	1.58 (1.54–1.61)	2.05 (1.95–2.16)
	71–80 years	2.11 (2.07–2.14)	3.46 (3.23–3.71)	1.23 (1.21–1.25)	3.99 (3.82–4.17)
	>80 years	1.21 (1.19–1.22)	5.84 (5.45–6.30)	1.72 (1.69–1.75)	7.79 (7.46–8.15)
Sex	Men	1	1	1	1
	Female	0.65 (0.64–0.66)	1.28 (1.24–1.32)	0.37 (0.36–0.38)	1.28 (1.25–1.32)
Charlson Index	0	1	1	1	1
	1–2	0.82 (0.81–0.83)	1.88 (1.82–1.95)	0.51 (0.50–0.53)	1.88 (1.83–1.92)
	≥3	0.20 (0.19–0.21)	2.64 (2.52–2.78)	0.09 (0.08–0.10)	2.76 (2.64–2.87)
Year	2001	0.75 (0.73–0.76)	1	0.93(0.92–0.95)	1
	2002	0.84(0.83–0.86)	1.03 (0.95–1.10)	1.01(0.99–1.02)	0.89 (0.85–0.94)
	2003	0.97(0.95–0.99)	0.90 (0.84–0.97)	1.00(0.99–1.02)	0.86 (0.82–0.90)
	2004	1	0.81 (0.76–0.87)	1	0.80 (0.76–0.84)
	2005	1.01(0.99–1.03)	0.82 (0.77–0.89)	0.99(0.97–1.00)	0.73 (0.70–0.77)
	2006	0.96(0.94–0.98)	0.76 (0.71–0.82)	0.97(0.96–0.98)	0.68 (0.65–0.72)
	2007	0.98(0.96–1.00)	0.73 (0.68–0.79)	0.97(0.96–0.98)	0.67 (0.64–0.71)
	2008	0.98(0.97–1.01)	0.69 (0.64–0.74)	0.98(0.96–0.99)	0.65 (0.62–0.68)
	2009	0.99(0.98–1.02)	0.63 (0.58–0.68)	0.97(0.95–0.98)	0.61 (0.58–0.65)
	2010	0.98 (0.96–1.01)	0.63 (0.58–0.68)	0.96(0.94–0.97)	0.61 (0.58–0.64)
PCI	Yes		1		1
	No		2,44 (2,32–2,56)		2,56 (2,42–2,66)

IHM: In-Hospital Mortality. PCI: Percutaneous Coronary Intervention.
*Calculated using multivariate Poisson regression: Incidence Rate Ratios (IRR).
†Calculate using logistic regression models: Odds Ratio (OR).
The logistic regression multivariate model and Poisson regression model were built using as dependent variables "death (yes/no)" and "Cumulative incidence of PCI" respectively, and as independent variables year, sex, Charlson comorbidity index, and age.

the corresponding figures were and 41.6% and 50.4%. The proportion of patients who had AMI and underwent PCI was significantly higher among those without diabetes in all the years studied.

As can be seen in Table 3, the mean age of a person with diabetes who underwent PCI was 65.7±10.2 years in 2001 and 67.8±11.1 years in 2010. The proportion of men varied from 68.9% in 2001 to 71.4% in 2010, and the prevalence of those with a CCI of ≥1 increased from 34.2% to 40.6% (p<0.05).

LOS after PCI decreased significantly during the study period in both groups of patients, showing higher values among those with diabetes in all the years analyzed (Table 3). IHM among those who underwent PCI decreased for patients without diabetes (3.9% to 3.0; p<0.05) but remained stable for those with diabetes (3.9% to 4.3%; p>0.05)

Multivariate analysis revealed that the cumulative incidence of discharge in patients with diabetes who underwent PCI increased significantly during the study period (IRR 3.49; 95%CI, 3.30–3.69) (Table 4).

After an adjusted multivariate analysis, the IHM among persons with diabetes who underwent a PCI did not change significantly over time. IHM was significantly greater in women than in men (OR 1.32; 95%CI, 1.20–1.46) and was higher in those with 1 or 2 diabetes-associated conditions (OR 2.39; 95%CI, 2.17–2.64) and

≥3 conditions (OR 3.19; 95%CI 2.73–3.73) than in those who had no associated comorbidities.

Discussion

Our results reveal that more than 30% of Spanish adults who experience AMI have an associated diagnosis of diabetes. These results are consistent with those of Gore *et al.* (2012) [15], who showed that 29% of patients admitted to hospital for AMI in the US had diabetes.

From 2004 to 2010, rates of hospitalization for AMI in patients with type 2 diabetes decreased, but not significantly. The results of a study in the UK showed a considerable decline in hospital discharge for AMI in patients with diabetes between 2004–2005 and 2009–2010 (OR, 0.95; 95%CI, 0.93–0.97) [9]. Our results are consistent with this finding: rates of hospitalization for AMI increased initially before leveling off in 2004 and finally declining slowly from 71 cases per 100,000 inhabitants in 2004 to 61.9 cases per 100,000 inhabitants in 2010, thus revealing the same tendency as in the UK. The changes in these rates can be attributed to favorable trends in physical activity levels and cigarette smoking and increased use of effective treatments (eg, antihypertensive agents, ACE inhibitors, and lipid-lowering drugs) [9]. We think that the lack in improvement of lifestyles among diabetic patients [16,17] and the absence of national prevention and treatment

Table 3. Characteristics and outcomes of hospital discharges after percutaneous coronary intervention among patients with and without type 2 diabetes in Spain, 2001–2010.

	2001	2002	2003	2004	2005	2006	2007	2008	2009	2010
Diabetes										
N*	1,467	2,206	2,885	3,640	4,439	4,781	5,474	6,067	6,645	6,727
%PCI*	11.9	15.9	18.1	22.2	26.7	30.3	34.1	37.4	40.5	41.6
Age, mean (SD)*	65.7	66.2	66.3	66.6	66.7	67.2	67.6	67.9	67.6	67.8
	(10.2)	(10.3)	(10.5)	(10.4)	(10.6)	(10.7)	(10.7)	(10.8)	(11.1)	(11.1)
Female, n (%)	457	702	861	1101	1304	1435	1691	1850	1980	1925
	(31.1)	(31.8)	(29.8)	(30.2)	(29.3)	(30.0)	(30.8)	(30.4)	(29.8)	(28.6)
CCI 0, n (%)	965	1420	1750	2226	2758	3086	3344	3524	3897	3994
	(65.7)	(64.3)	(60.6)	(61.1)	(62.1)	(64.5)	(61.1)	(58.1)	(58.6)	(59.3)
CCI 1–2, n (%)*	456	709	1004	1246	1442	1482	1846	2141	2265	2247
	(31.1)	(32.1)	(34.8)	(34.2)	(32.5)	(31.0)	(33.7)	(35.2)	(34.1)	(33.4)
CCI≥3, n (%)*	46	77	131	168	239	213	284	402	483	486
	(3.1)	(3.5)	(4.5)	(4.6)	(5.4)	(4.5)	(5.2)	(6.6)	(7.2)	(7.2)
LOS, mean (SE)*	11.3	10.9	10.5	9.8	9.7	9.3	9.1	9.0	8.6	8.2
	(0.23)	(0.21)	(0.18)	(0.13)	(0.12)	(0.12)	(0.11)	(0.1)	(0.1)	(0.1)
IHM, n (%)*	58	114	126	130	207	221	253	291	276	291
	(3.9)	(5.1)	(4.3)	(3.6)	(4.7)	(4.6)	(4.6)	(4.8)	(4.1)	(4.3)
No diabetes										
N*	5,715	7,624	8,882	10,252	12,249	13,216	14,807	16,325	17,499	17,637
%PCI*	16.7	20.6	24.1	28.1	33.8	37.1	41.6	45.6	49.5	50.4
Age, mean (SD)*	61.6	61.8	61.5	61.9	62.4	62.5	62.6	62.9	63.1	62.8
	(12.0)	(12.2)	(12.3)	(12.3)	(12.5)	(12.6)	(12.7)	(12.9)	(12.9)	(12.9)
Female, n (%)	1034	1363	1567	1808	2286	2526	2799	3115	3434	3473
	(18.0)	(17.8)	(17.6)	(17.6)	(18.6)	(19.1)	(18.9)	(19.0)	(19.6)	(19.6)
CCI 0, n (%)*	4188	5508	6367	7296	8675	9599	10548	11543	12438	12634
	(73.3)	(72.2)	(71.7)	(71.1)	(70.8)	(72.6)	(71.2)	(70.7)	(71.1)	(71.6)
CCI 1–2, n (%)*	1427	1968	2300	2688	3243	3262	3798	4208	4410	4339
	(24.9)	(25.8)	(25.9)	(26.2)	(26.4)	(24.6)	(25.6)	(25.7)	(25.2)	(24.6)
CCI≥3, n (%)*	100	148	215	268	331	355	461	574	651	664
	(1.7)	(1.9)	(2.4)	(2.6)	(2.7)	(2.6)	(3.1)	(3.5)	(3.7)	(3.7)
LOS, mean (SE)*	10.0	9.6	8.9	8.7	8.6	8.1	7.8	7.8	7.6	7.4
	(0.16)	(0.11)	(0.08)	(0.09)	(0.08)	(0.07)	(0.06)	(0.06)	(0.06)	(0.06)
IHM, n (%)*	227	238	297	324	379	367	422	497	566	531
	(3.9)	(3.1)	(3.3)	(3.1)	(3.0)	(2.7)	(2.8)	(3.0)	(3.2)	(3.0)

N:number of procedure; PCI:Percutaneous Coronary Intervention; SE:Standard Error;LOS:Length of stay; IHM:In-hospital mortality; CCI:Charlson comorbidity index; *p<0.05 Statistically significant differences were observed during 2001–2010.

program throughout the study period may explain the different behavior in the reduction of hospitalizations for AMI between our data and those reported by Vamos et al [9].

IHM as a consequence of AMI decreased both in patients with and in patients without type 2 diabetes. Recent studies showed that patients with and without diabetes who have experienced AMI have lower mortality rates over time, suggesting that management of AMI patients has improved in recent years [9,18–20]. More frequent and effective use of PCI, which reduced IHM in our study, has been observed by other investigators [18,20]. We found that IHM for patients who did not receive a PCI was very similar in 2001 and 2010 for both those with diabetes (14.4% to 13.6%) and those without diabetes (12.6% to 12.4%).

Consistent with the results of other studies, and after adjusting for age and gender, we found that IHM for patients with AMI was significantly greater for patients with type 2 diabetes than for those without diabetes (11.5% vs. 9.2%) [21–23], possibly because these patients have a worse clinical status or are at a greater risk of complications [9,18]. In our population, the proportion of patients with diabetes and a CCI≥3 was 10.0%, whereas the proportion for those without diabetes was 5.8% (p<0.05).

Our results are similar to those of studies reporting that women have a lower cumulative incidence of AMI than men [24,25]. However, after controlling for possible confounders, we found that women with diabetes had significantly higher IHM rates than men with diabetes. These results are consistent with those of other studies that analyze differences in diabetes between the sexes

Table 4. Multivariate analysis of the factors associated with cumulative incidence and mortality after percutaneous coronary intervention in patients with type 2 diabetes in Spain, 2001–2010.

		Incidence (IRR)*	In-hospital mortality (OR)†
Age (years)	35–60 years	1	1
	61–70 years	0.87 (0.85–0.89)	1.37 (1.16–1.61)
	71–80 years	0.70 (0.68–0.71)	2.56 (2.21–2.98)
	>80 years	0.33 (0.32–0.35)	3.31 (2.78–3.94)
Sex	Men	1	1
	Female	0.80 (0.79–0.82)	1.32 (1.20–1.46)
Charlson Index	0	1	1
	1–2	0.74 (0.73–0.76)	2.39 (2.17–2.64)
	≥3	0.51 (0.49–0.53)	3.19 (2.73–3.73)
Year	2001	1	1
	2002	1.32 (1.24–1.41)	1.27 (0.92–1.76)
	2003	1.53 (1.43–1.62)	1.04 (0.76–1.43)
	2004	1.86 (1.75–1.98)	0.83 (0.60–1.14)
	2005	2.25 (2.12–2.39)	1.08 (0.80–1.46)
	2006	2.52 (2.38–2.67)	1.07 (0.80–1.45)
	2007	2.86 (2.70–3.03)	1.03 (0.77–1.38)
	2008	3.16 (2.98–3.34)	1.02 (0.75–1.36)
	2009	3.40 (3.21–3.60)	0.89 (0.66–1.19)
	2010	3.49 (3.30–3.69)	0.92 (0.69–1.23)

*IRR: Incidence Rate Ratios calculated using multivariate Poisson regression.
†OR: Odds Ratio calculated using logistic regression models.
The logistic regression multivariate model and Poisson regression model were built using as dependent variables "death (yes/no)" and "Cumulative incidence of PCI" respectively, and as independent variables year, sex, Charlson comorbidity index, and age.

[3,24,25]. A recent study indicated that women with diabetes have a greater risk of mortality than men (3.44; 95%CI, 2.47–4.79), especially when diagnosed at a later stage [26]. These data suggest that factors such as the extent of treatment and monitoring, underuse of medications recommended by clinical guidelines, and reduced efficacy of active agents may be more common in women with diabetes than in men with diabetes [27,28].

Coronary revascularization

During the study period, the number of PCIs performed in patients with type 2 diabetes increased considerably from 11.9% in 2001 to 41.0% in 2010. This result is consistent with those of other studies [9,20,29], in which PCI rates increased significantly owing to marked advances in stent technology and adjunctive pharmacology. One report documented the rapid progress in PCI treatment options for patients with diabetes and indicated that PCI devices (drug-eluting stents) were used more often in patients with severe comorbidities and multivessel disease and were associated with more frequent prescription of recommended cardiac medications at discharge [30].

Successful PCI has probably improved in-hospital survival rates. Therefore, IHM was more likely to be associated with patient clinical status and medical treatment strategy. Vamos *et al.* [9] found significant increases in IHM rates for PCI, despite technological advances in interventional techniques and improve-

ments in periprocedural care. The authors explained their findings by referring to the increasing complexity of cases referred for PCI.

We found that IHM remained stable among diabetic patients with PCI. The higher comorbidity and older age can partially explain this lack of improvement.

In patients with AMI who had undergone PCI, women with type 2 diabetes had worse outcomes than men with diabetes. Our results are consistent with those of other studies, which suggest that the worse effect of diabetes on outcomes in women might be related to the onset mechanism of AMI, the success of the PCI procedure, and the higher burden of cardiovascular risk factors [20,24,31,32].

The strength of our investigation lies in its large sample size and standardized methodology, which has previously been used to investigate diabetes in Spain and elsewhere [33,34]. Nevertheless, our study is subject to a series of limitations. Our data source was the CMBD, an administrative database that contains discharge data for Spanish hospitalizations and uses information the physician has included in the discharge report; therefore, it does not include all the variables in the clinical history. Another limitation of this database is its anonymity (no identifying items such as number of the clinical history or the name of the hospital), which makes it impossible to detect whether the same patient was admitted more than once during the same year. In addition, patients who moved from one hospital to another would appear twice.

Nevertheless, this dataset, which was introduced in Spain in 1982, is a mandatory register, and its coverage is estimated to be more than 95% [10].

Unfortunately in Spain a validation study to assess the rate of unreported diagnosis of diabetes in administrative databases has not been conducted so far. However, a recent review and meta-analysis conducted by Leong A et al (2013) concluded that a commonly-used administrative database definition for diabetes had a pooled sensitivity of 82.3% (95%CI 75.8, 87.4) and specificity of 97.9% (95%CI 96.5, 98.8%), based on the findings of 6 studies with complete data available. While this definition appears to miss approximately one fifth of diabetes cases and wrongly classifies 2.1% of non-cases in the population as diabetes cases, it is likely sufficiently sensitive for monitoring prevalence trends in the general population if its accuracy remains reasonably stable over time [35].

We were unable to calculate diabetes-specific cumulative incidence rates, because no studies in Spain cover blood glucose measurements for the entire population; consequently, no precise estimation of the prevalence of diabetes is available [36]. Concerns have been raised about the accuracy of routinely collected datasets; however, these datasets are periodically audited. Consequently, the quality and validity of our dataset has been assessed and shown to be useful for health research [37].

In conclusion, we provide national data on changes in the burden of AMI events in Spain. Our results show that AMI hospitalization rates increased initially, before leveling off in 2004 and finally declining slowly in people with and without diabetes. Outcomes such as LOS and IHM are worse among persons with diabetes than without diabetes, although they improved over time for both groups. Higher comorbidity and female sex are associated with higher IHM.

The proportion of diabetic patients who undergo a PCI increased almost four-fold from 2001 to 2010. Older age and more comorbidity may explain why IHM among diabetic persons did not improve after a PCI during the study period.

Furthermore, given the rapid increase in prevalence of diabetes and the aging population, these findings emphasize the need for further improvement in the control of cardiovascular risk factors in people with diabetes.

Author Contributions

Conceived and designed experiments: AL RJG PCG. Performed the experiments: AL RJG PCG. Analyzed the data: AL RJG VHB PCG. Contributed reagents/materials/analysis tool: AL RJG VHB IJT CGP AGM PCG. Wrote the manuscript: AL RJG VHB PCG.

References

1. Lüscher TF, Creager MA, Beckman JA, Cosentino F (2003) Diabetes and vascular disease: pathophysiology, clinical consequences, and medical therapy: Part II. Circulation 108:1655–1661.
2. American Diabetes Association (2008) Economic costs of diabetes in the U.S. in 2007. Diabetes Care 31:596–615.
3. Svensson AM, Dellborg M, Abrahamsson P, Karlsson T, Herlitz J, et al. (2007) The influence of a history of diabetes on treatment and outcome in acute myocardial infarction, during two time periods and in two different countries. Int J Cardiol 119:319–325.
4. Ryden L, Standl E, Bartnik M, Van den Berghe G, Betteridge J, et al. (2007) Guidelines on diabetes, pre-diabetes, and cardiovascular diseases: executive summary. The Task Force on Diabetes and Cardiovascular Diseases of the European Society of Cardiology (ESC) and of the European Association for the Study of Diabetes (EASD). Eur Heart J 28:88–136.
5. Flahert JD, Davidson CJ (2005) Diabetes and coronary revascularization. JAMA 293: 1501–1508.
6. Aronson D, Edelman ER (2010) Revascularization for coronary artery disease in diabetes mellitus: angioplasty, stents and coronary artery bypass grafting. Rev Endocr Metab Disord 11:75–86.
7. Action to Control Cardiovascular Risk in Diabetes Study Group, Gerstein HC, Miller ME, Byington RP, Goff DC Jr, et al. (2008) Effects of intensive glucose lowering in type 2 diabetes. N Engl J Med 358:2545–2559.
8. Singh M, Holmes DR Jr, Gersh BJ, Frye RL, Lennon RJ, et al. (2013) Thirty-year trends in outcomes of percutaneous coronary interventions in diabetic patients. Mayo Clin Proc 88:22–30.
9. Vamos EP, Millett C, Parsons C, Aylin P, Majeed A, et al. (2012) Nationwide study on trends in hospital admissions for major cardiovascular events and procedures among people with and without diabetes in England, 2004–2009. Diabetes Care 35:265–272.
10. Ministry of Health Social Services and Equality. Conjunto Mínimo Básico de Datos. Available:http://www.msssi.gob.es/estadEstudios/estadisticas/estadisticas/estMinisterio/SolicitudCMBDdocs/Formulario_Peticion_Datos_CMBD.pdf. Accessed 23 Sep 2013.
11. Instituto Nacional de Gestión Sanitaria, Ministerio de Sanidad y Consumo. Conjunto Mínimo Básico de Datos, Hospitales del INSALUD. 2001; Available: http://www.ingesa.msc.es/estadEstudios/documPublica/CMBD- 2001.htm. Accessed 15 May 2013.
12. Instituto Nacional de Estadística (INE) Population estimates. 2010.Available: www.ine.es. Accessed 15 May 2013.
13. Charlson ME, Pompei P, Ales KL, MacKenzie CR (1987) A new method of classifying prognostic comorbidity in longitudinal studies: development and validation. J Chronic Dis 40:373–383.
14. Thomsen RW, Nielsen JS, Ulrichsen SP, Pedersen L, Hansen AM, et al. (2012) The Danish Centre for Strategic Research in Type 2 Diabetes (DD2) study: Collection of baseline data from the first 580 patients. Clin Epidemiol 4:43–48.
15. Gore MO, Patel MJ, Kosiborod M, Parsons LS, Khera A, et al. (2012) Diabetes mellitus and trends in hospital survival after myocardial infarction, 1994 to 2006: data from the national registry of myocardial infarction. Circ Cardiovasc Qual Outcomes 5:791–797.
16. Jiménez-García R, Hernández-Barrera V, Jiménez-Trujillo I, Garrido PC, López de Andrés A, et al. (2009)Trends in cardiovascular risk factors and lifestyle behaviors among Spanish adults with diabetes (1993–2003). J Diabetes Complications 23:394–400.
17. Jiménez Trujillo I, Jiménez García R, Vazquez-Fernandez del Pozo S, Hernández Barrera V, Carrasco Garrido P, et al. (2010) Trends from 1995 to 2006 in the prevalence of self-reported cardiovascular risk factors among elderly Spanish diabetics. Diabetes Metab 36:29–35.
18. Booth GL, Kapral MK, Fung K, Tu JV (2006) Recent trends in cardiovascular complications among men and women with and without diabetes. Diabetes Care 29:32–37
19. Degano IR, Elosua R, Marrugat J (2013) Epidemiology of acute coronary syndromes in Spain: Estimation of the number of cases and trends from 2005 to 2049. Rev Esp Cardiol 66:472–481.
20. Ouhoummane N, Abdous B, Louchini R, Rochette L, Poirier P (2010) Trends in postacute myocardial infarction managment and mortality in patients with diabetes. A population-based study from 1995 to 2001. Can J Cardiol 26(10):523–531.
21. Whiteley L, Padmanabhan S, Hole D, Isles C (2005) Should diabetes be considered a coronary heart disease risk equivalent? Results from 25 years of follow-up in the Renfrew and Paisley survey. Diabetes Care 28: 1588–1593.
22. Vaccaro O, Eberly LE, Neaton JD, Yang L, Riccardi G, et al. (2004) Impact of diabetes and previous myocardial infarction on long-term survival: 25-year mortality follow-up of primary screenees of the Multiple Risk Factor Intervention Trial. Arch Intern Med 164: 1438–1443.
23. Hirakawa Y, Masuda Y, Kuzuya M, Iguchi A, Kimata T, et al. (2007) Influence of diabetes mellitus on in-hospital mortality in patients with acute myocardial infarction in Japan: a report from TAMIS-II. Diabetes Res Clin Pract 75:59–64.
24. Norhammar A, Stenestrand U, Lindbäck J, Wallentin L, Register of Information and Knowledge about Swedish Heart Intensive Care Admission (RIKS-HIA) (2008) Women younger than 65 years with diabetes mellitus are a high-risk group after myocardial infarction: a report from the Swedish Register of Information and Knowledge about Swedish Heart Intensive Care Admission (RIKS-HIA). Heart 94:1565–1570.
25. Maier B, Thimme W, Kallischnigg G, Graf-Bothe C, Rohnisch JU, et al. (2006) Does diabetes mellitus explain the higher hospital mortality of women with acute myocardial infarction? Results from the Berlin Myocardial Infarction Registry. J Investig Med 54:143–151.
26. Roche MM, Wang PP (2013) Sex differences in all-cause and cardiovascular mortality, hospitalizations for individuals with and without diabetes, and patients with diabetes diagnosed early and late. Diabetes Care 36:2582–2590.
27. Gouni-Berthold I, Berthold HK, Mantzoros CS, Böhm M, Krone W (2008) Sex disparities in the treatment and control of cardiovascular risk factors in type 2 diabetes. Diabetes Care 31:1389–1391.
28. Ferrara A, Mangione CM, Kim C, Marrero DG, Curb D, et al. (2008) Sex disparities in control and treatment of modifiable cardiovascular disease risk factors among patients with diabetes: Translating Research Into Action for Diabetes (TRIAD) Study. Diabetes Care 31:69–74.
29. Bottle A, Millett C, Khunti K, Majeed A (2009) Trends in cardiovascular admissions and procedures for people with and without diabetes in England, 1996–2005. Diabetologia 52: 74–80.
30. Rana JS, Venkitachalam L, Selzer F, Mulukutla SR, Marroquin OC, et al. (2010) Evolution of percutaneous coronary intervention in patients with diabetes. A report from the National Heart, Lung, and Blood Institute-sponsored PTCA (1985-1986) and Dynamic (1997–2006) Registries. Diabetes Care 33:1976–1982.
31. Champney KP, Veledar E, Klein M, Samady H, Anderson D, et al. (2007) Sex-specific effects of diabetes on adverse outcomes after percutaneous coronary intervention: trends over time. Am Heart J 153:970–978.
32. Blöndal M, Ainla T, Marandi T, Baburin A, Eha J (2012) Sex-specific outcomes of diabetic patients with acute myocardial infarction who have undergone percutaneous coronary intervention: a register linkage study. Cardiovasc Diabetol 11:96.
33. López-de-Andrés A, Martínez-Huedo MA, Carrasco-Garrido P, Hernández-Barrera V, Gil-de-Miguel A, et al. (2011) Trends in lower-extremity amputations in people with and without diabetes in Spain, 2001–2008. Diabetes Care 34:1570–1576.
34. López –de-Andrés A, Jiménez-García R, Hernández-Barrera V, Gil-de-Miguel A, Jiménez-Trujillo MI, et al. (2013) Trends in utilization and outcomes of bariatric surgery in obese people with and without type 2 diabetes in Spain (2001–2010). Diabetes Res Clin Pract 99:300–306.
35. Leong A, Dasgupta K, Bernatsky S, Lacaille D, Avina-Zubieta A, et al. (2013) Systematic review and meta-analysis of validation studies on a diabetes case definition from health administrative records. PLoS ONE 8(10): e75256.
36. Ruiz-Ramos M, Escolar-Pujolar A, Mayoral-Sánchez E, Corral-San Laureano F, Fernández-Fernández I (2006) Diabetes mellitus in Spain: death rates, prevalence, impact, costs and inequalities. Gac Sanit 20:15–24.
37. Ferreira-González I, Cascant P, Pons JM, Mitjavila F, Salas T, et al. (2008) Predicting in-hospital mortality with coronary bypass surgery using hospital discharge data: comparison with a prospective observational study. Rev Esp Cardiol 61:843–852.

17

Outcomes in Patients with Acute and Stable Coronary Syndromes; Insights from the Prospective NOBORI-2 Study

Farzin Fath-Ordoubadi[1][9], **Erik Spaepen**[2][9], **Magdi El-Omar**[1][9], **Douglas G. Fraser**[1][9], **Muhammad A. Khan**[1], **Ludwig Neyses**[1][9], **Gian B. Danzi**[3][9], **Ariel Roguin**[4][9], **Dragica Paunovic**[5][9], **Mamas A. Mamas**[1,6]*[9]

1 Manchester Heart Centre, Manchester Royal Infirmary, Manchester, United Kingdom, 2 SBD Analytics, Hertstraat, Bekkevoort, Belgium, 3 Division of Cardiology, Fondazione IRCCS Cà Granda, Ospedale Maggiore Policlinico, Milan, Italy, 4 Department of Cardiology, Rambam Medical Center, Haifa, Israel, 5 European Medical and Clinical Division, Terumo Europe, Leuven, Belgium, 6 Cardiovascular Institute, University of Manchester, Manchester, United Kingdom

Abstract

Background: Contemporary data remains limited regarding mortality and major adverse cardiac events (MACE) outcomes in patients undergoing PCI for different manifestations of coronary artery disease.

Objectives: We evaluated mortality and MACE outcomes in patients treated with PCI for STEMI (ST-elevation myocardial infarction), NSTEMI (non ST-elevation myocardial infarction) and stable angina through analysis of data derived from the Nobori-2 study.

Methods: Clinical endpoints were cardiac mortality and MACE (a composite of cardiac death, myocardial infarction and target vessel revascularization).

Results: 1909 patients who underwent PCI were studied; 1332 with stable angina, 248 with STEMI and 329 with NSTEMI. Age-adjusted Charlson co-morbidity index was greatest in the NSTEMI cohort (3.78 ± 1.91) and lowest in the stable angina cohort (3.00 ± 1.69); $P < 0.0001$. Following Cox multivariate analysis cardiac mortality was independently worse in the NSTEMI vs the stable angina cohort (HR 2.31 (1.10–4.87), $p = 0.028$) but not significantly different for STEMI vs stable angina cohort (HR 0.72 (0.16–3.19), $p = 0.67$). Similar observations were recorded for MACE (< 180 days) (NSTEMI vs stable angina: HR 2.34 (1.21–4.55), $p = 0.012$; STEMI vs stable angina: HR 2.19 (0.97–4.98), $p = 0.061$).

Conclusions: The longer-term Cardiac mortality and MACE were significantly worse for patients following PCI for NSTEMI even after adjustment of clinical demographics and Charlson co-morbidity index whilst the longer-term prognosis of patients following PCI STEMI was favorable, with similar outcomes as those patients with stable angina following PCI.

Editor: Yan Gong, College of Pharmacy, University of Florida, United States of America

Funding: Terumo Europe N.V. Leuven, Belgium (www.terumo-europe.com/) provided a research grant but had no role in study design, data collection and analysis, decision to publish, or preparation of the manuscript.

Competing Interests: Dr Dragica Paunovic is affiliated to Terumo Europe N.V. Leuven, Belgium. There are no other conflicts of interest to report.

* E-mail: mamasmamas1@yahoo.co.uk

[9] These authors contributed equally to this work and take responsibility for all aspects of the reliability and freedom from bias of the data presented and their discussed interpretation.

Introduction

Percutaneous coronary intervention (PCI) has become the revascularisation therapy of choice in patients with both stable coronary artery disease and acute coronary syndromes. During the past few decades, multiple randomised controlled trials have been undertaken to assess the efficacy of both pharmacological, stent technology and adjunctive device developments on morbidity and mortality in both stable and acute coronary syndrome subgroups of patients [1,2]. However, despite this, contemporary data remains limited regarding mortality and major adverse cardiac events (MACE) outcomes when comparing across the spectrum of patients with different indications for PCI in a "real-life" setting.

For example, similar in-hospital mortality rates have been described in non ST-elevation myocardial infarction (NSTEMI) and ST-elevation myocardial infarction (STEMI) in some studies [3,4] whilst others have reported higher mortality rates amongst patients with STEMI [5,6]. In the longer term, some studies have suggested that the prognosis was worse in STEMI as compared to NSTEMI [7]. Other studies have reported the opposite in the long term [6] and only few studies have compared the outcome of these patient groups to those undergoing elective PCI [6]. Studies that have compared outcomes between STEMI and NSTEMI cohorts are often difficult to interpret since a significant proportion of NSTEMI patients may not have received revascularisation in these studies whilst the majority of patients presenting with

STEMI do [4,7]. Furthermore, in those studies bare-metal stent (BMS) and drug eluting stent (DES) usage which is known to influence MACE rates varies significantly amongst stable and acute coronary syndrome subgroups of patients [3,8]. This could further impact outcomes when comparing across the spectrum of patients with different indications for PCI in a "real-life" setting.

We have therefore evaluated early and late mortality and MACE outcomes in patients who have been treated with PCI for STEMI, NSTEMI and stable angina in an all-comer population through analysis of data derived from a large prospective multicenter study conducted in 125 centres across Europe and Asia using only DES - the Nobori-2 study.

Methods

Study Design and Patient Population

Nobori 2 is a prospective, multicenter study conducted in 125 centres across Europe and Asia to investigate the performance of the Nobori DES system in an all-comers clinical setting [9] with the only exclusion criterion used being the patient's refusal or inability to provide written informed consent. All patients that had at least one Nobori DES implanted or attempted were included in the analysis. All patients signed informed consent form reviewed and approved by the Institutional Review Board or Ethics Committee of each participating centres. Outcomes were stratified by indication for PCI; Stable Angina, NSTEMI and STEMI. Patients presenting with unstable angina were pooled with the NSTEMI cohort.

Outcomes and Study Definition

ACS was defined as typical symptoms with ischemic electrocardiographic changes including ST-segment elevation and non–ST-segment elevation and/or laboratory evidence of myocardial damage. All clinical, demographic and outcome data were collected into a Web-based data management system coordinated and analyzed by independent companies (KIKA Medical, Paris, France, and SBD Analytics, Bekkevoort, Belgium, respectively). Clinical follow-up data included the documentation of adverse events, in death, MI, repeat revascularisation, stent thrombosis, bleeding and angina status.

Follow-up was performed at 1 month, 6 months, and 12 months, and yearly up to 5 years. All clinical end points were adjudicated by an independent clinical events committee. Twelve-

month follow-up rate was 97% and at 2-years was 95%. The primary end point was cardiac mortality. MACE were defined as a composite of cardiac death, myocardial infarction (MI) and target vessel revascularization (TVR).

Statistical Analysis

Continuous variables are presented as mean±standard deviation and were compared using the non-parametric tests: the Kruskal-Wallis test to compare multiple groups (>2). All tests were 2-sided. Categorical variables are presented as frequencies and percentages, and were compared using Cochran–Mantel-Haenszel test or Fisher's exact test. Kaplan–Meier estimates were generated, and comparisons of MACE and mortality events were made using log-rank test. Cox proportional hazards regression was used to assess pair-wise hazard ratios (HR) of the 3 subgroups under investigation, either unadjusted (no other covariates) or adjusted for some selected covariates. The censoring time of a patient for these time-to-event analyses was defined as the patient's last observation time, i.e. follow-up or event time. The proportionality assumption for the Cox regression models was tested using the Supremum Test and cumulative score process plots (Cumulative martingale residuals). In case the proportional hazards assumption was violated for the main covariate (ACS status), the covariate was appropriately made time-dependent to maintain proportionality. Data analysis was performed by an independent statistical office (SBD Analytics, Bekkevoort, Belgium), using the statistical software package SAS V8.2 (The SAS Institute, Cary, NC).

Results

The Nobori-2 trial enrolled patients from 125 centres across the world and 1909 patients were included in this analysis. A total of 1332 patients who underwent PCI had a diagnosis of stable angina (69.7%) whilst 577 patients were diagnosed with ACS (30.3%). 248 of the patients with ACS presented with STEMI (43%) whilst 329 patients presented with NSTEMI (57%). Clinical demographics are presented in Table 1. The patients presenting with STEMI were significantly younger than those presenting with NSTEMI or stable angina and the age adjusted Charlson co-morbidity index was greatest in the NSTEMI cohort and lowest in the stable angina cohort.

Procedural demographics are presented in Table 2, which demonstrates that the mean number of lesions treated, mean stent

Table 1. Clinical Demographics.

Variable	Angina(n = 1,332)	NSTEMI (n = 329)	STEMI (n = 248)	P-Value
Age (mean ±SD)	64.4±10.5	65.0±11.8	61.3±11.8	<0.0001
Gender (% Male)	1023 (76.8%)	252 (76.6%)	194 (78.2%)	0.89
Hypercholesterolaemia	993 (74.5%)	220 (66.9%)	126 (50.8%)	<0.0001
Hypertension	996 (74.8%)	219 (66.6%)	119 (48.0%)	<0.0001
Diabetes	379 (28.5%)	99 (30.1%)	66 (26.6%)	0.64
Smoker	220 (16.5%)	101 (30.7%)	109 (44.0%)	<0.0001
History of Heart Failure	41 (3.1%)	13 (4.0%)	5 (2.0%)	0.47
Previous AMI	429 (32.2%)	113 (34.3%)	91 (36.7%)	0.35
Previous PCI	487 (37.2%)	70 (21.3%)	29 (11.7%)	P<0.0001
Charlson score (mean ±SD)	3.00±1.69	3.78±1.91	3.21±1.66	P<0.0001
*Charlson score (mean ±SD)	1.06±1.19	1.78±1.31	1.54±0.95	P<0.0001

*(without age scoring).

Table 2. Procedural Demographics.

Variable	Angina (n = 1,332)	NSTEMI (n = 329)	STEMI (n = 248)	P-Value
Glycoprotein IIb/IIIa	185 (14.7%)	92 (27.9%)	98 (39.5%)	0.0001
Radial Access	439 (33.2%)	145 (44.2%)	89 (35.8%)	0.001
Number of vessels diseased	1.73±0.78	1.77±0.75	1.68±0.72	0.42
Number of vessels treated	1.23±0.48	1.26±0.48	1.28±0.53	0.27
Number of lesions detected	1.97±1.11	2.10±1.11	2.01±1.07	0.076
Number of lesions treated	1.44±0.77	1.46±0.71	1.48±0.80	0.62
Number of stents	1.73±1.10	1.71±0.98	1.82±1.19	0.68
Stent Length	33.44±22.28	32.48±19.94	33.09±38.95	0.15

length and mean number of stents was similar across all 3 groups. Table 3 illustrates lesion characteristics and QCA analysis of lesions pre- and post-treatment. Lesion characteristics and type were similar across the 3 cohorts studied.

Figure 1 illustrates Kaplan-Meier unadjusted survival curves for cardiac death for all 3 cohorts. A statistically significant increase in cardiac death was observed in the NSTEMI cohort compared to the stable angina cohort (unadjusted HR 3.17, 95% CI 1.54–6.53, p = 0.0017) whereas survival was not statistically different the

STEMI group compared to the stable angina group (unadjusted HR 0.64 95%CI 0.15–2.78, p = 0.55). Figure 2 illustrates Kaplan-Meier unadjusted survival curves for MACE for all 3 cohorts. As the proportionality assumption was violated for the Cox model with MACE as outcome, Process Score plots were created. These indicated that a time cut-off around 180 days would reintroduce proportionality. That is, assessing the effects of ACS status before and after 180 days separately (but simultaneously model), will yield valid estimates for each of the time categories, for the ACS status.

Table 3. Lesion data (data presented per lesion.

Variable	Angina (n = 1,916)	NSTEMI (n = 479)	STEMI (n = 368)	P-Value
Target Vessel				
RCA	596 (31.1%)	128 (26.7%)	131 (35.6%)	0.021
LAD	746 (38.9%)	186 (38.8%)	167 (45.4%)	0.063
LCx	515 (26.9%)	150 (31.3%)	64 (17.4%)	<0.0001
Left Main	31 (1.62%)	3 (0.63%)	3 (0.82%)	0.199
SVG	28 (1.46%)	12 (2.51%)	3 (0.82%)	0.132
Lesion Characteristics				
	(n = 1,661)	(n = 438)	(n = 337)	
Ostial lesion	181 (10.9%)	49 (11.2%)	22 (6.5%)	0.037
Bifurcation	329 (19.8%)	87 (19.9%)	52 (15.4%)	0.163
Tortuous	131 (7.9%)	38 (8.7%)	17 (5.05%)	0.122
Calcified	432 (26.0%)	102 (23.3%)	85 (25.2%)	0.518
Lesion Type				
A	63 (3.8%)	13 (3.0%)	8 (2.4%)	0.404
B1	403 (24.3%)	93 (21.3%)	79 (23.4%)	0.44
B2	687 (41.3%)	193 (44.2%)	107 (31.8%)	0.001
C	508 (30.6%)	138 (31.6%)	142 (42.1%)	0.0002
QCA Results Pre				
Ref vessel diam (mm)	2.61±0.60 (1,528)	2.64±0.55 (398)	2.61±0.58 (252)	0.436
MLD (mm)	0.87±0.50 (1,655)	0.76±0.45 (436)	0.61±0.52 (335)	<0.0001
Lesion Length (mm)	15.61±9.93 (1,528)	16.19±8.66 (398)	16.44±9.71 (252)	0.0504
Diameter stenosis (%)	66.81±17.24 (1,655)	71.27±16.29 (437)	76.52±18.95 (335)	<0.0001
QCA Results Post				
Ref vessel diam (mm)	2.89±0.51 (1,604)	2.87±0.50 (429)	2.93±0.49 (321)	0.238
MLD (mm)	2.51±0.47 (1,604)	2.50±0.47 (429)	2.54±0.47 (321)	0.686
Stenosis in stent (%)	13.07±6.77 (1,604)	13.03±7.44 (429)	13.42±7.23 (321)	0.668

NOBORI - Cumulative Events, % patients
Kaplan-Meier curves - Cardiac Death

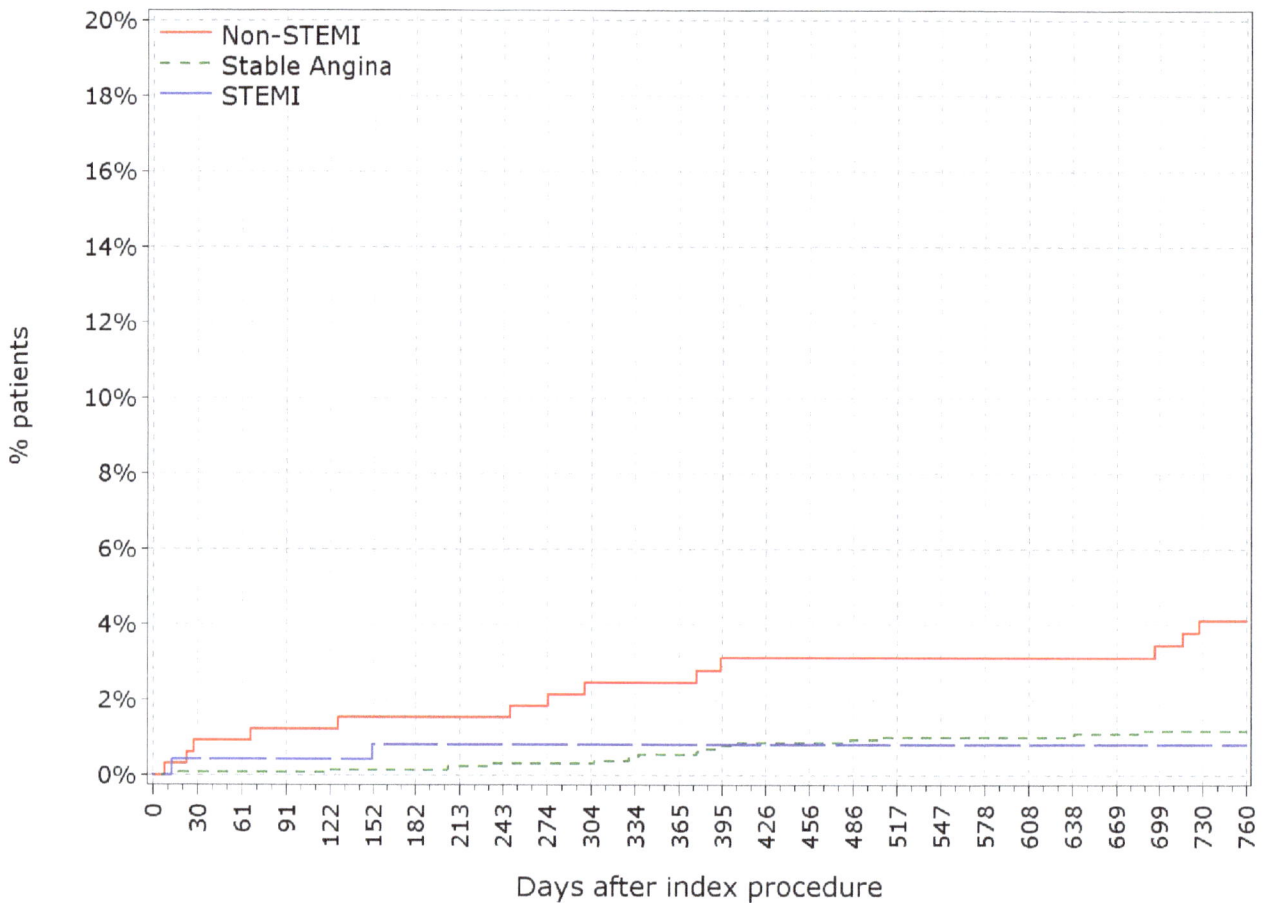

Figure 1. Kaplan-Meier curve for cardiac death.

Similarly, a statistically significant increase in MACE was observed in the NSTEMI cohort compared to the stable angina cohort (unadjusted HR ($\leq$180 days) 3.16, 95% CI 1.70–5.96; P = 0.0004) whereas MACE was not significantly different in the STEMI group compared to the stable angina group (unadjusted HR ($\leq$ 180 days) 5.44 95% CI 0.77–38.67; P = 0.09).

Table 4 illustrates mortality and MACE events for the stable angina, NSTEMI and STEMI groups at 30 days, 6 months, 1 year and 2 years. It can be seen that unadjusted 30-day cardiac mortality rates were higher in the NSTEMI and STEMI groups compared to the stable angina cohort (0.91%, 0.40% and 0.08% respectively; P = 0.021), although by two years cardiac mortality was similar in the STEMI and stable angina cohort but remained increased in the NSTEMI group (1.13%, 0.81% and 3.95% respectively; P = 0.0021). Similarly, 30-day unadjusted MACE events were greater in the NSTEMI and STEMI cohorts at baseline (2.4%, 1.6% compared to 0.8% in stable angina cohort; P = 0.039) although by 2 years follow up MACE events were similar in the stable angina and STEMI cohort but remained worse in the NSTEMI group (6.5%, 6.8% and 10.3% respectively; P = 0.048).

Multivariate analysis, using Cox regression, adjusted for clinical demographics and Charlson score for co-morbidity was performed for cardiac mortality and MACE events and this is summarized in

Table 5. This demonstrates that after multivariate adjustment, NSTEMI was independently associated with worse cardiac mortality compared to the stable angina cohort following adjustment of baseline clinical demographics and Charlson co-morbidity score, whilst cardiac mortality and MACE were not significantly different in the STEMI cohort when compared to the stable angina cohort.

Discussion

The current analysis was undertaken in patients undergoing PCI for different manifestations of coronary artery disease such as high risk acute coronary syndromes (STEMI and NSTEMI) and stable angina in an all-comer population through analysis of data derived from a prospective multicenter study conducted in 125 centres across Europe and Asia using a single DES platform. The main findings of the study were that cardiac mortality and MACE outcomes of patients following PCI for NSTEMI were significantly worse than patients undergoing PCI for stable angina, even after adjustment for baseline clinical demographics and comorbidities using the Charlson co-morbidity score, whereas longer cardiac mortality and MACE outcomes of patients following PCI for STEMI were similar to those following PCI with stable angina

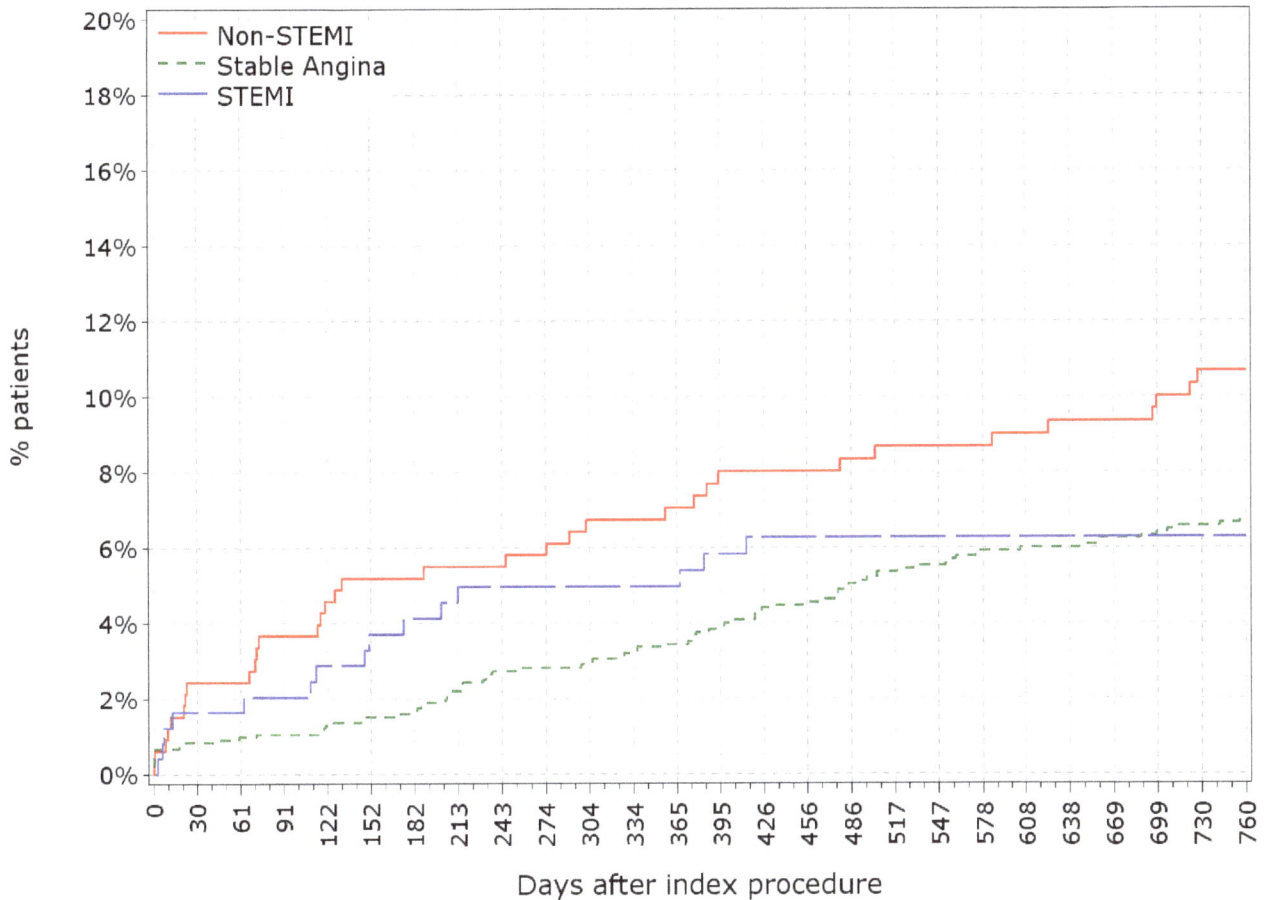

Figure 2. Kaplan- Meier curves for MACE.

following adjustment for baseline clinical demographics and co-morbidities.

To our knowledge this is one of the first studies that has compared short and longer-term outcomes in patients undergoing PCI for different manifestations of coronary artery disease using a single drug eluting stent platform. Previous studies have shown that in-hospital mortality rates have been greater in patients presenting with STEMI than those with NSTEMI [6,7,10,11] whilst other studies have reported similar in-hospital mortality rates [4,12]. Similarly at 6 years follow up mortality was greater in patients presenting with NSTEMI compared to those patients presenting with STEMI or stable angina in the study of Hirsch et al [6]. Other studies have shown either worse outcomes in NSTEMI cohort [11–13] or similar outcomes in STEMI and NSTEMI patients on longer term follow up [4]. Interpretation of many of these previous studies is complicated by the observation that they included patients with NSTEMI and STEMI acute coronary syndromes who were managed by both PCI or conservative treatment strategies [4,7,12] with significant differences in PCI rates in each respective cohort [4,7,12]. Such differences in the respective revascularisation rate amongst NSTEMI and STEMI patients has been shown to have significant implications on longer terms outcomes [7] and so would significantly bias outcomes previously reported for NSTEMI vs

STEMI cohorts. Furthermore, interpretation of previous studies comparing outcomes between NSTEMI, STEMI and stable angina cohorts following PCI are complicated by the fact that there were significant differences in DES/BMS use between the cohorts studied which will impact on outcomes [6]. For example, DES use was infrequent in the study of Hirsch et al. [6] (STEMI cohort 1%, NSTEMI 8% and stable angina 11%) with the majority of PCI procedures undertaken with BMS platforms which is not reflective of contemporary PCI practice where use of drug eluting stent platforms are much more widespread.

Our findings of worse cardiac mortality and MACE outcomes associated with patients undergoing PCI for NSTEMI compared to those with stable angina, with similar longer term MACE and mortality outcomes in the STEMI vs stable angina cohorts undergoing PCI is of interest. Whilst patients with NSTEMI undergoing PCI were older compared to both the STEMI and stable angina cohorts, which would in itself lend to worse outcomes in the NSTEMI cohort, the association between NSTEMI and adverse outcomes persisted even after multi-variate adjustment for age. Patients presenting with NSTEMI often have a higher prevalence of cardiovascular and non-cardiovascular co-morbidities compared to patients with STEMI [4,5,12,14,15] and the presence of such unmeasured confounders has been suggested to contribute to the adverse outcomes associated with NSTEMI in

Table 4. Clinical outcomes.

Timepoint	Angina (n = 1,332)	NSTEMI (n = 329)	STEMI (n = 248)	P-Value
Cardiac Mortality				
30-Day	1 (0.08%)	3 (0.91%)	1 (0.4%)	0.021
6 month	2 (0.15%)	5 (1.52%)	2 (0.81%)	0.0041
1 year	10 (0.75%)	10 (3.04%)	2 (0.81%)	0.0044
2 years	15 (1.13%)	13 (3.95%)	2 (0.81%)	0.0021
MACE				
30-Day	11 (0.8%)	8 (2.4%)	4 (1.6%)	0.0393
6 month	25 (1.9%)	17 (5.2%)	10 (4.0%)	0.0022
1 year	51 (3.8%)	26 (7.9%)	14 (5.7%)	0.008
2 years	86 (6.5%)	34 (10.3%)	15 (6.1%)	0.048
Myocardial Infarction				
30-Day	10 (0.8%)	6 (1.8%)	3 (1.2%)	0.164
6 month	11 (0.8%)	10 (3.0%)	5 (2.0%)	0.0039
1 year	17 (1.3%)	15 (4.6%)	5 (2.0%)	0.0012
2 years	27 (2.0%)	17 (5.2%)	6 (2.4%)	0.01
Target vessel revascularisation				
30-Day	2 (0.2%)	3 (0.9%)	2 (0.8%)	0.0328
6 month	14 (1.1%)	8 (2.4%)	7 (2.8%)	0.0288
1 year	32 (2.4%)	13 (4.0%)	11 (4.4%)	0.10
2 years	56 (4.2%)	18 (5.5%)	11 (4.4%)	0.57

previous studies. We have also confirmed that patients presenting with NSTEMI have a greater prevalence of co-morbid conditions compared to the STEMI and stable angina cohorts as evidenced by the greater Charlson co-morbidity score in the NSTEMI cohort. The Charlson co-morbidity score has been shown to be an

important independent predictor of mortality [16], stent thrombosis and major bleeding [17] in patients undergoing PCI. However, even following adjustment for the presence of co-morbidities through inclusion of the Charlson score in our multivariate analysis, NSTEMI was independently associated with worse cardiac mortality. The worse cardiac mortality outcomes associated with NSTEMI may relate to residual confounders that we may not have measured in the older NSTEMI group such as more severe coronary artery disease in non-revascularised areas of the coronary vasculature, greater frailty that is a strong predictor of mortality outcomes following PCI [16] or a greater prevalence of unmeasured co-morbid conditions that are not included in the Charlson co-morbidity score.

Whilst the current analysis provides insights into outcomes of patients undergoing PCI for different manifestations of coronary artery disease such as ACS (STEMI and NSTEMI) and stable angina, the findings of our study are not applicable to patients with stable angina or an ACS who are managed with a non-invasive strategy. Often these patients are more elderly and have significantly more cardiovascular and non-cardiovascular co-morbidities and so may have worse outcomes than reported here [7]. Indeed, an invasive PCI strategy was independently associated with a 36% and 49% reduction in 2- year mortality in NSTEMI and STEMI groups in the study of Polonski et al [7]. Secondly, information regarding the medical treatment of patients in the current analysis was not available and so we are unable to comment on adherence to evidence based therapies in these cohorts and so are unable to assess the influence of medical therapy on long-term outcomes. Thirdly, Due to the observational character of this study and the multitude of analyses performed, it was not feasible to adjust for multiple testing. As such, we have supplied nominal p-values, not adjusted for multiple testing. Finally, the possibility of selection bias cannot be excluded, as the patients were not consecutively recruited at the study centres.

In conclusion, current analysis undertaken in patients undergoing PCI for different manifestations of coronary artery disease such as acute coronary syndromes (STEMI and NSTEMI) and stable

Table 5. Unadjusted and adjusted Hazard Ratios and for cardiac death and MACE.

Endpoint	Unadjusted OR (95% CI)	Age, Gender adjusted OR (95% CI)	* Fully adjusted OR (95% CI)
Cardiac Mortality			
NSTEMI vs Stable Angina	3.17 (1.54–6.53), p = 0.0017**	2.84 (1.38–5.87), p = 0.0049**	2.31 (1.10–4.87), p = 0.028**
STEMI vs Stable Angina	0.64 (0.15–2.78), p = 0.55	0.75 (0.17–3.26), p = 0.70	0.72 (0.16–3.19), p = 0.67
NSTEMI vs STEMI	4.92 (1.11–21.74), p = 0.035**	3.77 (0.85–16.66), p = 0.081	3.21 (0.71–14.50), p = 0.13
MACE*			
≤180 days			
NSTEMI vs Stable Angina	3.16 (1.68–5.96), p = 0.0004**	3.06 (1.63–5.76), p = 0.0005**	2.34 (1.21–4.55), p = 0.012**
STEMI vs Stable Angina	2.49 (1.18–5.26), p = 0.017**	2.75 (1.30–5.82), p = 0.008*	2.19 (0.97–4.98), p = 0.061
NSTEMI vs STEMI	1.27 (0.58–2.78), p = 0.55	1.11 (0.51–2.43), p = 0.79	1.07 (0.45–2.54), p = 0.88
>180 days			
NSTEMI vs Stable Angina	1.07 (0.63–1.83), p = 0.80	1.04 (0.61–1.78), p = 0.87	0.86 (0.50–1.50), p = 0.60
STEMI vs Stable Angina	0.415 (0.17–1.03), p = 0.058	0.45 (0.18–1.13), p = 0.088	0.46 (0.18–1.14), p = 0.094
NSTEMI vs STEMI	2.59 (0.96–7.01), p = 0.062	2.30 (0.85–6.23), p = 0.10	1.89 (0.69–5.18), p = 0.22

OR corresponds to odds ratio,
*Adjusted for age, gender, hypertension, hypercholesterolaemia, diabetes and Charlson Index.
**equates to statistical significance.
***Time-dependent parameterization of ACS classification for MACE due to non-proportionality - cutoff at 180d.

angina in an all-comer ("real world") population has shown that NSTEMI presentation is associated with adverse cardiac mortality and MACE.

References

1. Levine GN, Bates ER, Blankenship JC, Bailey SR, Bittl JA, et al. (2011) ACCF/AHA/SCAI Guideline for Percutaneous Coronary Intervention. A report of the American College of Cardiology Foundation/American Heart Association Task Force on Practice Guidelines and the Society for Cardiovascular Angiography and Interventions. J Am Coll Cardiol. 58(24):e44–122.

2. Wijns W, Kolh P, Danchin N, Di Mario C, Falk V, et al. (2010) Task Force on Myocardial Revascularization of the European Society of Cardiology (ESC) and the European Association for Cardio-Thoracic Surgery (EACTS); European Association for Percutaneous Cardiovascular Interventions (EAPCI), Guidelines on myocardial revascularization. Eur Heart J. 31(20): 2501–55.

3. Ramcharitar S, Hochadel M, Gaster AL, Onuma Y, Gitt A, et al. (2008) An insight into the current use of drug eluting stents in acute and elective percutaneous coronary interventions in Europe. A report on the EuroPCI Survey. EuroIntervention. 3(4): 429–41.

4. Montalescot G, Dallongeville J, van Belle E, Rouanet S, Baulac C, et al. (2007) STEMI and NSTEMI are they so different? 1 year outcomes in acute myocardial infarction as defined by the ESC/ACC definition (the OPERA registry). Eur Heart J 28: 1409–17.

5. Nikus KC, Eskola MJ, Virtanen VK (2007) Mortality of patients with acute coronary syndromes still remains high: a follow-up study of 1188 consecutive patients admitted to a university hospital. Ann Med 39: 63–71.

6. Hirsch A, Verouden NJ, Koch KT, Baan J Jr, Henriques JP, et al. (2009) Comparison of long-term mortality after percutaneous coronary intervention in patients treated for acute ST-elevation myocardial infarction versus those with unstable and stable angina pectoris. Am J Cardiol. 104(3): 333–7.

7. Polonski L, Gasior M, Gierlotka M, Osadnik T, Kalarus Z, et al. (2011) A comparison of ST elevation versus non-ST elevation myocardial infarction outcomes in a large registry database: are non-ST myocardial infarctions associated with worse long-term prognoses? Int J Cardiol. 152(1): 70–7.

8. Lagerqvist B, James SK, Stenestrand U, Lindbäck J, Nilsson T, et al. (2007) Long-term outcomes with drug-eluting stents versus bare-metal stents in Sweden.N Engl J Med. 356(10): 1009–19.

9. Danzi GB, Chevalier B, Urban P, Fath-Ordoubadi F, Carrie D, et al. (2012) Clinical performance of a drug-eluting stent with a biodegradable polymer in an unselected patient population: the NOBORI 2 study. EuroIntervention. 8(1): 109–16.

10. García-García C, Subirana I, Sala J, Bruguera J, Sanz G, et al. (2011) Long-term prognosis of first myocardial infarction according to the electrocardiographic pattern (ST elevation myocardial infarction, non-ST elevation myocardial infarction and non-classified myocardial infarction) and revascularization procedures. Am J Cardiol. 108(8): 1061–7.

11. Chan MY, Sun JL, Newby LK, Shaw LK, Lin M, et al. (2009) Long-term mortality of patients undergoing cardiac catheterization for ST-elevation and non-ST-elevation myocardial infarction. Circulation. 119(24): 3110–7.

12. McManus DD, Gore J, Yarzebski J, Spencer F, Lessard D, et al. (2011) Recent trends in the incidence, treatment, and outcomes of patients with STEMI and NSTEMI. Am J Med. 124(1): 40–7.

13. Terkelsen CJ, Lassen JF, Norgaard BL, Gerdes JC, Jensen T, et al. (2005) Mortality rates in patients with ST-elevation acute myocardial infarction: observations from an unselected cohort. Eur Heart J 26(1): 18–26.

14. Balzi D, Di Bari M, Barchielli A, Ballo P, Carrabba N, et al. (2012) Should we improve the management of NSTEMI? Results from the population-based "acute myocardial infarction in Florence 2" (AMI-Florence 2) registry. Intern Emerg Med. Jul 10. (epub ahead of print)

15. Steg PG, Gooldberg RJ, Gore JM, Fox KA, Eagle KA, et al (2002) Baseline characteristics, management practices and in-hospital mortality of patients hospitalized with acute coronary syndromes in the Global Registry of Acute Coronary events (GRACE). Am J Cardiol 90: 358–63.

16. Singh M, Rihal CS, Lennon RJ, Spertus JA, Nair KS, et al. (2011) Influence of frailty and health status on outcomes in patients with coronary disease undergoing percutaneous revascularization. Circ Cardiovasc Qual Outcomes. 4(5): 496–502.

17. Urban P, Abizaid A, Banning A, Bartorelli AL, Baux AC, et al. (2011) Stent thrombosis and bleeding complications after implantation of sirolimus-eluting coronary stents in an unselected worldwide population: a report from the e-SELECT (Multi-Center Post-Market Surveillance) registry. J Am Coll Cardiol. 2011;57(13): 1445–54.

Author Contributions

Conceived and designed the experiments: FF ES MM. Analyzed the data: MK DP MM. Contributed reagents/materials/analysis tools: ME DF GD. Wrote the paper: ES AR DP MM. Recruited patients for study; edited manuscript for intellectual content: FF ME DF LN.

18

Systematic Review of Randomized Controlled Trials of Different Types of Patch Materials during Carotid Endarterectomy

Shiyan Ren[1]*, **Xianlun Li**[1]*, **Jianyan Wen**[2], **Wenjian Zhang**[2], **Peng Liu**[1]*

1 Cardiovascular Center, China-Japan Friendship Hospital, Beijing, People's Republic of China, 2 Clinical Research Institute, China-Japan Friendship Hospital, Beijing, People's Republic of China

Abstract

Background and Purpose: Carotid endarterectomy (CEA) with patch angioplasty produces greater results than with primary closure; however, there remains uncertainty on the optimal patch material in CEA. A systematic review of randomized controlled trials (RCTs) was performed to evaluate the effect of angioplasty using venous patch versus synthetic patch material, and Dacron patch versus polytetrafluoroethelene (PTFE) patch material during CEA.

Methods: A multiple electronic health database screening was performed including the Cochrane library, Pubmed, Ovid, EMBASE and Google Scholar on all randomized controlled trials (RCTs) published before November 2012 that compared the outcomes of patients undergoing CEA with venous patch versus synthetic patch. RCTs were included if they compared carotid patch angioplasty with autologus venous patch versus synthetic patch material, or compared one type of synthetic patch with another.

Results: Thirteen RCTs were identified. Ten trials, involving 1946 CEAs, compared venous patch with synthetic patch materials. Two trials, involving 400 CEAs in 380 patients, compared Dacron patch with PTFE patch. The hemostasis time in CEA with PTFE patch was significantly longer than with venous patch ($P<0.0001$), and longer than with Dacron patch ($P<0.0001$). There was no significant difference of mortality rate, stroke rate, restenosis, and operative time in CEA with venous patch versus synthetic patch material, or in CEA with Dacron patch versus PTFE patch (all $P>0.05$). One RCT of 95 CEAs in 92 patients compared bovine pericardium with Dacron patch, and demonstrated a statistically significant decrease in intraoperative suture line bleeding with bovine pericardium compared with Dacron patch ($P<0.001$).

Conclusions: The hemostasis time in CEA with PTFE patch was longer than with venous patch or Dacron patch. The overall perioperative and long-term mortality rate, stroke rate, restenosis, and operative time were similar when using venous patch versus synthetic patch material or Dacron patch versus PTFE patch material during CEA. More data are required to clarify differences between different patch materials.

Editor: Cordula M. Stover, University of Leicester, United Kingdom

Funding: This study was supported in part by National Sciences Foundation of China (grant 81070230). The funders had no role in study design, data collection and analysis, decision to publish, or preparation of the manuscript. No additional external funding received for this study.

Competing Interests: The authors have declared that no competing interests exist.

* E-mail: liupeng61@yahoo.com.cn (PL); lixianlun@hotmail.com (XL); shiyanr@yahoo.com (SR)

Introduction

Carotid endarterectomy (CEA) has been considered as one of the important procedures to treat patients with severe stenosis of carotid artery. However, patients may have postoperative restenosis of carotid artery [1] and subsequent recurrent ipsilateral ischemic stroke in high-grade recurrent stenosis. One solution to these problems is patch angioplasty in CEA [2,3]. Several systematic reviews have compared the results of the primary closure of arteriotomy with routine patch closure during CEA [4–6], and the outcomes favor patch angioplasty over primary closure in reducing risk of stroke and restenosis [4–6]. However, there remain reports that the difference was insignificant and that there was no benefit from the routine use of patch angioplasty in CEA [7].

A variety of patch materials for closure of the arteriotomy are available, including autologous venous patch and synthetic patch materials (Dacron, polytetrafluoroethelene (PTFE), bovine pericardium, and polyester urethane) [4–8]. Currently, selection of types of patch materials depends on the surgeon's preference, as there is no agreement on the priority of use of venous over synthetic patch materials during CEA [1]. Moreover, all randomized controlled trials (RCTs) on this issue so far have been underpowered because the number of patients involved was not large and the studies were unblinded. However, better evidence is not yet available; therefore, the aim of this paper is to update the review of RCTs via a meta-analysis to compare venous patch with synthetic patch materials, and different synthetic patch materials during CEA.

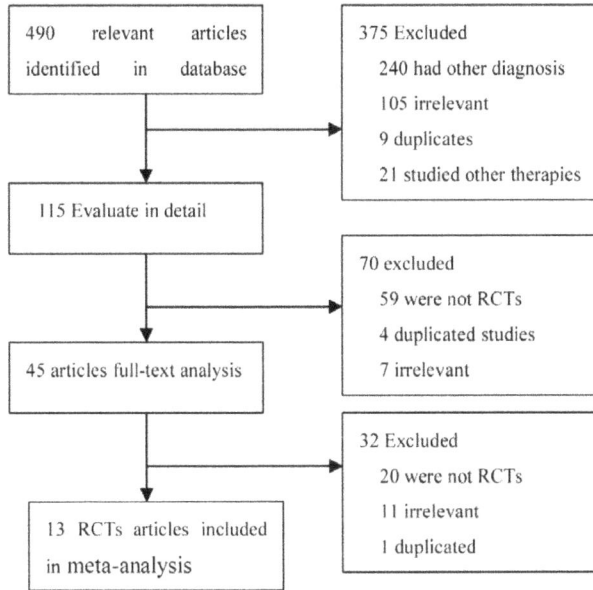

```
┌─────────────────────────┐      ┌─────────────────────────┐
│ 490    relevant articles│      │ 375 Excluded            │
│ identified  in database │      │   240 had other diagnosis│
└─────────────────────────┘      │   105 irrelevant         │
             │                   │   9 duplicates           │
             │                   │   21 studied other therapies│
             │                   └─────────────────────────┘
             ▼
┌─────────────────────────┐
│ 115 Evaluate in detail  │
└─────────────────────────┘      ┌─────────────────────────┐
             │                   │ 70 excluded             │
             │                   │   59 were not RCTs       │
             │                   │   4 duplicated studies   │
             ▼                   │   7 irrelevant           │
┌─────────────────────────┐      └─────────────────────────┘
│ 45 articles full-text   │
│ analysis                │
└─────────────────────────┘      ┌─────────────────────────┐
             │                   │ 32 Excluded             │
             │                   │   20 were not RCTs       │
             │                   │   11 irrelevant          │
             ▼                   │   1 duplicated           │
┌─────────────────────────┐      └─────────────────────────┘
│ 13 RCTs articles included│
│ in meta-analysis         │
└─────────────────────────┘
```

Figure 1. Flow diagram showing different steps of the systematic review. *RCTs:* randomized controlled trials.

Materials and Methods

Literature Search

The authors screened and identified various databases, including the Cochrane library, Pubmed, Ovid, Embase, and Google scholar, before November 2012. The following key words were used: "carotid artery stenosis, endarterectomy with venous patch or synthetic patch, saphenous vein patch, or jugular vein patch; and patch angioplasty". The reference lists of reviews and retrieved papers were searched manually. Language was not restricted in the literature search.

Inclusion Criteria and Exclusion Criteria

All RCTs papers that compared autologous venous patch versus synthetic patch material, or different types of synthetic patch during CEA were included. Exclusion criteria were RCTs comparing patch angioplasty with primary closure during CEA, non-RCT studies, abstracts or unpublished reports, case reports, and reviews.

Data Extraction

Titles and abstracts of all citations and searched papers were initially screened, and the eligible full-text articles were obtained. Two independent reviewers (Ren S, Li X) screened, selected, and cross-checked all the eligible papers, and discussed the disagreements on the eligibility of included papers in order to reach an agreement. In each trial, the number of patients and all the outcomes of treatment were identified. A greater than 50% restenosis or occlusion of the operated artery was defined by duplex ultrasound scan, or angiography.

The methodological quality of RCTs was assessed using the Jadad studies method [9], and any publication bias was assessed using funnel plots.

Statistical Analysis

Statistical analysis of categorical variables were performed using risk ratio (RR) as a summary statistic, mean differences were used for analysis of continuous data. An RR<1 favors the experimental (venous) patch group or the Dacron patch. The Software Review Manager (RevMan 5.1.7, Cochrane Collaboration, Oxford, UK) was used for statistical analysis. Heterogeneity among the RCTs results was evaluated with the standard Chi-square test to determine whether to use the fixed- or random-effects model. The Mantel-Haenszel method was used to combine the RR for the results of interest using a random-effects meta-analytical technique. P value less than 0.05 was considered statistically significant.

Table 1. Details of randomized controlled trials.

Trials	Year	No. of patients (no.operations)	Mean age(y)	Sex (% male)	Venous or synthetic patch	Synthetic patch type	FU time
Marien BJ [10]	2002	92 (95)	66	64.2	Dacron	BP	Perioperative
Grego F [11]	1996	160 (160)	70	72.5	EJV	PTFE	mean 4 y
O'Hara PJ [12]	1996	195 (207)	69	73.6	ASV	Dacron	18 mon
Hayes PD [13]	2001	274 (276)	70.5	66.3	SV	Dacron	30 days
AbuRahma AF [14]	1996	399 (357)	68	53	VPC (ankle)	PTFE	mean 30 mon
Lord RS [15]	1989	123 (140)	63	62	SV	PTFE	12 mon
Gonzalez-fajard JA [16]	1994	84 (95)	69.5	88.1	SV	PTFE	29 mon
Ricco JB [17]	1994	124 (141)	63	80	SV	PTFE	mean 53 mon
Katz SG [18]	1996	190 (207)	72	49.3	SV (thigh)	Dacron	Not mention
Naylor R [19]	2004	273 (276)	71	67	SV	Dacron	3 y
Meerwaldt R [20]	2008	87 (87)	67	79.6	SV (ankle)	Fluoropassiv	24 mon
AbuRahma AF [21]	2002	180 (200)	68.3	53	Dacron	PTFE	30 days
AbuRahma AF [22]	2003	180 (200)	68.3	53	Dacron	PTFE	36 months
AbuRahma AF [23]	2007	200 (200)	68	49.5	Dacron	PTFE	Perioperative

ASV ankle saphenous vein, *BP* bovine pericardium, *EJV* external jugular vein, *FU* follow up, *PTFE* polytetrafluoroethylene patch, *SV* saphenous vein, *VPC* vein patch closure, *Y* year, *Mon* month.

Study or Subgroup	Vein patch Events	Total	synthetic patch Events	Total	Weight	Risk Ratio M-H, Fixed, 95% CI	Risk Ratio M-H, Fixed, 95% CI
AbuRahma AF 1996	2	130	0	134	1.5%	5.15 [0.25, 106.31]	
AbuRahma AF 1998	18	130	18	134	52.6%	1.03 [0.56, 1.89]	
Carney WI Jr 1987	0	0	0	0		Not estimable	
Gonzalez-Fajardo JA 1994	2	45	2	50	5.6%	1.11 [0.16, 7.56]	
Grego F 2003	4	80	5	80	14.8%	0.80 [0.22, 2.87]	
Hayes PD 2001	3	139	1	137	3.0%	2.96 [0.31, 28.08]	
Katz SG 1996	1	100	0	107	1.4%	3.21 [0.13, 77.84]	
Meerwaldt R 2008	2	45	2	42	6.1%	0.93 [0.14, 6.33]	
Naylor R 2004	6	136	3	137	8.9%	2.01 [0.51, 7.89]	
O'Hara PJ 2002	1	106	1	101	3.0%	0.95 [0.06, 15.03]	
Ricco JB 1994	1	58	1	53	3.1%	0.91 [0.06, 14.25]	
Total (95% CI)		969		975	100.0%	1.23 [0.79, 1.89]	
Total events	40		33				

Heterogeneity: Chi² = 3.22, df = 9 (P = 0.96); I² = 0%
Test for overall effect: Z = 0.91 (P = 0.36)

0.01   0.1   1   10   100
Favours venous patch   Favours synthetic patch

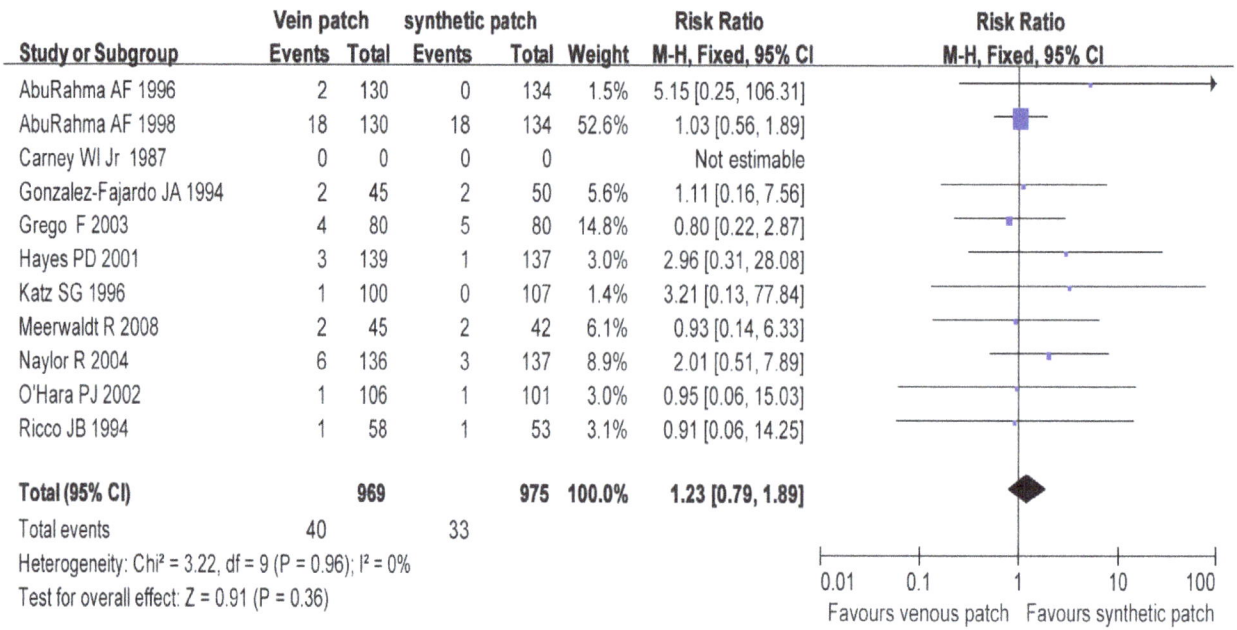

Figure 2. Mortality in both groups. Graphical representation of the results. *M-H* : Mantel-Haenszel.

Results

The significant complications after CEA included bleeding from or rupture of the patched artery, reoperation, wound infection, and wound hematoma. Initially, 490 papers were searched through the keyword search, and 445 papers were excluded after further reviewing the title and abstracts of the papers. The remaining 45 papers were carefully reviewed, and 14 articles conforming to the eligibility criteria were included in this study (Fig. 1, Table 1) [10–23]. Three of 14 articles compared results of Dacron patch with PTFE during CEA, of which two articles were the same RCT reporting the early and follow-up outcomes in different journals, thus these three studies had a subtotal of 380 patients who underwent 400 CEAs (Table 1). Ten of the 14 studies

selected compared outcomes of autologus venous patch with synthetic patch materials during CEA, and contained a combined total of 1909 subjects, of whom 1946 CEAs were performed. One RCT compared the outcomes of CEA using bovine pericardium with Dacron [10].

Table 1 shows the main outcomes and characteristics of each study. Two trials had three arms: primary closure, venous patch, and PTFE patch [15,17]. For the analysis of patients with bilateral carotid artery stenosis, the first CEA and contralateral CEA were counted (Table 1).

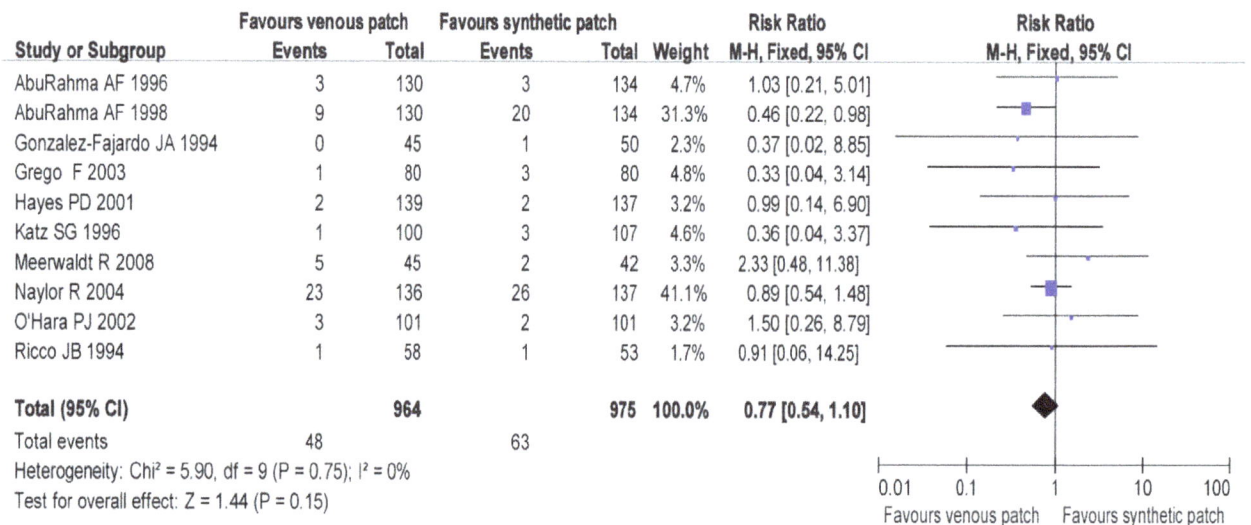

Study or Subgroup	Favours venous patch Events	Total	Favours synthetic patch Events	Total	Weight	Risk Ratio M-H, Fixed, 95% CI	Risk Ratio M-H, Fixed, 95% CI
AbuRahma AF 1996	3	130	3	134	4.7%	1.03 [0.21, 5.01]	
AbuRahma AF 1998	9	130	20	134	31.3%	0.46 [0.22, 0.98]	
Gonzalez-Fajardo JA 1994	0	45	1	50	2.3%	0.37 [0.02, 8.85]	
Grego F 2003	1	80	3	80	4.8%	0.33 [0.04, 3.14]	
Hayes PD 2001	2	139	2	137	3.2%	0.99 [0.14, 6.90]	
Katz SG 1996	1	100	3	107	4.6%	0.36 [0.04, 3.37]	
Meerwaldt R 2008	5	45	2	42	3.3%	2.33 [0.48, 11.38]	
Naylor R 2004	23	136	26	137	41.1%	0.89 [0.54, 1.48]	
O'Hara PJ 2002	3	101	2	101	3.2%	1.50 [0.26, 8.79]	
Ricco JB 1994	1	58	1	53	1.7%	0.91 [0.06, 14.25]	
Total (95% CI)		964		975	100.0%	0.77 [0.54, 1.10]	
Total events	48		63				

Heterogeneity: Chi² = 5.90, df = 9 (P = 0.75); I² = 0%
Test for overall effect: Z = 1.44 (P = 0.15)

0.01   0.1   1   10   100
Favours venous patch   Favours synthetic patch

Figure 3. Any stroke event is compared in both groups. Graphical representation of the results. *M-H:* Mantel-Haenszel.

Study or Subgroup	Favours venous patch Events	Total	Favours synthetic patch Events	Total	Weight	Risk Ratio M-H, Fixed, 95% CI	Risk Ratio M-H, Fixed, 95% CI
AbuRahma AF 1996	16	130	6	134	9.1%	2.75 [1.11, 6.81]	
AbuRahma AF 1998	11	130	3	134	4.5%	3.78 [1.08, 13.24]	
AbuRahma AF 2000	6	130	3	134	4.5%	2.06 [0.53, 8.07]	
Gonzalez-Fajardo JA 1994	0	45	2	50	3.6%	0.22 [0.01, 4.50]	
Grego F 2003	22	80	18	80	27.7%	1.22 [0.71, 2.10]	
Grego F 2001	0	29	0	29		Not estimable	
Hayes PD 2001	0	139	0	137		Not estimable	
Katz SG 1996	0	100	0	107		Not estimable	
Meerwaldt R 2008	0	45	0	42		Not estimable	
Naylor R 2004	22	136	28	137	42.9%	0.79 [0.48, 1.31]	
O'Hara PJ 2002	3	62	4	63	6.1%	0.76 [0.18, 3.27]	
Ricco JB 1994	1	69	1	66	1.6%	0.96 [0.06, 14.98]	
Total (95% CI)		**1095**		**1113**	**100.0%**	**1.26 [0.93, 1.70]**	
Total events	81		65				

Heterogeneity: Chi² = 11.34, df = 7 (P = 0.12); I² = 38%
Test for overall effect: Z = 1.52 (P = 0.13)

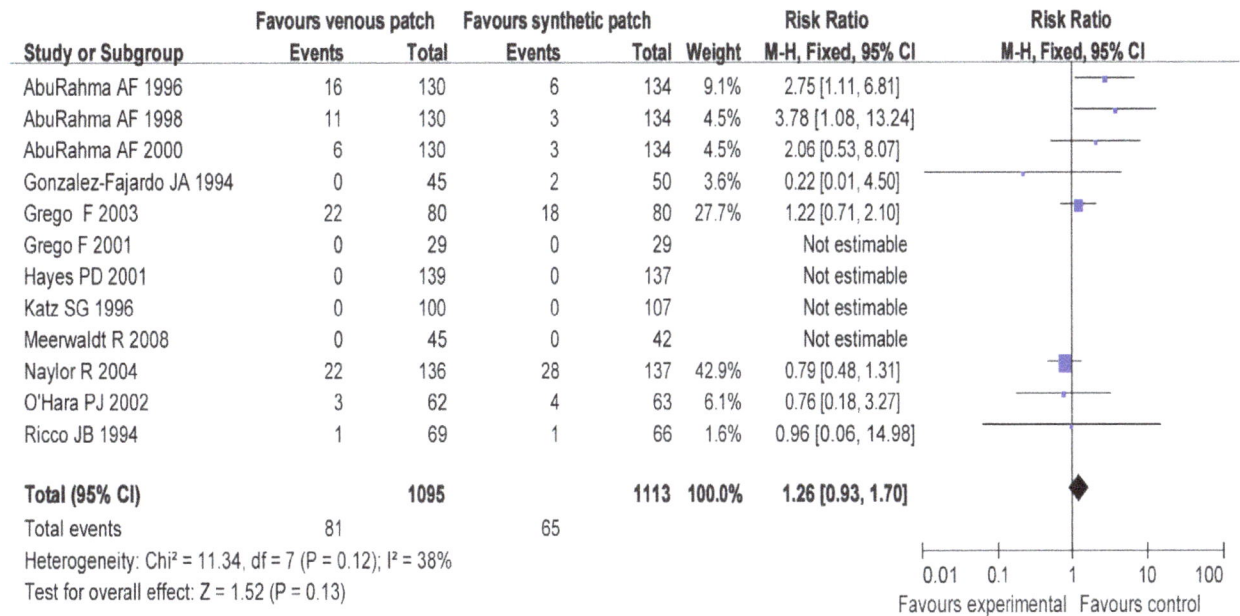

Figure 4. Restenosis of carotid artery in both groups. Graphical representation of the results. *M-H:* Mantel-Haenszel.

Trials of Venous Patch versus Synthetic Patch Materials during CEA

Figures 2–7 are the forest plots showing the outcomes of meta-analysis of the outcomes of CEA with venous patch versus synthetic patch material. There was no significant difference between CEA with venous patch versus synthetic patch material in the incidence of mortality (RR: 1.23; 95% CI: 0.79, 1.89; P=0.36; Fig. 2), any stroke events (RR: 0.77; 95% CI: 0.54, 1.10; P=0.15; Fig. 3), or restenosis of carotid artery (RR: 1.26; 95% CI: 0.93, 1.70; P=0.13; Fig. 4). Similarly, no significant difference between the two groups was observed in terms of incidence of postoperative wound infection (RR: 1.97; 95% CI: 0.70, 5.51; P=0.20; Fig. 5), incidence of reoperation for wound hematoma (RR: 0.67; 95% CI: 0.34, 1.32; P=0.24; Fig. 6); however, mean operative time (Mean difference: −0.45; 95% CI: −5.44, −3.57; P<0.00001; Fig. 7a), and the hemostasis time (Mean difference: −18.53; 95% CI: −20.87, −16.19; P<0.00001; Fig. 7b) in the synthetic patch group was significantly longer than in venous patch group.

Outcomes of RCTs Comparing Dacron Patch with PTFE

Fig. 8 demonstrates the incidence of transient ischemic attack (TIA) and stroke (RR: 4.45; 95% CI: 1.79, 11.06; P=0.001; Fig. 8b), 50% restenosis to occlusion of carotid artery (RR: 12.27;

95% CI: 5.26, 28.64; P<0.00001; Fig. 8c), and carotid thrombosis (RR: 8.00; 95% CI: 1.01, 63.38; P=0.05; Fig. 8d) after CEA were significantly higher in the Dacron patch group than in PTFE patch group, although incidence of mortality rate did not differ significantly (RR: 5.00; 95% CI: 0.24, 102.85; P=0.30; Fig. 8a). However, the hemostasis time in the PTFE patch cohort was significantly longer than in Dacron patch cohort (Mean difference: −2.71; 95% CI: −3.78, −1.64; P<0.00001; Fig. 9a), even though the operative times between both groups were similar (Mean difference: −3.23; 95% CI: −7.87, 1.41; P=0.17; Fig. 9b).

Results of RCT Comparing Bovine Pericardium with Dacron

One RCT [10] of 95 CEAs in 92 patients comparing bovine pericardium with Dacron patch observed bleeding at 3 and 4 minutes after removal of the carotid cross-clamp, and then objectively weighed the sponge used to tamponade bleeding during these time intervals. The incidence of suture line bleeding at 3 minutes was 14% (7/51) in the bovine pericardium group and 55% (24/44) in the Dacron group (P<0.001). Suture line bleeding at 4 minutes was present in 4% (2/51) in the bovine pericardium group and 30% (13/44) in the Dacron group (P=0.001). Weight of total intraoperative suture line bleeding (Net±SEM sponge

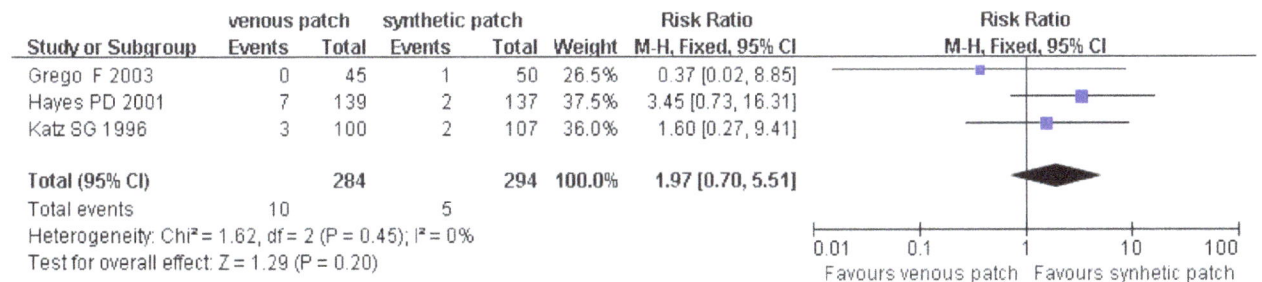

Study or Subgroup	venous patch Events	Total	synthetic patch Events	Total	Weight	Risk Ratio M-H, Fixed, 95% CI	Risk Ratio M-H, Fixed, 95% CI
Grego F 2003	0	45	1	50	26.5%	0.37 [0.02, 8.85]	
Hayes PD 2001	7	139	2	137	37.5%	3.45 [0.73, 16.31]	
Katz SG 1996	3	100	2	107	36.0%	1.60 [0.27, 9.41]	
Total (95% CI)		**284**		**294**	**100.0%**	**1.97 [0.70, 5.51]**	
Total events	10		5				

Heterogeneity: Chi² = 1.62, df = 2 (P = 0.45); I² = 0%
Test for overall effect: Z = 1.29 (P = 0.20)

Figure 5. Postoperative wound infection events in both groups. Graphical representation of the results. *M-H :* Mantel-Haenszel.

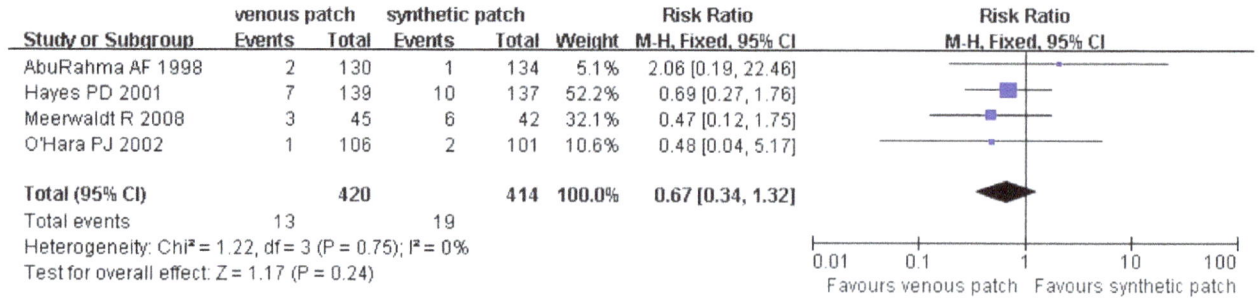

Figure 6. Reoperation for wound hematoma compared in both groups. Graphical representation of the results. *M-H:* Mantel-Haenszel.

weight) in the bovine pericardium group was significantly less than in Dacron group (6.25±0.55 g versus 16.34±1.85 g; *P*<0.001).

Methodological Quality of Included Studies

The study quality was assessed on the methods described by Jadad for randomized studies [9]. The randomization sequence in most trials was well concealed using sealed, opaque, sequentially-numbered envelopes. However, there were significant flaws in some trials, as no detailed randomization method was reported. Blinding is important in reducing bias in the detection of some operative results, yet the detailed blinding method was not mentioned in the reports.

The events of stroke and death were too few to determine whether there were significant differences between venous patch and synthetic patch during either the perioperative period or follow-up; thus, the results of trials were compared at the end of follow-up. One trial provided a definition of peudoaneurysm, but no ruptured pseudoaneurysm or related stroke was reported.

Publication Bias

Funnel plots were performed to test if publication bias existed within the studies included in the meta-analysis, none of the papers laid outside the limits of the 95% CI (Funnel plots were not shown).

Discussion

Several studies have showed that patch angioplasty is better than primary closure in CEA in lowering the risk of restenosis of carotid artery and stroke [2,3,5,24]. However, there is no consensus on the optimal patch material, and the available data do not support the use of venous patch over synthetic patch materials during CEA [4–6]. The present meta-analysis results indicate that the outcomes of CEA with venous patching was similar to that with synthetic patching in terms of reducing risks of stroke or death, and recurrent stenosis during the perioperative period and long-term follow-up, but the hemostasis time in CEA with synthetic patch was significantly longer than in CEA with

(a)

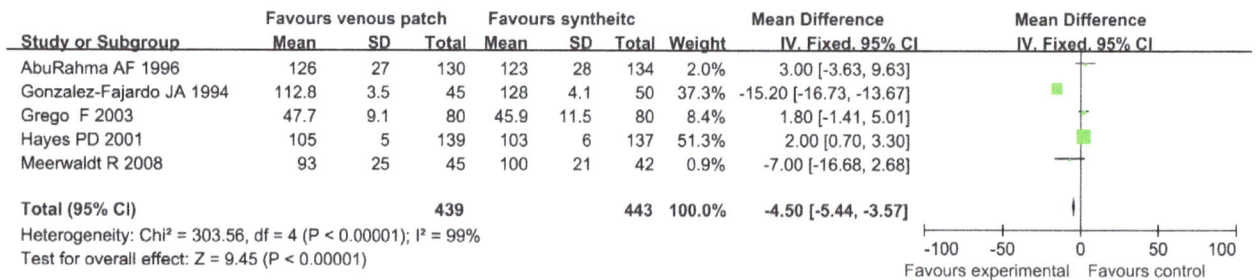

(b)

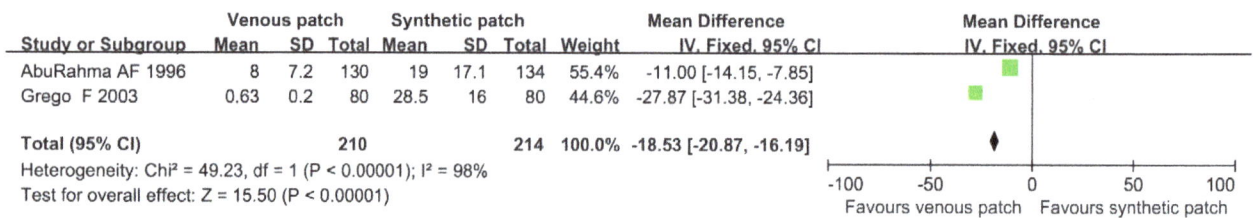

Figure 7. Mean operative time (a) and mean hemostasis time (b) in minutes are compared in both groups. Graphical representation of the results.

(a)

Study or Subgroup	Favours Dacron Events	Total	Favours PTFE Events	Total	Weight	Risk Ratio M-H, Fixed, 95% CI
AbuRahma AF 2002a	2	100	0	100	100.0%	5.00 [0.24, 102.85]
AbuRahma AF 2002b	0	0	0	0		Not estimable
AbuRahma AF 2007	0	0	0	0		Not estimable
Total (95% CI)		100		100	100.0%	5.00 [0.24, 102.85]
Total events	2		0			

Heterogeneity: Not applicable
Test for overall effect: Z = 1.04 (P = 0.30)

Risk Ratio M-H, Fixed, 95% CI — 0.01 0.1 1 10 100 — Favours Dacron Favours PTFE

(b)

Study or Subgroup	Dacron Events	Total	PTFE Events	Total	Weight	Risk Ratio M-H, Fixed, 95% CI
AbuRahma AF 2002a	12	100	3	100	54.5%	4.00 [1.16, 13.75]
AbuRahma AF 2002b	8	100	0	100	9.1%	17.00 [0.99, 290.62]
AbuRahma AF 2007	4	100	2	100	36.4%	2.00 [0.37, 10.67]
Total (95% CI)		300		300	100.0%	4.45 [1.79, 11.06]
Total events	24		5			

Heterogeneity: Chi² = 1.76, df = 2 (P = 0.41); I² = 0%
Test for overall effect: Z = 3.22 (P = 0.001)

Risk Ratio M-H, Fixed, 95% CI — 0.01 0.1 1 10 100 — Favours Dacron Favours PTFE

(c)

Study or Subgroup	Dacron Events	Total	PTFE Events	Total	Weight	Risk Ratio M-H, Fixed, 95% CI
AbuRahma AF 2002a	12	100	2	100	36.4%	6.00 [1.38, 26.12]
AbuRahma AF 2002b	51	100	3	100	54.5%	17.00 [5.49, 52.67]
AbuRahma AF 2007	4	100	0	100	9.1%	9.00 [0.49, 165.00]
Total (95% CI)		300		300	100.0%	12.27 [5.26, 28.64]
Total events	67		5			

Heterogeneity: Chi² = 1.27, df = 2 (P = 0.53); I² = 0%
Test for overall effect: Z = 5.80 (P < 0.00001)

Risk Ratio M-H, Fixed, 95% CI — 0.01 0.1 1 10 100 — Favours Dacron Favours PTFE

(d)

Study or Subgroup	Dacron Events	Total	PTFE Events	Total	Weight	Risk Ratio M-H, Fixed, 95% CI
AbuRahma AF 2002a	5	100	0	100	50.0%	11.00 [0.62, 196.33]
AbuRahma AF 2007	2	100	0	100	50.0%	5.00 [0.24, 102.85]
Total (95% CI)		200		200	100.0%	8.00 [1.01, 63.38]
Total events	7		0			

Heterogeneity: Chi² = 0.14, df = 1 (P = 0.71); I² = 0%
Test for overall effect: Z = 1.97 (P = 0.05)

Risk Ratio M-H, Fixed, 95% CI — 0.01 0.1 1 10 100 — Favours Dacron Favours PTFE

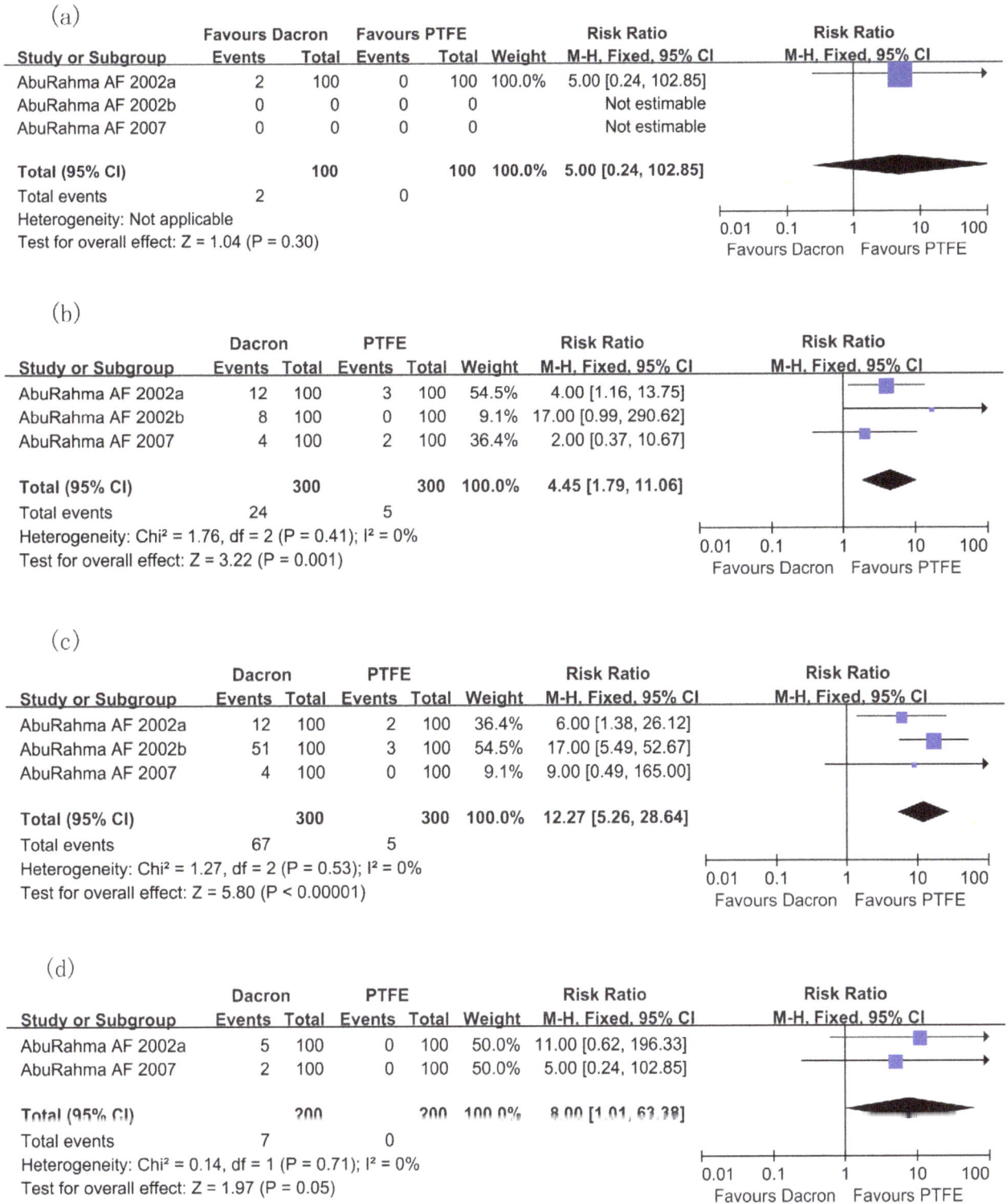

Figure 8. Meta-analysis of incidence of mortality rate (a), TIA and stroke (b), 50% restenosis to occlusion of carotid artery (c), and carotid thrombosis (d) after carotid endarterectomy, comparing Dacron and PTFE during CEA in randomized controlled trials. *CEA* carotid endarterectomy; *M-H* Mantel-Haenszel; *PTFE* polytetrafluoroethelene.

venous patch material. Due to the different types of synthetic patches used in the present study, and that different synthetic patch materials act variably, we further compared the outcomes of CEA using Dacron and PTFE materials. The data show that incidences of TIA and stroke, restenosis (from 50% to occlusion) of carotid artery, and carotid thrombosis after CEA were significantly

(a)

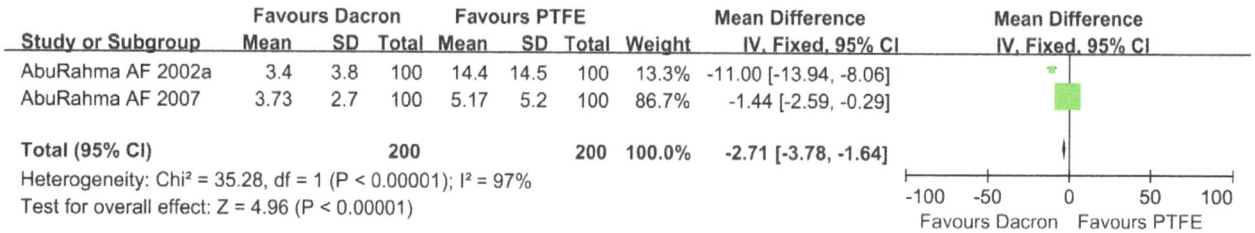

(b)

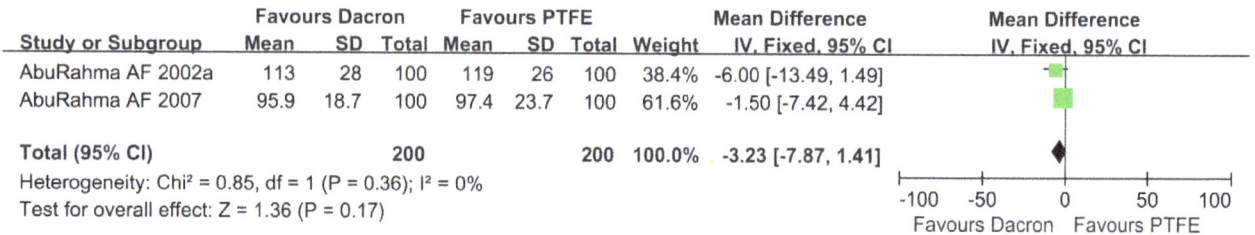

Figure 9. Meta-analysis of hemostasis time (a), and operative time (b) in minutes during carotid endarterectomy, comparing Dacron and PTFE during CEA in two randomized controlled trials. *CEA:* carotid endarterectomy; *PTFE:* polytetrafluoroethelene.

higher in Dacron patch group than in PTFE patch group ($P<0.05$), but the mortality rate was similar in both groups ($P=0.3$), and the hemostasis time in the PTFE group was significantly longer than in the Dacron group. Furthermore, bovine pericardium is superior to Dacron in reducing intraoperative suture line bleeding ($P<0.001$).

The benefit of patch angioplasty in CEA is clear in patients with narrow arteries [25]. Carotid patching plays a role in reducing risk of stroke, especially in the carotid artery with a narrow internal lumen or a long plaque [25]. However, there is no clear agreement on the size of the artery lumen required for patch angioplasty. Few authors have reported the size of internal carotid artery in RCTs [25]. However, it is generally accepted that a patch angioplasty is indicated for internal carotid artery diameter <4–5 mm to prevent perioperative stroke rates and occlusion, and [25].

There remains controversy on the choice of patch materials in CEA. Selection of patch material is affected by thrombogenicity, aneurismal formation, risk of patch rupture, availability of patch material, complications related to vein harvesting, and the resistance to infection. Some surgeons prefer harvesting autologous veins, including the saphenous vein, or the internal/external jugular vein and facial vein [8]. RCTs and animal studies support that using an intima-lined patch may potentially reduce the risk of perioperative thrombosis and infection [26]. Indeed, vein-patch walls did not develop a thickened intima [26]. However, complications with saphenous vein patch following CEA have been reported, including a longer operating time, a blow-out or patch rupture, potential risk of false aneurysm formation, thrombosis from dilated or aneurismal carotid dilation [4,27–29] in the postoperative period, and restenosis on long-term follow-up [30,31].

The benefits of synthetic patches, including the Dacron and PTFE, are easy availability, resistance to aneurismal formation

and patch rupture, lack of morbidity caused by vein harvesting, and preservation of vein conduits intact available for future potential coronary artery bypass grafting. However, it has been reported that Dacron synthetic patch is at risk of infection and thrombogenicity after CEA [18] and the PTFE patch causes a prolonged bleeding in CEA [18]. Our meta-analysis showed that the mean hemostasis time for the PTFE patch was significantly higher than for venous patch. We further compared the Dacron patch with the PTFE patch materials during CEA, and the results showed that the hemostasis time was still longer in CEA using PTFE patch than Dacron patch. Even using the new type of PTFE (Gore-Tex® Acuseal, W.L Fore & Associates Inc., Newark, USA), one RCT trial showed that hemostasis time in PTFE was longer than in Dacron patch group ($P=0.01$) [23]. Similarly, excessive intraoperative bleeding from needle holes in the conventional PTFE patch was reported in earlier studies [27,32]. Reduction of such blood loss has been found to be associated with a needle/suture diameter ratio of 1:1 [27]. It is reported that use of PTFE suture, CV-6 (Gore-Tex® Acuseal) and polypropylene sutures (prolene 5/0) with RB-1 needles (TT-9) could minimize hemostasis time [23,27]. Therefore, the hemostasis issue should be considered for the selection of the patching materials. In addition, the surgeon may prefer venous patching in the event that patients refuse to use the costly synthetic patch for CEA.

Limitations of this study include heterogeneity of synthetic patches, variety of follow-up periods, and statistically underpowered number of patients in each trial. Thus, these results may not be completely reliable and should be interpreted cautiously. In addition, a new type patch of PTFE (Gore-Tex® Acuseal) is reported to have a greater outcome than the conventional PTFE patch [23], and a new collagen-impregnated Dacron patch has been designed to restrict its thrombogenicity.

Conclusions

The hemostasis time in CEA with PTFE patch is longer than with venous patch or Dacron patch. The overall perioperative and long-term mortality rate, stroke rate, restenosis, and operative time are similar when using venous patch versus synthetic patch, or using Dacron patch versus PTFE patch during CEA. Nevertheless, larger cohorts of patients are warranted to demonstrate the optimal patch materials, and the priority of autologus venous patch versus synthetic patch.

Supporting Information

Table S1 PRISMA flow diagram of the meta-analysis.

Table S2 PRISMA checklist of the meta-analysis.

Acknowledgments

This paper is supported in part by National Sciences Foundation of China (Grant No. 81070230). Dr. Ren is the guarantor for this article, and takes responsibility for the integrity of the work as a whole.

Author Contributions

Conceived and designed the experiments: SR XL PL. Performed the experiments: SR XL. Analyzed the data: SR WZ JW. Contributed reagents/materials/analysis tools: SR. Wrote the paper: SR.

References

1. Ren S, Liu P, Ma G, Wang F, Qian S, et al. (2012) Long-term outcomes of synchronous carotid endarterectomy and coronary artery bypass grafting versus solely carotid endarterectomy. Ann Thorac Cardiovasc Surg 18: 228–35.
2. Counsell C, Salinas R, Warlow C, Naylor R (2000) Patch angioplasty versus primary closure for carotid endarterectomy. Cochrane Database Syst Rev CD000160.
3. Rerkasem K, Rothwell PM (2011) Carotid endarterectomy for symptomatic carotid stenosis. Cochrane Database Syst Rev CD001081.
4. Bond R, Rerkasem K, Naylor AR, Aburahma AF, Rothwell PM (2004) Patches of different types for carotid patch angioplasty. Cochrane Database Syst Rev (2): CD000071.
5. Rerkasem K, Rothwell PM (2010) Patches of different types for carotid patch angioplasty. Cochrane Database Syst Rev CD000071.
6. Rerkasem K, Rothwell PM (2011) Systematic review of randomized controlled trials of patch angioplasty versus primary closure and different types of patch materials during carotid endarterectomy. Asian J Surg 34: 32–40.
7. Louagie Y, Buche M, Eucher P, Goffinet JM, Laloux P, et al. (2011) Case-matched comparison of early and long-term outcomes of everted cervical vein and saphenous vein carotid patch angioplasty. Eur J Vasc Endovasc Surg 42: 766–74.
8. Mannheim D, Weller B, Vahadim E, Karmeli R (2005) Carotid endarterectomy with a polyurethane patch versus primary closure: a prospective randomized study. J Vasc Surg 41: 403–7.
9. Jadad AR, Moore RA, Carroll D, Jenkinson C, Reynolds DJ, et al. (1996) Assessing the quality of reports of randomized clinical trials: is blinding necessary? Controll Clin Trials 17: 1–12.
10. Marien BJ, Raffetto JD, Seidman CS, LaMorte WW, Menzoian JO (2002) Bovine pericardium vs dacron for patch angioplasty after carotid endarterectomy: a prospective randomized study. Arch Surg 137: 785–8.
11. Grego F, Antonello M, Lepidi S, Bonvini S, Deriu GP (2003) Prospective, randomized study of external jugular vein patch versus polytetrafluoroethylene patch during carotid endarterectomy: perioperative and long-term results. J Vasc Surg 38: 1232–40.
12. O'Hara PJ, Hertzer NR, Mascha EJ, Krajewski LP, Clair DG, et al. (2002) A prospective, randomized study of saphenous vein patching versus synthetic patching during carotid endarterectomy. J Vasc Surg 35: 324–32.
13. Hayes PD, Allroggen H, Steel S, Thompson MM, London NJ, et al. (2001) Randomized trial of vein versus Dacron patching during carotid endarterectomy: influence of patch type on postoperative embolization. J Vasc Surg 33: 994–1000.
14. AbuRahma AF, Khan JH, Robinson PA, Saiedy S, Short YS, et al. (1996) Prospective randomized trial of carotid endarterectomy with primary closure and patch angioplasty with saphenous vein, jugular vein, and polytetrafluoroethylene: perioperative (30-day) results. J Vasc Surg 24: 998–1006; discussion 1006–7.
15. Lord RS, Raj TB, Stary DL, Nash PA, Graham AR, et al. (1989) Comparison of saphenous vein patch, polytetrafluoroethylene patch, and direct arteriotomy closure after carotid endarterectomy. Part I. Perioperative results. J Vasc Surg 9: 521–9.
16. Gonzalez-Fajardo JA, Perez JL, Mateo AM (1994) Saphenous vein patch versus polytetrafluoroethylene patch after carotid endarterectomy. J Cardiovasc Surg 35: 523–8.
17. Ricco JB, Saliou C, Dubreuil F, Boin-Pineau MH (1994) Value of the prosthetic patch after carotid endarterectomy(In French). J Maladies Vasc 19 (Suppl A): 10–7.
18. Katz SG, Kohl RD (1996) Does the choice of material influence early morbidity in patients undergoing carotid patch angioplasty? Surgery 119: 297–301.
19. Naylor R, Hayes PD, Payne DA, Allroggen H, Steel S, et al. (2004) Randomized trial of vein versus dacron patching during carotid endarterectomy: long-term results. J Vasc Surg 39: 985–93; discussion 93.
20. Meerwaldt R, Lansink KW, Blomme AM, Fritschy WM (2008) Prospective randomized study of carotid endarterectomy with Fluoropassiv thin wall carotid patch versus venous patch. Euro J Vasc Endovasc Surg 36: 45–52.
21. AbuRahma AF, Hannay RS, Khan JH, Robinson PA, Hudson JK, et al. (2002) Prospective randomized study of carotid endarterectomy with polytetrafluoroethylene versus collagen-impregnated Dacron (Hemashield) patching: perioperative (30-day) results. J Vasc Surg 35: 125–30.
22. AbuRahma AF, Hopkins ES, Robinson PA, Deel JT, Agarwal S (2003) Prospective randomized trial of carotid endarterectomy with polytetrafluoroethylene versus collagen-impregnated dacron (Hemashield) patching: late follow-up. Ann Surg 237: 885–92; discussion 892–3.
23. AbuRahma AF, Stone PA, Flaherty SK, AbuRahma Z (2007) Prospective randomized trial of ACUSEAL (Gore-Tex) versus Hemashield-Finesse patching during carotid endarterectomy: early results. J Vasc Surg 45: 881–4.
24. Bond R, Rerkasem K, Naylor AR, Aburahma AF, Rothwell PM (2004) Systematic review of randomized controlled trials of patch angioplasty versus primary closure and different types of patch materials during carotid endarterectomy. J Vasc Surg 40: 1126–35.
25. Golledge J (2011) Carotid artery plaque composition–relationship to clinical presentation and ultrasound B-mode imaging commentary. Euro J Vasc Endovasc Surg 42 (Suppl 1): S39–40.
26. Stewart GW, Bandyk DF, Kaebnick HW, Storey JD, Towne JB (1987) Influence of vein-patch angioplasty on carotid endarterectomy healing. Arch Surg 122: 364–71.
27. AbuRahma AF, Robinson PA, Saiedy S, Kahn JH, Boland JP (1998) Prospective randomized trial of carotid endarterectomy with primary closure and patch angioplasty with saphenous vein, jugular vein, and polytetrafluoroethylene: long-term follow-up. J Vasc Surg 27: 222–32; discussion 233–4.
28. Clagett GP, Patterson CB, Fisher DF Jr, Fry RE, Eidt JF, et al. (1989) Vein patch versus primary closure for carotid endarterectomy. A randomized prospective study in a selected group of patients. J Vasc Surg 9: 213–23.
29. Carney WI, Lilly MP (1987) Intraoperative evaluation of PTFE, Dacron and autogenous vein as carotid patch materials. Ann Vasc Surg 1: 583–6.
30. Hans SS (1991) Late follow-up of carotid endarterectomy with venous patch angioplasty. Am J Surg 162: 50–4.
31. Ten Holter JB, Ackerstaff RC, Thoe Schwartzenberg CW, Eikelboom BC, Vermeulen FE, et al. (1990) The impact of vein patch angioplasty on long-term surgical outcome after carotid endarterectomy. A prospective follow-up study with serial duplex scanning. J Cardiovasc Surg 31: 58–65.
32. LeGrand DR, Linehan RL (1990) The suitability of expanded PTFE for carotid patch angioplasty. Ann Vasc Surg 4: 209–12.

19

The Association between Contrast Dose and Renal Complications Post PCI across the Continuum of Procedural Estimated Risk

Judith Kooiman[1], Milan Seth[2], David Share[3], Simon Dixon[4], Hitinder S. Gurm[2]*

1 Department of Thrombosis and Hemostasis and Department of Nephrology, Leiden University Medical Center, Leiden, Zuid-Holland, The Netherlands, 2 Department of Internal Medicine, Division of Cardiovascular Medicine, University of Michigan, Ann Arbor, Michigan, United States of America, 3 Blue Cross Blue Shield of Michigan, Detroit, Michigan, United States of America, 4 Beaumont Hospital, Royal Oak, Michigan, United States of America

Abstract

Background: Prior studies have proposed to restrict the contrast volume (CV) to <3x calculated creatinine clearance (CCC), to prevent contrast induced nephropathy (CIN) post percutaneous coronary interventions (PCI). The predictive value of this algorithm for CIN and therefore the benefit of this approach in high risk patients has been questioned. The aim of our study was to assess the association between contrast dose and the occurrence of CIN in patients at varying predicted risks of CIN and baseline CCC following contemporary PCI.

Methods: Consecutive patients undergoing PCI between 2010–2012 were included. Baseline risk of CIN was calculated using a previously validated risk tool. High contrast dose was defined as CV/CCC >3. Likelihood ratio tests were used to evaluate whether the effect of a high contrast dose on the risk of CIN and nephropathy requiring dialysis (NRD) varied across the spectrum of baseline predicted risk.

Results: Of the 82,120 PCI included in our analysis, 25% were performed using a high contrast dose. Patients treated with a high compared with a low contrast dose were at increased risks of CIN and NRD, throughout the entire range of baseline predicted risk and CCC in our population. The effect size of a high contrast dose on risks of both outcomes varied significantly with baseline predicted CIN risk and CCC (CIN p = 0.004, NRD p<0.001 for adding interactions), and was largest for patients with predicted CIN risk <10% and pre-existing chronic kidney disease.

Conclusions: The use of a high contrast dose is associated with increased risks of CIN and NRD across the continuum of baseline predicted risk and CCC. Efforts to reduce contrast dose may therefore be effective in preventing renal complications in all patients undergoing PCI.

Editor: Davide Capodanno, Ferrarotto Hospital, University of Catania, Italy

Funding: The BMC2 registry is funded by Blue Cross Blue Shield of Michigan. Hitinder S. Gurm receives research funding from the National Institutes of Health and Agency for Healthcare Research and Quality. The funders had no role in study design, data collection and analysis, decision to publish, or preparation of the manuscript.

Competing Interests: One of the co-authors, Dr. Share is currently employed by Blue Cross Blue Shield of Michigan. Hitinder S. Gurm has, in the interim, consulted for Osprey medical, a company that is developing devices for prevention of contrast induced kidney injury. No compensation was received for this work but the company made a donation to a local non-profit of his choice.

* E-mail: hgurm@med.umich.edu

Introduction

Contrast media induced renal complications are common among patients undergoing percutaneous coronary interventions (PCI) [1]. Contrast induced nephropathy (CIN) and the need for dialysis (NRD) post PCI have been associated with increased early and long-term mortality rates, and add significantly to healthcare expenses [1,2]. Current guidelines support multiple strategies for prophylaxis of CIN including adequate hydration, minimization of contrast dose and the use of iso-osmolar or certain low-osmolar contrast media[3–7].

Use of renal function based contrast dosing with the total contrast volume (CV) restricted to less than thrice the calculated creatinine clearance (CCC) has been suggested as a practical

strategy to reduce the risk of CIN [3]. However, the predictive value of this dosing algorithm for CIN and hence the benefit of this approach in patients at high risk of renal complications post PCI has been debated [8].

We recently reported an accurate prediction model for the risk of renal complications in patients undergoing PCI [9]. This model estimates the risk of CIN and NRD based on pre-procedural variables, has a higher discriminative power than other commonly used prediction models, and can therefore be used to study the effect of a high contrast dose on the occurrence of CIN in patients with varying baseline risks of renal complications.

The aim of our current study was to assess the impact of high contrast dose (CV/CCC >3) on the risk of renal complications across the continuum of pre-procedural predicted risk of CIN in a large cohort of patients undergoing contemporary PCI.

Methods

Our study population comprised consecutive patients undergoing PCI between January 2010 and September 2012 across 47 hospitals in Michigan participating in the Blue Cross Blue Shield of Michigan Cardiovascular Consortium (BMC2). Hence, this cohort consists of patients other than the population in which the effect of renal function-based contrast dosing on the risk of renal complications was originally assessed (who underwent PCI between 2007 and 2008) [3]. BMC2 is a quality improvement collaborative that tracks the inpatient outcome of consecutive patients undergoing PCI at all non-federal hospitals in the State of Michigan. The details of the BMC2 and its data collection and auditing process have been described previously [10,11]. Procedural data on all consecutive patients undergoing PCI at participating hospitals are collected using standardized data collection forms. Collected data include clinical and demographic patient characteristics, procedural, and angiographic characteristics, as well as medications used before, during, and after PCI, and in-hospital outcomes. All data elements have been prospectively defined, and the protocol is approved by local institutional review boards at each of the participating hospitals. In addition to a random audit in 2% of all PCI procedures, medical records of all patients undergoing multiple procedures or coronary artery bypass grafting and of patients who died in the hospital are reviewed routinely to ensure data accuracy.

Patients who were already on dialysis at the time of PCI, those with missing serum creatinine values pre or post procedurally, and those who died in the catheterization laboratory were excluded from outcome analysis. Patients with missing values for weight, gender, or CV were also excluded as these variables were needed to determine whether a patient received a high contrast dose. The type and volume of contrast media and hydration protocols used were as per the operator preference guided by institutional policy and practice.

Study Endpoints

CIN was defined as an acute decline in renal function post PCI resulting in an absolute increase in serum creatinine ≥ 0.5 mg/dL from baseline [12]. Baseline creatinine values were collected within a month prior to PCI. Among patients who had multiple assessments of serum creatinine in the month prior to PCI, the value closest to the time of the procedure was considered as the baseline value. Peak creatinine was defined as the highest value of creatinine in the week following the procedure or during the hospitalization following PCI and was ascertained as per local clinical practice. Time between PCI and peak creatinine was at least 1 day, and varied depending on length of hospital stay. The secondary endpoint for the study was NRD defined as a new, unplanned need for dialysis during hospitalization due to progression of chronic kidney disease post PCI.

High contrast dose was defined as administration of a CV thrice the CCC. CCC was calculated using the Cockgroft-Gault equation [13].

Statistical Analyses

Continuous variables are presented as mean with standard deviation and categorical variables as percentages, with standardized differences between groups presented for both types of variables as percentages. Unless otherwise stated, student t-tests for

continuous and Chi-squared tests for categorical variables were utilized for univariate comparisons.

Baseline estimated risk of CIN was calculated using the BMC2 CIN prediction tool [9]. Multivariate logistic regression models with CIN and NRD as outcomes were developed including high contrast dose, baseline estimated CIN risk, CCC, and other baseline clinical covariates as main effect terms. To investigate potential effect modification of baseline predicted CIN risk on CIN and NRD rates associated with a high contrast dose, regression models adding two and three way interaction terms involving baseline estimated CIN risk (logit transformed linear and quadratic terms) and CCC with high contrast dose were fitted to the data. A stepwise selection algorithm optimizing the Akaike Information Criteria was used to select an optimal model. The selected models including interactions were then compared to the base model using likelihood ratio tests to assess whether inclusion of interactions significantly improved the fit of the model.

Model predicted relative risks for CIN and NRD comparing high with low contrast dosages were plotted over a range of CCC and baseline predicted risk of CIN, to demonstrate the extent and implications of effect modification.

All analyses were performed in R version 2.14.1 using freely distributed contributed packages [14,15].

Results

Our study cohort comprised 82,120 (85%) of the 96,753 PCI procedures performed across Michigan between January 2010 through December 2012. Of the 14,633(15%) procedures that were excluded from the analysis, 2,251 (15%) patients were already on dialysis at the time of the procedure, 11,997 (82%) had missing serum creatinine values prior to (n = 2,229 (15%)) or following PCI (n = 9,907 (68%)), with 139 patients missing both pre and post procedural creatinine values. Additionally, 466 patients lacked information on CV, 99 on bodyweight, and 1 patient on gender. As all of these variables were needed to determine whether a patient received a high contrast dose, patients missing one or more of these data elements were excluded.

Table 1 reports characteristics at baseline of study patients categorized to the use of either a low or a high contrast dose at time of PCI (CV/CCC < = 3 and CV/CCC >3). In this cohort, 20,915(25.3%) patients received a high contrast dose who had a greater burden of comorbidities, a higher baseline estimated CIN risk, and were more likely to have preexisting chronic kidney disease.

The median predicted risk of CIN of the cohort was 0.54% (range = 0–80.4%, IQR = 0.08%–2.43%), and 90% of patients had a predicted risk of less than 7.92%. Patients at higher predicted risk of CIN were more likely to be treated with a high contrast dose (p<0.001, Figure 1).

CIN occurred in 2,146/82,120 (2.61%, 95% CI 2.51–2.72%) patients, and NRD in 308/82,120 (0.37%, 95% CI 0.33–0.42%). The median baseline CIN risk estimate, calculated using the risk tool, was 11.6% (IQR 3.1–25.5%) among patients developing CIN, and 24.9% (10.9–36.6%) among those with NRD. Of patients with CIN, 1,144/2,146 (53.3%, 95% CI 51.2–55.4%) received a high contrast doses, as did 211/308 (68.5%, 95% CI 63.0–73.7%) patients with NRD.

In regression models adjusting for baseline predicted CIN risk and CCC, high contrast dose was significantly associated with increased rates of both CIN (OR = 1.61, 95% CI 1.46–1.79, P< .001) and NRD (OR = 1.65, 95% CI 1.24–2.21, P<.001), indicating that high contrast dose is an independent predictor of these outcomes. Within a multivariate model adjusting for baseline

Table 1. Baseline characteristics of patients treated with high versus low contrast dose.

Characteristic	CV/CCC ≤3	CV/CCC >3	P-value	Standardized difference (%)
N (procedures)	61.205 (74.5%)	20.915 (25.5%)	NA	NA
BMI	31.48±7.83	27.89±5.63	<0.001	52.54
Age	62.16±11.36	73.26±10.53	<0.001	101.28
Creatinine clearance (CCC)	106.24±42.83	59.10±22.87	<0.001	137.31
Contrast volume (ml)	171.84±63.15	248.90±88.46	<0.001	100.28
Predicted CIN risk (%)	2.10±4.99	5.23±8.91	<0.001	43.32
Female gender	18.838/61.205 (30.8%)	9.039/20.915 (43.2%)	<0.001	25.98
Race - White	53.502/61.205 (87.4%)	17.725/20.915 (84.7%)	<0.001	7.71
Race - Black or African American	6.189/61.205 (10.1%)	2.655/20.915 (12.7%)	<0.001	8.13
Current/recent smoker (w/in 1 year)	20.138/61.178 (32.9%)	4.099/20.906 (19.6%)	<0.001	30.60
Hypertension	51.108/61.185 (83.5%)	18.726/20.905 (89.6%)	<0.001	17.79
Prior MI	20.910/61.196 (34.2%)	7.645/20.910 (36.6%)	<0.001	5.01
Prior heart failure	7.924/61.185 (13.0%)	4.696/20.907 (22.5%)	<0.001	25.11
Prior PCI	27.440/61.200 (44.8%)	9.087/20.913 (43.5%)	<0.001	2.79
Prior CABG	9.642/61.187 (15.8%)	5.668/20.912 (27.1%)	<0.001	27.92
Cerebrovascular disease	7.821/61.187 (12.8%)	4.652/20.907 (22.3%)	<0.001	25.11
Peripheral arterial disease	8.447/61.190 (13.8%)	4.937/20.909 (23.6%)	<0.001	25.35
Diabetes mellitus	22.697/61.198 (37.1%)	7.715/20.912 (36.9%)	0.614	0.40
CAD presentation/Evaluation				
No symptom. no angina	4.172/61.185 (6.8%)	1.329/20.906 (6.4%)	0.021	1.86
Symptom unlikely ischemic	1.352/61.185 (2.2%)	494/20.906 (2.4%)	0.197	1.03
Stable angina	9.701/61.185 (15.9%)	3.215/20.906 (15.4%)	0.102	1.31
Unstable angina	24.129/61.185 (39.4%)	7.957/20.906 (38.1%)	<0.001	2.82
Non-STEMI	12.223/61.185 (20.0%)	4.619/20.906 (22.1%)	<0.001	5.20
STEMI or equivalent	9.608/61.185 (15.7%)	3.292/20.906 (15.7%)	0.881	0.12
Cardiogenic shock w/in 24 hours	759/61.187 (1.2%)	592/20.909 (2.8%)	<0.001	11.28
Cardiac arrest w/in 24 hours	1.037/61.166 (1.7%)	460/20.901 (2.2%)	<0.001	3.66
PCI Indication				
Immediate PCI for STEMI	8.451/61.195 (13.8%)	2.912/20.909 (13.9%)	0.672	0.34
PCI for STEMI (unstable. >12 hrs from Sx onset)	421/61.195 (0.7%)	223/20.909 (1.1%)	<0.001	4.06
PCI for STEMI (Stable. >12 hrs from Sx onset)	218/61.195 (0.4%)	85/20.909 (0.4%)	0.301	0.82
Staged PCI	4.222/61.195 (6.9%)	870/20.909 (4.2%)	<0.001	12.00

Data are presented as mean (SD), or N (%) unless stated otherwise.
Abbreviations: BMI = body mass index, CIN = contrast induced nephropathy, CV/CCC = contrast volume/calculated creatinine clearance, MI = myocardial infarction, PCI = percutaneous coronary intervention, CABG = coronary artery bypass graft, CAD = coronary artery disease, STEMI = ST-elevation myocardial infarction.

clinical covariates (age, gender, recent heart failure, cardiogenic shock, cardiac arrest, CAD presentation, PCI status and indications), the effect of high contrast dose on the risk of CIN and NRD was consistent for both outcomes (CIN OR = 1.77, 95% CI 1.58–1.98, P<.001, NRD OR = 1.92, 95% CI 1.13–2.16, P<0.01).

Regression models were developed to investigate potential effect modification of baseline predicted CIN risk and baseline CCC on the association between high contrast dose and the risks of CIN and NRD. The fit of the models were significantly improved compared with the base models after adding of interaction terms involving baseline estimated CIN risk and CCC (Likelihood ratio test: LR 28 on 11 df, p = 0.004 for CIN, LR = 29 on 6 df, p<0.001 for NRD). This indicates that the effect of high contrast dose on

the risks of both CIN and NRD varied significantly across the spectrum of predicted CIN risk and baseline CCC.

Figure 2 depicts the model predicted relative risk of CIN (Figure 2A) and NRD (Figure 2B) for high versus a low contrast dose across the spectrum of baseline predicted risk and CCC. Both figures demonstrate an increased risk of renal complications post PCI associated with a high contrast dose regardless of a patient's baseline predicted risk or CCC, although the effect of a high contrast dose was most pronounced in those at lower predicted risk. The points on the graphed surfaces highlighted in red represent the estimated relative risks of high versus a low contrast dose at the median baseline risk and creatinine clearance values for patients with CIN (risk: 11.6%, CCC: 57 ml/min) and NRD (risk: 24.9%, CCC: 42.6 ml/min). The relative risk associated with

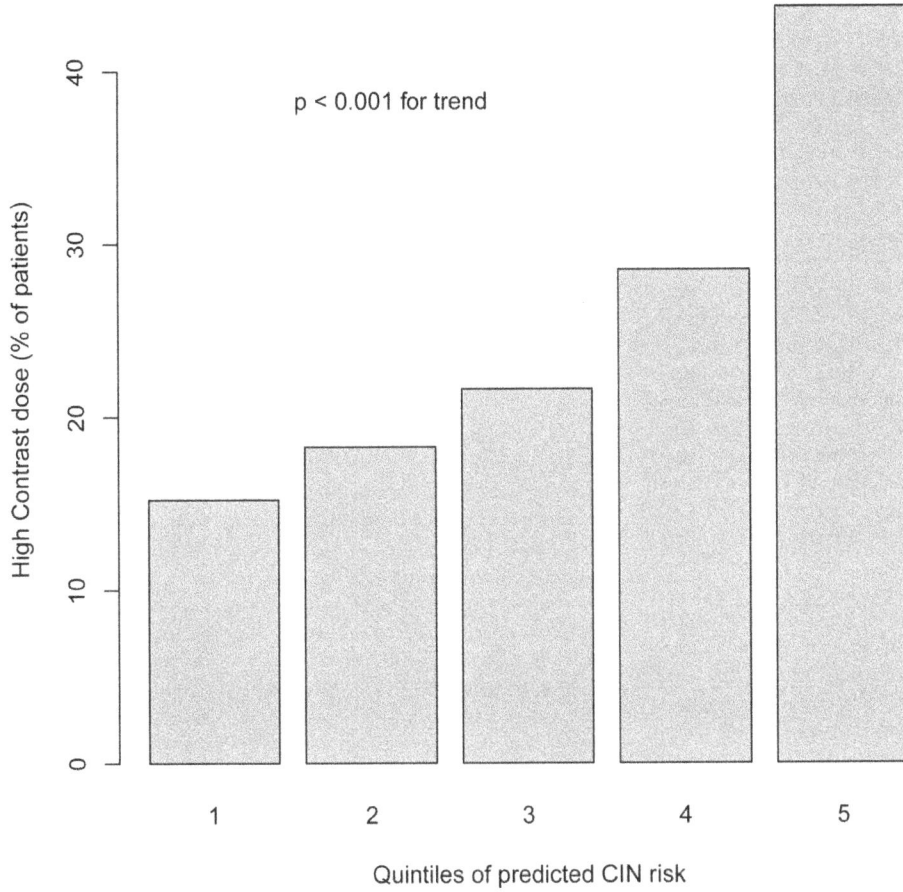

p < 0.001 for trend

Quintiles of predicted CIN risk

Figure 1. Proportions of patients treated with high dose contrast (Contrast volume/calculated creatinine clearance >3) across the quintiles of predicted risk of contrast induced nephropathy.

high a contrast dose at this point is 1.56 (95% CI 1.37–1.76) for CIN, and 2.05 (95% CI 1.35–2.75) for NRD.

Discussion

The key finding of our study is that the use of a high contrast dose is associated with increased risks of CIN and NRD across the

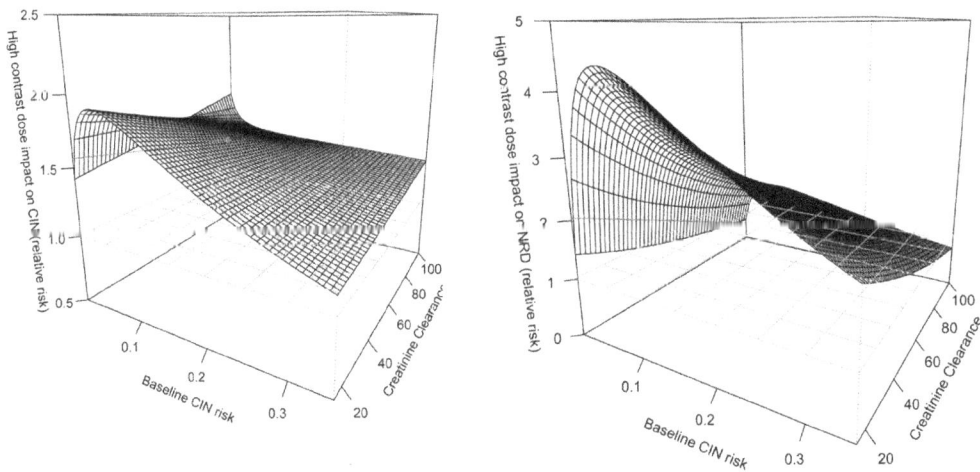

Figure 2. A. The relative risk of contrast induced nephropathy in association with high contrast dose across the continuum of predicted risk of contrast induced nephropathy among patients undergoing PCI. **B.** The relative risk of nephropathy requiring dialysis in association with high contrast dose across the continuum of predicted risk of contrast induced nephropathy among patients undergoing PCI.

continuum of predicted risk and CCC. Efforts to reduce the contrast dose may therefore be effective in preventing renal complications in all patients undergoing PCI. Especially in patients with pre-existing renal failure, restricting the contrast dose might result in lower rates of NRD.

Our findings significantly add to extend prior observations in this field. Work from many groups including ours has highlighted the role of high contrast dose as a risk factor for CIN and NRD in patients undergoing invasive cardiac procedures [3,16,17]. We have now demonstrated that regardless of baseline CCC and predicted risk of renal complications, the use of a high contrast dose is associated with increased risks of CIN and NRD post PCI. These results are in line with the results of two previous smaller studies concluding a high contrast dose to be associated with an increased risk of CIN throughout the continuum of baseline renal function [18,19]. These studies however, did not analyze the effect of baseline predicted risk on the association between a high contrast dose and renal complications post PCI. Our results demonstrated the effect of a high contrast dose on the risk of CIN and NRD to be most pronounced in those at lower predicted risk.

Efforts to improve outcomes of patients undergoing PCI for acute myocardial infarction or cardiogenic shock have traditionally focused on enhancing myocardial perfusion and hemodynamic support [20,21]. Restriction of contrast dose might be another important strategy to improve patient outcome after PCI, as our study findings suggest that the use of high contrast dosages is associated with an increased risk of CIN in all patients undergoing PCI. Limiting the CV to less than thrice the CCC may be even more important in patients at high risk of CIN, in terms of an absolute risk reduction, but also in those with pre-existing chronic kidney disease (i.e. eGFR <60 ml/min) in whom the effect of a high contrast dose on the risks of CIN was more profound compared to those without renal impairment. Our study findings also suggest that efforts to limit contrast dose in patients undergoing PCI may be helpful in reducing the risk of NRD, a complication which although rare, has not declined in the last few years among patients undergoing PCI, regardless of the introduction of less nephrotoxic contrast agents.

Patients at high predicted risk of CIN were more likely to receive a high contrast dose in our study. These patients might more frequently have comorbidity than patients receiving a low contrast dose, like peripheral artery disease, or an altered coronary vasculature due to prior PCI or prior coronary artery bypass graft resulting in more complex PCI procedures, requiring higher contrast volumes. Additionally, as a high contrast dose (CV/CCC >3) is also driven by impaired renal function, the frequent use of a high contrast dose in patients at high risk might also be explained by comorbidity associated with chronic kidney disease, increasing

the baseline predicted risk of CIN. Measures to reduce contrast dose are well recognized in literature but most of the work on contrast preservation has been performed in elective or stable patients, not those with acute myocardial infarction. Therefore, further research of the preventive effect of contrast preservation on the risk of renal complications in patients undergoing emergent PCI is warranted [22].

Our study findings must, however, be interpreted with certain qualifications. Our study associations, while strong do not support causality. However, it is unlikely that a randomized trial would ever be performed to evaluate the impact of high versus low contrast dose on the risk of renal complications. Since the findings appear biologically plausible and statistically robust, measures to limit contrast dose especially in high risk patients should be considered to reduce the risk of CIN and NRD. We have used the term CIN, although the role of contrast media in all patients who develop acute kidney injury after PCI remains debatable. It is likely that acute kidney injury after PCI is multifactorial and it may be preferable to use terms that do not assume that all renal dysfunction after PCI is secondary to contrast media. However, regardless of the term used, our study suggests that there is strong association between a high contrast dose and acute renal failure post PCI, even in high risk patients, implying that contrast media have an important contributory role towards the development of acute renal failure post PCI observed in this population. Only one post –procedure creatinine value was available and no follow up beyond the initial hospitalization was performed. Moreover, we lacked information on the timing of post-procedure serum creatinine measurements. No data on the type and amount of hydration used were available and this likely varied across institutions. However, we believe this makes our findings more generalizable to routine clinical care since it reflects observations from contemporary practice across multiple institutions.

To conclude, the use of a high contrast dose at time of PCI is associated with increased risks of CIN and NRD in all patients, regardless of their baseline predicted risk of these complications and renal function. Future research is needed to study whether the use of CV restricting measures decrease the risk of renal complications post PCI in patients with acute myocardial infarction. Until then, efforts to reduce CVs to less than thrice a patient's CCC should be encouraged for all patients undergoing PCI.

Author Contributions

Conceived and designed the experiments: HG JK MS. Analyzed the data: MS. Wrote the paper: JK. Provided critical review on study design and revision of the manuscript: SD DS.

References

1. Rihal CS, Textor SC, Grill DE, Berger PB, Ting HH, et. al. Incidence and prognostic importance of acute renal failure after percutaneous coronary intervention. Circulation 105: 2259–2264.

2. Gupta R, Gurm HS, Bhatt DL, Chew DP, Ellis SG (2005) Renal failure after percutaneous coronary intervention is associated with high mortality. Catheter Cardiovasc Interv 64: 442–448. 10.1002/ccd.20316 [doi].

3. Gurm HS, Dixon SR, Smith DE, Share D, Lalonde T, et al. (2011) Renal function-based contrast dosing to define safe limits of radiographic contrast media in patients undergoing percutaneous coronary interventions. J Am Coll Cardiol 58: 907–914. S0735–1097(11)02052–3 [pii];10.1016/j.jacc.2011.05.023 [doi].

4. Meier P, Ko DT, Tamura A, Tamhane U, Gurm HS (2009) Sodium bicarbonate-based hydration prevents contrast-induced nephropathy: a meta-analysis. BMC Med 7: 23. 1741-7015-7-23 [pii];10.1186/1741-7015-7-23 [doi].

5. Reed M, Meier P, Tamhane UU, Welch KB, Moscucci M, et al. (2009) The relative renal safety of iodixanol compared with low-osmolar contrast media: a meta-analysis of randomized controlled trials. JACC Cardiovasc Interv 2: 645–654. S1936-8798(09)00322-7 [pii];10.1016/j.jcin.2009.05.002 [doi].

6. Reed MC, Moscucci M, Smith DE, Share D, Lalonde T, et al. (2010) The relative renal safety of iodixanol and low-osmolar contrast media in patients undergoing percutaneous coronary intervention. Insights from Blue Cross Blue Shield of Michigan Cardiovascular Consortium (BMC2). J Invasive Cardiol 22: 467–472.

7. Stacul F, van der Molen AJ, Reimer P, Webb JA, Thomsen HS, et al. (2011) Contrast induced nephropathy: updated ESUR Contrast Media Safety Committee guidelines. Eur Radiol 21: 2527–2541. 10.1007/s00330-011-2225-0 [doi].

8. Kalra N, Fenster P (2012) Is renal function-based contrast dosing of radiographic contrast media in patients undergoing percutaneous coronary intervention sufficient to delineate safe limits of contrast dose? J Am Coll Cardiol 59: 432–433. S0735-1097(11)04825-X [pii];10.1016/j.jacc.2011.09.060 [doi].

9. Gurm HS, Seth M, Kooiman J, Share D (2013) A novel tool for reliable and accurate prediction of renal complications in patients undergoing percutaneous coronary intervention. J Am Coll Cardiol 61: 2242–2248. S0735-1097(13)01348-X [pii];10.1016/j.jacc.2013.03.026 [doi].

10. Kline-Rogers E, Share D, Bondie D, Rogers B, Karavite D, et al. (2002) Development of a multicenter interventional cardiology database: the Blue Cross Blue Shield of Michigan Cardiovascular Consortium (BMC2) experience. J Interv Cardiol 15: 387–392.

11. Moscucci M, Rogers EK, Montoye C, Smith DE, Share D, et.al. (2006) Association of a continuous quality improvement initiative with practice and outcome variations of contemporary percutaneous coronary interventions. Circulation 113: 814–822. CIRCULATIONAHA.105.541995 [pii];10.1161/CIRCULATIONAHA.105.541995 [doi].

12. Slocum NK, Grossman PM, Moscucci M, Smith DE, Aronow HD, et al. (2012) The changing definition of contrast-induced nephropathy and its clinical implications: insights from the Blue Cross Blue Shield of Michigan Cardiovascular Consortium (BMC2). Am Heart J 163: 829–834. S0002-8703(12)00095-6 [pii];10.1016/j.ahj.2012.02.011 [doi].

13. Cockcroft DW, Gault MH (1976) Prediction of creatinine clearance from serum creatinine. Nephron 16: 31–41.

14. Liaw A, Wiener M (2002) Classification and Regression by random Forest. R News 2: 18–22.

15. Robin X, Turck N, Hainard A, Tiberti N, Lisacek F, et.al. (2011) pROC: an open-source package for R and S+ to analyze and compare ROC curves. BMC Bioinformatics 12: 77. 1471-2105-12-77 [pii];10.1186/1471-2105-12-77 [doi].

16. Marenzi G, Assanelli E, Campodonico J, Lauri G, Marana I, et al. (2009) Contrast volume during primary percutaneous coronary intervention and subsequent contrast-induced nephropathy and mortality. Ann Intern Med 150: 170–177. 150/3/170 [pii].

17. Freeman RV, O'Donnell M, Share D, Meengs WL, Kline-Rogers E, et al. (2002) Nephropathy requiring dialysis after percutaneous coronary intervention and the critical role of an adjusted contrast dose. Am J Cardiol 90: 1068–1073. S0002914902027716 [pii].

18. Nyman U, Bjork J, Aspelin P, Marenzi G (2008) Contrast medium dose-to-GFR ratio: a measure of systemic exposure to predict contrast-induced nephropathy after percutaneous coronary intervention. Acta Radiol 49: 658–667. 792395239 [pii];10.1080/02841850802050762 [doi].

19. Brown JR, Robb JF, Block CA, Schoolwerth AC, Kaplan AV, et. al. (2010) Does safe dosing of iodinated contrast prevent contrast-induced acute kidney injury? Circ Cardiovasc Interv 3: 346–350. CIRCINTERVENTIONS.109.910638 [pii];10.1161/CIRCINTERVENTIONS.109.910638 [doi].

20. Mehran R, Aymong ED, Nikolsky E, Lasic Z, Iakovou I, et.al. (2004) A simple risk score for prediction of contrast-induced nephropathy after percutaneous coronary intervention: development and initial validation. J Am Coll Cardiol 44: 1393–1399. S0735-1097(04)01445-7 [pii];10.1016/j.jacc.2004.06.068 [doi].

21. McCullough PA (2008) Contrast-induced acute kidney injury. J Am Coll Cardiol 51: 1419–1428. S0735-1097(08)00353-7 [pii];10.1016/j.jacc.2007.12.035 [doi].

22. Nayak KR, Mehta HS, Price MJ, Russo RJ, Stinis CT, et al. (2010) A novel technique for ultra-low contrast administration during angiography or intervention. Catheter Cardiovasc Interv 75: 1076–1083. 10.1002/ccd.22414 [doi].

20

Culprit Vessel Only versus Multivessel Percutaneous Coronary Intervention in Patients Presenting with ST-Segment Elevation Myocardial Infarction and Multivessel Disease

Dongfeng Zhang, Xiantao Song*, Shuzheng Lv, Fei Yuan, Feng Xu, Min Zhang, Wei Li, Shuai Yan

Department of Cardiology, Capital Medical University affiliated Beijing Anzhen Hospital, Beijing Institute of Heart, Lung and Blood Vessel Disease, Beijing, China

Abstract

Background: The best strategy for ST-segment elevation myocardial infarction (STEMI) patients with multivessel disease (MVD), who underwent primary percutaneous coronary intervention (PCI) in the acute phase, is not well established.

Objectives: Our goal was to conduct a meta-analysis comparing culprit vessel only percutaneous coronary intervention (culprit PCI) with multivessel percutaneous coronary intervention (MV-PCI) for treatment of patients with STEMI and MVD.

Methods: Pubmed, Elsevier, Embase, and China National Knowledge Infrastructure (CNKI) databases were systematically searched for randomized and nonrandomized studies comparing culprit PCI and MV-PCI strategies during the index procedure. A meta-analysis was performed using Review Manager 5.1 (Cochrane Center, Denmark).

Results: Four randomized and fourteen nonrandomized studies involving 39,390 patients were included. MV-PCI strategy is associated with an increased short-term mortality (OR: 0.50, 95% CI: 0.32 to 0.77, $p = 0.002$), long-term mortality (OR: 0.52, 95% CI: 0.36 to 0.74, $p < 0.001$), and risk of renal dysfunction (OR: 0.77, 95% CI: 0.61 to 0.97, $p = 0.03$) compared with culprit PCI strategy, while it reduced the incidence of revascularization (OR: 2.65, 95% CI: 1.80 to 3.90, $p < 0.001$).

Conclusions: This meta-analysis supports current guidelines which indicate that the non-culprit vessel should not be treated during the index procedure.

Editor: Claudio Moretti, S.G.Battista Hospital, Italy

Funding: State Science and Technology Support Program (No. 2011BAI11B05) http://program.most.gov.cn/. The funders had no role in study design, data collection and analysis, decision to publish, or preparation of the manuscript.

Competing Interests: The authors have declared that no competing interests exist.

* E-mail: xiantao_song@163.com

Introduction

Acute ST-segment elevation myocardial infarction (STEMI) is a huge public health burden that affects many people worldwide every year. Approximately 40% to 65% of the patients presenting with STEMI have multivessel disease (MVD), which is associated with worse clinical outcomes than single-vessel disease (SVD) [1]. Percutaneous coronary intervention (PCI) is currently the favorable reperfusion treatment of choice in patients with STEMI. However, optimal strategies for STEMI patients with MVD during the index procedure, whether to treat non-culprit vessels, are still unclear.

2012 ESC guidelines [2] recommend that primary PCI should be limited to the culprit vessel with the exception of cardiogenic shock and persistent ischemia after PCI of the supposed culprit lesion while 2011 ACCF/AHA/SCAI PCI guidelines [3] suggest that PCI should not be performed in a non-culprit vessel at the time of primary PCI in patients with STEMI without hemodynamic compromise, where the classes and levels of evidence are IIaB and IIIB respectively. However, these suggestions were based

on some retrospective or small observational studies which did not have high evidence level. The main factors supporting these guidelines are summarized as follows: complications related to non-culprit vessel PCI, overvalued stenosis, renal insufficiency, and low success rates. The advancements in PCI technology and adjunctive pharmacotherapy have led some interventionalists to operate outside of established guidelines.

Several researches showed inconsistent outcomes. Our goal was to compare the safety and efficacy of culprit vessel only PCI (culprit PCI) and multivessel PCI (MV-PCI) during the index procedure in patients with STEMI and MVD quantitatively. Therefore, we conducted a meta-analysis of randomized and nonrandomized studies.

Methods

Search Strategy

Pubmed, Elsevier, Embase, and China National Knowledge Infrastructure (CNKI) databases were systematically searched by two independent investigators (S.Y and W.L) for all articles

Table 1. Main Characteristics of Included Studies.

	Primary Author	Year Published	Setting	Symptom Time, h	PCI strategies		Maximum Follow-Up
					Culprit PCI	MV-PCI	
Randomized studies							
1	Di Mario	2004	Multicenter	12	17	52	1 yr
2	Ochala	2004	Single-center	12	44	48	6 months
3	Politi	2010	Single-center	12	84	65	2.5±1.4 yrs
4	Wald	2013	Multicenter	–	231	234	23 months
Nonrandomized studies							
5	Abe	2013	Multicenter	12	220	54	1 yr
6	Bauer	2013	Multicenter	–	2118	419	In hospital
7	Carvender	2009	Multicenter	All	25802	3134	In hospital
8	Corpus	2004	Single-center	12	354	26	1 yr
9	Dziewierz	2010	Multicenter	–	707	70	1 yr
10	Hannan	2010	Multicenter	24	503	503	3.5 yrs
11	Jensen	2012	Multicenter	12	820	354	2 yrs
12	Khattab	2008	Single-center	12	45	28	1 yr
13	kornowski	2011	Multicenter	12	393	275	3 yrs
14	Mohamad	2011	Single-center	12	30	7	1 yr
15	Qarawani	2008	Single-center	12	25	95	1 yr
16	Roe	2001	Multicenter	–	61	68	6 months
17	Toma	2010	Multicenter	6	1984	217	3 months
18	Varani	2008	Single-center	24	156	147	1.7±1.0 yrs
Total					33594	5796	

published before 6 October 2013. The following keywords were used for the search: "percutaneous coronary intervention", "ST-segment elevation myocardial infarction", and "multivessel disease". Studies were excluded if they met any one of the following criteria: (1) duplicate publication, (2) ongoing or unpublished study, and (3) publication only as an abstract or as conference proceedings. References of retrieved studies were searched manually for additional potentially relevant articles. Authors of studies were contacted when results were unclear or when relevant data were not reported. Differences in investigator assessments of articles were resolved by discussing with a third investigator (D.F.Z). No language restrictions were enforced.

Study Selection

An initial screening of titles or abstracts was conducted, followed by full-text reviews. Studies' eligibility criteria included the followings: 1) a study population of STEMI patients with MVD; 2) PCI procedures included both culprit PCI and MV-PCI; 3) MV-PCI was performed during the index procedure; and 4) studies that reported quality assessment, data extraction, and endpoint data of interest. Randomized and nonrandomized studies were included. Exclusion criteria were: patient populations without concurrent STEMI and MVD, comparisons without culprit PCI or MV-PCI, and MV-PCI performed after the index procedure. Reviews, editorials, meeting abstracts, and commentaries were excluded from our analysis.

Quality Assessment

The quality of randomized studies was assessed using methods recommended by the Cochrane Collaboration based on the following six components: 1) sequence generation for allocation; 2) allocation concealment; 3) blinding of participants, personnel, and outcome assessors; 4) incomplete outcome data; 5) selective outcome reporting; and 6) other sources of bias. For nonrandomized studies, quality was assessed based on control of confounders, blinded assessment of angiography data, and preferred PCI strategy.

Data Extraction

Data were abstracted on prespecified forms by two reviewers (W.L and S.Y) that were not involved in any of the studies retrieved. Divergent assessments were resolved by discussing with a third investigator (D.F.Z). Study information was recorded as follows: study design, quality indicators, baseline clinical characteristics, and clinical outcomes.

Definition and Endpoints

The culprit PCI strategy was defined as PCI confined to culprit vessel lesions only. The MV-PCI strategy was defined as PCI in which lesions in the culprit vessel as well as ≥ 1 nonculprit vessel

lesions. All the interventions should have had taken place within the index procedure. MVD was defined as reported in each study. The primary endpoints were short-term (in hospital/30 days) and long-term mortality. Secondary endpoints included rates of renal dysfunction, reinfarction, and revascularization. Renal dysfunction as well as reinfarction and revascularization were defined as reported in each study. Mortality included both cardiac and no cardiac death.

Statistical Analysis

All statistical analysis was performed using Review Manager 5.1 (Cochrane Center, Denmark). Odds ratio (OR) and 95% confidence intervals (95% CI) were used as summary statistics. Heterogeneity across studies was analyzed using I^2 [$I^2 = (Q\text{-df})/Q$; where Q is the chi-square statistic and df is the degree of freedom]. Values of $I^2 > 50\%$ were considered statistically significant. Pooled estimates were first calculated using the Mantel-Haenszel fixed-effects model, whereas the DerSimonian and Lair random-effects model was used if there was heterogeneity.

The following methods were used to explore sources of heterogeneity: (1) subgroup analysis (randomized and nonrandomized studies); and (2) sensitivity analysis performed by excluding trials which potentially biased meta-analysis results.

Potential publication bias was examined by visual inspection of a funnel plot. All p values were 2-tailed, with statistical significance set at $p < 0.05$. This study was performed according to the MOOSE (Meta-Analysis of Observational Studies in Epidemiology) [4] statement.

Results

Eighteen studies including 39,390 patients comparing culprit PCI versus MV-PCI in patients with STEMI and MVD during the index procedure were identified finally (Table 1), four randomized [5,6,7,8] and fourteen nonrandomized studies [9,10,11,12,13,14,15,16,17,18,19,20,21,22] published between 2001 and 2013. Nine of the fourteen nonrandomized studies were subanalyses of prospective registries. Details of the screening process for eligible studies are shown in Fig. 1. Quality assessment results are detailed in Table 2 and Table 3.

Study Characteristics

Culprit PCI was the more frequently performed PCI strategy (33,594 of 39,390 patients, 85.3%). Baseline characteristics of the included studies are presented in Table 4. Compared with the culprit PCI group, patients in the MV-PCI group had a lower rate of diabetes, hypertension and hyperlipidemia. Six studies excluded the patients with cardiogenic shock [5,6,7,8,14,19], and three studies reported the rate of cardiogenic shock [11,16,21]. Ten studies gave information of the use of GP IIb/IIIa inhibitors.

Table 2. Quality of Randomized Studies.

Primary author	Adequate sequence generation of allocation	Allocation concealment	Blinding of participants, personnel, and outcome assessors	Complete outcome data	Free of selective outcome reporting	Free of other sources of bias
Di Mario	Unclear	Unclear	Unclear	Yes	Unclear	Unclear
Ochala	Unclear	Unclear	Unclear	Yes	Unclear	Unclear
Politi	Yes	Unclear	Unclear	Yes	Unclear	Unclear
Wald	Yes	Unclear	Yes	No	Yes	Unclear

Table 3. Quality of nonrandomized Studies.

Primary author	Control of confounders	Blinded assessment of angiography data	Preferred PCI strategy
Abe	±(subanalysis of prospective registry)	–	Operator decision
Bauer	±(subanalysis of prospective registry)	–	–
Carvender	±(subanalysis of prospective registry)	–	
Corpus	–	–	Operator decision
Dziewierz	±(subanalysis of prospective registry)	–	–
Hannan	±(subanalysis of prospective registry)	–	–
Jensen	±(subanalysis of prospective registry)	–	Operator decision
Khattab	Prospective observational	–	Operator decision
Kornowski	±(subanalysis of prospective registry)	–	Operator decision
Mohamad	–	–	–
Qarawani	–	–	Operator decision
Roe	–	–	Operator decision
Toma	±(subanalysis of prospective registry)	–	Operator decision
Varani	±(subanalysis of prospective registry)	–	Operator decision

Main Outcomes

Short-term mortality was reported in 15 studies including 36,687 patients. In-hospital or 30-day death occurred in 1,515 of 31,349 patients (4.83%) who underwent culprit PCI versus 370 of 5,338 patients (6.93%) who received MV-PCI. Signs of heterogeneity were found across trials ($I^2 = 70\%$) and a randomized model was used. Compared with culprit PCI, MV-PCI was associated with an increased short-term mortality (OR: 0.50, 95% CI: 0.32 to 0.77, p = 0.002). Pooled short-term outcome data are detailed in Fig. 2.

Long-term mortality for both strategies was reported in 16 studies including 7,905 patients. There were 362 long-term follow up deaths among 5,670 patients (6.38%) who received culprit PCI, whereas 245 deaths occurred among 2,235 (10.96%) patients who received MV-PCI. Heterogeneity was found across trials ($I^2 = 67\%$) and a randomized model was used. MV-PCI was associated with an obviously increased long-term mortality in comparison with culprit PCI strategy (OR: 0.52, 95% CI: 0.36 to 0.74, p<0.001). Pooled long-term outcome data are illustrated in Fig. 3.

Four studies are available of the short-term renal dysfunction detail. Politi et al. [7] defined renal dysfunction as an increase in serum creatinine values of 0.5 mg/dl or greater or a 25% or greater relative increase from baseline within 72 hours following PCI. Abe et al. [9] defined renal dysfunction as an increase in serum creatinine values of 0.5 mg/dl or greater or a 25% or greater relative increase from baseline within 1 week following exposure to contrast medium. Cavender et al. [11] defined renal dysfunction as a new requirement for dialysis or an increase in creatinine to >2 mg/dl and 2 times the baseline creatinine. Qarawani et al. [19] defined it as a rise of 30% and more in creatinine within 24 hours from the baseline value. To sum up, renal dysfunction occurred in 503 of 26,131 patients (1.92%) who underwent culprit PCI versus 93 of 3,348 patients (2.78%) who received MV-PCI. No heterogeneity was found among the studies ($I^2 = 0\%$) and a fixed effects model was used. The difference between two groups are significant (OR: 0.77, 95% CI: 0.61 to 0.97, p = 0.03), which indicates that the MV-PCI may increase the risk of renal dysfunction because of the high dose of contrast agent (Fig. 4).

Nine articles reported on long-term reinfarction, 1,449 cases in the culprit PCI group and 847 cases in the MV-PCI group. No heterogeneity was found among the studies ($I^2 = 41\%$) and a fixed effects model was used. No significant difference was found between the two groups (OR: 1.13, 95% CI: 0.76 to 1.67, p = 0.55) (Fig. 5).

Five studies gave the information of long-term revascularization, 421 cases in the culprit PCI group and 424 cases in the MV-PCI group. Signs of heterogeneity were not found across trials ($I^2 = 46\%$) and a fixed model was used. MV-PCI was associated with an obviously decreased long-term revascularization in comparison with culprit PCI strategy (OR: 2.65, 95% CI: 1.80 to 3.90, p<0.001) (Fig. 6).

Sensitivity Analysis

We performed sensitivity analyses by repeating analyses following removal of each study, one at a time (data not shown). No single study had excessive influence on the results for primary or secondary endpoints.

The results of randomized trials only and both randomized and nonrandomized trials are different which showed in Table 5. Assessment of funnel plots suggested no publication bias.

Discussion

Our analysis suggested that MV-PCI strategy is associated with an increased short-term mortality (OR: 0.50, 95% CI: 0.32 to 0.77, p = 0.002), long-term mortality (OR: 0.52, 95% CI: 0.36 to 0.74, p<0.001), and risk of renal dysfunction (OR: 0.77, 95% CI: 0.61 to 0.97, p = 0.03) compared with culprit PCI strategy, while it reduced the incidence of revascularization (OR: 2.65, 95% CI: 1.80 to 3.90, p<0.001). No significant difference was found between the two groups in terms of the rate of reinfarction.

MVD has been proved to be associated with a poor prognosis in STEMI patients. Appropriate management of these patients has always been a topic of debate. Current guidelines recommend that in the absence of hemodynamic compromise, PCI during STEMI should only focus on the culprit lesion. Other lesions are addressed during subsequent elective revascularization. Justifications for these guidelines include [23]: 1) the acute phase of STEMI is a

Table 4. Baseline Characteristics of Included Studies.

Primary Author	Year Published	GP IIb/IIIa, %		Age, mean, yrs		Male, %		Diabetes, %		Hypertension, %		Hyperlipidemia, %		Shock, %		Smoker, %	
		Culprit PCI	MV-PCI	Culprit PCI	MV-PCI	Culprit PCI	MV-PCI	Culprit PCI	MV-PCI	Culprit PCI	MV-PCI	Culprit PCI	MV-PCI	Culprit PCI	MV-PCI	Culprit PCI	MV-PCI
Randomized studies																	
1 Di Mario	2004	82.4	75	65.3±7.4	63.5±12.4	84.6	88.2	41.2	11.5	58.8	36.5	52.9	41.2	excl	excl	81	66.6
2 Ochala	2004	50.7	51.1	67±7.9	65±8.3	75	72.9	34.1	31.2	47.7	52.1	90.9	81.2	excl	excl	43.1	37.5
3 Politi	2010	100	100	66.5±13.2	64.5±11.7	76.2	76.9	23.8	13.8	59.5	49.2	N/A	N/A	excl	excl	N/A	N/A
4 Wald	2013	76	76	62(33–90)*	62(32–92)*	81	76	21	15	40	40	N/A	N/A	excl	excl	45	50
Nonrandomized studies																	
5 Abe	2013	N/A	N/A	68.6±11.7	72.0±11.7	77.3	77.8	43.2	50	65.9	62.9	52.7	48.1	N/A	N/A	60	57.4
6 Bauer	2011	48.9	60.2	65±12.2	62.8±12	73.8	76.1	23.1	22.4	60.7	62.4	44.6	52.5	N/A	N/A	55.4	55
7 Carvender	2009	N/A	N/A	62(53–73)*	60(52–72)*	72.1	71.5	23.4	24.7	63.2	60.4	58.6	56.5	10.3	13.8	64.8	63.2
8 Corpus	2004	N/A	N/A	N/A	N/A	N/A	N/A	N/A	N/A	N/A	N/A	N/A	N/A	N/A	N/A	N/A	N/A
9 Dziewierz	2010	N/A	N/A	N/A	N/A	N/A	N/A	N/A	N/A	N/A	N/A	N/A	N/A	N/A	N/A	N/A	N/A
10 Hannan	2010	N/A	N/A	N/A	N/A	78.7	75	21.4	23.7	N/A	N/A	N/A	N/A	excl	excl	N/A	N/A
11 Jensen	2013	79	61.3	N/A	N/A	79.8	76	10.1	10.7	27.4	21.5	N/A	N/A	N/A	N/A	62.4	46.9
12 Khattab	2008	44	36	65±13	69±12	78	75	16	7	82	75	80	79	4.4	3.6	40	36
13 Kornowski	2011	54.6	54.5	63.5	62	80.9	79.6	18.1	15.3	57.5	54.9	41.7	48	N/A	N/A	62.8	61.3
14 Mohamad	2011	N/A	N/A	N/A	N/A	N/A	N/A	N/A	N/A	N/A	N/A	N/A	N/A	N/A	N/A	N/A	N/A
15 Qarawani	2008	96	94.7	67±3.7	66±3.2	64	65	16	12.6	40	37.8	16	13.6	excl	excl	60	61
16 Roe	2001	N/A	N/A	N/A	N/A	N/A	N/A	N/A	N/A	N/A	N/A	N/A	N/A	N/A	N/A	N/A	N/A
17 Toma	2010	71.9	78.8	64(55–73)*	64(53–74)*	79.4	77.4	20	11.5	55.6	47.5	N/A	N/A	1.2	1.8	39.9	38.2
18 Varani	2008	N/A	N/A	69.8±13	68.7±13	75	67	N/A	N/A	N/A	N/A	N/A	N/A	N/A	N/A	N/A	N/A

*Median instead of mean; N/A = not available.

PRISMA 2009 Flow Diagram

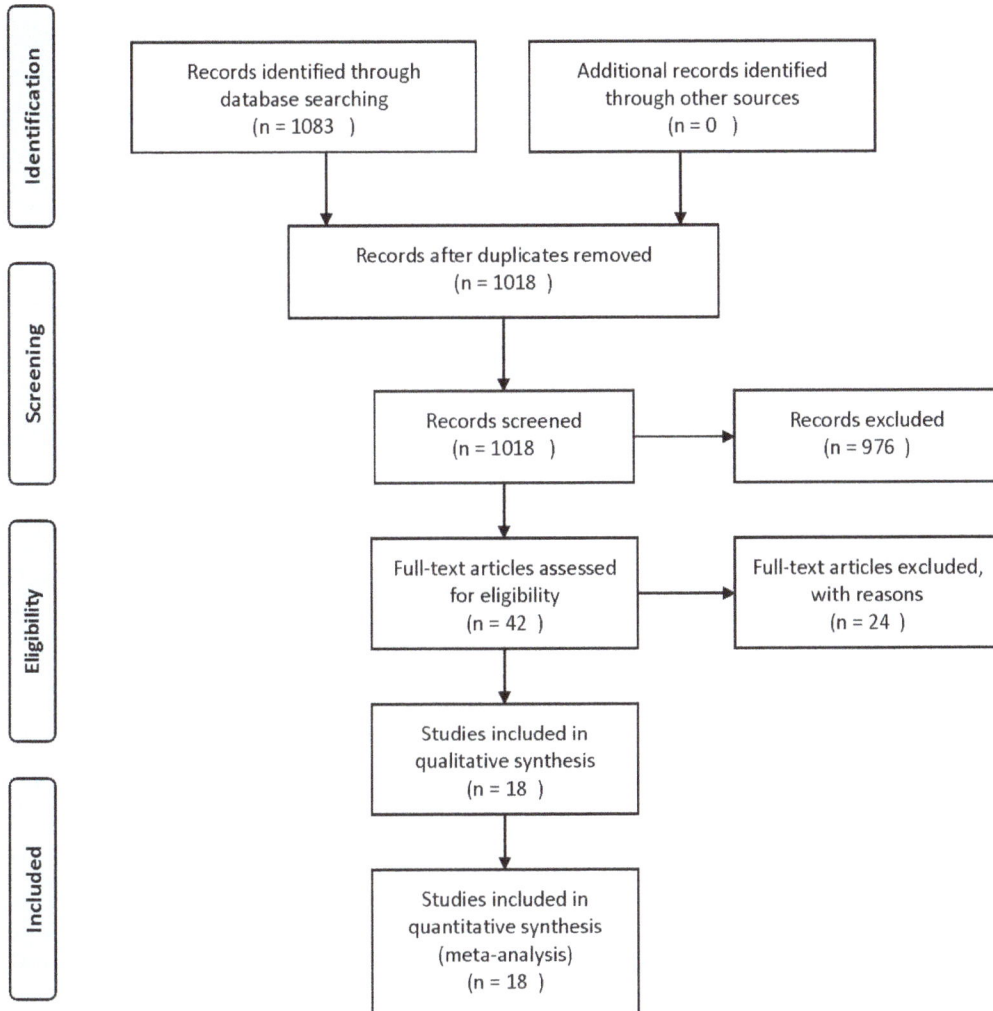

Identification

Records identified through
database searching
(n = 1083)

Additional records identified
through other sources
(n = 0)

Screening

Records after duplicates removed
(n = 1018)

Records screened
(n = 1018)

Records excluded
(n = 976)

Eligibility

Full-text articles assessed
for eligibility
(n = 42)

Full-text articles excluded,
with reasons
(n = 24)

Included

Studies included in
qualitative synthesis
(n = 18)

Studies included in
quantitative synthesis
(meta-analysis)
(n = 18)

From: Moher D, Liberati A, Tetzlaff J, Altman DG, The PRISMA Group (2009). *Preferred Reporting Items for Systematic Reviews and Meta-Analyses: The PRISMA Statement. PLoS Med 6(6): e1000097. doi:10.1371/journal.pmed1000097*

For more information, visit www.prisma-statement.org.

Figure 1. Flow diagram of study inclusion and exclusion.

highly unstable condition (haemodynamic instability, heart failure, arrhythmias, resuscitation, and patient stress among others) that does not favor performance of PCI, and additional intervention is probably safer after the patient is stabilized; 2) the acute phase of STEMI is extremely prothrombotic and inflammatory which contributes to a higher risk for additional PCI; 3) diffuse coronary spasms (either due to endothelial dysfunction or due to catecholamine use) are frequently present in the acute phase of STEMI, and this may lead to overestimation of stenosis severity in non-culprit vessels; 4) decisions to perform non-culprit vessel PCI during the acute phase of STEMI are usually not supported by objective evidence for the presence of myocardial ischemia in regions supplied by these non-culprit vessels; 5) MV-PCI increases the radiation dose, contrast overload, and risk of contrast-induced nephropathy. Counter arguments include concerns that plaque instability may be present in large areas of the coronary tree rather

Study or Subgroup	culprit-PCI Events	Total	MV-PCI Events	Total	Weight	Odds Ratio M-H, Random, 95% CI
1.1.1 prospective						
Di Mario 2004	0	17	1	52	1.6%	0.98 [0.04, 25.20]
Ochala 2004	0	44	0	48		Not estimable
Politi 2010	7	84	2	65	4.7%	2.86 [0.57, 14.27]
Subtotal (95% CI)		145		165	6.3%	2.32 [0.55, 9.79]
Total events	7		3			

Heterogeneity: Tau² = 0.00; Chi² = 0.34, df = 1 (P = 0.56); I² = 0%
Test for overall effect: Z = 1.15 (P = 0.25)

Study or Subgroup	culprit-PCI Events	Total	MV-PCI Events	Total	Weight	Odds Ratio M-H, Random, 95% CI
1.1.2 retrospective						
Abe 2013	12	220	11	54	8.6%	0.23 [0.09, 0.54]
Bauer 2011	72	2118	6	419	8.9%	2.42 [1.05, 5.61]
Cavender 2009	1321	25802	246	3134	13.1%	0.63 [0.55, 0.73]
Corpus 2004	23	354	5	26	7.4%	0.29 [0.10, 0.84]
Dziewierz 2010	42	707	9	70	9.4%	0.43 [0.20, 0.92]
Hannan 2010	10	503	17	503	9.2%	0.58 [0.26, 1.28]
Jensen 2013	4	820	25	354	7.4%	0.06 [0.02, 0.19]
Khattab 2008	2	45	1	28	2.5%	1.26 [0.11, 14.53]
Kornowski 2011	6	393	16	275	8.1%	0.25 [0.10, 0.65]
Qarawani 2008	1	25	4	95	2.9%	0.95 [0.10, 8.88]
Roe 2001	7	61	15	68	8.0%	0.46 [0.17, 1.21]
Varani 2008	8	156	12	147	8.3%	0.61 [0.24, 1.53]
Subtotal (95% CI)		31204		5173	93.7%	0.45 [0.29, 0.71]
Total events	1508		367			

Heterogeneity: Tau² = 0.36; Chi² = 39.33, df = 11 (P < 0.0001); I² = 72%
Test for overall effect: Z = 3.50 (P = 0.0005)

Study or Subgroup	culprit-PCI Events	Total	MV-PCI Events	Total	Weight	Odds Ratio M-H, Random, 95% CI
Total (95% CI)		31349		5338	100.0%	0.50 [0.32, 0.77]
Total events	1515		370			

Heterogeneity: Tau² = 0.37; Chi² = 43.09, df = 13 (P < 0.0001); I² = 70%
Test for overall effect: Z = 3.14 (P = 0.002)
Test for subgroup differences: Chi² = 4.52, df = 1 (P = 0.03), I² = 77.9%

Odds Ratio M-H, Random, 95% CI
0.005   0.1   1   10   200
Favours experimental   Favours control

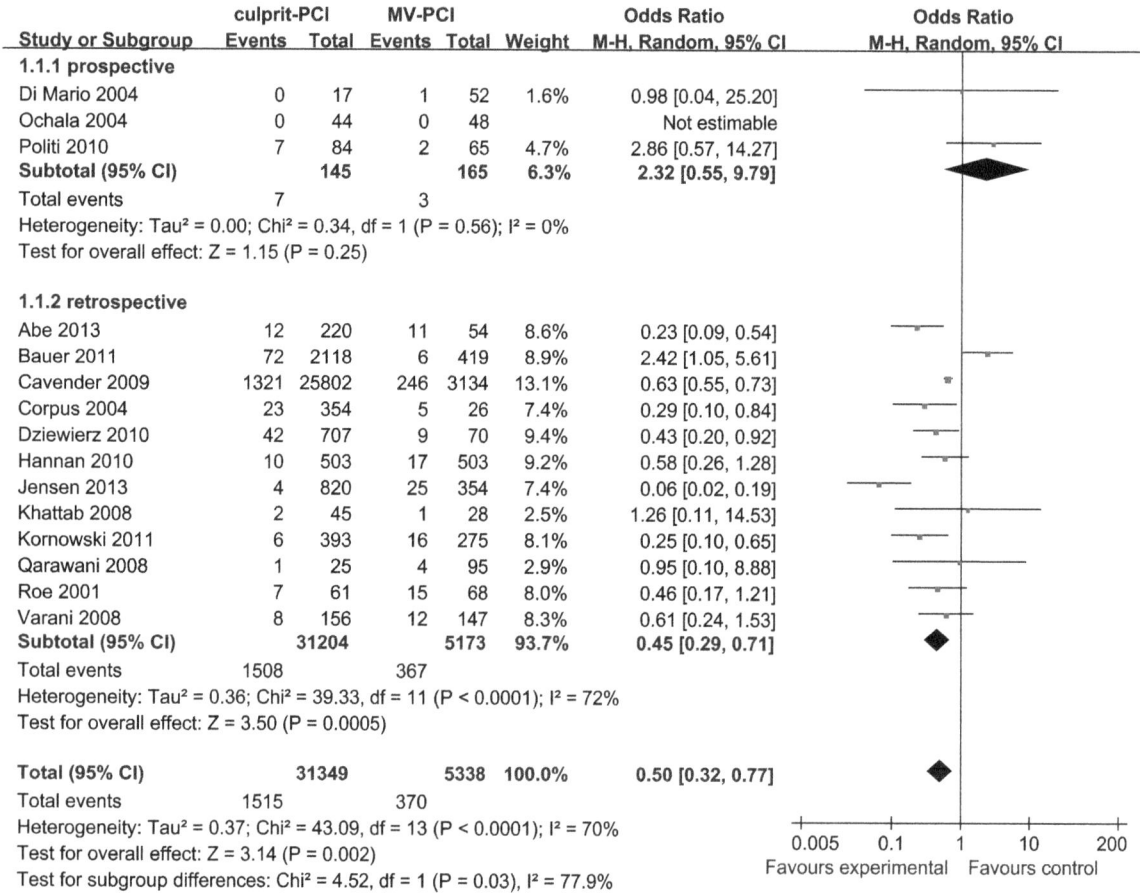

Figure 2. Culprit PCI Versus MV-PCI Short-Term Mortality.

than limited to the culprit lesion. Consequently, MV-PCI might achieve complete revascularization by treating secondary unstable lesions and thereby shorten cumulative hospital stays and costs. Patients may also be more comfortable following treatment of all lesions during index hospitalization.

The report was written in accordance to the PRISMA-statement (Checklist S1).Our findings support the current guidelines which indicate that the non-culprit vessel should not be treated during the index procedure. Although analysis of only the four small scaled randomized trials has different even opposite results. It is notable that the largest single-blind, randomized study, called the Preventive Angioplasty in Acute Myocardial Infarction (PRAMI) trail [8], enrolled 465 patients at five centers in the United Kingdom, with 231 assigned to the culprit PCI group and 234 to the MV-PCI group. The recruitment was stopped early after a recommendation from the data and safety monitoring committee that was based on a highly significant difference between groups (p<0.001) in the incidence of the primary outcome favoring MV-PCI. The combined rate of cardiac death, nonfatal myocardial infarction, or refractory angina was reduced by 65%, and absolute risk reduction of 14 percentage points over 23 months. The findings also suggest that MV-PCI may lead to less ischemia testing after the index procedure. Another randomized trial enrolled only 214 patients, with 84 patients in the culprit PCI group, 65 in the MV-PCI group, and 65 in the staged PCI group [7]. This study showed a significant benefit for MV-PCI, compared to culprit PCI, for long-term major adverse cardiac events (MACE) after a mean follow-up of 2.5 years. The

HEpacoat for cuLPrit or multivessel stenting for Acute Myocardial Infarction (HELP AMI) study [5] enrolled only 69 patients, with 17 patients in the culprit PCI group and 52 in the MV-PCI group. In this study, MV-PCI did not significantly increase in-hospital MACE (0 and 3.8% in culprit and MV-PCI groups, respectively, p = 0.164). Revascularization in the culprit PCI group at the 12 month follow-up was not statistically significant (35 vs 17%, p = 0.247). The trial's limitations included unequal randomization and use of heparin-coated stents which may be subject to bias.

A meta-analysis comparing culprit PCI, MV-PCI and staged PCI strategies found that MV-PCI was associated with highest mortality rates at both short- and long-term follow up, in which staged PCI strategy was defined as PCI confined to culprit vessel only, after which lesions in non-culprit vessel were treated during planned secondary procedures [24]. A proper analysis on the secondary endpoints was not possible because data were only available for a minority of the included studies. This meta-analysis included some patients with non-ST-segment elevation myocardial infarction (NSTEMI), and thus their included studies were different from ours. In addition, patients with STEMI or NSTEMI have different treating strategies.

Limitations

Only four studies were randomized. Consequently, the inclusion of nonrandomized studies introduces a potential selection bias, which means the benefit of culprit PCI shown in Table 5 may simply derive from selection bias towards patients with less severe

Study or Subgroup	culprit PCI Events	Total	MV-PCI Events	Total	Weight	Odds Ratio M-H, Random, 95% CI	Odds Ratio M-H, Random, 95% CI
2.1.1 prospective							
Di Mario 2004	0	17	0	52		Not estimable	
Ochala 2004	0	44	0	48		Not estimable	
Politi 2010	13	84	6	65	6.2%	1.80 [0.64, 5.03]	
Wald 2013	16	231	12	234	7.9%	1.38 [0.64, 2.98]	
Subtotal (95% CI)		**376**		**399**	**14.1%**	**1.52 [0.82, 2.81]**	
Total events	29		18				
Heterogeneity: Tau² = 0.00; Chi² = 0.17, df = 1 (P = 0.68); I² = 0%							
Test for overall effect: Z = 1.32 (P = 0.19)							
2.1.2 retrospective							
Abe 2013	24	220	17	54	8.3%	0.27 [0.13, 0.54]	
Corpus 2004	42	354	5	26	6.2%	0.57 [0.20, 1.58]	
Dziewierz 2010	57	707	11	70	8.4%	0.47 [0.23, 0.95]	
Hannan 2010	28	503	36	503	9.8%	0.76 [0.46, 1.27]	
Jensen 2013	26	820	52	354	10.0%	0.19 [0.12, 0.31]	
Khattab 2008	3	45	2	25	2.9%	0.82 [0.13, 5.28]	
Kornowski 2011	9	393	25	275	7.8%	0.23 [0.11, 0.51]	
Mohamad 2011	3	30	2	7	2.6%	0.28 [0.04, 2.11]	
Qarawani 2008	2	25	9	95	3.6%	0.83 [0.17, 4.11]	
Roe 2001	10	61	17	68	7.2%	0.59 [0.25, 1.41]	
Toma 2010	111	1984	27	217	10.3%	0.42 [0.27, 0.65]	
Varani 2008	18	152	24	142	8.7%	0.66 [0.34, 1.28]	
Subtotal (95% CI)		**5294**		**1836**	**85.9%**	**0.42 [0.31, 0.59]**	
Total events	333		227				
Heterogeneity: Tau² = 0.15; Chi² = 23.22, df = 11 (P = 0.02); I² = 53%							
Test for overall effect: Z = 5.17 (P < 0.00001)							
Total (95% CI)		**5670**		**2235**	**100.0%**	**0.52 [0.36, 0.74]**	
Total events	362		245				
Heterogeneity: Tau² = 0.28; Chi² = 38.97, df = 13 (P = 0.0002); I² = 67%							
Test for overall effect: Z = 3.56 (P = 0.0004)							
Test for subgroup differences: Chi² = 12.81, df = 1 (P = 0.0003), I² = 92.2%							

0.01   0.1   1   10   100
Favours experimental   Favours control

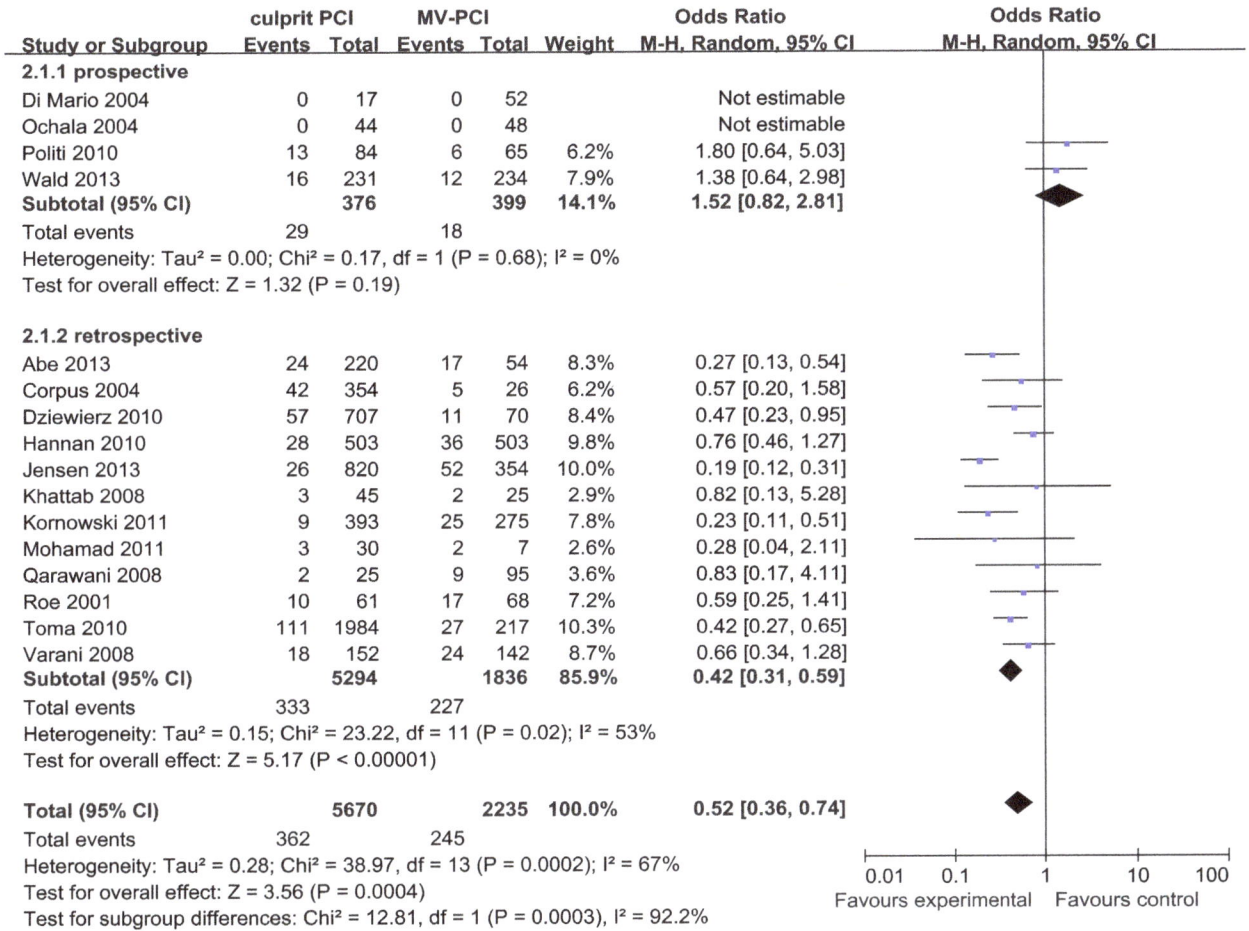

Figure 3. Culprit PCI Versus MV-PCI Long-Term Mortality.

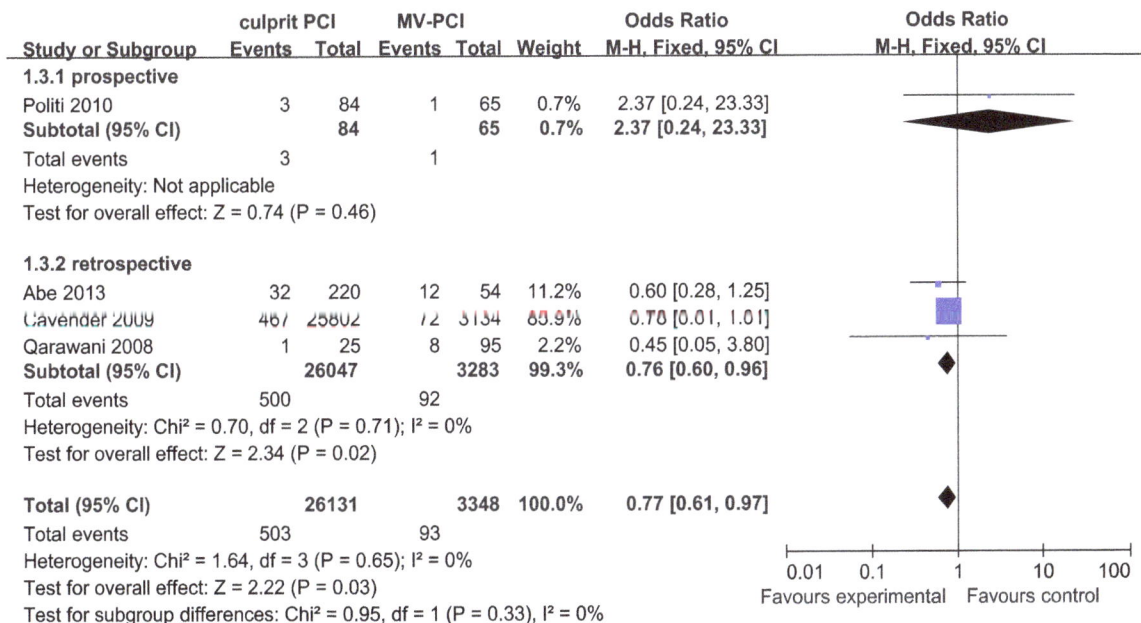

Study or Subgroup	culprit PCI Events	Total	MV-PCI Events	Total	Weight	Odds Ratio M-H, Fixed, 95% CI	Odds Ratio M-H, Fixed, 95% CI
1.3.1 prospective							
Politi 2010	3	84	1	65	0.7%	2.37 [0.24, 23.33]	
Subtotal (95% CI)		**84**		**65**	**0.7%**	**2.37 [0.24, 23.33]**	
Total events	3		1				
Heterogeneity: Not applicable							
Test for overall effect: Z = 0.74 (P = 0.46)							
1.3.2 retrospective							
Abe 2013	32	220	12	54	11.2%	0.60 [0.28, 1.25]	
Cavender 2009	467	25802	72	3134	85.9%	0.78 [0.01, 1.01]	
Qarawani 2008	1	25	8	95	2.2%	0.45 [0.05, 3.80]	
Subtotal (95% CI)		**26047**		**3283**	**99.3%**	**0.76 [0.60, 0.96]**	
Total events	500		92				
Heterogeneity: Chi² = 0.70, df = 2 (P = 0.71); I² = 0%							
Test for overall effect: Z = 2.34 (P = 0.02)							
Total (95% CI)		**26131**		**3348**	**100.0%**	**0.77 [0.61, 0.97]**	
Total events	503		93				
Heterogeneity: Chi² = 1.64, df = 3 (P = 0.65); I² = 0%							
Test for overall effect: Z = 2.22 (P = 0.03)							
Test for subgroup differences: Chi² = 0.95, df = 1 (P = 0.33), I² = 0%							

0.01   0.1   1   10   100
Favours experimental   Favours control

Figure 4. Culprit PCI Versus MV-PCI Renal Dysfunction.

Study or Subgroup	culprit PCI Events	Total	MV-PCI Events	Total	Weight	Odds Ratio M-H, Fixed, 95% CI	Odds Ratio M-H, Fixed, 95% CI
2.2.1 prospective							
Di Mario 2004	1	17	1	52	1.0%	3.19 [0.19, 53.91]	
Ochala 2004	4	44	3	48	5.5%	1.50 [0.32, 7.11]	
Politi 2010	7	84	2	65	4.3%	2.86 [0.57, 14.27]	
Wald 2013	20	231	7	234	13.4%	3.07 [1.27, 7.42]	
Subtotal (95% CI)		376		399	24.2%	2.68 [1.38, 5.23]	
Total events	32		13				

Heterogeneity: Chi² = 0.65, df = 3 (P = 0.89); I² = 0%
Test for overall effect: Z = 2.90 (P = 0.004)

2.2.2 retrospective							
Abe 2013	9	220	4	54	13.0%	0.53 [0.16, 1.80]	
Corpus 2004	10	354	1	26	3.8%	0.73 [0.09, 5.91]	
Khattab 2008	5	45	2	25	4.8%	1.44 [0.26, 8.01]	
Kornowski 2011	18	393	18	275	42.5%	0.69 [0.35, 1.34]	
Roe 2001	1	61	6	68	11.7%	0.17 [0.02, 1.47]	
Subtotal (95% CI)		1073		448	75.8%	0.63 [0.38, 1.05]	
Total events	43		31				

Heterogeneity: Chi² = 2.44, df = 4 (P = 0.66); I² = 0%
Test for overall effect: Z = 1.78 (P = 0.08)

Total (95% CI)		1449		847	100.0%	1.13 [0.76, 1.67]	
Total events	75		44				

Heterogeneity: Chi² = 13.67, df = 8 (P = 0.09); I² = 41%
Test for overall effect: Z = 0.59 (P = 0.55)
Test for subgroup differences: Chi² = 11.44, df = 1 (P = 0.0007), I² = 91.3%

Favours experimental   Favours control

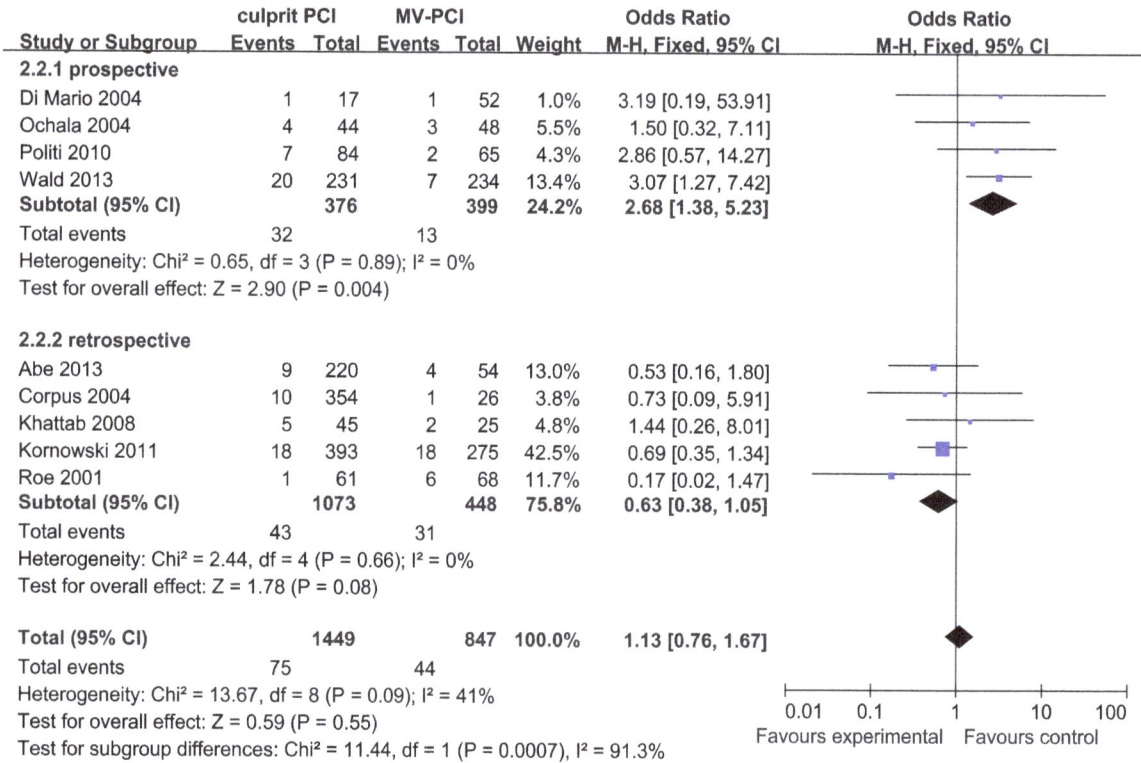

Figure 5. Culprit PCI Versus MV-PCI Long-Term Reinfarction.

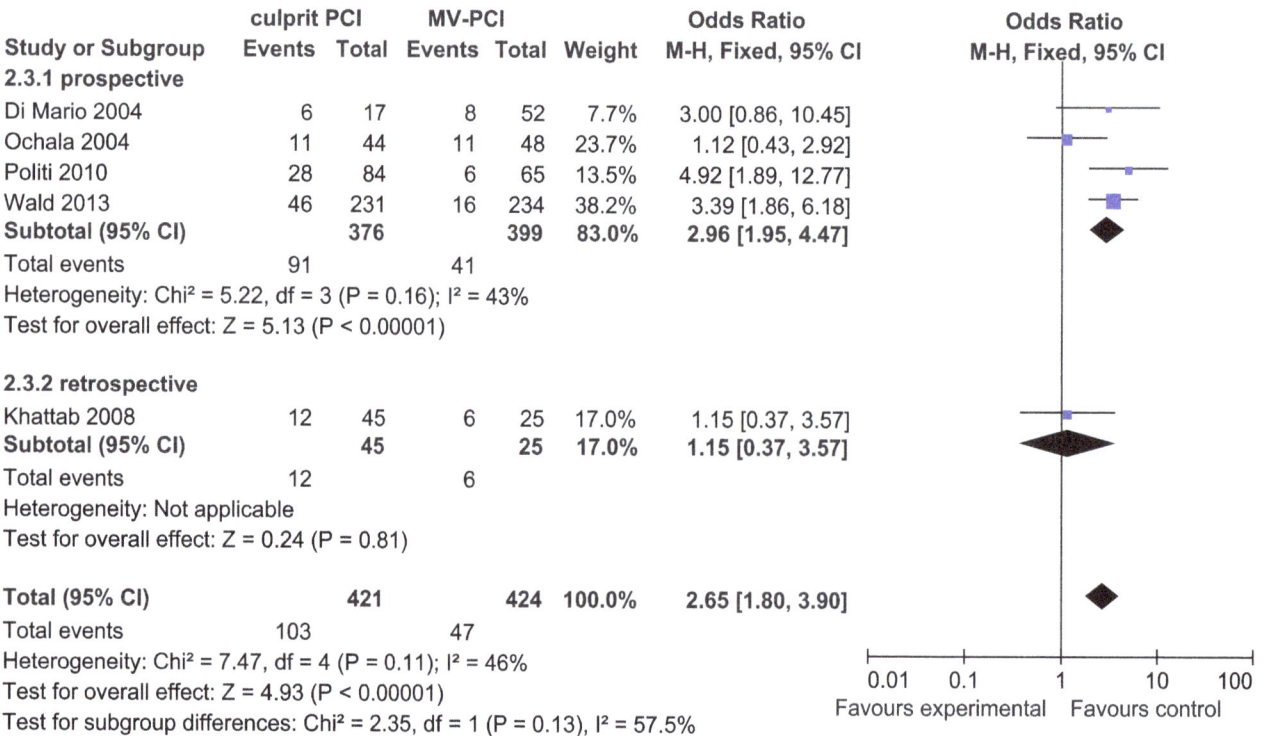

Study or Subgroup	culprit PCI Events	Total	MV-PCI Events	Total	Weight	Odds Ratio M-H, Fixed, 95% CI	Odds Ratio M-H, Fixed, 95% CI
2.3.1 prospective							
Di Mario 2004	6	17	8	52	7.7%	3.00 [0.86, 10.45]	
Ochala 2004	11	44	11	48	23.7%	1.12 [0.43, 2.92]	
Politi 2010	28	84	6	65	13.5%	4.92 [1.89, 12.77]	
Wald 2013	46	231	16	234	38.2%	3.39 [1.86, 6.18]	
Subtotal (95% CI)		376		399	83.0%	2.96 [1.95, 4.47]	
Total events	91		41				

Heterogeneity: Chi² = 5.22, df = 3 (P = 0.16); I² = 43%
Test for overall effect: Z = 5.13 (P < 0.00001)

2.3.2 retrospective							
Khattab 2008	12	45	6	25	17.0%	1.15 [0.37, 3.57]	
Subtotal (95% CI)		45		25	17.0%	1.15 [0.37, 3.57]	
Total events	12		6				

Heterogeneity: Not applicable
Test for overall effect: Z = 0.24 (P = 0.81)

Total (95% CI)		421		424	100.0%	2.65 [1.80, 3.90]	
Total events	103		47				

Heterogeneity: Chi² = 7.47, df = 4 (P = 0.11); I² = 46%
Test for overall effect: Z = 4.93 (P < 0.00001)
Test for subgroup differences: Chi² = 2.35, df = 1 (P = 0.13), I² = 57.5%

Favours experimental   Favours control

Figure 6. Culprit PCI Versus MV-PCI Long-Term Revascularization.

Table 5. Subgroup Analysis of Randomized Trails Compared with Overall Analysis.

Endpoints	Preferred strategy	
	Randomized and nonrandomized trails	Randomized trails
Short-term mortality	Culprit PCI	Equal
Long-term mortality	Culprit PCI	Equal
Renal dysfunction	Culprit PCI	Equal
Reinfarction	Equal	MV-PCI
Revascularization	MV-PCI	MV-PCI

or more stable coronary artery disease. There is the potential for ascertainment bias due to unequal follow-up.

Multiple combinations of angiographic and clinical findings, number of diseased vessels, location and type of occlusions, total chronic occlusions, Killip class, renal function, and other factors vary by individual. This introduces a level of complexity that is best addressed by individualized clinical decision-making.

Further, the operator's intent to perform culprit PCI or MV-PCI was not prospectively registered in a majority of the studies and may be influenced by important patient characteristics that we were unable to account for. Staged PCI was allowed for patients in culprit PCI group in some trials which may exaggerate the benefits of culprit PCI. As with many meta-analyses, we did not adjust our analyses for baseline confounders or unmeasured confounders, due to the lack of data in each trial.

Conclusions

This meta-analysis was based primarily on data derived from nonrandomized studies. It is suggested that culprit PCI is better than MV-PCI procedure in patients with STEMI and MVD. Large-scale randomized trials are urgently needed to further evaluate different revascularization procedures for patients with STEMI and MVD.

Author Contributions

Conceived and designed the experiments: DFZ XTS SZL. Performed the experiments: DFZ FX MZ WL SY. Analyzed the data: DFZ FX MZ WL SY. Wrote the paper: DFZ XTS FY.

References

1. Sorajja P, Gersh BJ, Cox DA, McLaughlin MG, Zimetbaum P, et al. (2007) Impact of multivessel disease on reperfusion success and clinical outcomes in patients undergoing primary percutaneous coronary intervention for acute myocardial infarction. Eur Heart J 28: 1709–1716.
2. Steg PG, James SK, Atar D, Badano LP, Blomstrom-Lundqvist C, et al. (2012) ESC Guidelines for the management of acute myocardial infarction in patients presenting with ST-segment elevation. Eur Heart J 33: 2569–2619.
3. Levine GN, Bates ER, Blankenship JC, Bailey SR, Bittl JA, et al. (2011) 2011 ACCF/AHA/SCAI Guideline for Percutaneous Coronary Intervention. A report of the American College of Cardiology Foundation/American Heart Association Task Force on Practice Guidelines and the Society for Cardiovascular Angiography and Interventions. J Am Coll Cardiol 58: e44–e122.
4. Stroup DF, Berlin JA, Morton SC, Olkin I, Williamson GD, et al. (2000) Meta-analysis of observational studies in epidemiology: a proposal for reporting. Meta-analysis Of Observational Studies in Epidemiology (MOOSE) group. JAMA 283: 2008–2012.
5. Di Mario C, Mara S, Flavio A, Imad S, Antonio M, et al. (2004) Single vs multivessel treatment during primary angioplasty: results of the multicentre randomised HEpacoat for culPrit or multivessel stenting for Acute Myocardial Infarction (HELP AMI) Study. Int J Cardiovasc Intervent 6: 128–133.
6. Ochala A, Smolka GA, Wojakowski W, Dudek D, Dziewierz A, et al. (2004) The function of the left ventricle after complete multivessel one-stage percutaneous coronary intervention in patients with acute myocardial infarction. J Invasive Cardiol 16: 699–702.
7. Politi L, Sgura F, Rossi R, Monopoli D, Guerri E, et al. (2010) A randomised trial of target-vessel versus multi-vessel revascularisation in ST-elevation myocardial infarction: major adverse cardiac events during long-term follow-up. Heart 96: 662–667.
8. Wald DS, Morris JK, Wald NJ, Chase AJ, Edwards RJ, et al. (2013) Randomized trial of preventive angioplasty in myocardial infarction. N Engl J Med 369: 1115–1123.
9. Abe D, Sato A, Hoshi T, Takeyasu N, Misaki M, et al. (2013) Initial culprit-only versus initial multivessel percutaneous coronary intervention in patients with ST-segment elevation myocardial infarction: results from the Ibaraki Cardiovascular Assessment Study registry. Heart Vessels.
10. Bauer T, Zeymer U, Hochadel M, Mollmann H, Weidinger F, et al. (2013) Prima-vista multi-vessel percutaneous coronary intervention in haemodynam-

ically stable patients with acute coronary syndromes: analysis of over 4.400 patients in the EHS-PCI registry. Int J Cardiol 166: 596–600.
11. Cavender MA, Milford-Beland S, Roe MT, Peterson ED, Weintraub WS, et al. (2009) Prevalence, predictors, and in-hospital outcomes of non-infarct artery intervention during primary percutaneous coronary intervention for ST-segment elevation myocardial infarction (from the National Cardiovascular Data Registry). Am J Cardiol 104: 507–513.
12. Corpus RA, House JA, Marso SP, Grantham JA, Huber KJ, et al. (2004) Multivessel percutaneous coronary intervention in patients with multivessel disease and acute myocardial infarction. Am Heart J 148: 493–500.
13. Dziewierz A, Siudak Z, Rakowski T, Zasada W, Dubiel JS, et al. (2010) Impact of multivessel coronary artery disease and noninfarct-related artery revascularization on outcome of patients with ST-elevation myocardial infarction transferred for primary percutaneous coronary intervention (from the EURO-TRANSFER Registry). Am J Cardiol 106: 342–347.
14. Hannan EL, Samadashvili Z, Walford G, Holmes DJ, Jacobs AK, et al. (2010) Culprit vessel percutaneous coronary intervention versus multivessel and staged percutaneous coronary intervention for ST-segment elevation myocardial infarction patients with multivessel disease. JACC Cardiovasc Interv 3: 22–31.
15. Jensen LO, Thayssen P, Farkas DK, Hougaard M, Terkelsen CJ, et al. (2012) Culprit only or multivessel percutaneous coronary interventions in patients with ST-segment elevation myocardial infarction and multivessel disease. EuroIntervention 8: 456–464.
16. Khattab AA, Abdel-Wahab M, Rother C, Liska B, Toelg R, et al. (2008) Multivessel stenting during primary percutaneous coronary intervention for acute myocardial infarction. A single-center experience. Clin Res Cardiol 97: 32–38.
17. Kornowski R, Mehran R, Dangas G, Nikolsky E, Assali A, et al. (2011) Prognostic impact of staged versus "one-time" multivessel percutaneous intervention in acute myocardial infarction: analysis from the HORIZONS-AMI (harmonizing outcomes with revascularization and stents in acute myocardial infarction) trial. J Am Coll Cardiol 58: 704–711.
18. Mohamad T, Bernal JM, Kondur A, Hari P, Nelson K, et al. (2011) Coronary revascularization strategy for ST elevation myocardial infarction with multivessel disease: experience and results at 1-year follow-up. Am J Ther 18: 92–100.
19. Qarawani D, Nahir M, Abboud M, Hazanov Y, Hasin Y (2008) Culprit only versus complete coronary revascularization during primary PCI. Int J Cardiol 123: 288–292.

20. Roe MT, Cura FA, Joski PS, Garcia E, Guetta V, et al. (2001) Initial experience with multivessel percutaneous coronary intervention during mechanical reperfusion for acute myocardial infarction. Am J Cardiol 88: 170–173, A6.
21. Toma M, Buller CE, Westerhout CM, Fu Y, O'Neill WW, et al. (2010) Non-culprit coronary artery percutaneous coronary intervention during acute ST-segment elevation myocardial infarction: insights from the APEX-AMI trial. Eur Heart J 31: 1701–1707.
22. Varani E, Balducelli M, Aquilina M, Vecchi G, Hussien MN, et al. (2008) Single or multivessel percutaneous coronary intervention in ST-elevation myocardial infarction patients. Catheter Cardiovasc Interv 72: 927–933.
23. Widimsky P, Holmes DJ (2011) How to treat patients with ST-elevation acute myocardial infarction and multi-vessel disease? Eur Heart J 32: 396–403.
24. Vlaar PJ, Mahmoud KD, Holmes DJ, van Valkenhoef G, Hillege HL, et al. (2011) Culprit vessel only versus multivessel and staged percutaneous coronary intervention for multivessel disease in patients presenting with ST-segment elevation myocardial infarction: a pairwise and network meta-analysis. J Am Coll Cardiol 58: 692–703.

21

Safety of Low-Dose Aspirin in Endovascular Treatment for Intracranial Atherosclerotic Stenosis

Ning Ma[1,9], Ziqi Xu[3,9], Dapeng Mo[1], Feng Gao[1], Kun Gao[1], Xuan Sun[1], Xiaotong Xu[1], Lian Liu[1], Ligang Song[1], Tiejun Wang[4], Xingquan Zhao[2], Yilong Wang[2], Yongjun Wang[2], Zhongrong Miao[1]*

1 Department of Interventional Neuroradiology, Beijing Tiantan Hospital, Capital Medical University, Beijing, China, 2 Department of Neurology, Beijing Tiantan Hospital, Capital Medical University, Beijing, China, 3 Department of Neurology, the First Affiliated Hospital of College of Medicine, Zhejiang University, Hangzhou, China, 4 Department of Neurology, the Daxing District Hospital of Beijing, Beijing, China

Abstract

Objectives: To evaluate the safety of low-dose aspirin plus clopidogrel versus high-dose aspirin plus clopidogrel in prevention of vascular risk within 90 days of duration of dual antiplatelet therapy in patients treated with intracranial endovascular treatment.

Methods: From January 2012 to December 2013, this prospective and observational study enrolled 370 patients with symptomatic intracranial atherosclerotic stenosis of $\geq$70% with poor collateral undergoing intracranial endovascular treatment. Antiplatelet therapy consists of aspirin, at a low-dose of 100 mg or high-dose of 300 mg daily; clopidogrel, at a dose of 75 mg daily for 5 days before endovascular treatment. The dual antiplatelet therapy continued for 90 days after intervention. The study endpoints include acute thrombosis, subacute thrombosis, stroke or death within 90 days after intervention.

Results: Two hundred and seventy three patients received low-dose aspirin plus clopidogrel and 97 patients received high-dose aspirin plus clopidogrel before intracranial endovascular treatment. Within 90 days after intervention, there were 4 patients (1.5%) with acute thrombosis, 5 patients (1.8%) with subacute thrombosis, 17 patients (6.2%) with stroke, and 2 death (0.7%) in low-dose aspirin group, compared with no patient (0%) with acute thrombosis, 2 patient (2.1%) with subacute thrombosis, 6 patients (6.2%) with stroke, and 2 death (2.1%) in high-dose aspirin group, and there were no significant difference in all study endpoints between two groups.

Conclusion: Low-dose aspirin plus clopidogrel is comparative in safety with high-dose aspirin plus clopidogrel within 90 days of duration of dual antiplatelet therapy in patients treated with intracranial endovascular treatment.

Editor: Mathias Gelderblom, University Hospital-Eppendorf, Germany

Funding: The following investigators have financial disclosure: Prof Z-R Miao - Contract grant sponsor from the National Natural Science Foundation of China (Contract grant number: 81371290) and from the Beijing High-level Personnel Funds (Contract grant number: 2013-2-19). Prof Ning Ma - Contract grant sponsor from the Clinical and Basic Medical Cooperation Project of Capital Medical University (Contract grant number: 13JL40). Prof X-Q Zhao - Contract grant sponsor from the Beijing Municipal Science and Technology Commission (Contract grant number: D111107003111007). The funders had no role in study design, data collection and analysis, decision to publish, or preparation of the manuscript.

Competing Interests: The authors have declared that no competing interests exist.

* Email: zhongrongm@163.com

[9] These authors contributed equally to this work.

Introduction

Intracranial atherosclerotic stenosis is one of the most common causes of ischaemic stroke worldwide [1]. Symptomatic intracranial atherosclerotic stenosis of $\geq$70% is associated with a high risk of recurrent stroke despite aggressive medical therapy [2,3,4]. As a means of preventing recurrent stroke, endovascular treatment remain to be considered potentially beneficial for patients with severe intracranial stenosis with insufficient collateral or with vulnerable plaque [5,6,7].

Aspirin in combination with clopidogrel preventing major thrombotic events has been the standard of care in patients undergoing intracranial endovascular treatment for more than a decade [8]. Despite its universal use, the optimal dose of aspirin from an efficacy and safety perspective remains unclear [9,10]. Based on the studies for patients who underwent percutaneous coronary intervention, high-dose aspirin ($\geq$300 mg daily) did not differ significantly from low-dose aspirin (75–100 mg daily) in prevention of cardiovascular death, myocardial infarction, or stroke, and stent thrombosis [11,12,13]. Given the high mortality of intracranial bleeding in intracranial endovascular treatment [14,15], a low-dose aspirin strategy is subsequently adopted when using low-dose aspirin is no harm compared with high-dose aspirin in prevention of periprocedural complications and major vascular events in duration of dual antiplatelet therapy. So we perform a prospective study to evaluate the effect and safety of low-dose aspirin plus standard-dose clopidogrel versus high-dose aspirin plus standard-dose clopidogrel in prevention of vascular risk in patients with symptomatic intracranial atherosclerotic stenosis of ≥70% with poor collateral undergoing intracranial endovascular treatment within 90 days of duration of dual antiplatelet therapy after intervention.

Methods

Standard protocol approval and patient consent

The protocol for this prospective, observational, single-center study was approved by the institutional ethics committee at Beijing Tiantan Hospital before screening any patients. The written informed consent was obtained from all patients participating in the study.

Patients

Patients were enrolled in this study according to the following criteria: 1. Primary or recurrent ischaemic stroke or transient ischaemic attack (TIA) in the target intracranial arterial territory within 90 days during the treatment with at least one antiplatelet drug. 2. Intracranial stenosis≥70%, lesion length<15 mm, target artery diameter≥2 mm, and a normal distal vessel bed on digital subtraction angiography (DSA). 3. No evidence of cardioembolism, including atrial fibrillation or recent myocardial infarction within one month. 4. Age≥30 years. 5. Two or more atherosclerotic risk factors including hypertension, hypercholesterolemia, diabetes mellitus, cigarette smoking, and obesity. Hypertension was defined as systolic blood pressure≥140 mmHg, diastolic blood pressure≥90 mmHg, or the patient is currently on an antihypertensive drug. Hypercholesterolemia was defined as a total cholesterol level ≥240 mg/dL or a low-density lipoprotein cholesterol level ≥160 mg/dL or current medication use for lowering the blood cholesterol level. Patients who used antidiabetic medications (insulin or oral hypoglycemics) were considered to have diabetes mellitus. Patients who smoked in the past or currently smoke were considered to have cigarette smoking history. Obesity was defined as a body mass index greater than 30 kg/m². 6. Poor collateral was determined by the following three methods: ASITN/SIR Collateral Flow Grading System score<3 confirmed by DSA [16]; ≥30% decrease in cerebral blood flow in the territory distal to the target lesion by computed tomography (CT) perfusion (The reference area for CT perfusion is the contralateral hemisphere for anterior circulation lesions and anterior circulation territory for posterior circulation lesions) [17]; hemodynamic ischaemic lesion by magnetic resonance imaging (MRI) or CT.

Patients with the following conditions were excluded: nonatherosclerosis vasculopathy such as vasculitis and arterial dissection, diagnosed by comprehensive laboratory work (such as erythrocyte sedimentation rate or C-reactive protein elevations, antinuclear antibody, or antiphospholipid antibody positivity), vascular imaging, and clinical evaluation.

Using a traditional clinical definition of ischaemic events, we defined ischaemic stroke as a new focal neurologic deficit of sudden onset lasting ≥24 hours with lesion detected by CT or MRI and not caused by hemorrhage and TIA was defined as acute onset of a focal neurologic deficit lasting <24 hours.

From January 2012 to December 2013, 370 consecutive patients with symptomatic ICAS ≥70% on vascular imaging were enrolled.

Medical treatment before procedure

All the enrolled patients received medical treatment. The dose of aspirin was used same as the dose recommended by the doctors in emergency or out-patient department. Other medical treatment consists of clopidogrel, at a dose of 75 mg daily for 5 days before procedure; and management of the atherosclerotic risk factors including elevated systolic blood pressure and elevated low-density lipoprotein cholesterol levels, and diabetes. Patients who have not been on dual antiplatelet therapy for five days prior to procedure are given a 300 mg loading dose of clopidogrel between 6 and 24 hours before the procedure.

Endovascular treatment protocol

The procedure was performed by experienced neurointerventionists, who had each done at least 100 endovascular procedures for intracranial atherosclerotic stenosis. Intravenous heparin was administered after placement of a 6-Fr sheath or a 5-Fr sheath by transfemoral artery or transradial artery (only for posterior circulation and tortuous arch) as a bolus (75 U/kg) followed by half the dose one hour later, and if the procedure last longer than 2 hours, a quarter of the initial dose was given at every hour thereafter. The guiding catheter was advanced into the cervical vertebral or internal carotid artery as high as the vessel tortuosity allowed.

Device selection depended on arterial access and lesion morphology. For patients with smooth arterial access and Mori A lesion [18], the Apollo balloon-mounted stent (MicroPort, Shanghai, China) was selected. For patients with tortuous arterial access and Mori B or C lesion, or lesion with a significant mismatch in the diameter between proximal and distal segment, angioplasty plus self-expanding stent (Gateway balloon plus Wingspan stent system [Styker, Maple Grove, Minnesota, USA]) is preferred. For patients with tortuous arterial access with a Mori A lesion, or small target vessel diameter (<2.5 mm), direct dilation with Gateway balloon was selected. If severe dissection or elastic recoil occurred after angioplasty, a balloon-mounted stent (for patients with less tortuous access) or Wingspan (for patients with severe tortuous access or small target vessel) stent were allowed to be implanted. Technical success rate of angioplasty was defined as complete coverage of the target lesion with the residual stent stenosis <50% and with thrombolysis in cerebral ischaemia (TICI) grade 3 [16]. Intraprocedural blood pressure was monitored every 5 minutes and postprocedural blood pressure was monitored from hourly to once every 4 hours for at least 1 day, and systolic blood pressure was kept between 100 and 120 mm Hg.

Medical management after procedure

After intervention, all patients were given a weight-based dose of 0.4 to 0.6 mL low molecular weight heparin every 12 hours subcutaneously for 3 days and monitored closely until discharge. Dual antiplatelet therapy consists of aspirin, at a dose same as the pre-procedural regimen, clopidogrel, at a dose of 75 mg daily, for 90 days after procedure. After 90 days, 100 mg aspirin or 75 mg clopidogrel daily is continuously used. Other medical therapies in follow-up are management of the atherosclerotic risk factors including elevated systolic blood pressure and elevated low-density lipoprotein cholesterol levels, diabetes, smoking, excess weight, and insufficient exercise.

Study endpoints

During the period of follow-up, patients were contacted monthly by phone to determine whether any events had occurred. At the first month after intervention and then every three months, patients were examined face-to-face by two neurologists. The study endpoints within 90 days below were collected. The study endpoint was acute thrombosis, subacute thrombosis, stroke (in any vascular territory) or death, non-stroke hemorrhage, and hyperperfusion symptoms within 30 days after intervention and stroke in the qualifying artery territory or death, and non-stroke hemorrhage beyond 30 days after intervention. Acute thrombosis was defined as thrombosis at 0 to 24 hours after intervention; Subacute thrombosis was defined as thrombosis at 24 hours to 30 days after intervention. All subacute thrombosis was confirmed by an emergency DSA. Stroke was defined as a new focal neurological deficit of sudden onset that lasted $\geq$24 hours. If a stroke is suspected during the follow-up period, the patient is examined by a neurologist, and the ischaemic or hemorrhagic stroke was diagnosed by brain MRI or CT. Non-stroke hemorrhage is defined as any subdural or epidural hemorrhage or a systemic hemorrhage. Hyperperfusion symptoms were defined as headache, seizure, delirium, or a neurologic deficit combined with a 100% increase of velocity by Transcranial Doppler compared with baseline [19].

Statistical Analysis

Continuous variables were presented as means$\pm$SD. Categorical variables were presented as percentages. Student's t-test or the Mann-Whitney U-test (when continuous variables had skewed distributions) was used to identify the difference in each of the variables between patients with low-dose aspirin and high-dose aspirin. The difference in each of the categorical variables between the two groups was tested with χ^2 or Fisher's exact tests (when the expected cell frequency was <5). A two-tailed P value less than 0.05 was considered statistically significant. All analyses were performed using the software SAS 9.2 (SAS Institute Inc., Cary, NC, USA).

Results

Patient Characteristics

Among 370 patients (mean age 59 years, range 37–80 years), 273 patients received aspirin at a low-dose of 100 mg and clopidogrel at a dose of 75 mg and 97 patients received aspirin at a high-dose of 300 mg and clopidogrel at a dose of 75 mg. The data on study endpoints presented below are based on all adverse events as of April 11, 2014, when the last patient enrolled completed the 90-day evaluation. The mean follow-up was 15 months (range from 1–28 months). Among all the patients, 10 patients had loss of follow-up within 90-day evaluation.

There were no significant differences with respect to any of the baseline characteristics of the patients between the two groups (Table 1). In low-dose aspirin group, there were 159 (159/273, 58.2%) patients treated with balloon-mounted stent, 89 (89/273, 32.6%) patients treated with balloon angioplasty plus expendable stent, and 22 (22/273, 8.1%) patients treated with balloon angioplasty alone. In high-dose aspirin group, there were 63 (63/97, 64.9%) patients treated with balloon-mounted stent, 24 (24/97, 24.7%) patients treated with balloon angioplasty plus expendable stent, and 6 (6/97, 6.2%) patients treated with balloon angioplasty alone. The procedure failed in 3 (3/273, 1.0%) patients in low-dose aspirin group and 4 (4/97, 4.1%) patients in high-dose aspirin group. There were no significant differences between the two groups in endovascular methods (Table 2).

Study endpoints

Within 30 days after intervention, there were 4 patients (4/273, 1.5%) with acute thrombosis and 5 patients (5/273, 1.8%) with subacute thrombosis compared with no patient (0/97, 0%) with acute thrombosis and 2 patient (2/97, 2.1%) with subacute thrombosis in high-dose aspirin group. There were 10 patients (10/273, 3.7%) with ischaemic stroke including 4 patients due to subacute thrombosis, 3 patients due to perforator infarction, 2 patients due to acute thrombosis, 1 patients due to embolization, in low-dose aspirin group, compared with 4 patients (2/97, 4.1%) including 2 patients due to perforator infarction and 2 patient due to subacute thrombosis in high-dose aspirin group. There were 3 patient (3/273, 1.1%) with hemorrhagic stroke including 2 patients due to guidewire perforation and 1 patient due to a delayed intraparenchymal hemorrhage related to hyperperfusion, compared with 1 patient (1/97, 1.0%) with a parenchymal hemorrhage out of the territory of qualifying artery in high-dose aspirin group. There were 1 death (1/273, 0.4%) due to subacute thrombosis in low-dose aspirin group, compared with 2 death (2/97, 2.1%) due to a delayed intraparenchymal hemorrhage related to hyperperfusion in high-dose aspirin group. There were 1 patient (1/273, 0.4%) with aural hemorrhage without requiring blood transfusion and surgery in low-dose aspirin group, compared with 1 patient (1/97, 1.0%) with urine hemorrhage without blood transfusion and surgery in high-dose aspirin group. Among all the patients, 14 patients (14/370, 3.7%) of with hyperperfusion symptoms was observed, including 9 patients in low-dose aspirin group in which 1 patient (1/9, 11%) evolved to hemorrhagic stroke, and 5 patients in high-dose aspirin group in which 3 patients (3/5, 60%) evolved to hemorrhagic stroke or death.

During the period of 30 days to 90 days after intervention, there were 4 (4/273, 1.5%) patients with ischaemic stroke due to in-stent restenosis, 1 non-stroke death (1/273, 0.4%) due to pneumonia and 1 patient (1/273, 0.4%) with nasal hemorrhage without requiring blood transfusion and surgery in low-dose aspirin group, and there was 1 patient (1/97, 1.0%) with ischaemic stroke due to in-stent restenosis in high-dose aspirin group. There were no significant differences in all study endpoints between two groups (Table 2).

All 11 patients with thrombosis were treated with a 10–20 mg dose of alteplase (Boehringer Ingelheim, Ingelheim, Germany) mixed as 1 mg per milliliter and/or a 6–10 ml tirofiban hydrochloride (Wuhan Grand Pharma, Wuhan, China) injected via guide catheter. There 2 patients with acute thrombosis remaining asymptomatic after the intervention and 1 death due to failure of intervention.

Discussion

To prevent periprocedural platelet emboli and thrombus formation, patients are typically treated for a variable number of days before the intracranial endovascular treatment with a combination of aspirin and clopidogrel [11,12,13]. The dose of each antiplatelet agent varies from operator to operator, and there is no consensus on the safety, dosage, or drug combination [11,12,13]. Particularly, the dose of aspirin varies greatly worldwide and it is given between 81 and 325 mg daily before the procedure [10]. This variation in practice is partly due to the fact that no comparisons of aspirin dose have been done in intracranial endovascular treatment since its routine use a decade ago. Based on the studies on percutaneous coronary intervention suggested high-dose aspirin did not differ significantly from low-dose aspirin in prevention of periprocedural complications [13], we want to evaluate wither there is the difference in safety and efficacy of the low-dose of aspirin plus standard-dose clopidogrel versus high-dose of aspirin plus standard-dose clopidogrel in intracranial endovascular treatment within the duration of dual antiplatelet therapy.

Our study suggested that in patients with severe symptomatic intracranial atherosclerotic stenosis with poor collateral, low-dose aspirin (100 mg daily) does not increase risk of ischaemic events compared with high-dose aspirin (300 mg daily). The risk of

Table 1. Comparison of baseline characteristics of patients receiving low-dose aspirin and patients receiving high- dose aspirin[*].

Characteristic	Patients receiving low-dose aspirin (N = 273)	Patients receiving high-dose aspirin (N = 97)	P value
Age — yr	59.2±8.1	58.2±9.3	0.39
Male sex — no. (%)	228(83.5)	75 (77.3)	0.22
Risk factors— no. (%)			
Hypertension	222 (81.3)	73 (75.3)	0.24
Hyperlipidemia	158 (57.9)	57 (58.8)	0.91
Diabetes mellitus	92 (33.7)	33 (34.0)	1.00
Smoking	164 (60.1)	47 (48.5)	0.07
Obesity	24 (8.8)	9 (9.3)	0.84
Qualifying ischaemic events — no. (%)			
TIA	149 (54.6)	64 (66.0)	0.06
Stroke	124 (45.4)	33 (34.0)	0.06
Symptomatic qualifying artery — no. (%)			
BA	109 (40.0)	38 (39.2)	1.00
Intracranial vertebral	101 (37.0)	35 (36.1)	0.90
MCA	34 (12.5)	15 (15.5)	0.49
Intracranial carotid	29 (10.6)	9 (9.3)	0.85
Cases with loading dose of clopidogrel	12 (4.4)	4 (4.1)	1.00
Time from qualifying event to endovascular treatment— days			0.52
Median	25	22	
Interquartile range	10–41	12–30	

[*]Plus–minus values are means ±SD. Baseline characteristics of the two groups were compared with the use of either an independent groups t-test (for means) or a chi-square test (for percentages). TIA denotes transient ischaemic attack; BA denotes basilar artery; MCA denotes middle cerebral artery.

hemorrhagic stroke or death evolving from hyperperfusion symptom (3/5, 60%) in high-dose aspirin group may be higher than that (1/9, 11%) in low-dose aspirin group. Considering an incidence of hyperperfusion symptoms was 3.7% (14/370) observed in this cohort with poor collateral, this finding may suggest that low-dose aspirin plus clopidogrel may be a reasonable option for intracranial endovascular treatment in patients with poor collateral.

The overall complications rate within 30 days after intervention in this study was lower than that reported in in the SAMMPRIS trial [4]. Aside from the different antiplatelet regimen, other factors are the following: 1.This study was performed a large volume stroke center. 2. The procedures were performed by operators with vast experience of intracranial endovascular treatment, who have long pasted the steep portion of the learning curve [20]. 3. A tailored endovascular treatment method was selected relying on individual access and lesion anatomy and it may be safe than using a single endovascular device for intracranial stenosis [21]. 4. The time from the last episodic event to the procedure was substantially longer than that in SAMM-PRIS. The longer waiting time may have allowed the plaque to stabilize and thrombus to dissolve, and probably reduced the risk of perforator infarction by snow plow effect during the procedure as well. 5. The difference of baseline characteristics may cause bias. This study only studied the Asia population. The rates of hypertension, hyperlipidemia, and diabetes mellitus except smoking are slightly lower than that in the SAMMPRIS study. The majority of qualifying event was TIA and the symptomatic qualifying artery was BA compared these was stroke and MCA in the SAMMRPIS study [4]. However, Concerns have been raised

to these explanations because the event rates in the registry are usually lower than randomized trial.

In this study, the subacute thrombosis rate in low-dose aspirin is 1.8% (5/273) which is low than 12.1% (4/33) in a previous study using 100 mg aspirin plus 75 mg clopidogrel 3 days before the procedure [22]. We thought that a 5 days dual antiplatelet regimen may be more efficacious than a 3 days dual antiplatelet regimen in achieving high levels of platelet inhibition.

In addition, the ischemic stroke within 30 days after intervention was ascribed to thrombosis and perforator stroke, compared that during the period of 30–90 days was due to in-stent restenosis. The high occurrence of thrombosis was different that observed in the SAMMPRIS study but similar with that found in a previous study on coronary artery disease [14,23].

Our study showed the risk of bleeding with dual antiplatelet therapy within 90 days after intervention is low. The overall non-stroke hemorrhage rate within 90 days after intervention was 0.8% (3/370) which is comparative with a previous study in which the incidence of minor bleeding events of patients with a 3-month dual antiplatelet therapy after implantation of zotarolimus-eluting stent for coronary artery disease was 1.5% [24].

There some limitations in this study. First, the sample size is small. Secondly, the dose of aspirins was not determined by randomization. Thirdly, this study did not focus on the mechanism of complications and the issues about antiplatelet drugs resistance or the effectiveness of the antiplatelet therapy by using lab tests. We try to improve these in the future study.

In summary, antiplatelet therapy consisting of low-dose aspirin plus clopidogrel is comparative in safety with high-dose aspirin plus clopidogrel for patients with severe symptomatic intracranial

Table 2. Comparison of endovascular treatment data and study endpoints within 30 days and 90 days after intervention of patients receiving low-dose aspirin and patients receiving high-dose aspirin*.

	Patients receiving low-dose aspirin (N = 273)	Patients receiving high-dose aspirin (N = 97)	P value
Endovascular treatment methods — no. (%)			
Balloon-mounted stenting	159 (58.2)	63 (64.9)	0.28
Balloon angioplasty + expendable stenting	89 (32.6)	24 (24.7)	0.16
Balloon angioplasty	22 (8.1)	6 (6.2)	0.66
Failure	3 (1.0)	4 (4.1)	0.08
Multi vessels treated — no. (%)	13 (4.8)	3 (3.1)	0.77
Loss of follow-up — no. (%)	6 (2.2)	4 (4.1)	0.30
Dual Antiplatelet drugs use within 90 days — no. (%)	270 (98.9)	96 (98.9)	1.00
Study endpoints within 30 days — no. (%)			
Acute thrombosis	4 (1.5)	0 (0)	0.58
Subacute thrombosis	5 (1.8)	2 (2.1)	1.00
Thrombosis	9 (3.3)	2 (2.1)	0.74
Ischaemic stroke	10(3.7)	4 (4.1)	0.77
Hemorrhagic stroke	3 (1.1)	1 (1.0)	1.00
Death	1 (0.4)	2 (2.1)	0.17
Non-stroke hemorrhage	1(0.4)	1 (1.0)	0.46
Hyperperfusion symptoms	9 (3.3)	5 (5.2)	0.54
Study endpoints within 90 days — no. (%)			
Ischaemic stroke	14 (5.1)	5 (5.2)	1.00
Hemorrhagic stroke	3 (1.1)	1 (1.0)	1.00
Death	2 (0.7)	2 (2.1)	0.28
Non-stroke hemorrhage	2 (0.7)	1 (1.0)	1.00

*Plus–minus values are means ±SD. Baseline characteristics of the two groups were compared with the use of either an independent groups t-test (for means) or a chi-square test (for percentages).

atherosclerotic stenosis with poor collateral undergoing intracranial endovascular treatment.

Acknowledgments

We thank Dr. Lin-Feng Zhang, MD, PhD at Department of Epidemiology, the Cardiovascular Institute, Fu Wai Hospital of the Chinese Academy of Medical Sciences and Peking Union Medical College, and the National Center for Cardiovascular Disease Control and Research, Beijing, China, 100037, for his help in statistics analysis.

Author Contributions

Conceived and designed the experiments: ZM. Performed the experiments: NM DM FG KG XS XX LL LS. Analyzed the data: NM ZX DM FG ZM. Contributed reagents/materials/analysis tools: NM ZX DM FG KG XS XX LL LS TW XZ Yilong Wang Yongjun Wang ZM. Wrote the paper: NM ZX ZM. Supervision of the quality of the study: XZ Yilong Wang Yongjun Wang ZM.

References

1. Wong LK (2006) Global burden of intracranial atherosclerosis. Int J Stroke 1: 158–159.
2. Chimowitz MI, Lynn MJ, Howlett-Smith H, Stern BJ, Hertzberg VS, et al. (2005) Warfarin-Aspirin Symptomatic Intracranial Disease Trial Investigators. Comparison of warfarin and aspirin for symptomatic intracranial arterial stenosis. N Engl J Med 352: 1305–16.
3. Kasner SE, Chimowitz MI, Lynn MJ, Howlett-Smith H, Stern BJ, et al. (2006) Predictors of ischemic stroke in the territory of a symptomatic intracranial arterial stenosis. Circulation 113: 555–563.
4. Chimowitz MI, Lynn MJ, Derdeyn CP, Turan TN, Fiorella D, et al. (2011) Stenting versus aggressive medical therapy for intracranial arterial stenosis. N Engl J Med 365: 993–1003.
5. Zaidat OO, Castonguay AC, Nguyen TN, Becker KJ, Derdeyn CP, et al. (2014) Impact of SAMMPRIS on the future of intracranial atherosclerotic disease management: polling results from the ICAD symposium at the International Stroke Conference. J Neurointerv Surg 6: 225–30.
6. Yu SC, Cheng HK, Cheng PW, Lui WM, Leung KM, et al. (2013) Angioplasty and stenting for intracranial atherosclerotic stenosis: position statement of the Hong Kong Society of Interventional and Therapeutic Neuroradiology. Hong Kong Med J 19: 69–73.
7. Chimowitz MI (2013) The Feinberg award lecture 2013: treatment of intracranial atherosclerosis: learning from the past and planning for the future. Stroke 44: 2664–2669.
8. SSYLVIA Study Investigators (2004) Stenting of symptomatic atherosclerotic lesions in the vertebral or intracranial arteries (SSYLVIA): study results. Stroke 35: 1388–1392.
9. Hussain MS, Fraser JF, Abruzzo T, Blackham KA, Bulsara KR, et al. (2012) Standard of practice: endovascular treatment of intracranial atherosclerosis. J Neurointerv Surg 4: 397–406.
10. Schumacher HC, Meyers PM, Higashida RT, Derdeyn CP, Lavine SD, et al. (2009) Reporting standards for angioplasty and stent-assisted angioplasty for intracranial atherosclerosis. Stroke 40:e348–65.
11. Peters RJ, Mehta SR, Fox KA, Zhao F, Lewis BS, et al. (2003) Effects of aspirin dose when used alone or in combination with clopidogrel in patients with acute coronary syndromes: observations from the Clopidogrel in Unstable angina to prevent Recurrent Events (CURE) study. Circulation 108: 1682–87.
12. Topol EJ, Easton D, Harrington RA, Amarenco P, Califf RM, et al. (2003) Randomized, double blind, placebo-controlled, international trial of the oral IIb/IIIa antagonist lotrafiban in coronary and cerebrovascular disease. Circulation 108: 399–406.

13. Mehta SR, Tanguay JF, Eikelboom JW, Jolly SS, Joyner CD, et al. (2010) Double-dose versus standard-dose clopidogrel and high-dose versus low-dose aspirin in individuals undergoing percutaneous coronary intervention for acute coronary syndromes (CURRENT-OASIS 7): a randomised factorial trial. Lancet 376: 1233–1243.

14. Derdeyn CP, Fiorella D, Lynn MJ, Rumboldt Z, Cloft HJ, et al. (2013) Mechanisms of stroke after intracranial angioplasty and stenting in the SAMMPRIS trial. Neurosurgery 72: 777–95.

15. Fiorella D, Derdeyn CP, Lynn MJ, Barnwell SL, Hoh BL, et al. (2012) Detailed analysis of periprocedural strokes in patients undergoing intracranial stenting in Stenting and Aggressive Medical Management for Preventing Recurrent Stroke in Intracranial Stenosis (SAMMPRIS). Stroke 43: 2682–2688.

16. Higashida R, Furlan A, Roberts H, Tomsick T, Connors B, et al. (2003) Trial design and reporting standards for intraarterial cerebral thrombolysis for acute ischemic stroke. J Vasc Interv Radiol 14:S493–S494.

17. Gao PY, Lin Y (2003) CT perfusion imaging and stages of regional cerebral hypoperfusion in pre-infarction period. Chin J Radiol (Chin) 37: 882–886.

18. Mori T, Fukuoka M, Kazita K, Mori K (1998) Follow-up study after intracranial percutaneous transluminal cerebral balloon angioplasty. AJNR Am J Neuroradiol 19: 1525–1533.

19. Sánchez-Arjona MB, Sanz-Fernández G, Franco-Macías E, Gil-Peralta A (2007) Cerebral hemodynamic changes after carotid angioplasty and stenting. AJNR Am J Neuroradiol. 28: 640–644.

20. Yu SC, Leung TW, Lee KT, Wong LK (2014) Learning curve of wingspan stenting for intracranial atherosclerosis: single-center experience of 95 consecutive patients. J Neurointerv Surg 6: 212–8.

21. Miao Z, Song L, Liebeskind DS, Liu L, Ma N, et al. (2014) Outcomes of tailored angioplasty and/or stenting for symptomatic intracranial atherosclerosis: a prospective cohort study after SAMMPRIS. J Neurointerv Surg. 2014 Apr 23. doi: 10.1136/neurintsurg-2014-011109.

22. Riedel CH, Tietke M, Alfke K, Stingele R, Jansen O (2009) Subacute stent thrombosis in intracranial stenting. Stroke 40: 1310–1314.

23. Mehran R, Baber U, Steg PG, Ariti C, Weisz G, et al. (2013) Cessation of dual antiplatelet treatment and cardiac events after percutaneous coronary intervention (PARIS): 2 year results from a prospective observational study. Lancet 382: 1714–1722.

24. Wada T1, Nakahama M, Toda H, Watanabe A, Hashimoto K, et al. (2013) Dual antiplatelet therapy can be discontinued at three months after implantation of zotarolimus-eluting stent in patients with coronary artery disease. ISRN Cardiol. 518968. doi: 10.1155/2013/518968.

22

High-Throughput Screening Identifies Idarubicin as a Preferential Inhibitor of Smooth Muscle versus Endothelial Cell Proliferation

Shakti A. Goel[1,9], Lian-Wang Guo[1*,9], Bowen Wang[1], Song Guo[2], Drew Roenneburg[1], Gene E. Ananiev[2], F. Michael Hoffmann[2], K. Craig Kent[1]

1 Department of Surgery, University of Wisconsin, Madison, Wisconsin, United States of America, **2** Small Molecule Screening & Synthesis Facility, UW Carbone Cancer Center, Madison, Wisconsin, United States of America

Abstract

Intimal hyperplasia is the cause of the recurrent occlusive vascular disease (restenosis). Drugs currently used to treat restenosis effectively inhibit smooth muscle cell (SMC) proliferation, but also inhibit the growth of the protective luminal endothelial cell (EC) lining, leading to thrombosis. To identify compounds that selectively inhibit SMC versus EC proliferation, we have developed a high-throughput screening (HTS) format using human cells and have employed this to screen a multiple compound collection (NIH Clinical Collection). We developed an automated, accurate proliferation assay in 96-well plates using human aortic SMCs and ECs. Using this HTS format we screened a 447-drug NIH Clinical Library. We identified 11 compounds that inhibited SMC proliferation greater than 50%, among which idarubicin exhibited a unique feature of preferentially inhibiting SMC versus EC proliferation. Concentration-response analysis revealed this differential effect most evident over an ~10 nM-5 µM window. *In vivo* testing of idarubicin in a rat carotid injury model at 14 days revealed an 80% reduction of intimal hyperplasia and a 45% increase of lumen size with no significant effect on re-endothelialization. Taken together, we have established a HTS assay of human vascular cell proliferation, and identified idarubicin as a selective inhibitor of SMC versus EC proliferation both *in vitro* and *in vivo*. Screening of larger and more diverse compound libraries may lead to the discovery of next-generation therapeutics that can inhibit intima hyperplasia without impairing re-endothelialization.

Editor: Bridget Wagner, Broad Institute of Harvard and MIT, United States of America

Funding: This work was supported by a Public Health Service Grant (R01-HL-068673 to K.C.K.) from the National Heart, Lung, and Blood Institute. The funders had no role in study design, data collection and analysis, decision to publish, or preparation of the manuscript.

Competing Interests: The authors have declared that no competing interests exist.

* E-mail: guo@surgery.wisc.edu

9 These authors contributed equally to this work.

Introduction

Atherosclerosis is the leading cause of death in the United States. Interventions for treating atherosclerosis including angioplasty, stenting and bypass frequently fail related to the development of recurrent disease (restenosis) [1]. The pathology of restenosis is primarily intimal hyperplasia, and central to this process is smooth muscle cell (SMC) proliferation. In response to the injury associated with arterial reconstructions, SMCs in the media transform from a differentiated to a proliferative and migratory phenotype leading to the formation of a highly cellular subintimal plaque that re-narrows the vessel lumen [2]. Diminished flow related to narrowed or occluded arteries gives rise to adverse outcomes such as heart attack, stroke, amputation and/or death.

Another key cell type integral to this process is the endothelial cell (EC). As a by-product of interventions to treat atherosclerosis, denudation of the endothelial layer of treated arteries or veins leads to deleterious consequences. First, ECs provide the vessel's anti-thrombotic lining. Without an EC layer, platelets accumulate on the vessel surface initiating thrombus that can cause sudden death [3]. Equally important, it has been shown that ECs and SMCs interact, such that a uniform EC layer lining the inner surface of a vessel inhibits underlying SMC growth and migration thus lessening the potential for the formation of hyperplastic plaque [4]. Third, an intact EC layer prevents transmigration of leukocytes into the arterial wall and leukocyte infiltration is one of many contributors to the process of intimal hyperplasia [5]. Lastly, recent clinical evidence indicates that endothelial dysfunction produced by rapamycin, a SMC inhibitor used to prevent the development of intimal hyperplasia, leads to impaired collateral flow [5] as well as paradoxical vasoconstriction in the arterial segment adjacent to the rapamycin-releasing stent [6]. Thus, following vascular reconstruction, it is essential that ECs be allowed to rapidly repopulate the vessel lumen [7,8].

Currently, the only clinically employed method for preventing restenosis is a stent coated with rapamycin or paclitaxel used in conjunction with angioplasty [9]. Unfortunately, both drugs inhibit EC proliferation, migration, and survival and thus impair the critically important process of re-establishing the vessel's protective endothelial lining [3]. Consequently, despite the success of drug-eluting stents, neo-intima plaque still leads to restenosis in approximately 15% of treated patients [10,11]. More importantly, impaired re-endothelialization leads to acute or late stent thrombosis which is associated with a 45% mortality [3]. Although dual antiplatelet therapy is used to reduce the incidence of stent thrombosis, the incidence of thrombosis still remains significant (1.3%), and antiplatelet agents are associated hemorrhage and additional cost in this patient population.

Thus, the optimal drug to prevent restenosis would be one that selectively inhibits SMC proliferation and intimal hyperplasia but has a minimally inhibitory effect on EC proliferation. Several such selective agents have been reported in the literature [12,13] [14–16] [17–19] but with various limitations, *e.g.* lack of effect *in vivo* or difficulty in delivery. Moreover, the scarceness of reports identifying agents that selectively inhibit SMCs versus ECs likely reflects the fact that ECs are generally more susceptible than SMCs to anti-proliferative drugs. Thus, in order to discover candidates for selective SMC inhibition, a high throughput screening campaign is necessary to screen large libraries of compounds. To the best of our knowledge, there has been a lack of such HTS studies with this goal in mind.

The purpose of this study is to establish a pilot HTS system that is amenable for screening larger chemical libraries with the goal of discovering new drugs that selectively retard human SMC proliferation while leaving the growth of endothelial cells unaffected. To circumvent the shortcomings in the aforementioned studies, we have developed accurate assays for proliferation of primary human aortic SMCs and human aortic ECs, which are more relevant to human restenotic disease than animal cells. In a pilot screen we have identified that idarubicin, an FDA-approved drug currently used for treating leukemia, inhibits the proliferation of SMCs to a much greater extent than ECs through a defined concentration window. Furthermore, for the first time, this drug has been shown through *in vivo* testing to be a potent inhibitor of injury-induced intimal hyperplasia. Our finding raise the possibility of repurposing idarubicin for the treatment of vascular restenosis and establish an efficient, low cost HTS that can be used through screening of large chemical libraries, to identify other candidate inhibitors of restenosis.

Materials and Methods

Ethics Statement

The experiments involving animal use were carried out in strict accordance with the recommendations in the Guide for the Care and Use of Laboratory Animals of the National Institutes of Health. The protocol (Permit Number: M02273) was approved by the Institutional Animal Care and Use Committee (IACUC) of the University of Wisconsin-Madison. All surgery was performed under isoflurane anesthesia, and all efforts were made to minimize suffering.

Materials

Alamar Blue was purchased from Invitrogen (Carlsbad, CA). Cell Titer Glo was from Promega (Madison, WI). Primary human aortic smooth muscle cells (HuAoSMCs) and primary human aortic endothelial cells (HuAoECs) at passage 3 were purchased from Lonza; their respective optimal culture media (SmGM-2 and EGM-2) were from the same commercial source. Cells were used at passage 5 after expansion. Trypsin/EDTA solution was from Clonetics (Walkersville, MD); and DPBS was from Gibco (Invitrogen, Carlsbad, CA). Microtiter tissue 96-well culture plates with transparent flat-bottoms and black-walled sides were from Costar (Corning, NY). Resveratrol and idarubicin were products of Sigma-Aldrich (St. Louis, MO). Stock solutions of these reagents

were prepared in DMSO (Thermo-Fisher). The library of NIH Clinical Collection composed of 447 unique compounds of known bioactivity was available at the Small Molecule Screening and Synthesis Facility (SMSSF) of the University of Wisconsin Carbone Cancer Center (UWCCC).

Cell Culture

Cryo-protected frozen HuAoSMCs and HuAoECs (Lonza, passage 3) were thawed and cultured in their respective media that are optimized for cell growth by the manufacturer. HuAoSMCs were grown in the SmGM-2 medium containing 5% FBS, and HuAoECs in the EGM-2 medium containing 2% FBS in a humidified incubator at 37°C with 5% CO_2. After expansion, cells at passage 5 were used for all the experiments.

Test of the Consistency of an Automated Cell Proliferation Assay System

Freshly collected HuAoSMCs (passage 5) were counted (>93% viability) by Cellometer AutoT4 (Nexelon Bioscience), and dispensed using Microflo Select (BioTek) to a final density of 2700 cells/200 µl/well in the SmGM-2 medium in a 96-well plate. After a 24 h incubation to allow cell attachment, 0.1 µl of DMSO (vehicle) or 0.1 µl of resveratrol (a known SMC growth inhibitor) stock in DMSO was robotically transferred using Biomek FX (Beckman) from a resveratrol stock plate into cell culture (final 50 µM resveratrol [20]. DMSO and resveratrol were added into alternate columns of wells (8 wells per column). We used a noncytotoxic and inexpensive reagent (Alama Blue) for proliferation assay. After incubation with resveratrol for 72 h, Alamar Blue dye was added using Matrix Hydra (Thermo-Fisher) and incubated with cells for another 24 h, and fluorescence was then determined using a Safir2 plate reader (Tecan, excitation/fluorescence: 530 nm/590 nm, bandwidth: 15 nm). The data from 40 wells of vehicle and 40 wells of resveratrol treatments were analyzed for assessment of well-well consistency in the assay. Background signal from the cell-free wells (medium only) was subtracted. In agreement with previous studies [21] we found that reading Alamar Blue fluorescence 24 h after incubation reduced variance compared to reading after shorter incubation (*e.g.* 4 h). To verify assay consistency with a additional method, Alamar Blue dye was removed and wells were gently washed, and Cell Titer Glo reagent was then added followed by a 10 min incubation and luminescence measured using Genios Pro.

HTS against the NIH Clinical Collection using HuAoSMCs and HuAoECs

The HTS assay of cell proliferation was performed to screen 447 compounds included in the NIH Clinical Collection using total six 96-well plates. Each compound was tested once by the addition of 0.1 µl of 10 mM stock dissolved in DMSO to yield a final concentration of 5 µM. Each plate contained 8 wells of negative controls added with DMSO (0.1 µl, final 0.05%) and 8 wells of positive controls added with resveratrol (final 50 µM). HTS assays against the same NIH Clinical Library were conducted with either SMCs or ECs. Cell growth, robotic liquid handling, and fluorescence reading were conducted as described in the preceding paragraph except that the test compounds were transferred (using Biomek FX) from preconfigured stock plates. Robustness of a HTS assay is estimated by the Z' value [22], which is calculated using the formula: $Z' = 1 - [3sdc^+ + 3sdc^-)/(mc^+ - mc^-)]$ where sd = standard deviation; m = mean; c^+ = positive control (resveratrol); c^- = negative control (DMSO). A Z' value of 0.5 is considered the minimal robustness for an assay to perform well in HTS [22].

Dose Responses of Proliferation of HuAoSMCs and HuAoECs

In order to compare differential effects of idarubicin on the proliferation of SMCs versus ECs, dose response experiments were carried out using the two cell types on the same 96-well plate. Assays were performed as described above except that idarubicin (or resveratrol) was added at serial dilutions into triplicate wells for each concentration. Curve fitting was performed with the Prism software (GraphPad).

Rat Balloon Angioplasty Model and Perivascular Drug Delivery

Balloon injury of the left common carotid artery was performed in Male Sprague-Dawley rats (300–350 g) following our previously described method [23]. Briefly, after induction of anesthesia with isoflurane, a 2F balloon catheter was inserted through the left external carotid artery into the common carotid artery, insufflated at 2 atm of pressure, pulled back to the bifurcation, and repeated 3 times. The external carotid artery was then ligated, and blood flow was resumed through the common and internal carotid arteries.

Immediately after re-establishment of flow, idarubicin (50 µg) or DMSO (vehicle, final 0.1%) dissolved in 300 µl of 25% F127 pluronic gel (Sigma-Aldrich) was applied around the injured segment of the carotid artery (5 animals in each group). The pluronic gel is a biodegradable polymer, which is soluble in water at 4°C but becomes a gel when in contact with tissues at 37°C [24]. Rats were euthanized 14 days after injury, and the injured segments of common carotid arteries were collected and fixed in 4% paraformaldehyde overnight for embedding in paraffin.

Morphometric Analysis of Intimal Hyperplasia and Restenosis

Nine evenly-spaced sections through each injured carotid artery were stained using routine hematoxylin and eosin (H&E) and images were collected with light microscopy. Intimal and medial areas, and circumferences were determined by measuring the internal elastic lamina (IEL), external elastic lamina (EEL), and lumen for each section using the ImageJ software (National Institutes of Health) [23,25]. Intimal hyperplasia is quantified by the area ratio of intima versus media; the extent of restenosis is reflected by a reduction in residual lumen [26], a ratio of intimal area versus IEL area.

Immunostaining of CD31, an Endothelial Cell Marker

To assess re-endothelialization, immunostaining of CD31 (an EC marker) was performed on carotid sections following our previous report. Briefly, a goat anti-CD31 primary antibody (R&D Sytems, 1:150) was incubated with the sections for 1 h followed by an incubation with a biotinylated rabbit-anti-goat secondary antibody for 30 min. Immunostaining of CD31 was then visualized by using streptavidin-HRP and DAB. Re-endothelialization was quantified following previously published methods [27,28]. Briefly, the percentage of the luminal perimeter that stained for CD31 versus total perimeter was measured using NIH Image J. Re-endothelialization was then scored from 1 to 5 (1: < 20%; 2:20 to 40%; 3:40 to 60%; 4:60 to 80%; 5:80%–100%) and the scores were averaged with the data from 5 rats (6 sections per rat) in each treatment group.

Statistical Analysis

All data are presented as mean ± standard error (SEM). Statistical analysis was performed using two-tailed unpaired Student's t-test. Data are considered statistically significant when a P value is <0.05.

Results

Development of a HTS System for the Evaluation of Human Vascular Smooth Muscle Cell and Human Vascular Endothelial Cell Proliferation

In order to establish a HTS system that produces consistent outcomes, we first set out to optimize assay conditions. We chose proliferation as an assay since SMC proliferation is the central event in the development of intimal hyperplasia and EC proliferation is essential to re-endothelialization of the vessel lumen and prevention of thrombosis. We chose to use primary human SMCs and ECs so that our findings would be readily translatable; human primary cells are most relevant to human diseases. For the proliferation assay we chose Alamar Blue which has been widely used for measurement of cell number as a surrogate of proliferation. This reagent is easy to use, noncytotoxic, inexpensive [29], and has been previously successfully applied in HTS projects. Moreover, this assay does not require washing or cell lysis thereby minimizing variability. To maximize cell growth rate, we used the complete SmGM-2 medium (supplemented with 5% serum) and EGM-2 medium (2% serum). Both are media optimized by Lonza for HuAoSMCs and HuAoECs, respectively. In preliminary studies, we varied seeding density and assay duration in order to maximize proliferation. We found that SMCs seeded at a density of 2000–3000 cells per well gave rise to maximal proliferation (Figure S1); higher seeding densities did not result in more significant growth (data not shown). Thus, we used for our HTS system a cell density of 2700 cells per well and an assay duration of 72 h. Optimization experiments were also performed for ECs resulting in a similar protocol except for the use of the EGM-2 medium and 2% serum (data not shown). Cell number was determined by quantifying fluorescence from the Alamar Blue reagent.

We then applied these optimized conditions to test the consistency of our automated HTS system for proliferation using resveratrol as a positive control. We chose resveratrol because this natural compound has been previously shown to inhibit SMC proliferation and angioplasty-induced intimal hyperplasia [20]. As shown in Figure 1, compared to vehicle control (DMSO), resveratrol inhibited SMC growth by ~65% with a very small SEM, indicating low well-to-well variation. The good well-to-well consistency achieved by this automated assay format with 96-well plates is also demonstrated by a Z' value of 0.63. The Z' factor is generally accepted as a measure to quantify the quality and hence suitability of a particular assay for use in a full-scale, high-throughput screen [22]. A Z'>0.4 is considered a good assay [22]. We also corroborated the Alamar Blue assay results using another established method, Cell Titer Glo assay, which quantifies ATP levels in cell lysates [30]. Cell Titer Glo assays using resveratrol for both SMCs and ECs also produced high Z' values (>0.7).

HTS of the NIH Clinical Collection Produces 11 Compounds that Inhibit HuAoSMC Growth Greater than 50%

We then utilized this HTS system to screen 447 FDA-approved drugs in the NIH Clinical Collection. All the compounds included in this collection are clinically used drugs with diverse bioactivities.

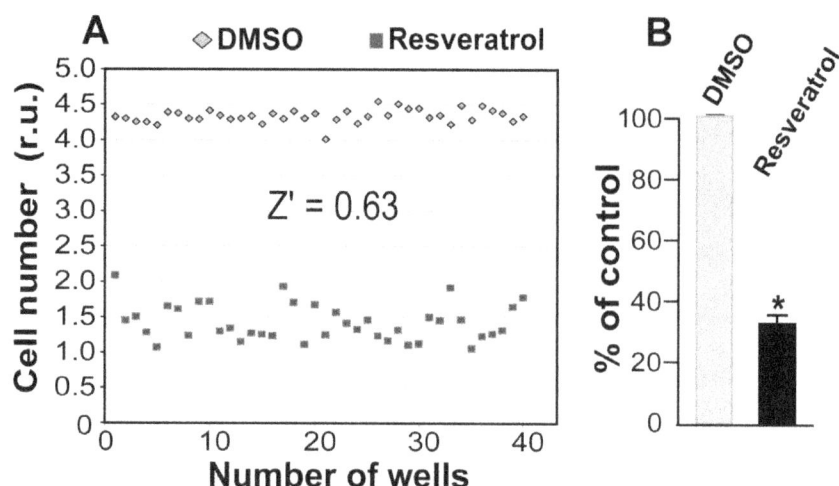

Figure 1. Test of reproducibility of the automated 96-well proliferation assay format. Experiments were performed as described in detail in Materials and Methods. DMSO (40 wells) and resveratrol (40 wells) were used as negative control and positive control, respectively. Data are presented either as Alamar Blue fluorescence reading from individual wells (A), or a mean ± SD (standard deviation) of 40 wells (B) (***P<0.001).

We used a compound concentration of 5 µM. Six 96-well plates were used with 8 wells of negative control (vehicle, DMSO) and 8 wells of positive control (resveratrol) per plate (Figure 2A). The overall signal to background ratio was 5.1±0.4 for all plates. A Z' value for each individual plate was calculated using the mean and SD (see Experimental Procedures) from the negative and positive controls. All of the Z' values were in the range of 0.71–0.89 (Figure 2B). The overall Z' calculated with the data from all six plates was 0.73. Thus the well-to-well and plate-to-plate consistency was high.

Among the 447 tested drugs, 11 inhibited human SMC proliferation more than 50%, producing a hit rate of ~2.5% (Figure 2A). We assumed that drugs providing more than 50% SMC inhibition have the greatest likelihood of inhibiting intimal hyperplasia. We then used the orthologous Cell Titer Glo assay to confirm the 11 positive hits. After removal of the Alamar Blue dye, wells were washed gently, and then subjected to the Cell Titer Glo assay. As shown in Figure S2, the Cell Titer Glo assay produced a pattern of inhibition that was similar to Almar Blue.

Idarubicin Preferentially Inhibits HuAoSMC Versus HuAoEC Proliferation

To identify drugs that selectively inhibit the growth of SMCs versus ECs, we performed the same HTS assay against the NIH Clinical Collection using ECs. Z' values for the endothelial assay calculated from six 96-well plates were all >0.7, indicating an excellent consistency. We then compared percent inhibition of EC proliferation to that of SMC proliferation for the 11 hits from the SMC assay. As shown in Figure 3A, 5 of the compounds inhibited ECs more than SMCs. We concurrently also evaluated rapamycin, a clinicially used inhibitor of intimal hyperplasia (Figure 3B). Consistent with the propensity for rapamycin-coated stents to induce thrombosis secondary to inhibition of re-endothelialization, rapamycin also inhibited EC proliferation to a much greater degree than SMC proliferation. Four of the 11 compounds (cervistatin, triptolide, dactinomycin, and SDM25N) inhibited EC and SMC proliferation to an approximately equal degree. However, two of the 11 compounds inhibited EC proliferation to a lesser degree than that of SMCs. The first of these compounds, homoharringtonine, was associated with a small,

approximately 10% advantage for ECs. In contrast to the other 10 hits, idarubucin stood out as a unique drug that demonstrated significant selectivity between SMCs and ECs. That is, idarubicin reduced SMC proliferation by ~60% but suppressed EC growth by only ~20% (Figure 3A). Since the HTS assays were conducted at a single drug concentration (5 µM) which is conventionally used for primary screens, we created idarubicin dose-response curves for proliferation of both SMCs and ECs using the protocol from our HTS assays. Resveratrol dose-response curves were also generated for comparison. Blending together dose response curves for the two cell types (Figure 4A) revealed a concentration window of ~10 nM-5 µM, where idarubicin preferentially inhibited SMC (IC50 = 0.13 µM) versus EC proliferation (IC50 = 0.61 µM). In contrast, within a concentration range of 1 nM–100 µM resveratrol did not produce differential inhibition of SMC versus EC proliferation (Figure 4B).

Locally Administered Idarubicin Inhibits Intimal Hyperplasia but not Re-endothelialization in Rat Carotid Arteries Following Balloon Injury

Idarubincin is a drug used for treating leukemia, but whether it has an inhibitory effect on intimal hyperplasia has not been reported. Prompted by its favorable property of selectively inhibiting SMC proliferation, we evaluated the ability of idarubicin to suppress intimal hyperplasia using an established rat carotid angioplasty model of restenosis (which mimics the post-angioplasty pathology in humans). In order to minimize undesirable side effects that could result from systemic drug delivery, we administered idarubicin locally around the common carotid artery following injury by balloon angioplasty. The morphometric data show that on day 14 after angioplasty, an aggressive neointimal plaque develops (see vehicle control, Figure 5A). However, arteries treated with idarubicin were found to have an 80% reduction in intimal hyperplasia (Figure 5B and C) compared to vehicle control. Moreover, the relative lumen size (calculated as a ratio of luminal area versus IEL area [26]) of arteries treated with idarubicin was substantially increased compared to vehicle control (approximately 45%, Figure 5D). No significant effect of idarubicin on arterial remodeling (EEL length) was observed (Figure 5E).

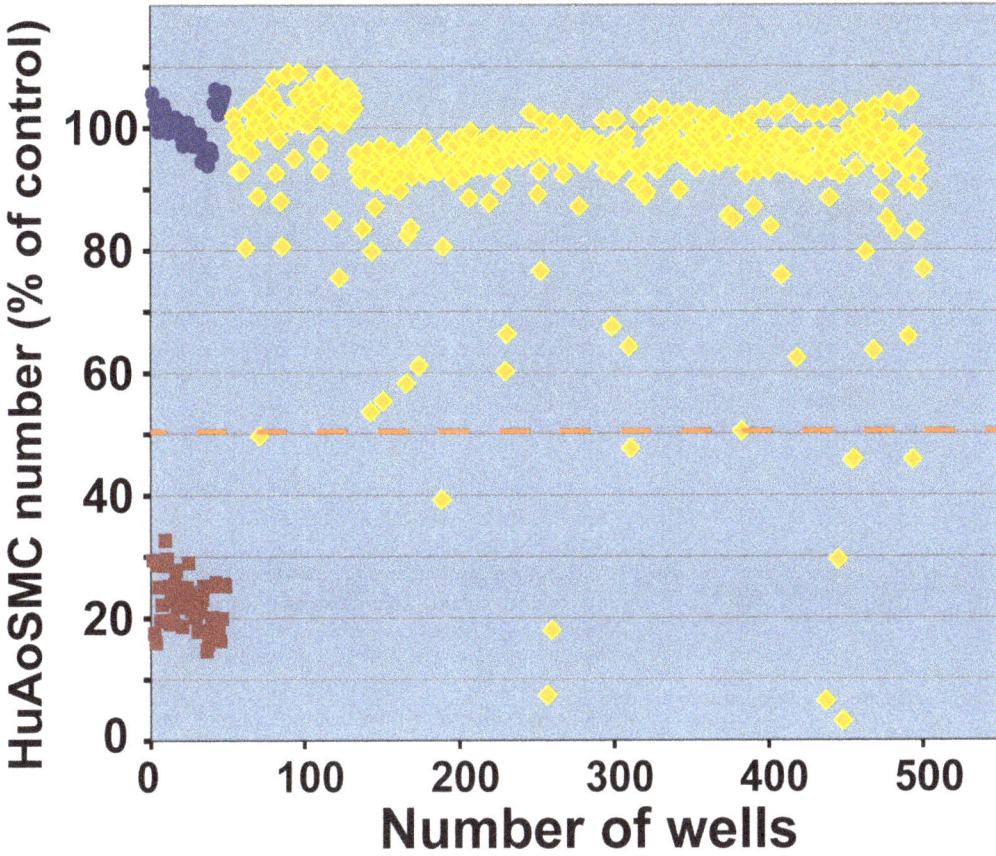

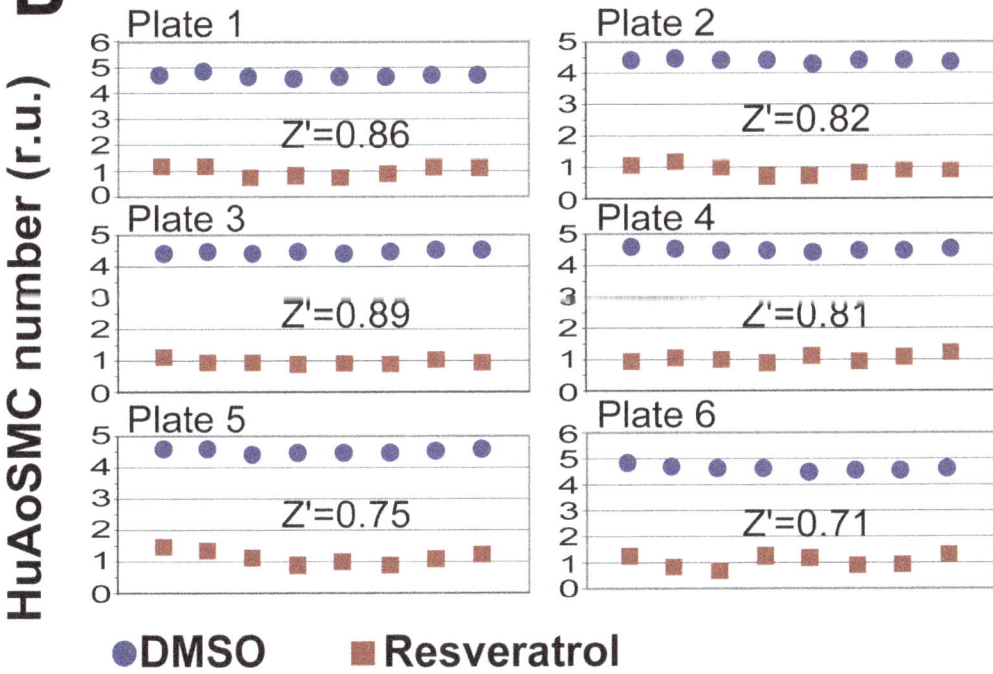

Figure 2. HTS against the NIH Clinical Collection for HuAoSMC proliferation. Assays were performed with SMCs using the automated assay system as described in detail in Materials and Methods. DMSO (blue, final 0.05% in each of 8 wells) and resveratrol (red, final 50 µM in each of 8 wells) served as negative control and positive control, respectively, on each of six 96-well plates. Total 447 compounds in the NIH Clinical Collection (yellow) were tested at a final concentration of 5 µM (1 well for each drug). *For confirmation of the hits with a different method (Cell Titer Glo), please see Figure S2.* **A**). Percent Alamar Blue fluorescence reading. The dashed line marks 50% inhibition of SMC proliferation. **B**). Consistency of HTS assay on each of six 96-well plates.

In our *in vitro* experiments idarubicin differentially inhibited SMC proliferation with a lesser effect on ECs (Figures 3 and 4). With this in mind, we further explored whether idarubicin could spare the endothelial layer while attenuating the growth of the neointima. Using the carotid artery sections collected on day 14 following angioplasty, we performed immunostaining for CD31 (Figure 6, A–C), a commonly used marker for assessment of the endothelium. Quantification of CD31 staining indicated that a similar extent of re-endothelialization was achieved in idarubicin-treated arteries compared to that in vehicle-treated arteries (Figure 6D). This result suggests that idarubicin as a potent inhibitor of SMC proliferation and intimal hyperplasia does not impose a significant inhibitory effect on the endothelial recovery after angioplasty denudation.

Discussion

The anti-restenosis drugs currently available for clinical use inhibit vascular SMC proliferation, migration and survival, but also suppress growth, mobility and survival of ECs [31]. The latter results in adverse side effects, such as delayed re-endothelialization and late stent thrombosis, compromising the long-term efficacy of these treatments [8,32]. Despite the efficacy of these drugs in preventing restenosis, 15% of patients still develop recurrent disease. The lack of an endothelial lining has been shown to propagate intimal hyperplasia. Thus drugs that do not inhibit re-endothelialization may be more effective in preventing restenosis. The ideal drug designed to prevent restenosis should have a selective anti-proliferative effect on SMCs, but be inert toward ECs. Such candidate drugs could be identified through cellular assay-based high throughput screening (HTS). However, in PubChem or the literature there is a lack of reports of HTS campaigns with the goal of identifying compounds that differentially inhibit SMC versus EC proliferation.

In this study, using relevant primary human SMCs and ECs, we have demonstrated good reproducibility of an automated HTS assay system. We have used this system to screen the NIH Clinical Collection of 447 compounds and identified 11 that produced greater than 50% inhibition of SMC proliferation. Among these hits idarubicin exhibited the unique feature of preferentially inhibiting SMC versus EC proliferation. Moreover, idarubicin had a profound effect on intimal hyperplasia without affecting re-endothelialization, a novel role for a drug that is currently clinically used to treat leukemia. Our study demonstrates the feasibility of using HTS to identify compounds that inhibit the proliferation of SMCs while minimally affecting EC growth. In addition, our HTS format is scalable to large compound libraries, opening the pathway for discovery of additional compounds that differentially affect SMC and EC function.

Vascular SMCs and ECs share many similarities. However, there is also evidence in the literature supporting the existence of pathways and targets that are differentially important to proliferation of SMCs versus ECs. For example, the oligo inhibitors of miRNA-221/222 have been reported to inhibit rat aortic SMC proliferation but stimulate human umbilical vein endothelial cell (HUVEC) growth [18]. Following delivery through intraluminal infusion and also periadventitial administration, these inhibitors

were found to suppress post-angioplasty intimal hyperplasia but not re-endothelialization in rats [18]. Different expression levels of the target genes of miR-221/222 in SMCs and ECs might account for differential cellular effects of miR221/222 in these two cell types. In another report, local gene transfer of p85αPKA reduced neointimal formation without affecting endothelial regeneration after balloon injury in rats [33]. The authors found that cAMP inhibits vascular SMC proliferation through the phosphorylation of (Ser83) p85α, which forms an inhibitory complex with p21^{ras}, preventing ERK1/2 activation. However, cAMP-induced cell cycle inhibition of ECs is independent of cAMP/PKA modification of p85α. In addition, activation of AMPK has been shown to inhibit SMC proliferation and intimal hyperplasia in a mouse wire injury model while preserving the endothelial layer [34]. Interestingly, expressing AMPK in ECs in a cell type-specific manner stimulates EC growth through up-regulation of HO-1 [35], suggesting differential pathways targeted by AMPK in these two cell types. Aside from differential signaling pathways in SMCs and ECs, differential drug uptake by these two cell types could also explain the varying effects of a particular drug on growth. Since idarubicin inhibits cell growth by intercalating DNA (a universal pathway in all cells) it is likely that differential uptake of idarubicin rather than differential targets/pathways in SMCs and ECs is responsible for the selective inhibition of SMC versus EC proliferation.

These findings suggest that it is possible to identify drugs that differentially inhibit SMCs versus ECs. To this end, we have established a 96-well HTS format through test assays using resveratrol as a control drug and pilot screens using human SMCs and ECs. We began by optimizing cell number, treatment times and liquid handling protocols to maximize the signal to background ratio and Z' (See Figure S1). The Alamar Blue method has been successfully applied in HTS studies with the major advantage of reducing cost per well [21,29]. Our findings with Alamar Blue were confirmed with Cell Titer Glo assay, uniformly demonstrating more significant inhibition of SMC proliferation with each of the compounds tested (Figure S2) [30]. Thus for future scale-up screens it is advisable to use Alamar Blue for the primary assay and Cell Titer Glo as the orthologous assay to confirm hits. Although the results reported herewith are with a 96-well format we have recently shown that the assay can be readily converted to a format using 384-well plates [36,37]. Alternatively, as indicated by the high reproducibility of assays in this study, HTS of larger libraries can be implemented using the 96-well format.

While a HTS format of one well per compound is widely used in the literature, the rationale for using this format in our HTS study is several fold. First, prior to HTS we used 40 wells for each of the positive and negative controls to specifically determine well-to-well variation. A value of Z' (0.65) above 0.5 indicated an excellent well-to-well consistency. Second, upon HTS assays we again confirmed a low variation between wells on each plate using 8 wells for each of the positive and negative controls (Z'>0.7, Figure 2B). Thus the high Z's suggest that possible errors in negative or positive hits were minor. Moreover, we performed parallel HTS of the same library with ECs to effectively narrow

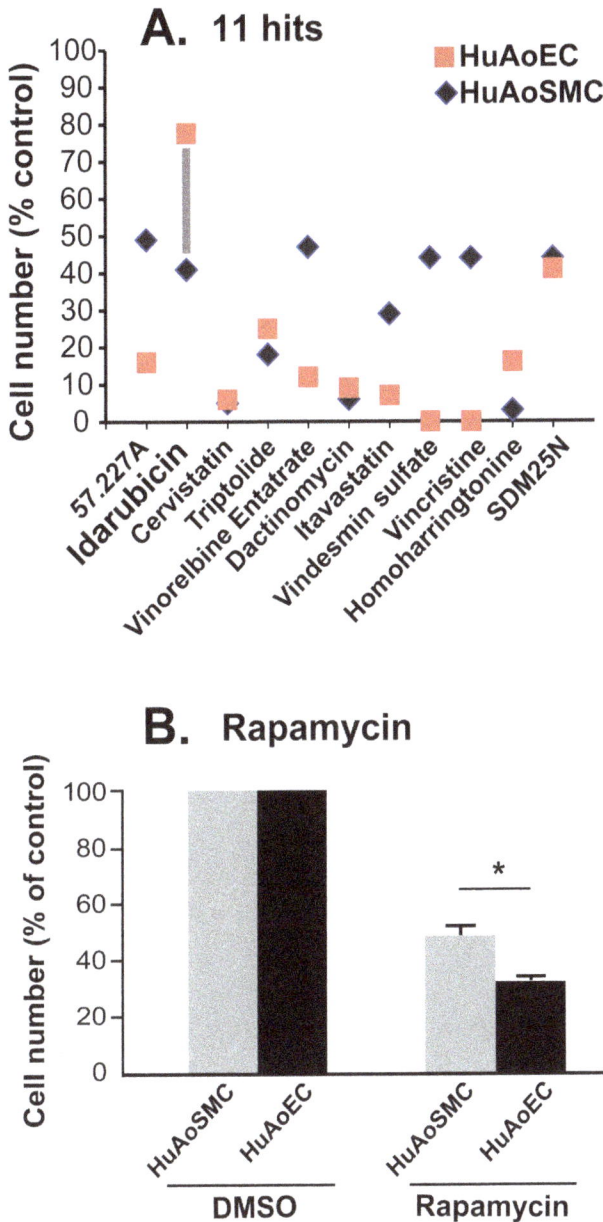

Figure 3. Differential inhibition of HuAoSMC versus HuAoEC proliferation by the 11 hits selected from the NIH Clinical Collection. A). HTS of the NIH Clinical Collection was performed using SMCs as well as ECs, as described for Figure 2. Percent inhibition of SMC proliferation (Black) by the 11 hits was compared with that of EC proliferation (red). The vertical bar highlights greater inhibition of SMC versus EC proliferation by idarubicin, which is opposite to the effect of most of the other hits. **B).** Inhibition of cell proliferation by rapamycin was compared between HuAoSMCs and HuAoECs. The experiment was performed using the automated assay system as described in Figure 1. Rapamycin was added to a final concentration of 200 nM. Cell number was assessed by Cell Titer Glo assay. Each bar represents a mean ± SD (*P<0.05).

Figure 4. Dose-responses of HuAoSMCs and HuAoECs to idarubicin treatment. Proliferation of SMCs or ECs in the presence of various concentrations of idarubicin or resveratrol was assayed in a 96-well plate and handled by the same robotic system as described in Materials and Methods. Each data point is a mean ± SD of triplicates, *P<0.05.

down the number of hits thus minimizing potential positive hit errors (Figure 3A). Finally, dose response determination provided a definitive measure to confirm a preferential effect of the lead hit (idarubicin) on inhibition of SMC versus EC proliferation in a range of concentrations (Figure 4A).

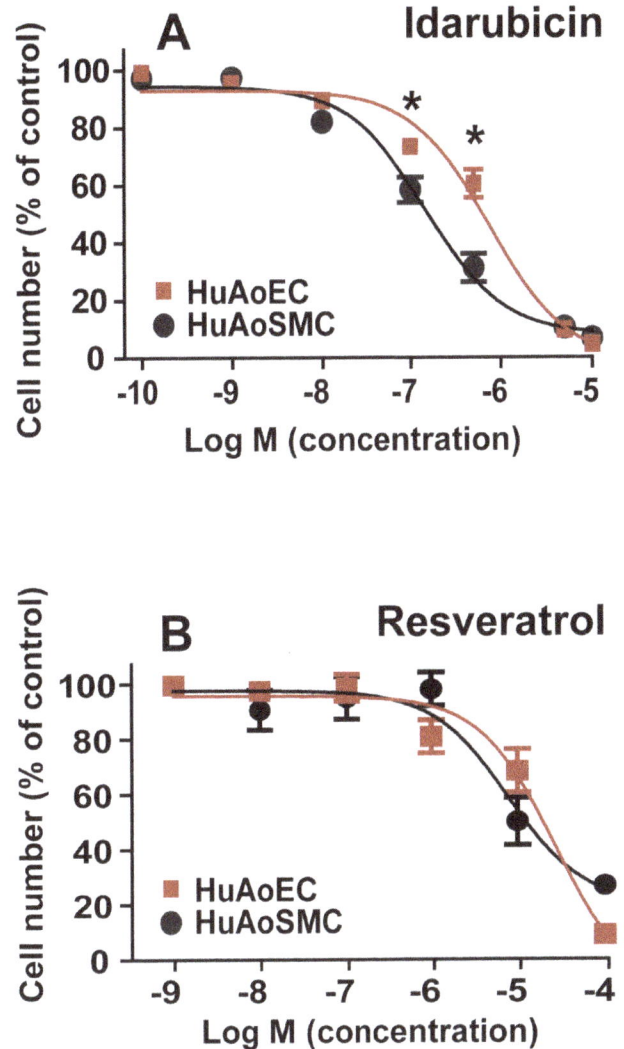

In our screening of the NIH clinical collection our initial hit rate was 2.5%. Factors contributing to the initial hit rate include final concentration of tested compounds, the chosen library, sensitivity of assay method, and the threshold for selecting hits etc. In the primary screen we used a relatively low drug concentration (5 μM) to minimize nonspecific drug effects. In addition, 50% inhibition of SMC proliferation measured by Alamar Blue (equal to ~80% if measured by Cell Titer Glo, see Figure S2) is a quite stringent threshold. Although we identified only 11 compounds with significant inhibition of SMC proliferation, this rate could easily have been increased by increasing the drug concentration or lowering the threshold or stringency. Another important component of this evaluation is the determination of dose response curves. A given compound's ability to differentially inhibit SMC and EC proliferation will most likely be dependent upon drug concentration. For most compounds extremely high concentrations are likely to produce cytotoxicity regardless of the cell type.

Likewise extremely low concentrations will have only a minimal effect. Thus it is important to search the middle range of concentrations of a given compound for a differential effect on SMC versus EC proliferation. We chose to further evaluate idarubicin because at a concentration of 5 μM there was a differential effect on SMC versus EC proliferation and we found this differential effect persisted through a range of ~10 nM− 5 μM. Other two tested compounds, homoharrinytonine and triptolide, also exhibited a greater inhibition of SMC versus EC proliferation, although the differential effect was only 10% and 3%, respectively. Nevertheless, this differential inhibition may have been more significant at a lesser or greater concentration of these compounds. Thus by creating concentration response curves for all hit compounds one would avoid eliminating hits that inhibit the growth of both cell types at a single concentration but have a differential effect at a concentration other than the one used in the initial screening [38]. Although not necessarily practical for screening large numbers of compounds, the ideal method of evaluating a compound is to perform and compare full concentration response curves for both EC and SMC proliferation.

Through HTS against the NIH Clinical Collection, idarubicin has emerged as an examplary compound demonstrating selective inhibition of SMC versus EC proliferation. Considering that generally inhibitors of proliferation including the clinically used drug, rapamycin, impose a more profound effect on ECs than SMCs (Figure 3B), the findings of a more potent inhibitory effect of idarubicin on SMCs versus EC proliferation is highly desirable. Importantly, in our in vivo study idarubicin proved to be effective in reducing intimal hyperplasia in an established rat carotid angioplasty model of restenosis which mimics post-angioplasty pathology in humans. Idarubicin is an analog of daunorubicin with improved properties over other anthracyclines, including higher lipophilicity and hence better cellular uptake. This drug is FDA-approved for treating childhood acute lymphoblastic leukemia. Recently, idarubincin has entered clinical trials for adult patients with acute myeloid leukemia. Although there is evidence of cardiotoxic effects of idarubicin following systemic delivery [39], its use in the prevention of restenosis would be achieved through local delivery (drug-coated stent [10,40] or balloon [41,42]). Importantly, despite its profound inhibitory effect on intimal

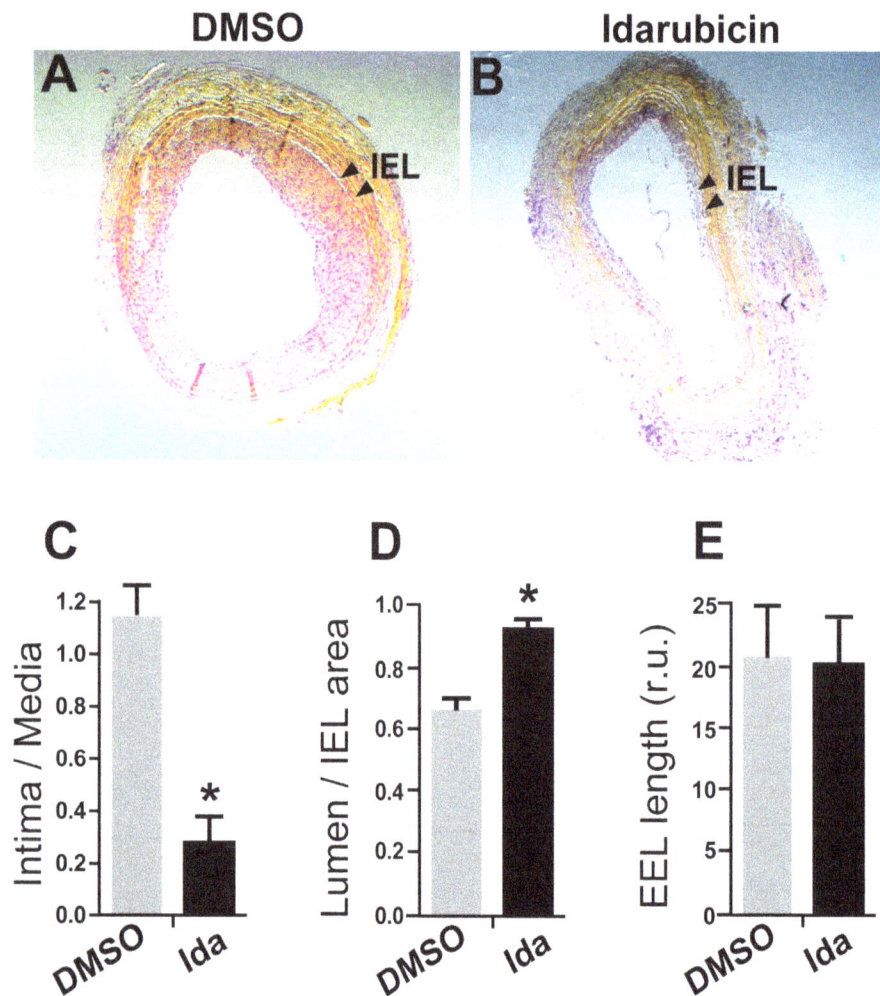

Figure 5. Inhibitory effect of idarubicin on intimal hyperplasia in balloon-injured rat carotid arteries. Following balloon angioplasty, idarubicin was applied locally around the injured arteries. Morphometric analysis was performed on the sections of carotid arteries collected on day 14 post angioplasty, as described in detail in Materials and Methods. Shown in A and B are representative H&E-stained sections from the arteries treated with vehicle (DMSO) and idarubicin, respectively. Arrow heads point to IEL. Statistics of the area ratio of intima versus media (C), residual lumen (the ratio of lumen area versus IEL area) (D), and EEL length (E) were calculated with the data pooled from 5 rats in each treatment group. Each bar represents a mean ± SEM (*P<0.05).

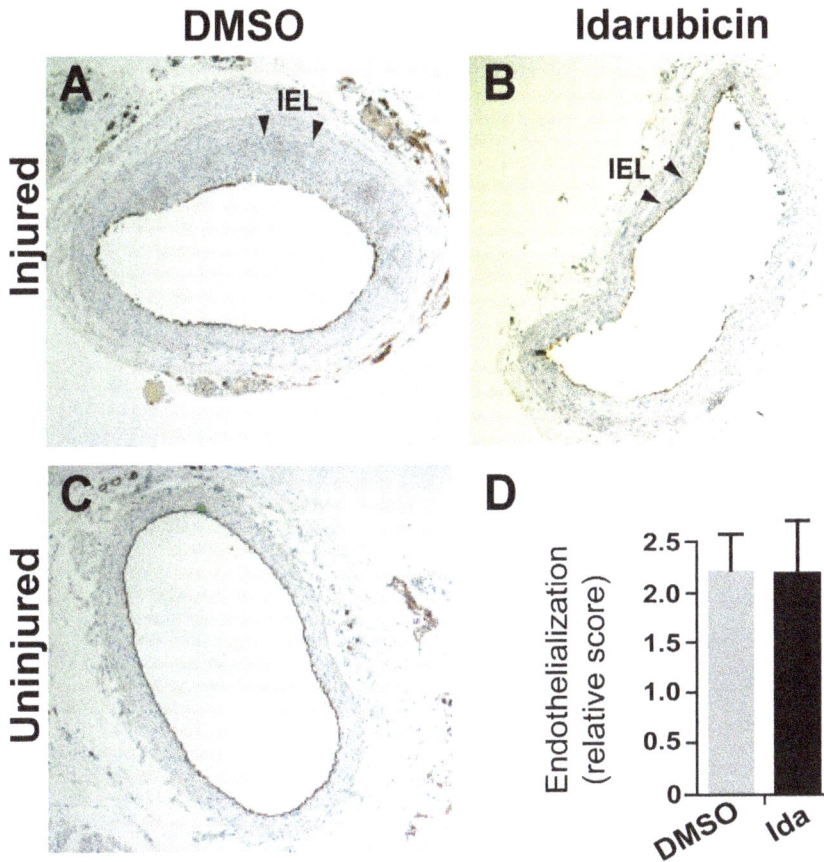

Figure 6. Lack of effect of idarubicin on re-endothelialization in balloon-injured rat carotid arteries. Following balloon angioplasty, idarubicin was applied locally around the injured arteries. For determination of re-endothelialization, immunostaining of CD31 was performed on the sections of carotid arteries collected on day 14 post angioplasty, as described in detail in Materials and Methods. Shown in A and B are representative immunostained sections from the arteries treated with vehicle (DMSO) and idarubicin, respectively. Arrow heads point to IEL. A section of uninjured right carotid artery (C) shows CD31 staining of the undisrupted endothelial layer (see the brown circle). The relative score of re-endothelialization (stained versus total circumference) was quantified with the data pooled from 5 rats in each treatment group (D). Each bar represents a mean ± SEM.

hyperplasia, idarubicin did not have a significant effect on re-endothelialization, which is consistent with our *in vitro* findings demonstrating preferential inhibition of SMC versus EC proliferation (Figure 4A). Thus, further characterization of idarubicin for its potential in treating restenosis is warranted.

While the HTS approach with two human cell types is promising for discovering novel functions of known drugs or potential novel drugs, there are limitations in the current study. A major one is the complexity to translate *in vitro* results into desired *in vivo* outcomes. For example, it is not readily practical to recapitulate the SMC/EC interactions *in vitro* in order to precisely understand their *in vivo* functions or differential responses to drug treatment. Moreover, considering drug diffusion to the greater perivascular space, tissue barriers for drug permeability into SMCs, and drug decomposition over time *etc.*, majority of the perivascularly administered drug would not be able to reach SMCs in the vessel wall. Thus an *in vivo* dose in great excess over an effective dose derived from *in vitro* studies may be necessary. Ideally, different amounts of drug would be tested *in vivo* for finding an optimal dose. Even though we have obtained a favorable effect of idarubicin on inhibition of intimal hyperplasia in the rat carotid injury model, it remains a question whether this outcome can be translated to human patients. In future studies, it will be necessary to use a porcine coronary model [42] which is

close to human restenotic conditions to further examine the anti-restenotic efficacy of idarubicin. Nevertheless, combined use of our HTS system and an established rat restenosis model constitutes a viable platform for identifying lead compounds that may potentially develop into effective therapeutics.

In sum, using human vascular cells we have established the first HTS format that is adaptable to large-scale screening with a specific goal of discovering novel compounds that selectively inhibit SMC versus EC proliferation. We have demonstrated the validity of this HTS assay, through a screen against the NIH Clinical Library and Idarubicin was identified as a selective drug that preferentially suppresses SMC versus EC growth both *in vitro* and *in vivo*. The HTS protocol developed herewith can be used to screen large libraries for compounds that inhibit SMC proliferation with no or reduced effect on ECs. The hits from these screens may generate new compounds that can be translated into therapeutics for the prevention of intimal hyperplasia while allowing re-endothelialization (the desired properties for the next-generation anti-restenotic drugs). Since mechanisms for selective inhibition of SMC versus EC proliferation are not well understood [18], new selective drugs will provide valuable tools for elucidating the intracellular pathways and targets that are differentially important for proliferation of human vascular SMCs versus ECs. Moreover, by screening more diverse libraries we may identify compounds that have properties more favorable than idarubicin, *e.g.* a wider concentration window for selective inhibition of SMCs versus ECs. Ultimately, further screening studies based on our HTS format using human SMCs and ECs will allow the discovery of highly selective and potent small molecule drugs for the purpose of developing safe, efficacious treatments for vascular restenosis.

Supporting Information

Figure S1   Time courses of the growth of HuAoSMCs seeded at different densities. SMCs were seeded at 1000 (blue), 2000 (green), or 3000 (red) cells/well on a 96-well plate, and cultured in SmGM-2 supplemented with 5% serum. Alamar Blue dye was added at different time points (to separate wells) and after a 24 h continued incubation fluorescence was read. A background reading from cell-free wells was subtracted.

Figure S2   Re-test of the initial hits from the HTS using Cell Titer Glo assay. Following the HTS assay of HuAoSMC proliferation, Alamar Blue dye was removed and the wells were gently washed by the automated system. The plates were then subjected to Cell Titer Glo assay, and percent inhibition of SMC proliferation by some of the initial 11 hits was compared between these two different assay methods.

Acknowledgments

We thank Dr. Xu-Dong Shi, Dr. Daniel DiRenzo, Dr. Toshio Takayama, and Dr. Bo Liu for helpful discussions.

Author Contributions

Conceived and designed the experiments: LWG S. Goel FMH KCK. Performed the experiments: S. Goel LWG BW S. Guo DR. Analyzed the data: LWG S. Goel GA FMH KCK. Contributed reagents/materials/ analysis tools: FMH. Wrote the paper: LWG KCK.

References

1. Mills B, Robb T, Larson DF (2012) Intimal hyperplasia: slow but deadly. Perfusion 27: 520–528.
2. Suwanabol PA, Kent KC, Liu B (2011) TGF-beta and restenosis revisited: a Smad link. J Surg Res 167: 287–297.
3. Iakovou I, Schmidt T, Bonizzoni E, Ge L, Sangiorgi GM, et al. (2005) Incidence, predictors, and outcome of thrombosis after successful implantation of drug-eluting stents. JAMA: the journal of the American Medical Association 293: 2126–2130.
4. Curcio A, Torella D, Coppola C, Mongiardo A, Cireddu M, et al. (2002) Coated stents: a novel approach to prevent in-stent restenosis. Italian heart journal: official journal of the Italian Federation of Cardiology 3 Suppl 4: 16S–19S.
5. Simon DI (2012) Inflammation and vascular injury. Circulation journal: official journal of the Japanese Circulation Society 76: 1811–1818.
6. Togni M, Windecker S, Cocchia R, Wenaweser P, Cook S, et al. (2005) Sirolimus-eluting stents associated with paradoxic coronary vasoconstriction. J Am Coll Cardiol 46: 231–236.
7. Mills B, Robb T, Larson DF (2012) Intimal Hyperplasia: slow but deadly. Perfusion.
8. Curcio A, Torella D, Indolfi C (2011) Mechanisms of smooth muscle cell proliferation and endothelial regeneration after vascular injury and stenting: approach to therapy. Circulation journal: official journal of the Japanese Circulation Society 75: 1287–1296.
9. Windecker S, Remondino A, Eberli FR, Juni P, Raber L, et al. (2005) Sirolimus-eluting and paclitaxel-eluting stents for coronary revascularization. The New England journal of medicine 353: 653–662.
10. Mehilli J, Byrne RA, Tiroch K, Pinieck S, Schulz S, et al. (2010) Randomized trial of paclitaxel- versus sirolimus-eluting stents for treatment of coronary restenosis in sirolimus-eluting stents: the ISAR-DESIRE 2 (Intracoronary Stenting and Angiographic Results: Drug Eluting Stents for In-Stent Restenosis 2) study. J Am Coll Cardiol 55: 2710–2716.
11. Inoue T, Croce K, Morooka T, Sakuma M, Node K, et al. (2011) Vascular inflammation and repair: implications for re-endothelialization, restenosis, and stent thrombosis. JACC Cardiovascular interventions 4: 1057–1066.
12. Giordano A, Romano S, Monaco M, Sorrentino A, Corcione N, et al. (2012) Differential effect of atorvastatin and tacrolimus on proliferation of vascular smooth muscle and endothelial cells. Am J Physiol Heart Circ Physiol 302: H135–142.
13. Sun L, Zhao R, Zhang L, Zhang T, Xin W, et al. (2012) Salvianolic acid A inhibits PDGF-BB induced vascular smooth muscle cell migration and proliferation while does not constrain endothelial cell proliferation and nitric oxide biosynthesis. Molecules 17: 3333–3347.
14. Vallieres K, Petitclerc E, Laroche G (2009) On the ability of imatinib mesylate to inhibit smooth muscle cell proliferation without delaying endothelialization: an in vitro study. Vascular pharmacology 51: 50–56.
15. Hacker TA, Griffin MO, Guttormsen B, Stoker S, Wolff MR (2007) Platelet-derived growth factor receptor antagonist STI571 (imatinib mesylate) inhibits human vascular smooth muscle proliferation and migration in vitro but not in vivo. J Invasive Cardiol 19: 269–274.
16. Yoon JW, Cho BJ, Park HS, Kang SM, Choi SH, et al. (2012) Differential effects of trimetazidine on vascular smooth muscle cell and endothelial cell in response to carotid artery balloon injury in diabetic rats. International journal of cardiology.
17. Forte A, Grossi M, Turczynska KM, Svedberg K, Rinaldi B, et al. (2013) Local inhibition of ornithine decarboxylase reduces vascular stenosis in a murine model of carotid injury. International journal of cardiology 168: 3370–3380.
18. Liu X, Cheng Y, Yang J, Xu L, Zhang C (2012) Cell-specific effects of miR-221/222 in vessels: molecular mechanism and therapeutic application. J Mol Cell Cardiol 52: 245–255.
19. Yao EH, Fukuda N, Ueno T, Matsuda H, Nagase H, et al. (2009) A pyrrole-imidazole polyamide targeting transforming growth factor-beta1 inhibits restenosis and preserves endothelialization in the injured artery. Cardiovasc Res 81: 797–804.
20. Breen DM, Dolinsky VW, Zhang H, Ghanim H, Guo J, et al. (2012) Resveratrol inhibits neointimal formation after arterial injury through an endothelial nitric oxide synthase-dependent mechanism. Atherosclerosis 222: 375–381.
21. Nociari MM, Shalev A, Benias P, Russo C (1998) A novel one-step, highly sensitive fluorometric assay to evaluate cell-mediated cytotoxicity. Journal of immunological methods 213: 157–167.
22. Zhang JH, Chung TD, Oldenburg KR (1999) A Simple Statistical Parameter for Use in Evaluation and Validation of High Throughput Screening Assays. Journal of biomolecular screening 4: 67–73.
23. Kundi R, Hollenbeck ST, Yamanouchi D, Herman BC, Edlin R, et al. (2009) Arterial gene transfer of the TGF-beta signalling protein Smad3 induces adaptive remodelling following angioplasty: a role for CTGF. Cardiovasc Res 84: 326–335.
24. Ji R, Cheng Y, Yue J, Yang J, Liu X, et al. (2007) MicroRNA expression signature and antisense-mediated depletion reveal an essential role of MicroRNA in vascular neointimal lesion formation. Circ Res 100: 1579–1588.
25. Kingston PA, Sinha S, Appleby CE, David A, Verakis T, et al. (2003) Adenovirus-mediated gene transfer of transforming growth factor-beta3, but not transforming growth factor-beta1, inhibits constrictive remodeling and reduces luminal loss after coronary angioplasty. Circulation 108: 2819–2825.
26. Nugent HM, Rogers C, Edelman ER (1999) Endothelial implants inhibit intimal hyperplasia after porcine angioplasty. Circ Res 84: 384–391.
27. Tian W, Kuhlmann MT, Pelisek J, Scobioala S, Quang TH, et al. (2006) Paclitaxel delivered to adventitia attenuates neointima formation without compromising re-endothelialization after angioplasty in a porcine restenosis model. Journal of endovascular therapy: an official journal of the International Society of Endovascular Specialists 13: 616–629.
28. Brown MA, Zhang L, Levering VW, Wu JH, Satterwhite LL, et al. (2010) Human umbilical cord blood-derived endothelial cells reendothelialize vein grafts and prevent thrombosis. Arterioscler Thromb Vasc Biol 30: 2150–2155.
29. Antczak C, Shum D, Escobar S, Bassit B, Kim E, et al. (2007) High-throughput identification of inhibitors of human mitochondrial peptide deformylase. Journal of biomolecular screening 12: 521–535.
30. Sachsenmeier KF, Hay C, Brand E, Clarke L, Rosenthal K, et al. (2012) Development of a novel ectonucleotidase assay suitable for high-throughput screening. Journal of biomolecular screening 17: 993–998.
31. Wessely R, Schomig A, Kastrati A (2006) Sirolimus and Paclitaxel on polymer-based drug-eluting stents: similar but different. J Am Coll Cardiol 47: 708–714.
32. Hofma SH, van der Giessen WJ, van Dalen BM, Lemos PA, McFadden EP, et al. (2006) Indication of long-term endothelial dysfunction after sirolimus-eluting stent implantation. European heart journal 27: 166–170.
33. Torella D, Gasparri C, Ellison GM, Curcio A, Leone A, et al. (2009) Differential regulation of vascular smooth muscle and endothelial cell proliferation in vitro and in vivo by cAMP/PKA-activated p85alphaPI3K. Am J Physiol Heart Circ Physiol 297: H2015–2025.
34. Song P, Wang S, He C, Liang B, Viollet B, et al. (2011) AMPKalpha2 deletion exacerbates neointima formation by upregulating Skp2 in vascular smooth muscle cells. Circ Res 109: 1230–1239.

35. Li FY, Lam KS, Tse HF, Chen C, Wang Y, et al. (2012) Endothelium-selective activation of AMP-activated protein kinase prevents diabetes mellitus-induced impairment in vascular function and reendothelialization via induction of heme oxygenase-1 in mice. Circulation 126: 1267–1277.

36. Ewald JA, Peters N, Desotelle JA, Hoffmann FM, Jarrard DF (2009) A high-throughput method to identify novel senescence-inducing compounds. Journal of biomolecular screening 14: 853–858.

37. Tomasini-Johansson BR, Johnson IA, Hoffmann FM, Mosher DF (2012) Quantitative microtiter fibronectin fibrillogenesis assay: use in high throughput screening for identification of inhibitor compounds. Matrix biology: journal of the International Society for Matrix Biology.

38. Mukadam S, Tay S, Tran D, Wang L, Delarosa EM, et al. (2012) Evaluation of time-dependent cytochrome p450 inhibition in a high-throughput, automated assay: introducing a novel area under the curve shift approach. Drug metabolism letters 6: 43–53.

39. Volkova M, Russell R 3rd (2011) Anthracycline cardiotoxicity: prevalence, pathogenesis and treatment. Current cardiology reviews 7: 214–220.

40. Gertz ZM, Wilensky RL (2011) Local drug delivery for treatment of coronary and peripheral artery disease. Cardiovascular therapeutics 29: e54–66.

41. Werk M, Langner S, Reinkensmeier B, Boettcher HF, Tepe G, et al. (2008) Inhibition of restenosis in femoropopliteal arteries: paclitaxel-coated versus uncoated balloon: femoral paclitaxel randomized pilot trial. Circulation 118: 1358–1365.

42. Cremers B, Schmitmeier S, Clever YP, Gershony G, Speck U, et al. (2013) Inhibition of neo-intimal hyperplasia in porcine coronary arteries utilizing a novel paclitaxel-coated scoring balloon catheter. Catheterization and cardiovascular interventions: official journal of the Society for Cardiac Angiography & Interventions.

23

Improvement in Prediction of Coronary Heart Disease Risk over Conventional Risk Factors Using SNPs Identified in Genome-Wide Association Studies

Jennifer L. Bolton[1]*, Marlene C. W. Stewart[1], James F. Wilson[1,2], Niall Anderson[1], Jackie F. Price[1]

1 Centre for Population Health Sciences, Medical School, Teviot Place, University of Edinburgh, Edinburgh, United Kingdom, 2 MRC Institute of Genetics and Molecular Medicine, University of Edinburgh, Western General Hospital, Edinburgh, United Kingdom

Abstract

Objective: We examined whether a panel of SNPs, systematically selected from genome-wide association studies (GWAS), could improve risk prediction of coronary heart disease (CHD), over-and-above conventional risk factors. These SNPs have already demonstrated reproducible associations with CHD; here we examined their use in long-term risk prediction.

Study Design and Setting: SNPs identified from meta-analyses of GWAS of CHD were tested in 840 men and women aged 55–75 from the Edinburgh Artery Study, a prospective, population-based study with 15 years of follow-up. Cox proportional hazards models were used to evaluate the addition of SNPs to conventional risk factors in prediction of CHD risk. CHD was classified as myocardial infarction (MI), coronary intervention (angioplasty, or coronary artery bypass surgery), angina and/or unspecified ischaemic heart disease as a cause of death; additional analyses were limited to MI or coronary intervention. Model performance was assessed by changes in discrimination and net reclassification improvement (NRI).

Results: There were significant improvements with addition of 27 SNPs to conventional risk factors for prediction of CHD (NRI of 54%, $P<0.001$; C-index 0.671 to 0.740, $P=0.001$), as well as MI or coronary intervention, (NRI of 44%, $P<0.001$; C-index 0.717 to 0.750, $P=0.256$). ROC curves showed that addition of SNPs better improved discrimination when the sensitivity of conventional risk factors was low for prediction of MI or coronary intervention.

Conclusion: There was significant improvement in risk prediction of CHD over 15 years when SNPs identified from GWAS were added to conventional risk factors. This effect may be particularly useful for identifying individuals with a low prognostic index who are in fact at increased risk of disease than indicated by conventional risk factors alone.

Editor: Momiao Xiong, University of Texas School of Public Health, United States of America

Funding: The EAS was supported by the British Heart Foundation (BHF RG/98002 - R34429). Genotyping for this project was funded by a project grant from the Chief Scientist Office of Scotland (CZB/4/672). Jennifer Bolton was supported by a PhD studentship from the College of Medicine and Veterinary Medicine at the University of Edinburgh, and an Overseas Research Students Award. The funders had no role in study design, data collection and analysis, decision to publish, or preparation of the manuscript.

Competing Interests: The authors have declared that no competing interests exist.

* E-mail: J.Bolton@ed.ac.uk

Introduction

There has been much discussion of personalised medicine and the use of genetic risk scores for identifying people at increased risk for chronic diseases including coronary heart disease (CHD). The expectation is that such individuals might benefit from targeted interventions, thereby reducing their risk of developing disease. The Framingham risk score [1] is the most commonly used method of CHD risk prediction, and has been widely assessed for validity. However, the accuracy of this score differs between populations, commonly over-estimating risk in European countries [2], and overall accuracy is generally low for individuals not at the extremes of risk distributions. Alternative risk prediction models have been developed which incorporate a range of additional risk factors, such as biomarkers [3], socio-economic indicator, or family history [4], but these still have limited predictive power.

Family history is predictive of CHD after adjusting for other conventional risk factors [5,6], and CHD is estimated to be approximately 40–50% heritable [7,8]. Despite this, genetic information has so far generally not resulted in appreciable improvements in prediction over non-genetic risk factors, (apart from monogenic disease). This is likely due in part to the small effects exerted by individual single nucleotide polymorphisms (SNPs) relative to established risk factors; but the selection of SNPs for evaluation, and methods of inclusion in a predictive model, are also likely contributors. Previous genetic risk prediction models have often relied on candidate SNPs that have a known biological role in, or association with, CHD or atherosclerosis [9]. The publication of genome-wide association studies (GWAS) has provided another method for identification of SNPs, independent of known biological function, but based on statistical evidence of association. Models have often used genetic risk scores, basically a sum of the number of risk alleles, which do not take into account the individual effect sizes and assume independence of these alleles.

The primary aim of this analysis was to determine whether a systematically selected panel of SNPs, already found individually to be reproducibly associated with CHD through GWAS, could improve prediction of CHD over and above well established conventional risk factors, thereby contributing additional clinical utility. Since the majority of coronary events occur in individuals with Framingham based risk scores of less than 20% [10], the inclusion of genetic information has the potential to create a more personalised and accurate risk evaluation.

Methods

Study Population

Details of the Edinburgh Artery Study (EAS), have been published previously [11,12]. In brief, the EAS enrolled 1592 men (809) and women (783) aged 54–75 years living in Edinburgh, Scotland. Recruitment used an age-stratified random sample from ten general practices, resulting in a geographical and socio-economic representation of the population of Edinburgh. Clinical examinations were held during 1987/8, and DNA samples were collected at a five year follow-up examination (attended by 1165 (73%) subjects). At time of genotyping for the current study (2009), DNA was available for 856 subjects, of which 840 were successfully genotyped (409 men, 431 women). Reasons for not having a DNA sample included refusal to provide a blood sample or allow genotyping at the 5-year examination, or insufficient sample remaining. Baseline characteristics of the full EAS population and the population used for the current analysis were very similar (Table 1).

Data collection for identification and validation of coronary events at baseline and throughout follow-up included the WHO chest pain questionnaire, ECG (coded using Minnesota Classification Code), self-reported doctor diagnosis of disease, record linkage to hospital discharge data and death certificates, and scrutiny of general practitioner records [12]. Conventional risk factors mea-

sured at baseline included lipids and blood pressure. Complete follow-up was available until June 2003, a mean follow-up of 15 years.

The classification of CHD used in the current analyses was based on validated events and comprised of fatal or non-fatal myocardial infarction (MI), angioplasty, coronary artery bypass surgery, angina and/or unspecified ischaemic heart disease as a cause of death. To reduce the potential for mis-classification, further analyses were restricted to fatal or non-fatal MI or coronary intervention (angioplasty or coronary artery bypass surgery). Family history was also collected at baseline, but was limited to unconfirmed self-reports of MI or angina in a parent.

Ethical Approvals

Ethical approval for the EAS was granted by the Lothian Health Board Medical Research Ethics Committee. Written informed consent was obtained from all participants.

SNP Identification

Selection of SNPs used recent large scale meta-analyses of GWAS of CHD to identify SNPs that have demonstrated reproducible associations with CHD [13,14]. This provided 36 SNPs, of which six were not available on Metabochip (rs10953541, rs1412444, rs17609940, rs216172, rs46522, rs964184) and no proxy was available; rs4977574 was replaced with rs133049 ($r^2 = 0.97$, D' = 1.0). Three SNPs were removed because they were in LD ($r^2 > 0.85$) with other included SNPs (rs646776, rs1199338, rs12526453). Details of SNPs used in prediction models are presented in Table 2 (detailed in Table S1).

Additional SNPs for use in a secondary, exploratory analysis were selected based on nominal significance ($P < 1 \times 10^{-5}$) in GWAS of CVD, significant associations with lipids in GWAS, and/or biological plausibility. This provided an additional 44 SNPs (detailed in Table S2) that were available and successfully genotyped in the study population, resulting in a total set of 74

Table 1. Comparison of baseline characteristics of the EAS population used in genetic risk prediction models and full study population.

	Study population (1592)	Genotyped population (840)
	Mean (95%CI)	Mean (95%CI)
Age at baseline	64.9 (64.6,65.1)	64.4 (64.0,64.8)
Body Mass Index	25.6 (25.4,25.8)	25.5 (25.3,25.8)
Systolic Blood Pressure	144 (143,146)	143 (142,145)
Diastolic Blood Pressure	77 (77,78)	77 (77,78)
Total Cholesterol	7.03 (6.97,7.10)	7.00 (6.99,7.02)
HDL Cholesterol	1.44 (1.42,1.46)	1.45 (1.42,1.50)
LDL Cholesterol	5.28 (5.22,5.34)	5.33 (5.25,5.40)
log(Triglycerides)	0.15 (0.14,0.16)	0.14 (0.13,0.20)
	n (%)	n (%)
Sex Male	809 (51)	409 (49)
Diabetes	288 (18.1)	136 (16.2)
Family History in parent	576 (36.2)	257 (38.0)
Current Smoker	404 (25.4)	182 (21.7)
Previous Smoker	582 (36.6)	315 (37.5)
Never Smoked	561 (35.2)	328 (39.0)

Table 2. SNPs identified from meta-analysis of GWAS of CHD used in risk prediction models.

SNP	Chr	Position (b37)	Gene(s)	Alleles	Minor allele	MAF
rs11206510	1	55,268,627	PCSK9	C/T	C	0.16
rs17114036	1	56,735,409	PPAP2B	A/G	G	0.11
rs599839	1	109,623,689	SORT1	A/G	G	0.28
rs17011666	1	220,865,588	MIA3	A/G	G	0.17
rs17465637	1	220,890,152	MIA3	A/C	A	0.27
rs6725887	2	203,454,130	WDR12	C/T	C	0.16
rs2306374	3	139,602,642	MRAS	C/T	C	0.18
rs1332844	6	12,996,990	PHACTR1	C/T	C	0.39
rs12190287	6	134,256,218	TCF21	C/G	G	0.40
rs3798220	6	160,881,127	LPA	C/T	C	0.00
rs11556924	7	129,450,732	ZC3HC1	C/T	T	0.39
rs1333049	9	22,115,503	CDKN2A,	C/G	C	0.46
rs579459	9	135,143,989	ABO	C/T	C	0.20
rs2505083	10	30,375,128	KIAA1462	C/T	C	0.43
rs1746048	10	44,095,830	CXCL12	C/T	T	0.15
rs12413409	10	104,709,086	CYP17A1, CNNM2, NT5C2	A/G	A	0.08
rs974819	11	103,165,777	PDGFD	C/T	T	0.22
rs3184504	12	110,368,991	SH2B3	C/T	T	0.45
rs4773144	13	109,758,713	COL4A1, COL4A2	A/G	G	0.42
rs2895811	14	99,203,695	HHIPL1	C/T	C	0.42
rs3825807	15	76,876,166	ADAMTS7	A/G	G	0.45
rs4380028	15	76,898,148	ADAMTS7-MORF4L1	C/T	T	0.41
rs12936587	17	17,484,447	RASD1, SMCR3, PEMT	A/G	G	0.47
rs1122608	19	11,024,601	LDLR	G/T	T	0.26
rs2228671	19	11,071,912	LDLR	C/T	T	0.11
rs9982601	21	34,520,998	MRPS6	C/T	T	0.21
rs7278204	21	34,543,235	SLC5A3-MRPS6-KCNE2	A/G	G	0.17

SNPs for use in secondary analysis. This was a more subjectively selected and therefore potentially biased set of SNPs.

Genotyping

Genotyping used the Illumina MetaboChip, from which the chosen SNPs were extracted. Quality control was carried out on the full MetaboChip results, 16 samples with call rates below 75% were excluded. Table S1 reports: call rates, mean genotypic call rate of 97.7% (range 85.5–99.5); Hardy Weinberg Equilibrium (HWE), one SNPs showed deviation from HWE (rs4773144); and minor allele frequencies (MAF), range 3–49%.

Statistical Analysis

Statistical analysis used R version 2.14.0 [15], all p-values were two-sided. Prediction of coronary risk used multivariate adjusted Cox proportional hazards in the *survival* library [16], the assumption of proportional hazards was satisfied for all models. Conventional risk factors were based on the Framingham model [1], and included: sex, baseline age, systolic blood pressure, smoking (Yes/No), diabetes and/or glucose intolerance (Yes/No), and total cholesterol/HDL cholesterol. SNPs were added as covariates to the conventional risk factors, assuming an additive model. This was thought preferable to creation of a single genetic risk score as it allows more influential SNPs to exert more of an

effect on the model, whereas a composite risk score assumes all SNPs have the same effect size. The derived ß coefficients were used to calculate prognostic indices, thereby creating weighted prediction models. Prognostic indices were converted to predicted probabilities as $1-S_0(t)^{exp(PI)}$ [1].

Model performance was evaluated by C-indices, net reclassification indices (NRI), integrated discrimination improvement (IDI), and plotted ROC curves. ROC curves were plotted using the *ROCR* library [17], C-indices, NRI, and IDI used the *Hmisc* library [18]. The C-index used in survival analysis is analogous to area under the ROC curve used in logistic regression, simply it is a measure of the concordance in predicted and observed survival times between subjects [19]. NRI was based on event specific reclassification and used continuous measures rather than categories, which increases statistical power. NRI can be used to compare the clinical impact of different models, simply, it is a comparison of the proportion of subjects with disease who have appropriately increased risk scores with the new model, and the proportion of subjects without disease who have appropriately decreased risk scores with the new model [20]. IDI represents desired improvements in average sensitivity corrected for undesirable increases in 1-specificity, it therefore compared whether the new models improved sensitivity without affecting specificity, as described in Pencina *et al.* (2008). ROC curves are plots of 1-

specificity vs sensitivity, allowing visualisation of changes in discrimination over different sensitivities.

All analyses used first incident events only, subjects with a diagnosis of prevalent CHD at baseline were excluded, as appropriate. Time to event was determined individually for both CHD and fatal or non-fatal MI or coronary intervention, based on appropriate diagnostic criteria. Since models based on different subjects could differ, risk prediction models that were compared contained identical population groups. Power was calculated using the *gap* library [21]. Though underpowered to detect significant associations for individual SNPs, it was hypothesised that a set of SNPs with high prior probability could jointly have a sufficiently large effect size. There was 80% power to detect an effect size of 1.5 with a minor allele frequency (MAF) of 30% in a multiplicative model, at 5% significance with a disease prevalence of 20%.

An exploratory method of selecting SNPs used regression trees in the *rpart* library [22]. To identify SNPs that were informative after conventional risk factors, the residuals of a model containing conventional risk factors were used as the dependent variable. This analysis included the full collection of 74 SNPs as potential covariates. Tree development used the Gini Index as the splitting rule, SNPs were treated as ordinal, and splitting was only considered as dominant or recessive models. Regression trees sequentially selected SNPs that best partitioned subjects into the appropriate group [23]; the sets of SNPs that were identified by the regression trees were then used to develop prediction models.

Results

Risk Prediction Using SNPs with Confirmed Associations with CHD

27 SNPs identified in meta-analysis of GWAS of CHD were successfully genotyped in the EAS population (Table 2), and results of prediction models are summarised in Table 3 (hazard ratios given in Tables S3 and S4). Addition of the 27 SNPs to conventional risk factors in prediction of CHD increased the C-index from 0.671 to 0.740 ($P = 0.001$) and NRI was 54% (95%CI 35–74; $P<0.001$). When restricted to fatal or non-fatal MI or coronary intervention the C-index increased from 0.717 to 0.750 ($P = 0.256$), and NRI was 44% (95%CI 20–67; $P<0.001$). The results were almost identical when family history of CHD was also included in the models.

Plotted ROC curves (Figure 1) showed that addition of SNPs improved prediction over much of the curve for CHD, however for fatal or non-fatal MI or coronary intervention the models performed differently at different sensitivities when SNPs were added; here the addition of SNPs better improved discrimination when the sensitivity of conventional risk factors was lower, translating to improved identification of an individual with a low prognostic index in fact at increased risk of an event. This was mirrored in density plots, in which a second distribution of higher risk scores for subjects with events emerged upon addition of SNPs (Figure S1). Addition of SNPs to conventional risk factors moved 10 subjects to predicted risk ≥20%, and increased the OR of having any CHD given a ≥20% predicted risk increased from 3.86 (95%CI 2.52,5.93) to 5.42 (95%CI 3.54,8.38). When restricted to fatal or non-fatal MI or coronary intervention, 16 subjects moved to predicted risk ≥20%., and the odds ratio of having an event given a ≥20% predicted risk increased from 4.42 (95%CI 1.78,10.46) to 12.18 (95%CI 6.30,24.03).Reclassification tables are presented in Table S5.

Risk Prediction Using SNPs Identified from Regression Trees

The use of regression trees to identify SNPs that explained the remaining variance after consideration of conventional risk factors was a secondary, exploratory approach to developing prediction models. Of the potential 74 SNPs, seven SNPs were found to explain some of the remaining risk of CHD: rs1122608 (*SMARCA1*), rs3798220 (*LPA*), rs780094 (*GCKR*), rs1332844 (*PHACTR1*), rs11668477 (*LDLR*), rs3184504 (*SH2B3*), rs2505083 (*KIAA1462*). When done for fatal or non-fatal MI or coronary intervention, the list of nine predictive SNPs differed: rs780094 (*GCKR*), rs17011666 (*MIA3*), rs11556924 (*ZC3HC1*), rs3798220 (*LPA*), rs4939883 (*LIPG*), rs12413409 (*CNNM2*), rs17145738 (*TBL2/MLXIPL*), rs174570 (*FADS1/2*), rs173539 (*CETP*). Regression trees are shown in Figure S2, model results in Table 3, and ROC curves in Figure S3. Addition of regression tree SNPs to conventional risk factors increased the C-index for prediction of CHD from 0.668 to 0.709, ($P = 0.027$), had a NRI of 42% (95%CI 25,58; $P<0.001$), and moved six subjects with CHD to predicted risk ≥20%. The SNPs predictive of fatal or non-fatal MI or coronary intervention increased the C-index from 0.694 to 0.718 ($P = 0.463$), had a NRI of 43% (95%CI 22,63; $P<0.001$), and moved 15 subjects to predicted risk ≥20%.

Discussion

In this prospective, population-based cohort of men and women from Edinburgh, Scotland, a systematically-selected set of SNPs improved prediction of CHD over 15 years, over-and-above conventional risk factors. A total of 27 SNPs that were significantly associated with CHD, when added to the Framingham-based conventional risk factors of age, sex, SBP, total cholesterol/HDL cholesterol, diabetes and/or glucose intolerance, and smoking, improved prediction as indicated by significant improvements in NRI and C-indices. NRI were used to evaluate the clinical impact of addition of SNPs. Given that an estimated 15–20% of MI occur in individuals considered as lower risk based on conventional risk factors [24], the ability of this genetic model to identify such subjects and increase their predicted risk indicates potential clinical utility. The highest risk category of at least 20% CHD risk was of interest as individuals in this category are often considered suitable for clinical intervention, and the risk of mis-classification is decreased [25]. The appropriate reclassification of subjects to ≥20% predicted risk on addition of SNPs to conventional risk factors suggests that such a model could affect treatment decisions for a number of individuals.

Regression trees were used to evaluate whether a smaller collection of SNPs was sufficient to improve prediction, to account for the possibility that not all SNPs contribute to prediction. This allowed for selection of additional SNPs as it was not expected that GWAS would have sufficient power to identify all associated and/or predictive SNPs. Though regression trees are prone to over-fitting, they were an exploratory method to limit the number of SNPs included in the models. They also provided branching patterns that may show that an effect at one SNP may only occur in the presence of another SNP. This would indicate that only SNPs with independent effects should be included, in order to get more accurate population based risk associated with the SNP.

Previous studies that added candidate SNPs to conventional risk factors, using either genetic risk scores (a count of the number or risk alleles) or weighting of SNPs, have generally not significantly improved model discrimination as measured by C-index. They have however indicated through NRI [26] and/or increased hazard ratios that SNPs could improve risk prediction

Table 3. Incidence, Discrimination, and Calibration Estimates of Models Using Conventional Risk Factors* and GWAS or Regression Tree SNPs in the EAS.

	Concordance	R^2	C-index	NRI (95% CI)	NRI event/ nonevent	IDI (95% CI)
SNPs identified through GWAS of CHD						
CHD (n = 508, 131 incident events)						
Conventional risk factors	0.658	0.081	0.671			
Conventional risk factors & SNPs	0.712	0.137	0.740	54.4 (34.5,74.3)	17.6/36.9	0.04 (0.02,0.06)
Conventional risk factors & Family history	0.658	0.082	0.671			
Conventional risk factors, Family history & SNPs	0.712	0.138	0.741	54.4 (34.5,74.3)	17.6/36.9	0.04 (0.02,0.06)
Fatal or non-fatal MI or coronary intervention (n = 590, 81 incident events)						
Conventional risk factors	0.701	0.062	0.717			
Conventional risk factors & SNPs	0.731	0.106	0.750	43.5 (20.1,67.0)	11.1/32.4	0.05 (0.02,0.08)
Conventional risk factors & Family history	0.702	0.063	0.718			
Conventional risk factors, Family history & SNPs	0.734	0.107	0.753	42.7 (19.3,66.2)	11.1/31.6	0.05 (0.02,0.07)
SNPs identified through Regression Trees						
CHD (n = 663, 180 incident events)						
Conventional risk factors	0.652	0.077	0.686			
Conventional risk factors & SNPs	0.686	0.124	0.709	41.5 (24.6,58.4)	21.5/20.0	0.04 (0.02,0.05)
Fatal or non-fatal MI or coronary intervention (n = 768, 107incident events)						
Conventional risk factors	0.679	0.050	0.694			
Conventional risk factors & SNPs	0.704	0.077	0.718	42.9 (22.5,63.3)	14.0/28.9	0.03 (0.01,0.04)

*Conventional risk factors = Age, Sex, SBP, Total Cholesterol/HDL Cholesterol, Diabetes and/or glucose intolerance, Smoking.
Each analysis used only subjects without a diagnosis at baseline, as appropriate to investigate incident events, and with full genotypic data for included SNPs.

[27,28,29,30,31]; with significant associations reported between incident CHD and genetic risk scores [26,27,28]. Humphries *et al.* (2007) [32] found a significant improvement in C-index in the Northwick Park Heart Study II ($P<0.001$), which was further improved after inclusion of an interaction with smoking ($P = 0.01$).

More recently there have been other studies that used GWAS-identified SNPs in prospective cohorts; these contained many but not all of the GWAS SNPs used in the present analyses. Paynter *et al.* (2010) [6] assessed the predictive ability of adding genetic risk scores to conventional risk factors for prediction of any CVD (MI, stroke, arterial revascularization, and cardiovascular death) in a large

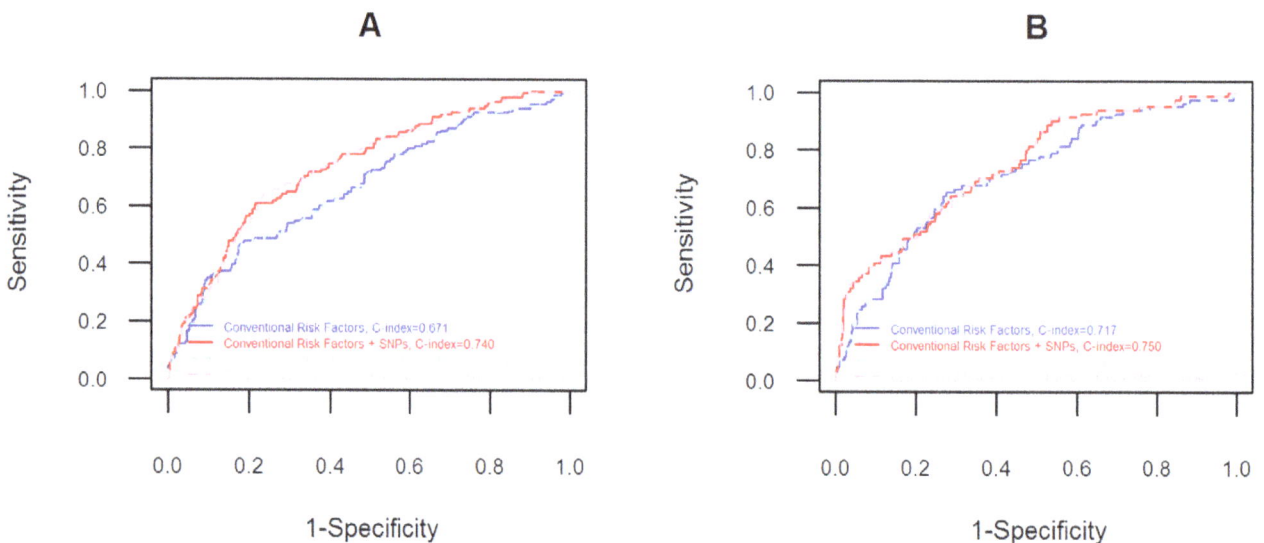

Figure 1. ROC curves of prediction of coronary heart disease when GWAS significant SNPs were added to conventional risk factors.
A: ROC curves for CHD, comprised of fatal or non-fatal MI, angioplasty, coronary artery bypass surgery, angina and/or unspecified ischaemic heart disease as a cause of death; B: ROC curves for diagnoses limited to fatal or non-fatal MI or coronary intervention (angioplasty or coronary artery bypass surgery).

cohort, and found no improvement in discrimination or reclassification. Additionally the investigators found that the genetic risk score alone was not associated with risk of CVD; this may be due to the use of a broader phenotype. Davies *et al.* (2010) [33] assessed the predictive utility for CHD and found a significant improvement in the C-index when SNPs were added to conventional risk scores, from 0.801 to 0.809, ($P = 0.0073$). They additionally found that weighting SNPs led to models that performed better than un-weighted models. Ripatti et al. (2010) [34] also reported an association between incident CHD and genetic risk score after adjusting for conventional risk factors, however this was observed through improvements in IDI and NRI, and did not lead to significant changes in C-index. They also reported that though family history was associated with increased risk of CVD, adjustment for family history did not change the risk estimates of the genetic risk score.

The use of a genetic risk score results in equal weighting of all SNPs, possibly missing relevant information on the relative effects of each SNP within the model [32]. Also, in the development of a model in which covariates are not unrelated, the ß coefficients need to be adjusted to account for the impact covariates have on each other to prevent distortion of the model. ROC curves measure discrimination but are 'insensitive to change' [19,35], however as our curves showed, the changes in risk prediction did not always change consistently over the full range of sensitivities, a large change in one portion of the curve may be clinically relevant but not represented in summary measures. The clinical value was demonstrated by the increased NRI, and subsequent increased odds of subjects with CHD to have predicted risk ≥20%, showing that addition of GWAS SNPs can have clinical applicability.

There were a number of strengths and weaknesses of the current study. A strength of the EAS population was the long follow-up of 15 years, and the prospective method that included regular contact with study participants and general practitioners, as well as use of hospital discharge records and death certificates. This enabled confirmation of reported events, providing accurate phenotypic data and minimising misclassification bias; as well as detailed and accurate records for subjects that died during follow-up, thereby removing survivor bias. Here we found that genetic data was more informative than self-reported family history of CHD. This was possibly due to the difficulty in collecting accurate reports of family history in epidemiological studies, which would also exist clinically and therefore not result in accurate risk prediction.

As the cohort was recruited from Edinburgh only and was primarily white, the risk of population stratification was low. However, the EAS study population was small for a genetic study. There may also have been temporal trends that affected CHD risk and consequently risk prediction, such as smoking habits and primary prevention of CHD. At baseline, medications for CHD risk factors were not as commonly used as recently, and during follow-up a considerable portion of the population were prescribed anti-hypertensive, lipid lowering, and/or diabetes treatments. With such a long follow-up this may have been a confounder that was not accounted for.

This is not a definitive list of predictive SNPs. Further analysis of GWAS and fine mapping is necessary to identify causal SNPs that will be more accurate in risk prediction. There remains the possibility that some of the GWAS significant SNPs did not contribute to risk prediction. It is also likely that there are gene-environment and gene-gene interactions that were not accounted for, for example Humphries *et al.* (2007) found an interaction with smoking [32], and *HMGCR* genotypes may affect lipid lowering responses to statins [36]. Though use of GWAS results removed sources of bias associated with the inclusion of candidate gene

study results, there remain problems specifically associated with GWAS, such as poor representation of low MAF SNPs, that debatably have larger effect sizes [37]. However, we have shown that use of a systematically selected panel of SNPs can significantly improve prediction of CHD risk over-and-above conventional risk factors, indicating that this approach to incorporating genotypic data into prediction models has potential clinical utility.

Supporting Information

Figure S1 Density plots of risk scores in prediction of CHD with addition of GWAS SNPs to conventional risk factors. A: Plots for CHD, comprised of fatal or non-fatal MI, angioplasty, coronary artery bypass surgery, angina and/or unspecified ischaemic heart disease as a cause of death; B: Plots for diagnoses limited to fatal or non-fatal MI or coronary intervention (angioplasty or coronary artery bypass surgery). Solid lines represent density curves of risk scores using conventional risk factors, dotted lines represent density curves of risk scores using conventional risk factors and SNPs.

Figure S2 Regression trees to explain residual variance from models with conventional risk factors in prediction of CHD in the EAS. A: Regression tree derived for CHD, comprised of fatal or non-fatal MI, angioplasty, coronary artery bypass surgery, angina and/or unspecified ischaemic heart disease as a cause of death; B: Regression tree derived for diagnoses limited to fatal or non-fatal MI or coronary intervention (angioplasty or coronary artery bypass surgery).

Figure S3 ROC curves derived from SNPs identified by regression trees to explain residual variance from models with conventional risk factors in prediction of CHD in the EAS. A: ROC curve for CHD, comprised of fatal or non-fatal MI, angioplasty, coronary artery bypass surgery, angina and/or unspecified ischaemic heart disease as a cause of death; B: ROC curve for diagnoses limited to fatal or non-fatal MI or coronary intervention (angioplasty or coronary artery bypass surgery).

Table S1 SNPs with confirmed associations with CHD used in risk prediction models.

Table S2 Additional SNPs Associated with CVD used in regression trees.

Table S3 Hazard ratios for conventional risk factors and SNPs in prediction of fatal or non-fatal MI or coronary intervention.

Table S4 Hazard ratios for conventional risk factors and SNPs in prediction of coronary heart disease.

Table S5 Reclassification of subjects based on a predicted risk of 20%.

Author Contributions

Statistical support: NA. Genetic support: JFW. Conceived and designed the experiments: JFP. Analyzed the data: JLB. Contributed reagents/materials/analysis tools: MCWS. Wrote the paper: JLB.

References

1. Wilson PWF, D'Agostino RB, Levy D, Belanger AM, Silbershatz H, et al. (1998) Prediction of Coronary Heart Disease Using Risk Factor Categories. Circulation 97: 1837–1847.
2. Eichler K, Puhan MA, Steurer J, Bachmann LM (2007) Prediction of first coronary events with the Framingham score: A systematic review. American Heart Journal 153: 722–731.
3. Ridker PM, Brown NJ, Vaughan DE, Harrison DG, Mehta JL (2004) Established and Emerging Plasma Biomarkers in the Prediction of First Atherothrombotic Events. Circulation 109: IV-6-19.
4. Martin C, Taylor P, Potts H (2008) Construction of an odds model of coronary heart disease using published information: the Cardiovascular Health Improvement Model (CHIME). BMC Medical Informatics and Decision Making 8: 49.
5. Schunkert H, Erdmann J, Samani NJ (2010) Genetics of myocardial infarction: a progress report. European Heart Journal 31: 918–925.
6. Paynter NP, Chasman DI, Pare G, Buring JE, Cook NR, et al. (2010) Association Between a Literature-Based Genetic Risk Score and Cardiovascular Events in Women. JAMA 303: 631–637.
7. Zdravkovic S, Wienke A, Pedersen NL, de Faire U (2007) Genetic influences on angina pectoris and its impact on coronary heart disease. Eur J Hum Genet 15: 872–877.
8. Fischer M, Broeckel U, Holmer S, Baessler A, Hengstenberg C, et al. (2005) Distinct Heritable Patterns of Angiographic Coronary Artery Disease in Families With Myocardial Infarction. Circulation 111: 855–862.
9. Humphries SE, Drenos F, Ken-Dror G, Talmud PJ (2010) Coronary Heart Disease Risk Prediction in the Era of Genome-Wide Association Studies: Current Status and What the Future Holds. Circulation 121: 2235–2248.
10. Brindle P, Emberson J, Lampe F, Walker M, Whincup P, et al. (2003) Predictive accuracy of the Framingham coronary risk score in British men: prospective cohort study. BMJ 327: 1267-.
11. Fowkes FGR, Housley E, Cawood EHH, Macintyre CCA, Ruckley CV, et al. (1991) Edinburgh Artery Study: Prevalence of Asymptomatic and Symptomatic Peripheral Arterial Disease in the General Population. Int J Epidemiol 20: 384–392.
12. Price JF, Lee AJ, Rumley A, Lowe GDO, Fowkes FGR (2001) Lipoprotein (a) and development of intermittent claudication and major cardiovascular events in men and women: The Edinburgh Artery Study. Atherosclerosis 157: 241–249.
13. Peden J, Hopewell J, Saleheen D, Chambers J, Hager J, et al. (2011) A genome-wide association study in Europeans and South Asians identifies five new loci for coronary artery disease. Nature Genetics 43: 339–344.
14. Schunkert H, Konig IR, Kathiresan S, Reilly MP, Assimes TL, et al. (2011) Large-scale association analysis identifies 13 new susceptibility loci for coronary artery disease. Nature Genetics 43: 4.
15. R Development Core Team (2010) R: A language and environment for statistical computing. In: Computing RFfS, editor. Vienna, Austria.
16. Therneau T, Lumley T (2010) survival: Survival analysis R package. R package.
17. Sing T, Sander O, Beerenwinkel N, Lengauer T (2009) ROCR: Visualizing the performance of scoring classifiers. R package.
18. Harrell FEJ (2010) Hmisc: Harrell Miscellaneous. R package.
19. Pencina MJ, D' Agostino RBS, D' Agostino RBJ, Vasan RS (2008) Evaluating the added predictive ability of a new marker: From area under the ROC curve to reclassification and beyond. Statistics in Medicine 27: 157–172.
20. Pencina MJ, D'Agostino RB, Steyerberg EW (2011) Extensions of net reclassification improvement calculations to measure usefulness of new bio-markers. Statistics in Medicine 30: 11–21.
21. Zhao JH, Hornik K, Ripley B (2010) gap: Genetic analysis package. R package.
22. Therneau T, Atkinson B, Ripley B (2010) rpart: Recursive Partitioning. R package.
23. Foulkes AS (2009) Applied Statistical Genetics in R; Gentleman R, Hornik K, Parmigiani G, editors. Amherst: Springer.
24. Thanassoulis G, Vasan RS (2010) Genetic Cardiovascular Risk Prediction: Will We Get There? Circulation 122: 2323–2334.
25. NICE (2010) Lipid Modification: Cardiovascular risk assessment and the modification of blood lipids for the primary and secondary prevention of cardiovascular disease. National Institute for Health and Clinical Excellence clinical guideline 67.
26. Talmud PJ, Cooper JA, Palmen J, Lovering R, Drenos F, et al. (2008) Chromosome 9p21.3 Coronary Heart Disease Locus Genotype and Prospective Risk of CHD in Healthy Middle-Aged Men. Clin Chem 54: 467–474.
27. Morrison AC, Bare LA, Chambless LE, Ellis SG, Malloy M, et al. (2007) Prediction of Coronary Heart Disease Risk using a Genetic Risk Score: The Atherosclerosis Risk in Communities Study. Am J Epidemiol 166: 28–35.
28. Bare LAP, Morrison ACP, Rowland CMMS, Shiffman DP, Luke MMMBAP, et al. (2007) Five common gene variants identify elevated genetic risk for coronary heart disease. Genetics in Medicine 9: 682–689.
29. Kathiresan S, Melander O, Anevski D, Guiducci C, Burtt NP, et al. (2008) Polymorphisms Associated with Cholesterol and Risk of Cardiovascular Events. N Engl J Med 358: 1240–1249.
30. Zee RYL, Cook NR, Cheng S, Reynolds R, Erlich HA, et al. (2004) Polymorphism in the P-selectin and interleukin-4 genes as determinants of stroke: a population-based, prospective genetic analysis. Hum Mol Genet 13: 389–396.
31. Zee RYL, Cook NR, Cheng S, Erlich HA, Lindpaintner K, et al. (2006) Multi-locus candidate gene polymorphisms and risk of myocardial infarction: a population-based, prospective genetic analysis. Journal of Thrombosis and Haemostasis 4: 341–348.
32. Humphries SE, Cooper JA, Talmud PJ, Miller GJ (2007) Candidate Gene Genotypes, Along with Conventional Risk Factor Assessment, Improve Estimation of Coronary Heart Disease Risk in Healthy UK Men. Clin Chem 53: 8–16.
33. Davies RW, Dandona S, Stewart AFR, Chen L, Ellis SG, et al. (2010) Improved Prediction of Cardiovascular Disease Based on a Panel of Single Nucleotide Polymorphisms Identified Through Genome-Wide Association Studies/Clinical Perspective. Circulation: Cardiovascular Genetics 3: 468–474.
34. Ripatti S, Tikkanen E, Orho-Melander M, Havulinna AS, Silander K, et al. (2010) A multilocus genetic risk score for coronary heart disease: case-control and prospective cohort analyses. The Lancet 376: 1393–1400.
35. Hlatky MA, Greenland P, Arnett DK, Ballantyne CM, Criqui MH, et al. (2009) Criteria for Evaluation of Novel Markers of Cardiovascular Risk: A Scientific Statement From the American Heart Association. Circulation 119: 2408–2416.
36. Medina MW, Krauss RM (2009) The Role of HMGCR Alternative Splicing in Statin Efficacy. Trends in Cardiovascular Medicine 19: 173–177.
37. Iles MM (2008) What Can Genome-Wide Association Studies Tell Us about the Genetics of Common Disease? PLoS Genet 4: e33.

24

Cardiovascular Events in Patients with Atherothrombotic Disease: A Population-Based Longitudinal Study in Taiwan

Wen-Hsien Lee[1,2], Po-Chao Hsu[1], Chun-Yuan Chu[1], Ho-Ming Su[1,2,3]*, Chee-Siong Lee[1,3], Hsueh-Wei Yen[1,3], Tsung-Hsien Lin[1,3], Wen-Chol Voon[1,3], Wen-Ter Lai[1,3], Sheng-Hsiung Sheu[1,3]

1 Division of Cardiology, Department of Internal Medicine, Kaohsiung Medical University Hospital, Kaohsiung Medical University, Kaohsiung, Taiwan, 2 Department of Internal Medicine, Kaohsiung Municipal Hsiao-Kang Hospital, Kaohsiung Medical University, Kaohsiung, Taiwan, 3 Faculty of Medicine, College of Medicine, Kaohsiung Medical University, Kaohsiung, Taiwan

Abstract

Background: Atherothrombotic diseases including cerebrovascular disease (CVD), coronary artery disease (CAD), and peripheral arterial disease (PAD), contribute to the major causes of death in the world. Although several studies showed the association between polyvascular disease and poor cardiovascular (CV) outcomes in Asian population, there was no large-scale study to validate this relationship in this population.

Methods and Results: This retrospective cohort study included patients with a diagnosis of CVD, CAD, or PAD from the database contained in the Taiwan National Health Insurance Bureau during 2001–2004. A total of 19954 patients were enrolled in this study. The atherothrombotic disease score was defined according to the number of atherothrombotic disease. The study endpoints included acute coronary syndrome (ACS), all strokes, vascular procedures, in hospital mortality, and so on. The event rate of ischemic stroke (18.2%) was higher than that of acute myocardial infarction (5.7%) in our patients (P = 0.0006). In the multivariate Cox regression analyses, the adjusted hazard ratios (HRs) of each increment of atherothrombotic disease score in predicting ACS, all strokes, vascular procedures, and in hospital mortality were 1.41, 1.66, 1.30, and 1.14, respectively (P ≦ 0.0169).

Conclusions: This large population-based longitudinal study in patients with atherothrombotic disease demonstrated the risk of subsequent ischemic stroke was higher than that of subsequent AMI. In addition, the subsequent adverse CV events including ACS, all stroke, vascular procedures, and in hospital mortality were progressively increased as the increase of atherothrombotic disease score.

Editor: Yan Li, Shanghai Institute of Hypertension, China

Funding: The authors have no support or funding to report.

Competing Interests: The authors have declared that no competing interests exist.

* E-mail: cobeshm@seed.net.tw

Introduction

Atherothrombotic diseases including cerebrovascular disease (CVD), coronary artery disease (CAD), and peripheral arterial disease (PAD), contribute to the major causes of death in the world. Meanwhile, in Taiwan, the CAD and CVD rank as the second and third leading causes of death and possess a great budget on healthcare system in recent years [1–3]. In the future, the atherothrombotic disease will still be predicted as the leading cause of death worldwide by 2020 [4].

The REduction of Atherothrombosis for Continued Health (REACH) Registry was an international and observational study which enrolled patients with established atherosclerotic arterial disease or multiple risk factors of atherothrombosis and evaluated the medical management and risks of cardiovascular (CV) events in these patients [5]. It demonstrated patients with polyvascular disease were associated with a significantly higher risk of adverse CV events [6–8]. Although the REACH Registry included 69,055

patients, there were only 13.5% patients enrolled from the Asia. In patients with atherothrombotic disease, the most occurred CV event was CAD in Western population, but was CVD in Asian population [9–12]. Although several studies showed the association between polyvascular disease and poor CV outcomes in Asian population [13,14], there was no large-scale study to evaluate the relationship between polyvascular disease and adverse CV events in Taiwanese. Therefore, we conducted this large study to assess whether patients with polyvascular disease were independently associated with increased CV events in Taiwanese.

Methods

Ethics statement

The retrospective study protocol was approved by the institutional review board of the Kaohsiung Medical University Hospital (KMUH-IRB-EXEMPT-20130049). Because patient records and information was anonymized and de-identified prior to analysis, the written informed patient consent was waived by the IRB.

Data source

The data was analyzed from the National Health Insurance Research Dataset (NHIRD), published by the National Health Research Institute (NHI) in Taiwan, which provided a database of 1,000,000 random subjects. The NHI program has been implemented in Taiwan since 1995, offering a comprehensive, unified, and universal health insurance program to all citizens. All citizens who have established a registered domicile for at least 4 months in the Taiwan area should be enrolled in NHI. The coverage provides outpatient service, inpatient care, Chinese medicine, dental care, childbirth, physical therapy, preventive health care, home care, and rehabilitation for chronic mental illness. The coverage rate was 96% of whole population in 2000 and was elevated to 99% at the end of 2004. The NHI medical claim database included ambulatory care, hospital inpatient care, dental services, and prescription drugs. Therefore, the NHIRD is one of the largest and most complete nationwide population-based datasets in Taiwan and there were no statistically significant differences in age, sex, and average insured payroll-related amount between the sample group and all enrollees.

Study sample

This study population consisted of all patients with more than two-time outpatient or inpatient claims with a diagnosis of CVD, CAD, or PAD between July 1, 2001 and December 31, 2004. Initially, these patients with CVD, CAD, or PAD were enrolled by their disease code of international classification of diseases 9th revision clinical modification (ICD-9-CM) or their vascular location related procedure codes of ICD-9-CM during study period [15-18]. Therefore, the patients with CVD were enrolled by ICD-9-CM (433–438) or its related procedures, such as carotid angioplasty and carotid endarterectomy (procedure codes: 00.61, 00.63, 38.1). The patients with CAD were enrolled by ICD-9-CM (410–414) or its related procedures, such as coronary angioplasty/ stenting and coronary artery bypass grafting (procedure codes: 36.01–36.02, 36.05 to 36.07, 36.10–36.20). The patients with PAD were enrolled by ICD-9-CM (250.7, 443, 443.81, 443.9, 785.4, and 444.2) or its related procedures, such as peripheral angioplasty and lower extremity amputation (procedure codes: 84.1, 84.10-84.18). Then, the data of the first claim with a CVD, CAD or PAD diagnosis was considered the index date. The patients who were younger than 45 years old and had a diagnosis of CVD, CAD or PAD before index date were excluded. Finally, these patients with newly diagnosed CVD, CAD or PAD who received any antithrombotic or antiplatelet agents, such as aspirin, clopidogrel, ticlopidine, warfarin, or cilostazol, ≥ 30 days after each patient's index date were finally identified to form our study patients [19]. Based on these claim data, the patients were then classified according to the number or location of vascular disease. Baseline characteristics including age, sex, treatment information, and comorbidities were extracted from all claims within 180 days before the index data. Baseline comorbidities included diabetes mellitus (DM) (ICD-9-CM: 250), hypertension (ICD-9-CM: 401–405), hyperlipidemia (ICD-9-CM: 272.0–272.4), congestive heart failure (ICD-9-CM: 428), atrial fibrillation (ICD-9-CM: 427.31), chronic obstructive pulmonary disease (ICD-9-CM: 491, 492, 496), chronic kidney disease (ICD-9-CM: 585), aortic and mitral valve stenosis (ICD-9-CM: 394–396), peptic ulcer disease (ICD-9-CM: 531–534), monthly income (New Taiwan [NT] $0, NT $1-20000, NT $>20000), using of anti-thrombotic agents (aspirin, clopidogrel, ticlopidine, warfarin, and cilostazol), using of anti-

hypertensive agents (angiotensin converting enzymes, angiotensin II receptor blockers, β blockers, calcium channel blockers, diuretics, hydralazine, α blockers, and central α-2 adrenergic agonist), using of anti-diabetic agents (sulfonylureas, meglitinide, biguanides, thiazolidinediones, acarbose, and insulins), using of lipid-lowing agents (statins, fibrates, acipimox, and cholestyramine), using of proton pump inhibitors, urbanization level (ranging from most urbanized [level 1] to least urbanized level [level 5]), and hospital level (including medical center, regional hospital, district hospital and clinics). Patients with the single vascular disease were defined as those with CVD, CAD, or PAD. Patients with the double vascular disease were defined as those with CVD and CAD, CVD and PAD, or CAD and PAD. Patients with the triple vascular disease were defined as those with CVD, CAD, and PAD.

Study outcomes

The study endpoints included acute myocardial infarction (AMI) (ICD-9-CM: 410), unstable angina (ICD-9-CM: 411.1), acute coronary syndrome (ACS) including AMI and unstable angina, hemorrhagic stroke (ICD-9-CM: 430–432), ischemic stroke (ICD-9-CM: 433–436), other strokes including undetermined types of stroke and stroke sequela (ICD-9-CM: 437–438), all strokes including ischemic, hemorrhagic, and other strokes, vascular procedures, and in hospital mortality. The vascular procedures included carotid angioplasty and endarterectomy, coronary angioplasty/stenting and coronary artery bypass grafting surgery, and peripheral angioplasty and lower extremity amputation. In patients reaching the study endpoints, they were followed until the first episode of adverse CV events. The other patients were followed until December 2008.

Statistical analysis

Categorical variables among groups were compared by Chi-square analysis. Continuous variables among groups were compared by one-way analysis of variance. Time to CV events was assessed by Cox regression analysis. The atherothrombotic disease score was defined according to the number of athero-thrombotic disease, i.e. 1, 2, and 3 points were defined for single, double, and triple vascular diseases, respectively. Gender and significant variables in the univariate analysis were selected into the multivariate Cox regression analysis. Significance was set at p<0.05. All the data processing and statistical analyses were performed with SAS 9.3 software.

Results

Of the 73,744 patients diagnosed as CVD, CAD or PAD from January 2001 to December 2004, 19,954 patients (53.5% male) met all the inclusion criteria (Fig. 1). The mean follow-up period was 1198±8 days. Table 1 shows the comparison of baseline characteristics in patients with single, double, and triple vascular diseases. There were significant differences in age, the prevalence of DM, hypertension, hyperlipidemia, atrial fibrillation, chronic obstructive pulmonary disease, and peptic ulcer disease, using of anti-hypertensive agents, anti-diabetic agents, lipid-lowing agents, and proton pump inhibitors, monthly income, and hospital level in patients with single, double, and triple vascular diseases.

Table 2 shows the hazard ratios (HRs) of each increment of atherothrombotic disease score in predicting adverse CV events in all patients. The event rates of all strokes (26.5%) and ischemic stroke (18.2%) were higher than those of ACS (9.3%) and AMI (5.7%) in all study patients (P≤0.0028). After adjustment for gender and significant variables in the univariate analysis, the

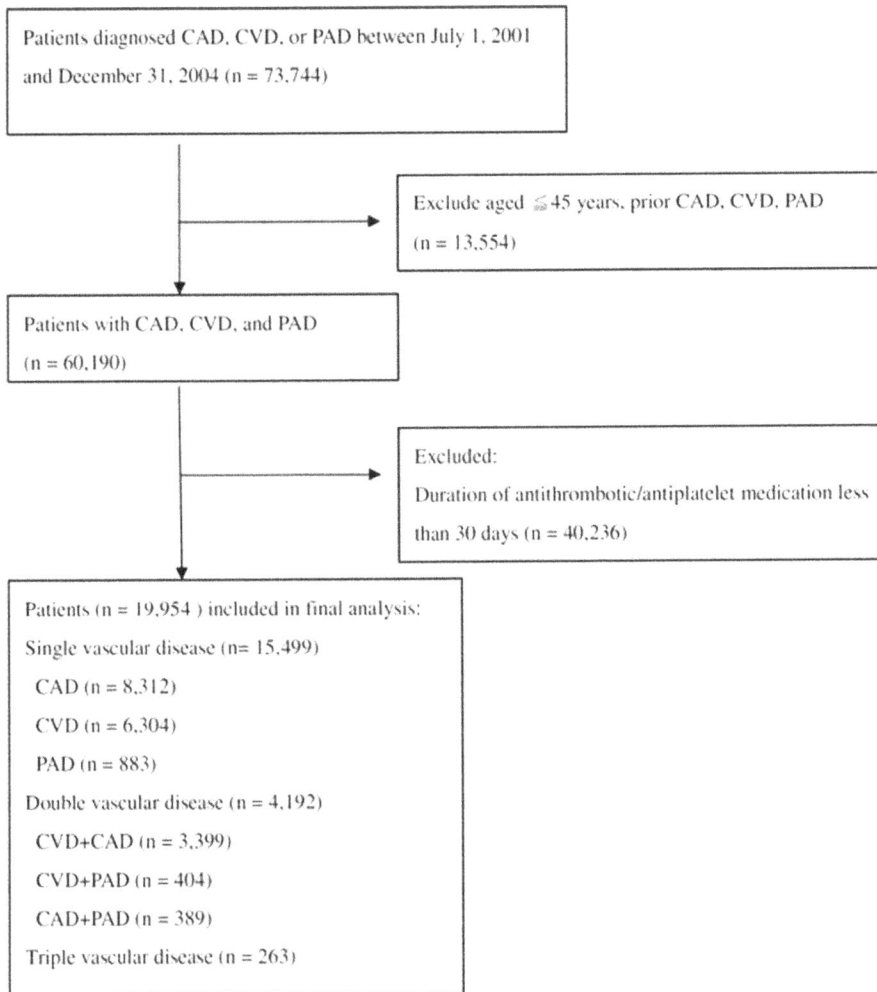

Figure 1. Flow chart of study participants. CVD, cerebrovascular disease; CAD, coronary artery disease; PAD, peripheral arterial disease.

adjusted HRs of each increment of atherothrombotic disease score in predicting ACS, all strokes, vascular procedures, and in hospital mortality were 1.41, 1.66, 1.30, and 1.14, respectively (P≦0.0169). Figure 2 demonstrates the Kaplan-Meier cumulative risk curves for the ACS, all strokes, vascular procedures, and in hospital mortality in patients with single, double, and triple vascular diseases. There were significant differences in these four CV outcomes in patients with single, double, and triple vascular diseases (all Log-rank P<0.0001) (Figure 2A to 2D).

We also performed subgroup analyses in patients with age between 45 and 64 years old and age ≥ 65 years old and in patients with different gender. Table 3 shows the adjusted HRs of each increment of atherothrombotic disease score in predicting adverse CV events in subgroup patients. In female patients, the adjusted HRs of each increment of atherothrombotic disease score in predicting ACS, all strokes, and vascular procedures were 1.53, 1.67, and 1.41, respectively (P≦0.0001). In male patients, the adjusted HRs of each increment of atherothrombotic disease score in predicting ACS, all strokes, vascular procedures, and in hospital mortality were 1.35, 1.66, 1.26, and 1.23, respectively (P≦0.0033). In patients with age between 45 and 64 years old, the adjusted HRs of each increment of atherothrombotic disease score predicting ACS, all strokes, and vascular procedures were 1.21, 1.84, and 1.20, respectively (P≦0.0160). In patients with age ≥

65 years old, the adjusted HRs of each increment of atherothrombotic disease score in predicting ACS, all strokes, vascular procedures, and in hospital mortality were 1.53, 1.59, 1.36, and 1.13, respectively (P≦0.0384).

Discussion

In the relatively large population-based longitudinal study in patients with atherothrombotic disease, we demonstrated that the risk of subsequent ischemic stroke was higher than that of subsequent AMI. In addition, the subsequent adverse CV events including ACS, all stroke, vascular procedures, and in hospital mortality were progressively increased as the increase of atherothrombotic disease score.

Previous studies showed that stroke mortality and incidence were higher in Asian population than in Western population [9,11]. In the REACH Registry, the ethnic comparison of 1-year CV outcomes showed that the event rate of non-fatal myocardial infarction was higher in North American (1.29%) than in Asia (0.82%), but the event rate of non-fatal stroke was higher in Asian (2.60%) than in North American (1.18%) [5]. A large-scale project, the Asia Pacific Cohort Studies Collaboration (APCSC), which included 44 separate cohorts and data from over 650,000 individuals, showed that hypertension, smoking, and DM were

Table 1. Comparison of baseline characteristics in patients with single, double, and triple vascular diseases.

Variables/Groups, N (%)	Total patients N = 19954	Single vascular disease N = 15499 (77.7)	Double vascular disease N = 4192 (21.0)	Triple vascular disease N = 263 (1.3)	P value
Gender (male)	10666 (53.5)	8286 (53.5)	2233 (53.3)	147 (55.9)	0.7091
Age (mean ± SD)	66.05±10.32	65.71±10.46	67.16±9.75	68.27±9.42	<0.0001
Age ≥65 years old	11465 (57.5)	8660 (55.9)	2628 (62.7)	177 (67.3)	<0.0001
Diabetes mellitus	5569 (29.9)	4203 (27.1)	1262 (30.1)	104 (39.5)	<0.0001
Hypertension	12481 (62.5)	9613 (62.0)	2687 (64.1)	181 (68.8)	0.0051
Hyperlipidema	4171 (20.9)	3209 (20.7)	889 (21.2)	73 (27.8)	0.0176
Congestive heart failure	1360 (6.8)	1035 (6.7)	303 (7.2)	22 (8.4)	0.2753
Atrial fibrillation	448 (2.2)	330 (2.1)	115 (2.7)	3 (1.1)	0.0280
Chronic kidney disease	608 (3.0)	448 (2.9)	151 (3.6)	9 (3.4)	0.0555
Chronic obstructive pulmonary disease	2393 (14.7)	2199 (14.2)	684 (16.3)	50 (19.0)	0.0004
Aortic and mitral valve stenosis	291 (1.5)	238 (1.5)	49 (1.2)	4 (1.5)	0.2128
Peptic ulcer disease	4114 (20.6)	3122 (20.1)	937 (22.4)	55 (20.9)	0.0073
Medication					
Anti-thrombotic agents	19889(99.7)	15449(99.7)	4178(99.7)	262(99.6)	0.9814
Anti-hypertensive agents	18870 (94.6)	14559 (93.9)	4056 (96.8)	255 (97.0)	<0.0001
Anti-diabetic agents	7111 (35.6)	5360 (34.6)	1617 (38.6)	134 (51.0)	<0.0001
Lipid-lowering agents	9550 (47.9)	7306 (47.1)	2104 (50.2)	140 (53.2)	<0.0001
Proton pump inhibitors	6979 (35.0)	5169 (33.4)	1678 (40.0)	132 (50.2)	<0.0001
Monthly income					0.0008
0	6851 (34.3)	5300 (34.2)	1466 (35.0)	86 (32.7)	
NT$ 1-20000	10894 (54.6)	8407 (54.2)	2331 (55.6)	156 (59.3)	
NT$ >20000	2208 (11.1)	1792 (11.6)	395 (9.4)	21 (8.0)	
Urbanization level					0.1544
1	4379 (21.9)	3452 (22.3)	874 (20.8)	53 (20.2)	
2	1434 (7.2)	1145 (7.4)	271 (6.5)	19 (7.2)	
3	839 (4.2)	665 (4.3)	164 (3.9)	10 (3.8)	
4	8842 (44.3)	6800 (43.9)	1927 (46.0)	115 (43.7)	
5	4411 (22.1)	3398 (21.9)	947 (22.6)	66 (25.1)	
Hospital level					0.0480
Medical center	1189 (6.0)	908 (5.9)	261 (6.2)	20 (7.6)	
Regional hospital	1127 (5.6)	859 (5.5)	254 (6.1)	14 (5.3)	
District hospital	3787 (19.0)	2885 (18.6)	843 (20.1)	59 (22.4)	
Clinics	13851 (69.4)	10847 (70.0)	2834 (67.6)	170 (64.6)	

Abbreviations: NT, new Taiwan; SD, standard deviation. Urbanization level is ranging from the most urbanized (level 1) to the least urbanized level (level 5).

the major risk factors for fatal and non-fatal stroke [20–23]. The high event rate of stroke in Asian countries may be explained by a high prevalence of hypertension, low level of serum total cholesterol, and low proportion of effective risk-reducing treatment [9,11]. Our present study similarly showed that the event rate of ischemic stroke was higher than that of AMI in Taiwanese patients with atherothrombotic disease.

In the REACH Registry, all major CV event rates increased with the number of vascular disease, ranging from 12.6% for patients with single, 21.1% for patients with double, and 26.3% for patients with triple vascular disease during 1-year follow up [6]. Furthermore, among patients with atherothrombosis, those with a

prior history of myocardial infarction or stroke at baseline had the higher rate of subsequent ischemic events (18.3%) than those with a stable CAD, CVD, or PAD at baseline (12.2%) during 4-year follow up [7]. In the present study, in Taiwanese patients with atherothrombotic disease, we consistently found the subsequent adverse CV events including ACS, all stroke, vascular procedures, and in hospital mortality were progressively increased as the increase of atherothrombotic disease score.

Several reasons may illustrate that polyvascular disease is a strong predictor for future CV events. Although CAD, CVD, and PAD shared common risk factors, poor controlled risk factors including current smoking, high blood pressure, fasting glucose,

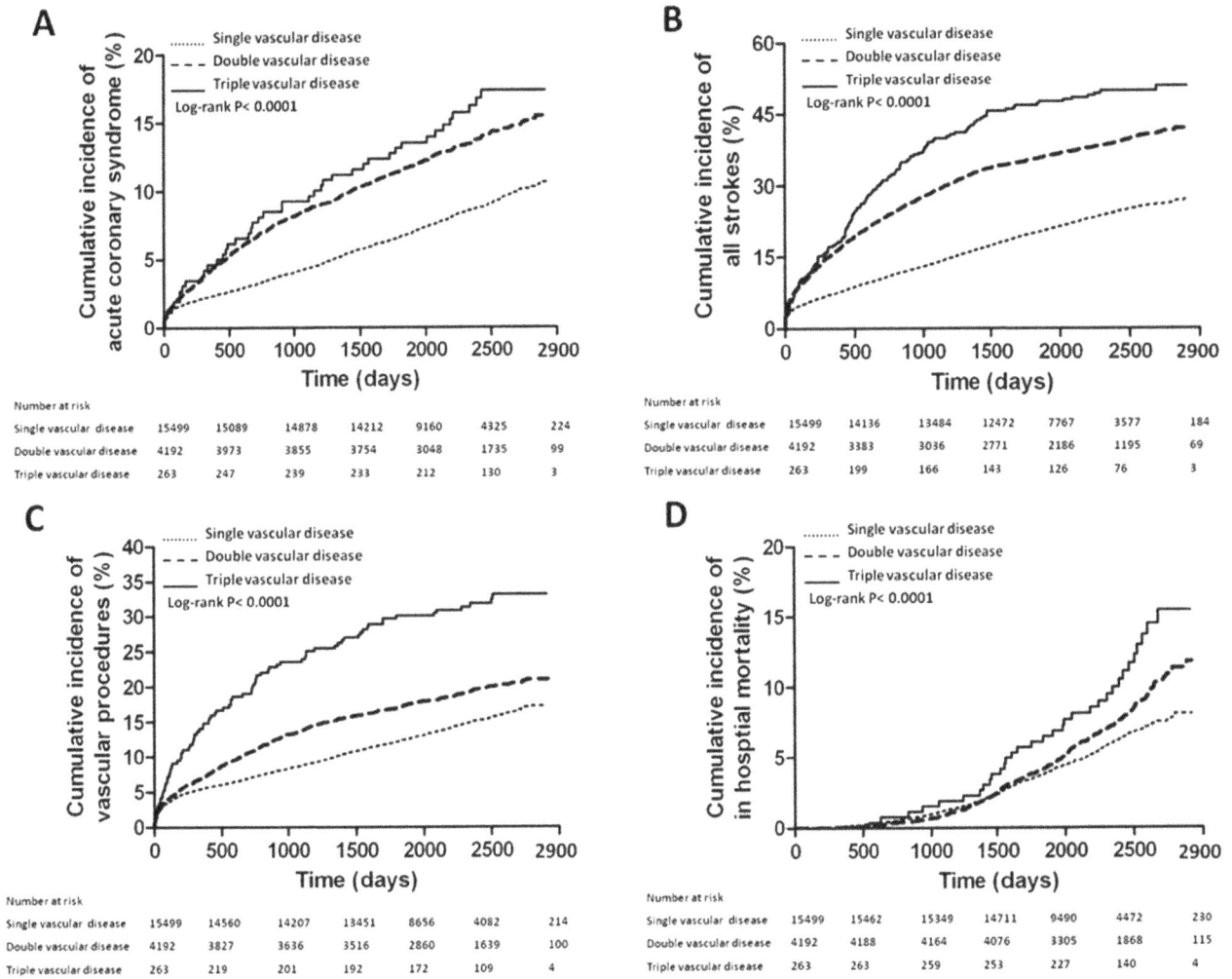

Figure 2. Kaplan-Meier cumulative risk curves for adverse cardiovascular events in patients with single, double, and triple vascular diseases. Kaplan-Meier cumulative risk curves for acute coronary syndrome (A), all strokes (B), vascular procedures (C), and in hospital mortality (D) in patients with single, double, and triple vascular diseases. All strokes included ischemic, hemorrhagic, and other strokes. Vascular procedures included carotid angioplasty and endarterectomy, coronary angioplasty/stenting and coronary artery bypass grafting surgery, and peripheral angioplasty and lower extremity amputation.

Table 2. The HRs of each increment of atherothrombotic disease score in predicting adverse cardiovascular events in all patients.

Events	Number (%)	Unadjusted HR (95%CI)	P value	Adjusted HR (95%CI)	P value
Acute coronary syndrome	1857 (9.3)	1.54 (1.41–1.68)	<0.0001	1.41(1.30–1.54)	<0.0001
AMI	1134 (5.7)	1.13(1.20–1.60)	<0.0001	1.30(1.16–1.45)	<0.0001
Unstable angina	1173 (5.9)	1.13(1.08–1.19)	<0.0001	1.06(1.01–1.12)	0.0123
All strokes	5297 (26.5)	1.78(1.70–1.87)	<0.0001	1.66(1.58–1.74)	<0.0001
Hemorrhagic stroke	837 (4.2)	1.76(1.56–1.99)	<0.0001	1.65(1.46–1.86)	<0.0001
Ischemic stroke	3640 (18.2)	1.71(1.61–1.81)	<0.0001	1.58(1.48–1.68)	<0.0001
Other stroke	3200 (16.0)	1.75 (1.64–1.86)	<0.0001	1.62(1.52–1.72)	<0.0001
Vascular procedures	3106 (15.6)	1.40 (1.31–1.50)	<0.0001	1.30(1.21–1.39)	<0.0001
In hospital mortality	1218 (6.1)	1.32(1.19–1.47)	<0.0001	1.14 (1.02–1.27)	0.0169

Abbreviations: AMI, acute myocardial infarction; CI, confidence interval; HR, hazard ratio.
Other strokes included undetermined types of stroke and stroke sequel.
In above multivariate Cox regression models, covariates included gender and the significant variables in the univariate analysis (age, diabetes, hypertension, hyperlipidemia, atrial fibrillation, chronic obstructive pulmonary disease, peptic ulcer disease, using of anti-hypertensive agents, anti-diabetic agents, lipid-lowing agents, and proton pump inhibitors, monthly income, and hospital level.).

Table 3. The adjusted HRs of each increment of atherothrombotic disease score in predicting adverse cardiovascular events in subgroup patients.

Events	Female, number = 9288		Male, number = 10666		Age between 45–64 years old, number = 8489		Age ≥ 65 years old, number = 11465	
	Adjusted HR (95%CI)	P value	Adjusted HR (95%CI)	P value	Adjusted HR (95%CI)	P value	Adjusted HR (95%CI)	P value
Acute coronary syndrome	1.53(1.34–1.75)	0.0001	1.35(1.21–1.51)	<0.0001	1.21(1.04–1.40)	0.0160	1.53(1.38–1.70)	<0.0001
AMI	1.52(1.28–1.82)	<0.0001	1.19(1.03–1.38)	0.0179	1.10(0.91–1.36)	0.3085	1.41(1.23–1.62)	<0.0001
Unstable angina	1.07(0.99–1.15)	0.0769	1.06(1.00–1.13)	0.0685	1.12(1.03–1.22)	0.0088	1.04(0.98–1.11)	0.1671
All strokes	1.67(1.54–1.80)	<0.0001	1.66(1.55–1.77)	<0.0001	1.84(1.68–2.02)	<0.0001	1.59(1.50–1.69)	<0.0001
Hemorrhagic stroke	1.64(1.34–2.01)	<0.0001	1.65(1.41–1.92)	<0.0001	2.01(1.64–2.47)	<0.0001	1.49(1.28–1.73)	<0.0001
Ischemic stroke	1.56(1.42–1.72)	<0.0001	1.59(1.47–1.72)	<0.0001	1.78(1.61–1.98)	<0.0001	1.49(1.39–1.60)	<0.0001
Other stroke	1.62(1.47–1.79)	<0.0001	1.62(1.49–1.76)	<0.0001	1.85(1.64–2.08)	<0.0001	1.54(1.42–1.66)	<0.0001
Vascular procedures	1.41(1.26–1.59)	<0.0001	1.26(1.15–1.37)	<0.0001	1.20(1.07–1.34)	0.0016	1.36(1.25–1.49)	<0.0001
In hospital mortality	1.03(0.86–1.23)	0.7766	1.23(1.07–1.40)	0.0033	1.18(0.91–1.53)	0.2091	1.13(1.01–1.28)	0.0384

Abbreviations: AMI, acute myocardial infarction; CI, confidence interval; HR, hazard ratio.
Other strokes included undetermined types of stroke and stroke sequel.
In multivariate Cox regression models, covariates included gender and the significant variables in the univariate analysis.

and total cholesterol were more frequently in patients with polyvascular diseases than those with single vascular disease [24]. The ACS patients with prior atherothrombotic disease had higher in hospital mortality than those without prior atherothrombotic disease [25,26]. In addition, inflammation may be an important factor for the initiation, progression, and linkage among CAD, CVD, and PAD [27,28]. The inflammation triggered from the affected arterial bed may activate the endothelium at distant arterial beds. Patients with polyvascular diseases were reported to have higher levels/concentrations of inflammation makers, such as high sensitivity C reactive protein, neutrophil myeloperoxidase content, interleukin 6, intercellular adhesion molecule 1, vascular cell adhesion molecule 1, matrix metalloproteinase 9, cellular fibronectin, and so on [27–29]. In the present study, we similarly demonstrated polyvascular disease was significantly associated with an increase in future adverse CV events.

There were several limitations in our population-based longitudinal investigation. First, the database provided by NHI might have possible disease misclassifications and inadequate diagnostic codes for increasing payment to hospitals and administration of certain medications [30]. Second, we did not know the real data of ankle-brachial index, carotid intima-media thickness, National Institutes of Health Stroke Scale, and modified Rankin Scale. The education status, personal history of smoking and alcohol habits, and body mass index were also lacking in the NHI database. These factors might affect the subsequent CV events [13,14,31,32]. Additionally, we did not know the severity of vascular diseases and devices of vascular intervention, which might also affect the subsequent CV outcomes [33–35]. Third, we did not enroll patients who were younger than 45 years old. In young patients, the etiologies of premature CAD or CVD were more heterogeneous than those in older patients [36–37]. Therefore, our results can not be applied in young patients with atherothrombotic disease. Finally, despite of the population based database, this study did not have any randomization which might have some selection bias.

Conclusion

This large population-based longitudinal study in patients with atherothrombotic disease demonstrated the risk of subsequent ischemic stroke was higher than that of subsequent AMI. In addition, the subsequent adverse CV events including ACS, all stroke, vascular procedures, and in hospital mortality were progressively increased as the increase of atherothrombotic disease score.

Acknowledgments

This study is based in part on data from the National Health Insurance Research Database provided by the Bureau of National Health Insurance, Department of Health and managed by National Health Research Institutes (Registered number 98178). The interpretation and conclusions contained herein do not represent those of Bureau of National Health Insurance, Department of Health or National Health Research Institutes. The authors also thank the help from the Statistical Analysis Laboratory, Department of Internal Medicine, Kaohsiung Medical University Hospital.

Author Contributions

Conceived and designed the experiments: W-HL T-HL P-CH. Performed the experiments: C-YC H-MS C-SL. Analyzed the data: H-MS W-HL C-SL. Contributed reagents/materials/analysis tools: H-WY W-CV W-TL S-HS. Wrote the paper: H-MS W-HL.

References

1. Directorate-general of budget, accounting and statistics executive yuan, republic of china (2010) Statistical Yearbook of the Republic of China. Health. 114.
2. Chen CL, Chen L, Yang WC (2008) The influences of taiwan's generic grouping price policy on drug prices and expenditures: Evidence from analysing the consumption of the three most-used classes of cardiovascular drugs. BMC Public Health 8: 118.
3. Chang KC, Tseng MC (2003) Costs of acute care of first-ever ischemic stroke in taiwan. Stroke 34: e219–221.
4. Murray CJ, Lopez AD (1997) Alternative projections of mortality and disability by cause 1990-2020: Global burden of disease study. Lancet 349: 1498–1504.
5. Bhatt DL, Steg PG, Ohman EM, Hirsch AT, Ikeda Y, et al. (2006) International prevalence, recognition, and treatment of cardiovascular risk factors in outpatients with atherothrombosis. JAMA 295: 180–189.
6. Steg PG, Bhatt DL, Wilson PW, D'Agostino R Sr, Ohman EM, et al. (2007) One-year cardiovascular event rates in outpatients with atherothrombosis. JAMA 297: 1197–1206.
7. Bhatt DL, Eagle KA, Ohman EM, Hirsch AT, Goto S, et al. (2010) Comparative determinants of 4-year cardiovascular event rates in stable outpatients at risk of or with atherothrombosis. JAMA 304: 1350–1357.
8. Uchiyama S, Goto S, Matsumoto M, Nagai R, Origasa H, et al. (2009) Cardiovascular event rates in patients with cerebrovascular disease and atherothrombosis at other vascular locations: Results from 1-year outcomes in the japanese reach registry. J Neurol Sci 287: 45–51.
9. Reddy KS (2004) Cardiovascular disease in non-western countries. N Engl J Med 350: 2438–2440.
10. van den Hoogen PC, Feskens EJ, Nagelkerke NJ, Menotti A, Nissinen A, et al. (2000) The relation between blood pressure and mortality due to coronary heart disease among men in different parts of the world. Seven countries study research group. N Engl J Med 342:1–8.
11. Ueshima H, Sekikawa A, Miura K, Turin TC, Takashima N, et al. (2008) Cardiovascular disease and risk factors in asia: A selected review. Circulation 118: 2702–2709.
12. Bild DE, Detrano R, Peterson D, Guerci A, Liu K, et al. (2005) Ethnic differences in coronary calcification: The multi-ethnic study of atherosclerosis (MESA). Circulation 111: 1313–1320.
13. Chien KL, Su TC, Jeng JS, Hsu HC, Chang WT, et al. (2008) Carotid artery intima-media thickness, carotid plaque and coronary heart disease and stroke in chinese. PLoS One 3: e3435.
14. Li C, Wang H, Chen S, Chen Y, Chiang Y, et al. (2012) High risk for future events in acute stroke patients with an ankle-brachial index less than 0.9. Acta Cardiol Sin 28: 17–24.
15. Wen HC, Tang CH, Lin HC, Tsai CS, Chen CS, et al. (2006) Association between surgeon and hospital volume in coronary artery bypass graft surgery outcomes: A population-based study. Ann Thorac Surg 81: 835–842.
16. Chen JJ, Lee CH, Lin LY, Liau CS (2011) Determinants of lower extremity amputation or revascularization procedure in patients with peripheral artery diseases: A population-based investigation. Angiology 62: 306–309.
17. Lee WH, Chu CY, Hsu PC, Su HM, Lin TH, et al. (2013) Comparison of antiplatelet and antithrombotic therapy for secondary prevention of ischemic stroke in patients with peripheral artery disease: Population-based follow-up study in taiwan. Circ J 77: 1046–1052.
18. Lee WH, Chu CY, Hsu PC, Su HM, Lin TH, et al. (2013) Cilostazol for primary prevention of stroke in peripheral artery disease: A population-based longitudinal study in Taiwan. Thromb Res 132: 190–195.
19. Cheng CL, Kao YH, Lin SJ, Lee CH, Lai ML (2011) Validation of the national health insurance research database with ischemic stroke cases in Taiwan. Pharmacoepidemiol Drug Saf 20: 236–242.
20. Lawes CM, Rodgers A, Bennett DA, Parag V, Suh I, et al. (2003) Blood pressure and cardiovascular disease in the Asia Pacific region. J Hypertens 21: 707–716.
21. Woodward M, Lam TH, Barzi F, Patel A, Gu D, et al. (2005) Smoking, quitting, and the risk of cardiovascular disease among women and men in the Asia-Pacific region. Int J Epidemiol 34: 1036–1045.
22. Woodward M, Zhang X, Barzi F, Pan W, Ueshima H, et al. (2003) The effects of diabetes on the risks of major cardiovascular diseases and death in the Asia-Pacific region. Diabetes Care 26: 360–366.
23. Zhang X, Patel A, Horibe H, Wu Z, Barzi F, et al. (2003) Cholesterol, coronary heart disease, and stroke in the Asia Pacific region. Int J Epidemiol 32: 563–572.
24. Suarez C, Zeymer U, Limbourg T, Baumgartner I, Cacoub P, et al. (2010) Influence of polyvascular disease on cardiovascular event rates. Insights from the REACH registry. Vasc Med 15: 259–265.
25. Brilakis ES, Hernandez AF, Dai D, Peterson ED, Banerjee S, et al. (2009) Quality of care for acute coronary syndrome patients with known atherosclerotic disease: Results from the get with the guidelines program. Circulation 120: 560–567.
26. Mukherjee D, Eagle KA, Kline-Rogers E, Feldman LJ, Juliard JM, et al. (2007) Impact of prior peripheral arterial disease and stroke on outcomes of acute coronary syndromes and effect of evidence-based therapies (from the global registry of acute coronary events). Am J Cardiol 100: 1–6.
27. Brevetti G, Giugliano G, Brevetti L, Hiatt WR (2010) Inflammation in peripheral artery disease. Circulation 122: 1862–1875.
28. Lombardo A, Biasucci LM, Lanza GA, Coli S, Silvestri P, et al. (2004) Inflammation as a possible link between coronary and carotid plaque instability. Circulation 109: 3158–3163.
29. Blanco M, Sobrino T, Montaner J, Medrano V, Jimenez C, et al. (2010) Stroke with polyvascular atherothrombotic disease. Atherosclerosis 208: 587–592.
30. Assaf AR, Lapane KL, McKenney JL, Carleton RA (1993) Possible influence of the prospective payment system on the assignment of discharge diagnoses for coronary heart disease. N Engl J Med 329: 931–935.
31. Nakano T, Ohkuma H, Suzuki S (2004) Measurement of ankle brachial index for assessment of atherosclerosis in patients with stroke. Cerebrovasc Dis 17: 212–217.
32. Wang TD, Goto S, Bhatt DL, Steg PG, Chan JC, et al. (2010) Ethnic differences in the relationships of anthropometric measures to metabolic risk factors in asian patients at risk of atherothrombosis: Results from the reduction of athero-thrombosis for continued health (REACH) registry. Metabolism 59: 400–408.
33. Lin MS, Lin LC, Li HY, Lin CH, Chao CC, et al. (2008) Procedural safety and potential vascular complication of endovascular recanalization for chronic cervical internal carotid artery occlusion. Circ Cardiovasc Interv 1: 119–125.
34. Chang SH, Chen CC, Hsieh MJ, Wang CY, Lee CH, et al. (2013) Lesion length impacts long term outcomes of drug-eluting stents and bare metal stents differently. PLoS One 8: e53207.
35. Huang HL, Chou HH, Wu TY, Chang SH, Tsai YJ, et al. (2013) Endovascular intervention in Taiwanese patients with critical limb ischemia: Patient outcomes in 333 consecutive limb procedures with a 3-year follow-up. Journal of the Formosan Medical Association 1–8.
36. Ji R, Schwamm LH, Pervez MA, Singhal AB (2013) Ischemic stroke and transient ischemic attack in young adults: Risk factors, diagnostic yield, neuroimaging, and thrombolysis. JAMA Neurol 70:51–57.
37. Klein LW, Nathan S (2003) Coronary artery disease in young adults. J Am Coll Cardiol 41:529–531.

25

CYP2C19 Phenotype, Stent Thrombosis, Myocardial Infarction, and Mortality in Patients with Coronary Stent Placement in a Chinese Population

Xiang Xie[1], Yi-Tong Ma[1]*, Yi-Ning Yang[1], Xiao-Mei Li[1], Xiang Ma[1], Zhen-Yan Fu[1], Ying-Ying Zheng[1], Bang-Dang Chen[2], Fen Liu[2]

1 Department of Cardiology, First Affiliated Hospital of Xinjiang Medical University, Urumqi, P.R. China, 2 Xinjiang Key Laboratory of Cardiovascular Disease Research, Urumqi, P.R. China

Abstract

Background: Several studies have indicated that CYP2C19 loss-of-function polymorphisms have a higher risk of stent thrombosis (ST) after percutaneous coronary interventions (PCIs). However, this association has not been investigated thoroughly in a Chinese population. In this study, we aimed to determine the effect of CYP2C19*2 and CYP2C19*3 loss-of-function polymorphisms on the occurrence of ST and other adverse clinical events in a Chinese population.

Methods: We designed a cohort study among 1068 consecutive patients undergoing intracoronary stent implantation after preloading with 600 mg of clopidogrel. CYP2C19*2 and CYP2C19*3 were genotyped by using polymerase chain reaction-restriction fragment length polymorphism analysis. The adverse clinical events recorded were ST, death, myocardial infarction (MI), and bleeding events. The primary end point of the study was the incidence of cumulative ST within 1 year after PCI. The secondary end point was other adverse clinical outcomes 1 year after the procedure.

Results: The cumulative 1-year incidence of ST was 0.88% in patients with extensive metabolizers (EMs) (CYP2C19*1/*1 genotype), 4.67% in patients with intermediate metabolizers (IMs) (CYP2C19*1/*2 or *1/*3 genotype), and 10.0% in patients with poor metabolizers (PMs) (CYP2C19*2/*2, *2/*3, or *3/*3 genotype) ($P<0.001$). The one-year event-free survival was 97.8% in patients with EMs, 96.5% in patients with IMs, and 92.0% in patients with PMs ($P=0.014$). Multivariate analysis confirmed the independent association of CYP2C19 loss-of-function allele carriage with ST ($P=0.009$) and total mortality ($P<0.05$).

Conclusion: PM patients had an increased risk of ST, death, and MI after coronary stent placement in a Chinese population.

Editor: Alberico Catapano, University of Milan, Italy

Funding: This study was funded by the National Natural Science Foundation of China (grant number 81160017) and the Urumqi City Science and Technology Projects (grant number Y101310008). The funders had no role in study design, data collection and analysis, decision to publish, or preparation of the manuscript.

Competing Interests: The authors have declared that no competing interests exist.

* E-mail: myt-xj@163.com

Introduction

Stent thrombosis (ST) and other adverse clinical events, including myocardial infarction (MI) and bleeding events, are life-threatening complications of percutaneous coronary intervention (PCI). Dual antiplatelet treatment with aspirin and clopidogrel is routinely administered to prevent thrombotic events, including ST and MI, after PCI. However, this therapy significantly increases the risk of bleeding events and related death [1]. Clopidogrel is an inactive prodrug and requires metabolization and activation by the CYP2C19 to generate its active thiol metabolite, which can significantly inhibit platelet aggregation by binding to the ADP P2Y12 receptor [2]. Recent reports suggest that two loss-of-function variants in CYP2C19 are associated with an increased rate of recurrent cardiovascular events, including ST [3–5]. These two main enzyme loss-of-function alleles are CYP2C19*2 and CYP2C19*3. CYP2C19*2 is a single base pair

G681A mutation in Exon 5 of CYP2C19. CYP2C19*3 is a single base pair G636A mutation in Exon 4 of CYP2C19, which results in a premature stop codon [6,7].

Sibbing et al. [3] enrolled 2485 consecutive patients undergoing coronary stent placement after pretreatment with 600 mg of clopidogrel and found that the cumulative 30-day incidence of ST was significantly higher in subjects with the CYP2C19*2 allele vs. CYP2C19 wild-type homozygotes (1.5% vs. 0.4%). Harmsze et al. [4] also reported that carriage of the loss-of-function alleles CYP2C19*2 and CYP2C9*3 increases the risk of ST after PCI. In these studies, the enrolled participants were Europeans, whose minor allele frequency (MAF) of CYP2C19*3 was <1%. Therefore, in these two studies, CYP2C19*3 was not found to be associated with the incidence of ST. However, in our previous study, the frequency of CYP2C19*3 was noted to be 6.250% in coronary artery disease (CAD) patients in a Chinese population [5]. Therefore, more attention should be paid to those populations that have a high frequency of CYP2C19*3, especially in China, where there are about 1.3 billion people, which indicates that there are about 50 million people who carry CYP2C19*3. With regard to CYP2C19*2, MAF was significantly higher in Chinese people (28.4%) than in other ethnicities, such as Europeans (15.3%), Sub-Saharan Africans (14.4%), and African-Americans (10.0%), according to a report from the NCBI database (http://www.ncbi.nlm.nih.gov/pubmed/SNP). However, the associations of the CYP2C19 genotypes with the risk of ST and other adverse clinical events after PCI have not been thoroughly investigated.

In this study, we aimed to determine the effect of CYP2C19 loss-of-function polymorphisms on the occurrence of ST and other adverse clinical events in a Chinese population.

Methods

Ethics Statement

The present study complies with the Declaration of Helsinki and was approved by the Ethics Committee of the Fist Affiliated Hospital of Xinjiang Medical University. All patients gave written informed consent before study inclusion.

Patients

A total of 1068 patients with CAD undergoing PCI in the First Affiliated Hospital of Xinjiang Medical University from January 2008 to March 2010 were enrolled in the present study. Figure 1 presents the flowchart of the study population. All the patients included in this study were pretreated with a loading dose of 600 mg of clopidogrel for ≥ 2 h before the procedure. Coronary interventions were done according to the current standard guidelines as described previously [8]. Intravenous anticoagulative treatment with unfractionated heparin was administered to the majority of patients. A small subset of the patients ($<10\%$) received intravenous antiplatelet therapy with glycoprotein IIb/IIIa inhibitor, in addition to a reduced dose of heparin. During the

time period after the procedure, the patients were treated and discharged with a dual antiplatelet regimen of 75 mg of clopidogrel (once daily) and 100 mg of aspirin (once daily) for at least 12 months.

The inclusion criterion was clopidogrel-naive patients with CAD, including non–ST-segment elevation acute coronary syndrome (ACS) patients undergoing coronary angiography. The exclusion criteria [3] were as follows: age >75 years, primary PCI for ST-segment elevation acute MI, severe anemia or platelet count $<70\times10^9/L$, uncoalesced peptic ulcer, high risk of active bleeding, cerebrovascular accident <3 months, history of malignancy, and severe liver disease or chronic renal failure (serum creatinine >2 mg/dL).

Systemic arterial hypertension was defined as a systolic blood pressure (SBP) of ≥ 140 mm Hg and/or a diastolic blood pressure (DBP) of ≥ 90 mm Hg on at least two separate occasions, or antihypertensive treatment [9]. Hypercholesterolemia was defined as a documented total cholesterol value of ≥ 240 mg/dL (≥ 6.2 mmol/L) or current treatment with cholesterol-lowering medication [9]. The smoking status classifications were current smokers, former smokers, and never-smokers. Alcohol drinking was classified as current drinking, former drinking, and never-drinking. Diabetes mellitus was defined according to the American Diabetes Association (ADA) 2009 criteria [10] (fasting plasma glucose ≥ 7.0 mmol/L [≥ 126 mg/dL]) or self-reported current diabetes treatments.

Biochemical Analysis

Serum and plasma collected for measurement were immediately frozen at $-80°C$ until analysis. We measured the serum concentration of total cholesterol, triglyceride, blood urea nitrogen (BUN), creatinine (Cr), low-density lipoprotein (LDL), high-density lipoprotein (HDL), uric acid, and fasting glucose with the chemical analysis equipment (Dimension AR/AVL Clinical Chemistry System, Newark, NJ, USA) used by the Clinical Laboratory

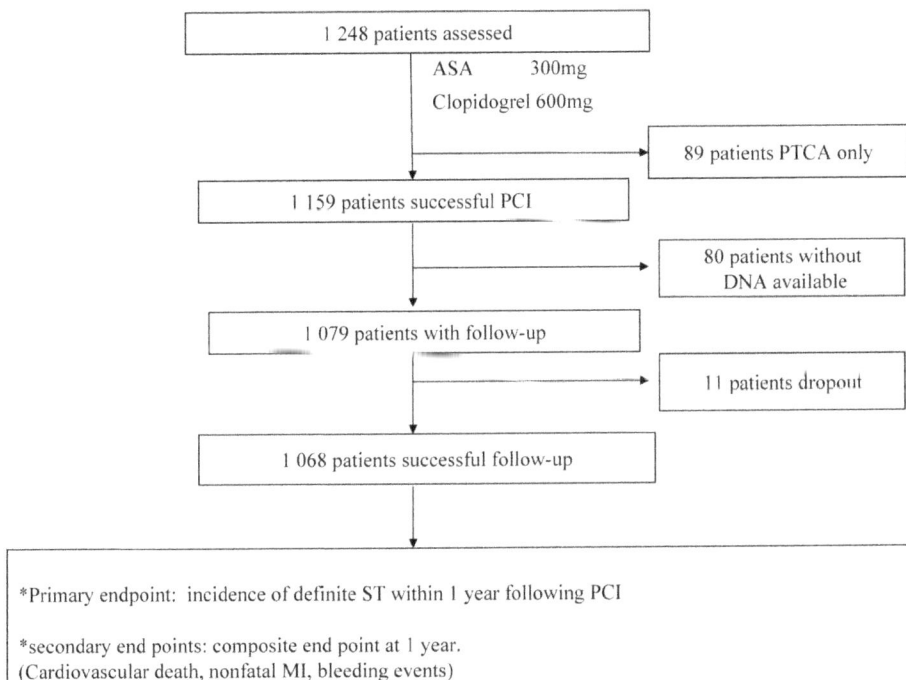

Figure 1. **Study flow chart.** DNA:desoxy-ribonucleic acid; PTCA, conventional balloon angioplasty.

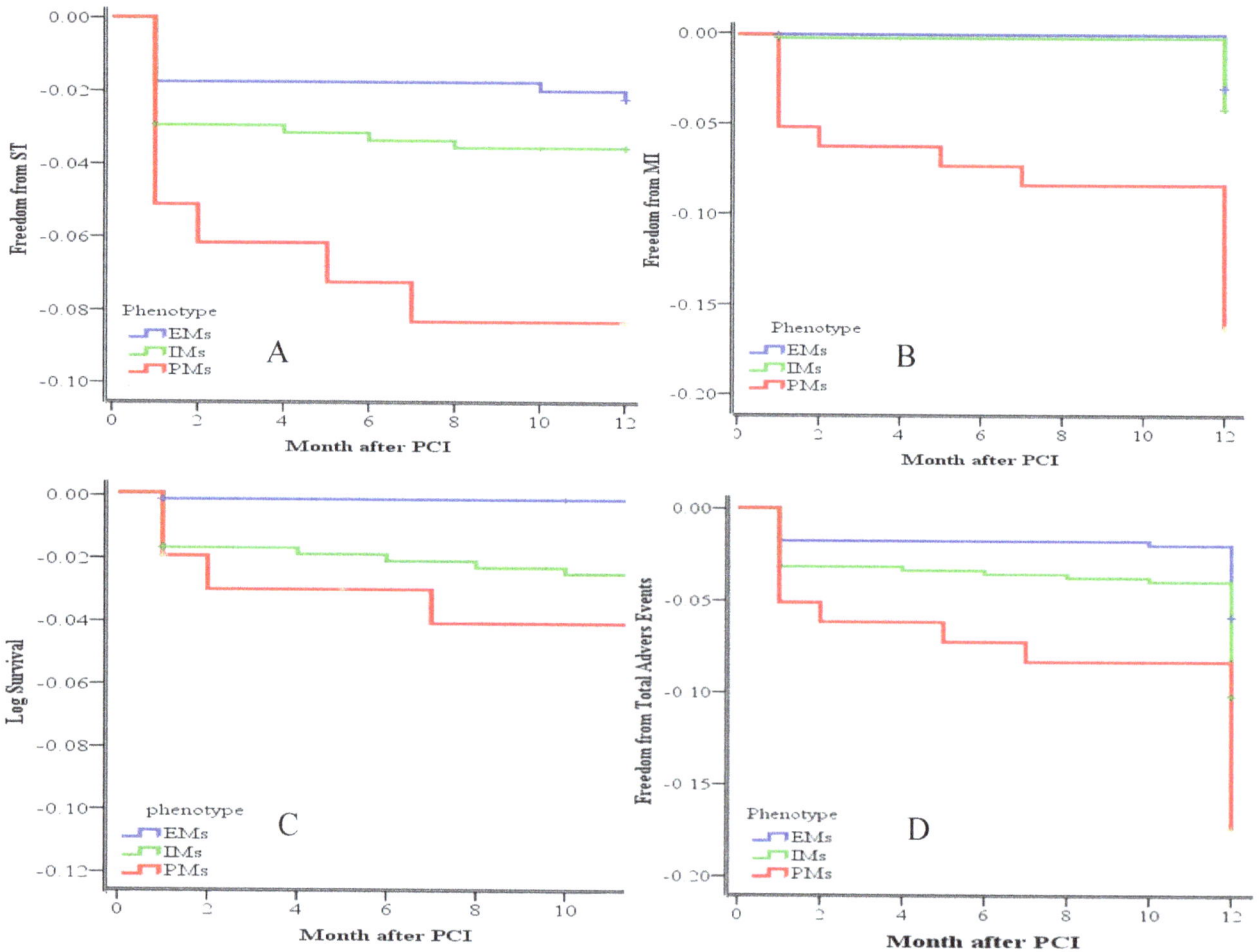

Figure 2. Kaplan – Meier Curves for Event free Survival According to CYP2C19 Loss-of-Function Allele Carrier Status among Chinese Patients with CAD following PCI.

Department of the First Affiliated Hospital of Xinjiang Medical University, as described previously [11,12].

Blood sampling and genotyping

Whole blood for genotyping was obtained from the arterial sheath of all patients directly after diagnostic angiography and before PCI. Genomic DNA was extracted from blood leukocytes with the use of a DNA extraction kit [Tiangen Biotech (Beijing) Co. Ltd], according to the manufacturer's instructions. Genotyping was confirmed by polymerase chain reaction (PCR)-restriction fragment length polymorphism (RFLP) analysis, as described previously [5]. To verify our results, we used sequenced genomic DNAs as positive controls in our assays. To control for correct sample handling, genotyping was repeated in 10% of the patients. All the repeated experiments revealed identical results when compared with the initial genotyping.

Individuals can be divided into three groups according to the CYP2C19 genotype. Those who inherit two mutant CYP2C19 alleles (*2 and/or *3) have a reduced capacity to metabolize CYP2C19 substrates and are defined as poor metabolizers (PMs). Individuals who are homozygous (*1/*1) for wild-type CYP2C19*1 have efficient enzymes to metabolize CYP2C19 substrates and are defined as extensive metabolizers (EMs). Subjects who are heterozygous (*1/*2, *1/*3) for wild-type CYP2C19*1 are defined as intermediate metabolizers (IMs) [13–

15]. Patients who carry a loss-of-function CYP2C19 allele have 1.53- to 3.69-fold increased risk of major cardiovascular events compared with noncarriers [16,17].

Study end points and definitions

The primary end point of this study was the cumulative incidence of ST during a 1-year follow-up period. The secondary end point was the other adverse clinical outcomes, including death, MI, and bleeding events, 1 year after the procedure. We defined ST according to the Academic Research Consortium (ARC) 2007 criteria [18] and classified it by the level of certainty (definite, probable, or possible) and the timing of the event (early [0–30 days] or late [31 days to 1 year]). Definite ST was defined as an angiographically or pathologically confirmed thrombus, along with ischemic symptoms or signs. Probable ST was defined as any unexplained deaths within 30 days or acute MI of the target vessel territory without angiographic evidence. Possible ST included any unexplained deaths after more than 30 days. In the present study, we defined the cumulative incidence of ST, including these three categories. MI was defined as new Q waves and an increase in the creatine kinase MB concentration to greater than five times the upper limit of the normal range, if occurring within 48 h after the procedure, or as new Q waves or an increase in creatine kinase MB concentration to greater than the upper limit of the normal range, plus ischemic symptoms or signs, if

Table 1. Baseline characteristics of the study population.

Variables	Overall (n = 1068)	Genotypes			P value
		EMs (n = 454)	IMs (n = 514)	PMs (n = 100)	
Age (year)	59.46±11.04	59.44±11.35	59.58±10.85	59.02±10.71	0.897
BMI (Kg/m²)	25.93±6.20	25.53±3.72	26.25±3.72	26.05±4.11	0.202
SBP (mmHg)	135.94±26.34	138.00±27.79	134.89±25.46	131.65±23.05	0.074
DBP (mmHg)	83.50±16.53	84.63±17.63	83.11±14.97	79.97±19.08	0.060
Pulse (beats/min)	73.53±10.89	73.49±11.51	73.42±10.26	74.22±11.14	0.803
BUN (mmol/L)	5.15±1.98	5.23±1.90	5.1±2.1	5.06±1.78	0.577
Cr (mmol/L)	79.41±21.13	79.19±21.73	80.40±20.29	75.25±22.37	0.091
URIC (mmol/L)	325.63±89.32	327.39±94.86	327.45±83.29	308.77±93.19	0.154
GLU (mmol/L)	6.22±2.50	6.32±2.49	6.16±2.57	6.14±2.19	0.598
HbA1c (mmol/L)	2.34±3.79	2.2±0.65	2.5±5.41	2.08±0.47	0.411
TG (mmol/L)	2.06±1.62	2.0±1.42	2.09±1.76	2.11±1.68	0.694
TC (mmol/L)	4.23±1.13	4.23±1.21	4.25±1.07	4.13±0.98	0.640
HDLC (mmol/L)	1.06±0.36	1.05±0.3	1.07±0.41	1.07±0.25	0.511
LDLC (mmol/L)	2.44±.940	2.5±0.96	2.42±0.93	2.34±0.88	0.231
APOA (mmol/L)	1.20±.32	1.18±0.31	1.21±0.35	1.17±0.23	0.242
APOB (mmol/L)	0.98±3.11	0.86±0.42	1.1±0.405	0.87±0.234	0.513

occurring >48 h after the procedure, as described previously [19]. Bleeding events were defined according to the Bleeding Academic Research Consortium (BARC) criteria [20]. All the events were adjudicated by an event adjudication committee blinded to the genotype of the patients.

Follow-up

All the patients stayed in hospital for at least 48 h after inclusion and PCI. The patients were interviewed after 30 days (±3 days) and 1 year (±7 days), respectively. All the patients were recommended to have a follow-up coronary angiography in 9 months.

The investigators followed the patients either by office visits or telephone calls as necessary. Compliance of the drugs and adverse events were assessed at every visit for clinical follow-up. Those patients with cardiac symptoms received complete clinical, electrocardiographic, and laboratory check-up in the outpatient clinic. A standardized questionnaire was used in the present study to collect information on each subject's medical history, medication status, and lifestyle characteristics.

Table 2. Baseline characteristics of the study population.

Variables	Overall (n = 1068)	Phenotypes			P value
		EMs (n = 454)	IMs (n = 514)	PMs (n = 100)	
Sex, Female, n (%)	854 (20.0)	95 (20.9)	98 (19.07)	21 (21.0)	0.747
Smoking, n (%)					
Never smoking	456 (42.7)	184 (40.52)	226 (43.97)	46 (46.0)	0.779
Former smoking	26 (2.4)	11 (2.42)	13 (2.53)	2 (2.0)	
Current smoking	586 (54.9)	259 (57.05)	275 (53.50)	52 (52.0)	
Drinking, n (%)					
Never drinking	654 (61.2)	283 (62.33)	302 (58.75)	69 (69.00)	0.080
Former drinking	361 (33.8)	152 (33.48)	186 (36.19)	23 (23.00)	
Current drinking	53 (5.0)	19 (4.19)	26 (5.06)	8 (8.0)	
DM, n (%)	330 (30.90)	154 (33.92)	148 (28.79)	28 (28.0)	0.177
Hp, n (%)	647 (60.6)	284 (62.56)	309 (60.11)	54 (54.00)	0.323
Obesity, n (%)	236 (22.1)	91 (20.0)	122 (23.74)	23 (23.00)	0.375
Hypertriglyceridemia, n (%)	473 (44.3)	193 (42.51)	234 (45.53)	46 (36.0)	0.601
Hypercholesterolemia, n (%)	178 (16.7)	76 (16.7)	87 (16.9)	15 (15.0)	0.893

Table 3. Angiographic and procedural characteristics.

Variables	Phenotypes			P value
	EMs (n = 454)	IMs (n = 514)	PMs (n = 100)	
Target vessel, n (%)				
Left main	19 (4.19)	27 (5.25)	3 (3.00)	0.362
LAD	325 (71.59)	336 (65.37)	70 (70.00)	
LCX	59 (13.00)	73 (14.20)	11(11.00)	
RCA	51 (11.23)	78 (15.18)	16 (16.00)	
Stent type, n (%)				
Taxus®	70 (15.42)	75 (14.59)	12 (12.00)	0.247
Firebird®	86 (18.94)	111 (21.60)	20 (20.00)	
EXCEL®	37 (8.15)	36 (7.00)	13 (13.00)	
Cypher®	127 (27.97)	132 (25.68)	24 (24.00)	
Partner®	74 (16.30)	68 (13.23)	15 (15.00)	
Endeaver®	29 (6.39)	28 (5.45)	4 (4.00)	
Others	31 (6.83)	64 (12.45)	12 (12.00)	

Table 4. Distribution of genotypes of CYP2C19.

Subjects	EMs (n, %)	IMs (n, %)		PMs (n, %)		
	*1/*1	*1/*2	*1/*3	*2/*2	*2/*3	*3/*3
Total	454 (42.51)	493 (46.16)	21 (1.97)	81 (7.58)	8 (0.75)	11 (1.03)
Men	359 (33.61)	400 (37.45)	16 (1.50)	65 (6.10)	6 (0.56)	8 (0.75)
Women	95 (8.90)	93 (8.70)	5 (0.47)	16 (1.50)	2 (0.19)	3 (0.28)

The cumulative incidence of ST, death, MI, and total adverse events was significantly higher in PMs than in EMs (10.0% vs. 0.88%, 8.0% vs. 2.2%, 15.0% vs. 2.28%, and 16.0% vs.3.52%, respectively). However, there was no difference in the incidence of bleeding events among the three phenotypes ($P = 0.187$; Table 5).

The results of the multivariate Cox proportional hazards model showed that PM carriers were an independent predictor of 1-year ST (HR = 5.268, 95% CI = 1.528–18.164, $P = 0.009$). Table 6 shows the detailed results of the multivariate analysis. There was a decreased adverse-event–free survival rate (including ST, MI, death, and total adverse events) among patients carrying the CYP2C19 PM phenotypes when compared with the EMs (Fig. 2).

Discussion

In the present study, we reported the associations of CYP2C19 loss-of-function polymorphisms with the incidences of adverse outcomes of CAD patients after PCI. We found that patients with PMs have much higher incidences of ST, MI, and death when compared with EMs of CYP2C19.

Several studies have provided evidences linking CYP2C19 genetic variation to reduced exposure to the active drug metabolite, lower platelet inhibition, and less protection from recurrent ischemic events in people receiving clopidogrel [21]. According to previous reports, common polymorphisms in the CYP2C19 gene were approximately 30% in whites, 40% in blacks, and >55% in East Asians [22]. As described earlier, according to CYP2C19 genotype, individuals can be divided into three groups: PMs, IMs, and EMs. Our results indicate that PMs accounted for 9.36% and IMs for 48.12% of the Chinese CAD patients. Our result is in line with that reported in previous studies [22].

Although several studies have shown that CYP2C19*2 and CYP2C19*3 polymorphisms influence the platelet response to

Statistical Analysis

All analyses were carried out using SPSS version 17.0 (SPSS Inc., Chicago, IL, USA). The Hardy-Weinberg equilibrium was assessed using chi-square analysis. Discrete variables, expressed as counts or percentages, were compared by chi-square or Fisher's exact test, as appropriate. Continuous variables were expressed as mean ± standard deviation (SD). Normally distributed continuous variables were compared by t-test, and non-normally distributed data were compared by nonparametric test. The independent association between the presence of the CYP2C19*2 or *3 allele and its outcome was assessed after adjusting for other potential confounding factors by using multivariate Cox regression analysis and a Cox proportional hazards model for event-free survival. All variables associated with $P < 0.1$ in the univariate analysis were entered into the multivariate model as covariates. A value of $P < 0.05$ was considered as statistically significant.

Results

Patient Characteristics and CYP2C19 Genotype

Among the 1068 patients, there were 524 (49.06%) with wild homozygous, 465 (43.54%) with heterozygous, and 79 (7.40%) with mutant homozygous CYP2C19*2, and there were 947 (88.67%) with wild homozygous, 100 (9.36%) with heterozygous, and 11 (1.97%) with mutant homozygous CYP2C19*3. We divided these 1068 patients into three phenotypes based on CYP2C19*2 and CYP2C19*3 genotypes. Accordingly, there were 454 (42.51%) EMs, 514 (48.13%) IMs, and 100 (9.36%) PMs in the present study. Table 1 and Table 2 describe the baseline characteristics of the studied population according to CYP2C19 phenotype. All these variables were well balanced among these three groups (all $P > 0.05$). Table 3 shows the angiographic and procedural characteristics, which were also well balanced among the three groups (all $P > 0.05$).

Genotyping and outcomes

Table 4 shows the characteristics of the CYP2C19 genotype. After 1 year of follow-up, the total cumulative incidence of ST, death, MI, and bleeding events was 3.56% (38 of 1068), 3.37% (36 of 1068), 4.49% (48 of 1068), and 1.12% (12 of 1068), respectively.

Table 5. Accumulated Major Adverse Events During the One-year Period After Intervention.

Clinical outcomes	Phenotypes			P value
	EMs (n = 454)	IMs (n = 514)	PMs (n = 100)	
ST, n (%)	4 (0.88)	24 (4.67)	10 (10.00)	<0.001
Death, n (%)	10 (2.20)	18 (3.50)	8(8.00)	0.014
MI, n (%)	13 (2.86)	20 (3.89)	15 (15.00)	<0.001
Any of the above events, n (%)	26 (3.52)	50 (9.73)	16 (16.00)	<0.001
Bleeding events, n (%)	8 (1.76)	4 (0.78)	0 (0)	0.187

Table 6. Results of a multivariable Cox proportional hazards model.

Variables	B	SE	P value	Hazard ratio (95.0% CI)
Sex	0.247	0.379	0.514	1.280 (0.609–2.690)
Age	0.052	0.016	0.001	1.054 (1.021–1.087)
Stent type	0.701	0.377	0.063	2.015 (0.963–4.217)
DM	0.299	0.359	0.406	1.348 (0.666–2.727)
HP	0.704	0.394	0.074	2.021 (0.934–4.374)
Hypertriglyceridemia	0.272	0.357	0.447	1.312 (0.651–2.645)
Hypercholesterolemia	0.565	0.415	0.173	1.759 (0.781–3.964)
Phenotype			0.019	
IMs	0.818	0.563	0.146	2.266 (0.751–6.834)
PMs	1.662	0.632	0.009	5.268 (1.528–18.164)

clopidogrel [23–28], clinical data concerning the relevance of CYP2C19*2 and CYP2C19*3 carrier status in patients with CAD after PCI are limited, especially in China. Tang et al. [29] observed 267 CAD patients with PCI. After 1 year of follow-up, the researchers did not find an increased risk of ST among patients with CYP2C19*2, although they observed that the incidence of combined end point was higher in patients with CYP2C19*2 than in patients with CYP2C19*1/*1. Luo et al. [30] reported the relationship between CYP2C19*2 and the incidence of 180-day ST in Chinese Han and found the presence of at least one CYP2C19*2 allele, which was significantly associated with increased ST risk (CYP2C19*2/*2 or *1/*2 patients [2.4%] vs. CYP2C19*1/*1 patients [0.75%]). The risk of definite ST was highest in patients with the CYP2C19*2/*2 genotype. Chen et al. [31] reported that the homozygous CYP2C19*2/*2 genotype is an independent determinant of adverse vascular events in Chinese patients with CAD (HR = 5.191; 95% CI = 1.936–13.917; $P=0.001$). Oh et al. [32] also reported that the CYP2C19*2 genetic variant may be associated with worse outcome in Korean patients treated exclusively with DES and dual-antiplatelet therapy due to a significant increase in cardiac death, MI, or ST. However, Galiavich et al. [33] found that CYP2C19 gene polymorphism does not influence the prognosis for the next 6 months if patients follow medical recommendations, including regular use of clopidogrel. In their studies, they only selected CYP2C19*2 for examination. Although Tazaki et al. [34] selected not only CYP2C19*2 but also CYP2C19*3, they only described that a test can rapidly detect CYP2C19 PMs and predict low responders to clopidogrel. In addition, Tello-Montoliu et al. [35] examined CYP2C19*2 and *17 and found that even though the CYP2C19 genotype is associated with a variable on clopidogrel platelet reactivity, it has no significant clinical influence. In our study, we selected two loss-of-function polymorphisms (CYP2C19*2 and CYP2C19*3), observed 1068 CAD patients, and conducted 12-month follow-up. In our analysis, we divided the participants into three groups (EMs, IMs, and PMs). We observed that the PMs have higher incidences of MI, ST, and death compared with the EMs. After adjusting for other confounders, the PMs were found to remain as an independent risk factor for ST. Our finding is not only in line with the work carried out by Sibbing et al. [3] but also consistent with pharmacodynamic [25,26] and pharmacokinetic [23,24] investigations showing the strongest attenuation of platelet response to clopidogrel treatment among patients homozygous (*2/*2) for the mutant CYP2C19 allele. In addition, we also found that other clinical end points, such as MI and death, were associated with PMs. This result is not in line with Sibbing et al. and Trenk et al. [27], both of which only examined CYP2C19*2 and compared the clinical outcomes between

subjects carrying the CYP2C19*2 allele and those carrying CYP2C19*1/*1. The strength of our study is the selection of two loss-of-function polymorphisms (CYP2C19*2 and CYP2C19*3) and the division of the subjects into three groups, which may assist in finding the association between clinical outcomes and the combined effects of CYP2C19*2/*2, CYP2C19*3/*3, and CYP2C19*2/*3. However, our result is in line with a meta-analysis, which revealed that CYP2C19*2 carriers have not only higher ST incidence (OR = 3.03, $P<0.001$) but also higher cardiovascular mortality (OR = 1.79, $P=0.019$) [36].

In our results, the total incidence of ST is 3.56%, which appears higher than that in a previous report (0.8–2.0%). Many factors, including diabetes, active smoking, prior or ongoing MI, heart failure, recent cancer, renal insufficiency [37], and angiographic characteristics, such as small arteries, long lesions, bifurcations, thrombotic or ulcerated lesions, or low TIMI flow, influence the prevalence of ST [36]. However, pieces of evidence have been accumulated to suggest that the strongest factor associated with ST is the discontinuation of clopidogrel treatment and CYP2C19 genetic polymorphisms. In coronary patients who are carriers of a genetic variant associated with a loss of function of the CYP2C19 enzyme, the risk of ST on clopidogrel treatment was noted to be 3- to 6-fold higher depending on the population [38,39,3,4,29,30,36,37]. Our results indicate that after adjustment for other confounders in CAD patients with PMs, the risk of ST increased by 4.268-fold (HR = 5.268; 95% CI = 1.528–18.164).

Limitation

Due to the absence of some angiographic characteristics, such as vessel diameter, lesion length, and blood flow status, we only included target vessels, stent type, and other clinical characteristics in the multivariate Cox regression model. As a result, overestimation of the effect of CYP2C19 loss-of-function polymorphisms on ST may have occurred.

Conclusions

PM patients in a Chinese population had an increased risk of ST, death, and MI after coronary stent placement.

Author Contributions

Conceived and designed the experiments: XX YTM. Performed the experiments: YNY XML XX YYZ. Analyzed the data: FL BDC XX. Contributed reagents/materials/analysis tools: ZYF XM. Wrote the paper: XX.

References

1. Yusuf S, Zhao F, Mehta SR, Chrolavicius S, Tognoni G, et al. (2001) Effects of clopidogrel in addition to aspirin in patients with acute coronary syndromes without ST-segment elevation. N Engl J Med; 345: 494–502.
2. Savi P, Pereillo JM, Uzabiaga MF, Combalbert J, Picard C, et al. (2000) Identification and biological activity of the active metabolite of clopidogrel. Thromb Haemost; 84: 891–896.
3. Sibbing D, Stegherr J, Latz W, Koch W, Mehilli J, et al. (2009) Cytochrome P450 2C19 loss-of-function polymorphism and stent thrombosis following percutaneous coronary intervention. Eur Heart J; 30: 916–22.
4. Harmsze AM, van Werkum JW, Ten Berg JM, Zwart B, Bouman HJ, et al. (2010) CYP2C19*2 and CYP2C9*3 alleles are associated with stent thrombosis: a case-control study. Eur Heart J; 31: 3046–53.
5. Yang YN, Wang XL, Ma YT, Xie X, Fu ZY, et al. (2010). Association of interaction between smoking and CYP 2C19*3 polymorphism with coronary artery disease in a Uighur population. Clin Appl Thromb Hemost. 2010; 16: 579–83.
6. Fuchshuber-Moraes M, Carvalho RS, Rimmbach C, Rosskopf D, Carvalho MA, et al. (2011) Aminoglycoside-induced suppression of CYP2C19*3 premature stop codon. Pharmacogenet Genomics; 21: 694–700.
7. Holmes MV, Perel P, Shah T, Hingorani AD, Casas JP (2011) CYP2C19 genotype, clopidogrel metabolism, platelet function, and cardiovascular events: a systematic review and meta-analysis. JAMA. 2011; 306: 2704–14.
8. Sibbing D, Braun S, Morath T, Mehilli J, Vogt W, et al. (2009) Platelet reactivity after clopidogrel treatment assessed with point-of-care analysis and early drug-eluting stent thrombosis. J Am Coll Cardiol; 53: 849–856.
9. Xie X, Ma YT, Yang YN, Li XM, Liu F, et al. (2010) Alcohol consumption and ankle-to-brachial index: results from the Cardiovascular Risk Survey. PLoS One; 5(12): e15181.
10. American Diabetes Association (2009) Diagnosis and classification of diabetes mellitus. Diabetes Care; 32 Suppl 1: S62–67.
11. Xie X, Ma YT, Yang YN, Fu ZY, Li XM, et al. (2010) Polymorphisms in the SAA1/2 gene are associated with carotid intima media thickness in healthy Han Chinese subjects: the Cardiovascular Risk Survey. PLoS One; 5: e13997.
12. Xie X, Ma YT, Yang YN, Fu ZY, Li XM, et al. (2011) Polymorphisms in the SAA1 gene are associated with ankle-to-brachial index in Han Chinese healthy subjects. Blood Press; 20: 232–238.
13. Mega JL, Close SL, Wiviott SD, Shen L, Hockett RD, et al. (2009) Cytochrome p-450 polymorphisms and response to clopidogrel. N Engl J Med; 360: 354–62.
14. Caraco Y (2004) Genes and the response to drugs.N Engl J Med; 351: 2867–9.
15. Shi WX, Chen SQ (2004) Frequencies of poor metabolizers of cytochrome P450 2C19 in esophagus cancer, stomach cancer, lung cancer and bladder cancer in Chinese population. World J Gastroenterol; 10: 1961–1963.
16. Collet JP, Hulot JS, Pena A, Villard E, Esteve JB, et al. (2009) Cytochrome P450 2C19 polymorphism in young patients treated with clopidogrel after myocardial infarction: a cohort study. Lancet; 373: 309–17.
17. Shuldiner AR, O'Connell JR, Bliden KP, Gandhi A, Ryan K, et al. (2009) Association of cytochrome P450 2C19 genotype with the antiplatelet effect and clinical efficacy of clopidogrel therapy. JAMA; 302: 849–57.
18. Cutlip DE, Windecker S, Mehran R, Boam A, Cohen DJ, et al. (2007) Clinical end points in coronary stent trials: a case for standardized definitions. Circulation; 115: 2344–2351.
19. Thygesen K, Alpert JS, White HD (2007) Joint ESC/ACCF/AHA/WHF Task Force for the Redefinition of Myocardial Infarction.Universal definition of myocardial infarction. Eur Heart J; 28: 2525–38.
20. Ndrepepa G, Schuster T, Hadamitzky M, Byrne RA, Mehilli J, et al. (2012) Validation of the bleeding academic research consortium definition of bleeding in patients with coronary artery disease undergoing percutaneous coronary intervention. Circulation; 125(11): 1424–31.
21. Paré G, Mehta SR, Yusuf S, Anand SS, Connolly SJ, et al. (2010) Effects of CYP2C19 genotype on outcomes of clopidogrel treatment. N Engl J Med; 363(18): 1704–14.
22. Desta Z, Zhao X, Shin JG, Flockhart DA (2002) Clinical significance of the cytochrome P450 2C19 genetic polymorphism. Clin Pharmacokinet; 41: 913–58.
23. Brandt JT, Close SL, Iturria SJ, Payne CD, Farid NA, et al. (2007) Common polymorphisms of CYP2C19 and CYP2C9 affect the pharmacokinetic and pharmacodynamic response to clopidogrel but not prasugrel. J Thromb Haemost; 5: 2429–2436.
24. Umemura K, Furuta T, Kondo K (2008) The common gene variants of CYP2C19 affect pharmacokinetics and pharmacodynamics to an active metabolite of clopidogrel in healthy subjects. J Thromb Haemost; 6: 1439–1441.
25. Hulot JS, Bura A, Villard E, Azizi M, Remones V, et al. (2006) Cytochrome P450 2C19 loss-of-function polymorphism is a major determinant of clopidogrel responsiveness in healthy subjects. Blood; 108: 2244–2247.
26. Giusti B, Gori AM, Marcucci R, Saracini C, Sestini I. et al. (2007) Cytochrome P450 2C19 loss-of-function polymorphism, but not CYP3A4, IVS10+12G/A and P2Y12 T744C polymorphisms, is associated with response variability to dual antiplatelet treatment in high risk vascular patients. Pharmacogenet Genomics; 17: 1057–1064.
27. Trenk D, Hochholzer W, Fromm MF, Chialda LE, Pahl A, et al. (2008) Cytochrome P450 2C19 681G>A polymorphism and high on-clopidogrel platelet reactivity associated with adverse 1-year clinical outcome of elective percutaneous coronary intervention with drug-eluting or bare-metal stents. J Am Coll Cardiol;51: 1925–1934.
28. Frere C, Cuisset T, Morange PE, Quilici J, Camoin-Jau L, et al. (2008) Effect of cytochrome p450 polymorphisms on platelet reactivity after treatment with clopidogrel in acute coronary syndrome. Am J Cardiol; 101: 1088–1093.
29. Tang XF, He C, Yuan JQ, Meng XM, Yang YJ, et al. (2011) Impact of cytochrome P450 2C19 polymorphisms on outcome of cardiovascular events in clopidogrel-treated Chinese patients after percutaneous coronary intervention. Zhonghua Xin Xue Guan Bing Za Zhi. 2011; 39: 617–20.
30. Luo Y, Zhao YT, Verdo A, Qi WG, Zhang DF, et al. (2011) Relationship between cytochrome P450 2C19*2 polymorphism and stent thrombosis following percutaneous coronary intervention in Chinese patients receiving clopidogrel. J Int Med Res; 39: 2012–9.
31. Chen M, Liu XJ, Yan SD, Peng Y, Chai H, et al. (2012) Association between cytochrome P450 2C19 polymorphism and clinical outcomes in Chinese patients with coronary artery disease. Atherosclerosis. 220(1): 168–71.
32. Oh IY, Park KW, Kang SH, Park JJ, Na SH, et al. (2012) Association of cytochrome P450 2C19*2 polymorphism with clopidogrel response variability and cardiovascular events in Koreans treated with drug-eluting stents. Heart. 98(2): 139–44.
33. Galiavich AS, Valeeva DD, Minnetdinov RSh, Arkhipova AA, Akhmetov II, et al. (2012) CYP2C19 gene polymorphism in patients with myocardial infarction who use clopidogrel. Kardiologiia. 52(4): 20–4.
34. Tazaki J, Jinnai T, Tada T, Kato Y, Makiyama T, et al. (2012) Prediction of clopidogrel low responders by a rapid CYP2C19 activity test. J Atheroscler Thromb. 19(2): 186–93.
35. Tello-Montoliu A, Jover E, Marin F, Bernal A, Lozano ML, et al. (2012) Influence of CYP2C19 polymorphisms in platelet reactivity and prognosis in an unselected population of non ST elevation acute coronary syndrome. Rev Esp Cardiol (Engl Ed). 2012; 65(3): 219–26.
36. Montalescot G, Hulot JS, Collet JP (2009) Stent thrombosis: who's guilty? Eur Heart J; 30: 2685–8.
37. Van Werkum JW, Heestermans AA, Zomer AC, Kelder JC, Suttorp MJ, et al. (2009) Predictors of coronary stent thrombosis: the Dutch Stent Thrombosis Registry. J Am Coll Cardiol; 53: 1399–1409.
38. Simon T, Verstuyft C, Mary-Krause M, Quteineh L, Drouet E, et al. (2009) Acute ST-Elevation and Non–ST-Elevation Myocardial Infarction (FAST-MI) Investigators. Genetic determinants of response to clopidogrel and cardiovascular events. N Engl J Med; 360: 363–375.
39. Bauer T, Bouman HJ, van Werkum JW, Ford NF, ten Berg JM, et al. (2011) Impact of CYP2C19 variant genotypes on clinical efficacy of antiplatelet treatment with clopidogrel: systematic review and meta-analysis. BMJ; 343: d4588.

26

Optimal Oral Antithrombotic Regimes for Patients with Acute Coronary Syndrome

Yicong Ye*, Hongzhi Xie, Yong Zeng, Xiliang Zhao, Zhuang Tian, Shuyang Zhang

Department of Cardiology, Peking Union Medical College Hospital, Peking Union Medical College and Chinese Academy of Medical Sciences, Beijing, China

Abstract

Objective: We performed a network meta-analysis to investigate the optimal antithrombotic regime by indirectly comparing new antithrombotic regimes (new P2Y12 inhibitors plus aspirin or novel oral anticoagulants on top of traditional dual antiplatelet therapy [DAPT]) in patients with acute coronary syndrome (ACS).

Methods: A systematic search of MEDLINE, EMBASE, and the Cochrane databases was performed to identify all phase 3 randomized controlled trials (RCTs) involving novel oral anticoagulants or oral $P2Y_{12}$ inhibitors in patients with ACS. Major adverse cardiac events (MACE) were regarded as the efficacy endpoint, and thrombolysis in myocardial infarction (TIMI) major bleeding events were used as the safety endpoint. The net clinical benefit was calculated as the sum of MACE and TIMI major bleeding events.

Results: Five phase 3 RCTs with 64,476 ACS patients were included. Although there were no significant differences among new antithrombotic regimes, rivaroxaban 5 mg twice daily plus traditional DAPT might be the most effective in reducing the incidence of MACE, accompanying the highest risk of TIMI major bleeding. Ticagrelor plus aspirin presented slight advantage on the net clinical benefit over other new antithrombotic regimes, with the highest probability of being the best regimes for net clinical benefit (35.0%), followed by prasugrel plus aspirin (28.0%), and rivaroxaban 2.5 mg twice daily plus traditional DAPT (19.5%).

Conclusion: Novel antithrombotic regime with ticagrelor plus aspirin brings a larger clinical benefit in comparison with other regimes, suggesting that it may be the optimal antithrombotic regime for patients with ACS.

Editor: Adrian V Hernandez, Universidad Peruana de Ciencias Aplicadas (UPC), Peru

Funding: The authors have no support or funding to report.

Competing Interests: The authors have declared that no competing interests exist.

* E-mail: Zhangebmg@gmail.com

Introduction

It is well known that the formation of thrombosis is the major pathophysiologic mechanism of acute coronary syndrome (ACS), and thus traditional dual antiplatelet therapy (DAPT) (aspirin in combination with thienopyridines, predominantly clopidogrel) has become the mainstay of treatment in patients with ACS. Nevertheless, there remains about 10% risk of recurrent thrombotic events within one year after percutaneous coronary intervention (PCI), even after the use of traditional DAPT [1].

Recently, more intensive antithrombotic regimes have been developed in order to overcome this issue, and the safety and efficacy of these therapies have been verified by a series of randomized clinical trials (RCTs). Newly developed antiplatelet agents ($P2Y_{12}$ receptor inhibitors, e.g. Cangrelor [intravenous], Elinogrel [intravenous], prasugrel [oral] and ticagrelor [oral]) have been shown to have more potent therapeutic effect and have faster onset of action, as well as significantly decrease cardiovascular mortality after PCI as compared to clopidogrel [2]. These advantages make P2Y12 inhibitors particularly attractive to patients with ACS. On the other hand, novel oral anticoagulants, such as rivaroxaban, apixaban, darexaban and dabigatran, have also been developed. A recent meta-analysis in ACS patients has demonstrated that use of the novel oral anticoagulant agents, on top of single antiplatelet regimens, or DAPT in ACS is associated with 30% reduction in recurrent ischemic events, but a substantial increase in bleeding, which is most pronounced when novel oral anticoagulants are prescribed in addition to DAPT [3].

Based on the above clinical evidence, new antithrombotic agents, in addition to DAPT, have been recommended in specific subsets among ACS patients in the current clinical practice guidelines [4]. However, to date there is not any large scale head-to-head trial to compare the clinical utility of these new antithrombotic agents. It is also unclear whether the new DAPT using ticagrelor or prasugrel has superiority to novel oral anticoagulants on top of traditional DAPT in ACS subjects.

We therefore conducted a network meta-analysis based on the available data from published RCTs to investigate the efficacy and safety of these new antithrombotic agents in patients with ACS.

Methods

Data Sources and Searches

We conducted a computerized literature search of MEDLINE (1950 to April 2013), EMBASE (1966 to April 2013), and the

Cochrane Central Register of Controlled Trials (until April 2013) to identify the eligible studies. An extensive manual search of the literature using the references of the original manuscripts, reviews, and meta-analyses was performed. No language restrictions were imposed. The search strategy was presented in *Text S1*.

Selection criteria

The clinical trials were eligible for inclusion if 1) study design (phase 3 RCTs) involved patient randomization; 2) participants were diagnosed with ACS; and 3) comparisons were made between new oral P2Y12 receptor inhibitors with clopidogrel and novel anticoagulants with placebo in addition to DAPT. Trials would be excluded if the control group used single antiplatelet treatment, or if the sample size was less than 500.

Data Extraction

Two authors (Y. Y. and H. X.) independently determined the study eligibility and extracted the following data from the included studies: (1) study design; (2) participant and intervention characteristics; (3) treatment (including novel oral anticoagulants or new oral P2Y12 inhibitors); and (4) clinical outcomes (including major adverse cardiac events [MACE] and Thrombolysis in Myocardial Infarction [TIMI] major bleeding). MACE was defined as a composite endpoint of cardiovascular death, myocardial infarction, or stroke. The net clinical benefit was calculated as the sum of MACE and TIMI major bleeding events. Any disagreements were resolved by consensus, and the principal investigators resolved any disagreements.

Risk of Bias Assessment

The internal validity of the eligible studies was assessed according to the Cochrane Collaboration risk of bias tool [5]. The risk of bias was described and assessed in seven specific domains: 1) random sequence generation; 2) allocation concealment; 3) blinding of participants, personnel; 4) blinding of outcome assessment; 5) incomplete outcome data; 6) selective reporting; and 7) other sources of bias. The judgments involved using the answers "yes" (indicating a low risk of bias), "no" (indicating a high risk of bias), and "unclear" (if risk of bias is unknown, or if an entry is not relevant to the study).

Data Synthesis and Analysis

The κ statistic was used to assess the agreement between reviewers for study selection. In the pair-wise meta-analysis, the pooled odd ratio (OR) was calculated for each outcome using the Mantel-Haenszel method for random effects [6]. The heterogeneity across the included studies was assessed using the Cochrane Q test via a χ^2 test and was quantified with the I^2 test [7].

A network meta-analysis was conducted to compare the efficacy and safety among these new antithrombotic regimes. Due to indirect comparison among these antithrombotic regimes, it was not feasible to use an inconsistency model or a node-splitting model to statistically identify inconsistencies. We assumed the included studies were consistent based on the criteria of study selection and analysis using a consistency random effects model. This model was implemented in the Bayesian framework and estimated using Markov chain Monte Carlo (MCMC) methods [8], which was recommended by the National Institute for Health and Clinical Excellence (NICE) Decision Support Unit technical support documenton evidence synthesis [9]. The models were run for 300,000 iterations, after which convergence was assessed using the Brooks-Gelman-Rubin diagnostic [9]. Specifically, convergence was assessed by comparing within-chain and between-chain variance to calculate the Potential Scale Reduction Factor (PSRF) [10]. If the PSRF is large, it means that the between-chains variance can be decreased by running additional iterations. If the PSRF is close to 1, it indicates approximate convergence has been reached.

Sensitivity analysis, including both phase 2 and phase 3 studies, was conducted to test how robust the final ranking of these new antithrombotic regimes was relative to eligibility criteria. Publication bias was assessed by the Begg's funnel plot and the Egger weighted regression statistic where a value of $p<0.10$ indicates a significant publication bias among the included studies.

All analyses were performed using STATA (version 11.0) and ADDIS (AggregateData Drug Information System,version 1.16.3). The meta-analysis was prepared in accordance with the PRISMA (Preferred Reporting Items for Systematic Reviews and Meta-Analyses) statement [11].

Results

Characteristics of included studies

Four-hundred and sixty-three records were retrieved from the initial search. Seventeen studies were reviewed in full-text. Five phase 3 randomized control trials (TRITON-TIMI 38 [12], TRILOGY ACS [13], PLATO [14], APPRAISE 2 [15], and ATLAS ACS2-TIMI 51 [16]) comparing 5 new antithrombotic regimes with traditional DAPT were included in the meta-analysis (Figure 1 and Figure 2). The inter-reviewer agreement for the study selection was high ($\kappa = 0.98$).

Basically, all of the studies included ACS patients with moderate-to-high risk, although the reporting detail of criteria in each study is different (Table S1). The baseline characteristics of the study population were presented in Table 1 and Table S2. A total of 64,476 ACS patients were included in the 5 trials. Of them, 34,864 were randomized to receive new antithrombotic regimes and 29,612 to receive traditional DAPT. The mean or median age of the enrolled patients ranged from 61 to 67 years, and each trial predominantly enrolled men. The median follow-up periods ranged from 8 to 17.1 months. The TRITON-TIMI 38 [12] and TRILOGY ACS trials [13] compared prasugrel plus aspirin with traditional DAPT (clopidogrel plus aspirin) in ACS patients undergoing PCI and non-ST segment elevation ACS patients without PCI, respectively, while the PLATO trial [14] compared ticagrelor plus aspirin with traditional DAPT (clopidogrel plus aspirin) in ACS patients. In APPRAISE 2 [15] and ATLAS ACS2-TIMI 51 trials [16], apixaban and rivaroxaban (two dose regimes: 2.5 mg and 5 mg twice daily) plus traditional DAPT were compared with traditional DAPT (predominately clopidogrel plus aspirin), respectively.

Risk of bias assessment

All trials were high quality multiple-center RCTs with pre-specified protocols, making them low risk of reporting bias (FigureS1).All trials used center randomization and double-blinded methods, and thus had low risk of selection bias and performance bias. The primary and secondary outcomes in all studies were adjudicated with the use of pre-specified criteria by an independent clinical events committee and therefore had a low risk of detection bias. In these included studies, the proportion of missing outcomes was not enough to have a clinically relevant impact on the intervention effect estimate, or missing outcome data balanced in numbers across intervention groups with similar reasons.

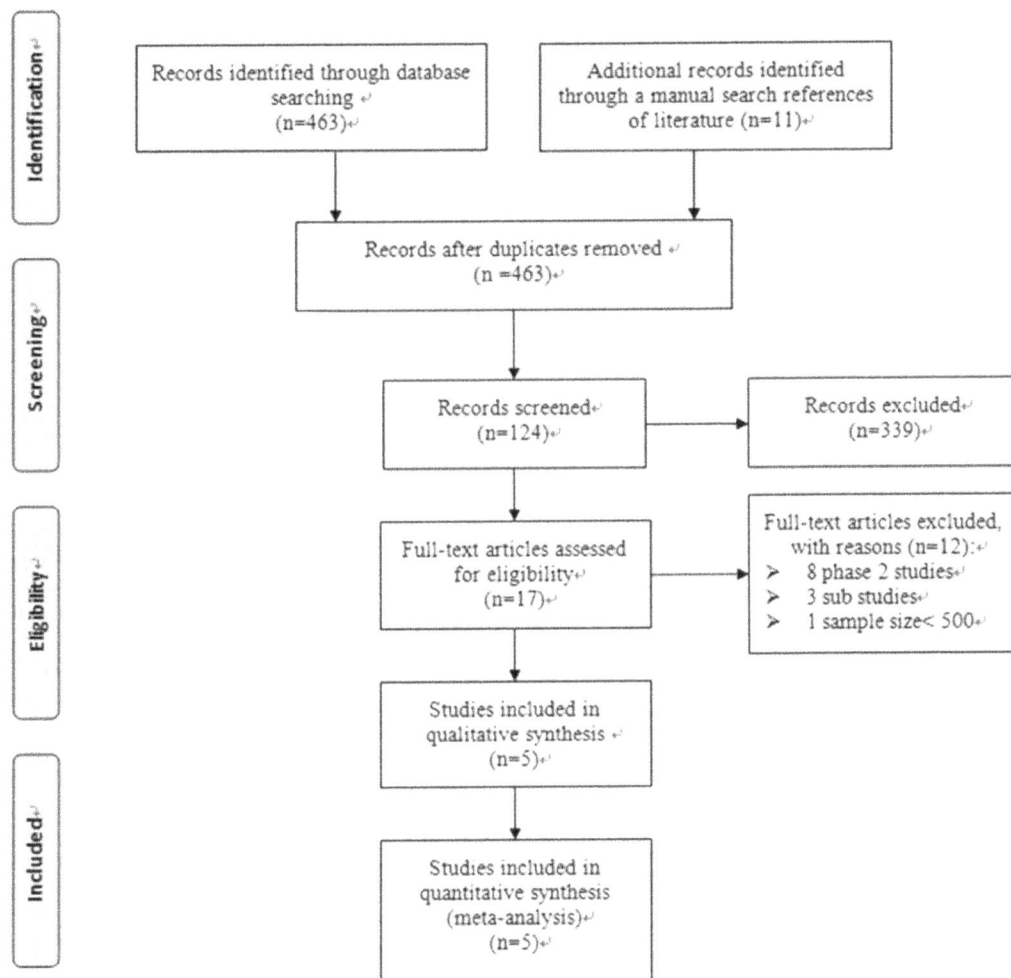

Figure 1. PRISMA flow diagram of study selection.

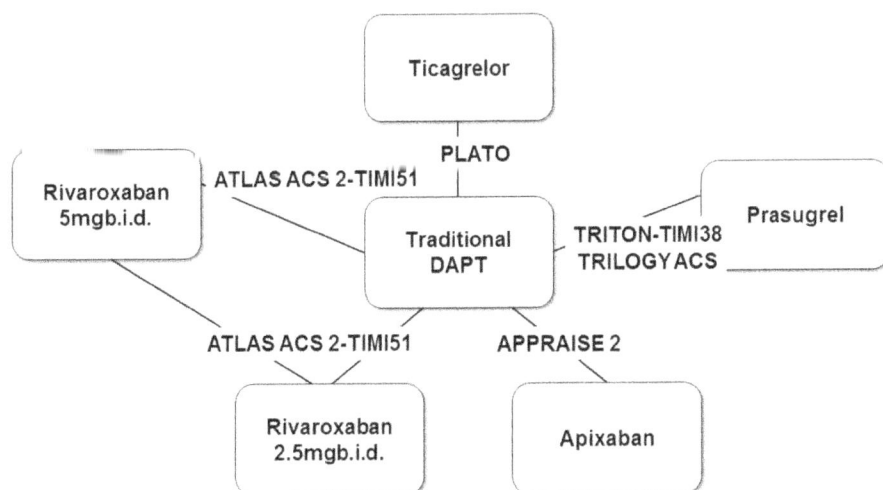

Figure 2. Studies and treatments included in the network meta-analysis.

Table 1. Characteristics of included studies.

Studies	Year	Study population	Sample size	Age yr	Male%	STEMI%*	Duration Months	Active group — New P2Y$_{12}$ inhibitors or novel oral anticoagulants	Thienopyridine %	ASA%	Control group — Thienopyridine %	ASA %
TRITON -TIMI38	2007	ACS with PCI	13,608	61	74	26	14.5	Prasugrel 60 mg(LD)+10 mg daily	0	99	100	99
PLATO	2009	ACS	18,624	62	71.7	37.7	9.2	Ticagrelor 180 mg(LD)+90 mg b.i.d	0	97.4	82.8	97.5
APPRAISE 2	2011	ACS	7392	67	67.8	39.6	8	Apixaban 5 mg b.i.d	81	97	81	97
ATLAS ACS2-TIMI 51	2012	ACS	15526	61.7	74.7	50.3	13	Rivaroxaban 2.5/5.0 mg b.i.d	98.7	98.6	92.9	98.7
TRILOGY ACS	2012	NSTEACS without PCI	9326	66	60.8	0	17.1	Prasugrel 30 mg(LD)+5/10 mg daily	0	94	100	93.4

ACS = acute coronary syndrome; ASA = aspirin; LD = loading dose; NSTEACS = Non-ST segment elevation acute coronary syndrome; PCI = percutaneous coronary intervention; STEMI = ST elevation myocardial infarction

Pair-wise meta-analysis

The use of new antithrombotic agents resulted in significantly reduced risk of MACE compared with traditional DAPT (OR = 0.860; 95% CI, 0.803 to 0.921; p<0.001) with modest heterogeneity ($\chi^2 = 6.35$, p for $\chi^2 = 0.175$; $I^2 = 37.0\%$). However, an increased risk of TIMI major bleeding was identified in new antithrombotic treatment group (OR1.702; 95% CI, 1.125–2.573; $p = 0.012$) with significant heterogeneity ($\chi^2 = 40.99$, p for $\chi^2 < 0.001$; $I^2 = 90.2\%$). To take the benefit and the bleeding risk together, we found that the use of new antithrombotic agents was associated with a net benefit compared with traditional DAPT (OR = 0.934; 95% CI, 0.888 to 0.983; $p = 0.009$). No significant heterogeneity was identified across the included studies ($\chi^2 = 4.48$, p for $\chi^2 = 0.345$; $I^2 = 10.6\%$; Figure 3)

Network meta-analysis

In the consistency model, convergence of the model was achieved by extending the number of iterations to 100,000. The ORs and the 95% CIs for all treatments relative to each other under the consistency model were presented in Table 2. Rivaroxaban, either at the dose of 5 mg or 2.5 mg twice daily, presented a beneficial effect of reducing the risk of MACE compared with other agents. However, rivaroxaban was associated with the higher risk of TIMI major bleeding events, especially at the dose of 5 mg twice daily. In addition, ticagrelor seemed likely to have a greater net benefit compared with other antithrombotic agents.

The distribution of probabilities of each treatment being ranked at each of the possible six positions was presented in Table S3. The cumulative probabilities of being among the two most efficacious regimes in reducing MACE were: 27.0% for rivaroxaban 5 mg twice daily, 26.5% for rivaroxaban 2.5 mg twice daily, 23.5% for ticagrelor, 14.5% for prasugrel, 8.5% for apixaban, and 0% for traditional DAPT. The cumulative probabilities of reducing TIMI major bleeding were: 43.0% for traditional DAPT, 36.5% for ticagrelor, 13% for prasugrel, 4.0% for apixaban, 2.0% for rivaroxaban 2.5 mg twice daily, and 1.0% for rivaroxaban 5 mg twice daily. The cumulative probabilities of net benefit were: 35.0% for ticagrelor, 28.0% for prasugrel, 19.5% for rivaroxaban 2.5 mg twice daily, 9.5% for rivaroxaban 5 mg twice daily, 6.5% for apixaban, and 1.0% for traditional DAPT (Figure 4).

In the sensitivity analysis, we included all the phase 2 trials investigating these antithrombotic regimes in patients with ACS. DISPERSE-2 (ticagrelor) [17], APPRAISE (apixaban) [18], and ATLAS ACS-TIMI46 (rivaroxaban) [19] were included in the sensitivity analysis, while JUMBO-TIMI 26 [20] was excluded, which investigated prasugrel both in ACS and stable coronary disease. The cumulative probabilities of the two most efficacious regimes in net benefit were similar with the result above: 35.0% for ticagrelor, 30.0% for prasugrel, 21.0% for rivaroxaban 2.5 mg twice daily, 8.0% for rivaroxaban 5 mg twice daily, 5.0% for apixaban, and 1.5% for traditional DAPT. In addition, neither the Egger's nor the Begg's tests, which assessed publication bias, showed statistical significance (both p>0.10).

Discussion

The finding of this analysis demonstrated that the use of new antithrombotic agents resulted in significant reduction in MACE with an increased risk of major bleeding. There was a significant net benefit towards new antithrombotic regimes compared with traditional DAPT. Although no statistical significance was identified, the new P2Y$_{12}$ receptor inhibitor, ticagrelor, showed a trend toward achieving the greatest beneficial effect compared to

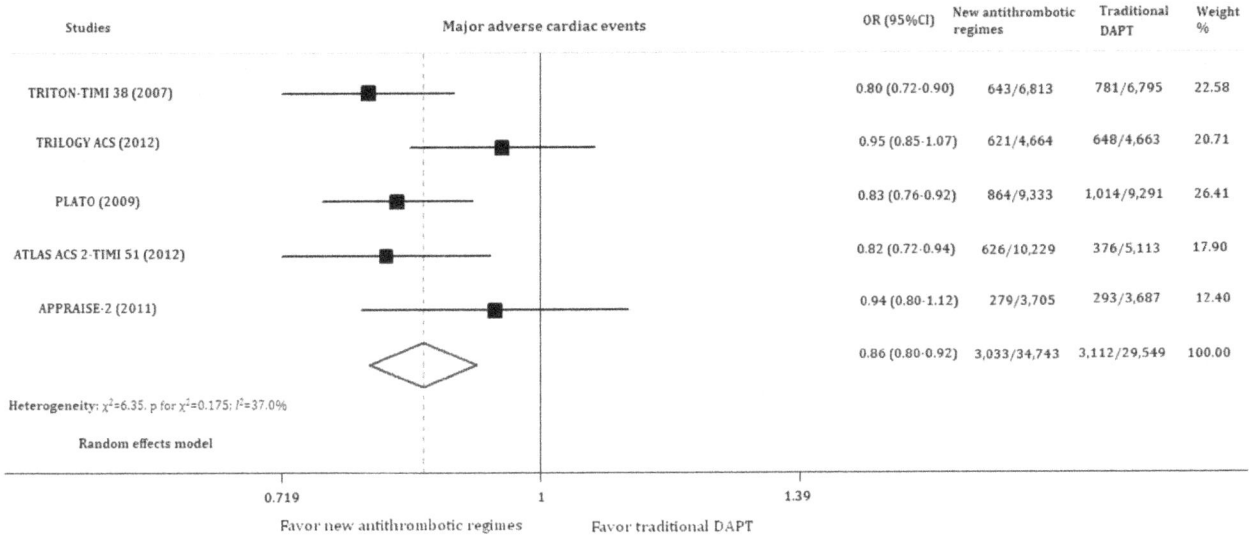

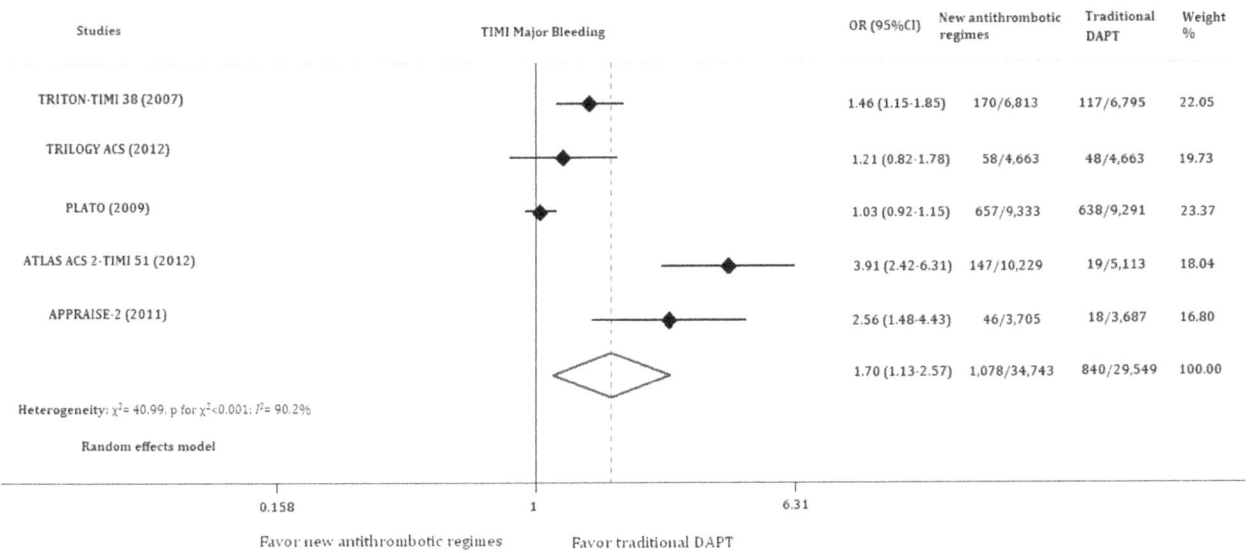

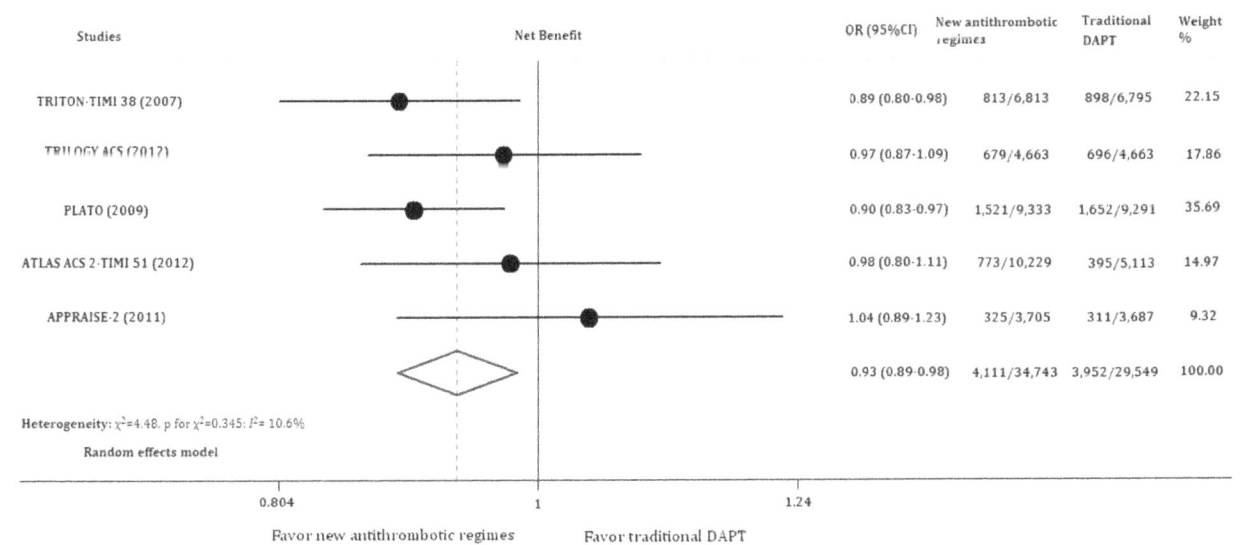

Figure 3. Forest plots of comparisons between new antithrombotic therapy and traditional DAPT in major cardiac adverse events, TIMI major bleeding events and net clinical benefit. DAPT: dual antiplatelet therapy; OR: odd ratio; CI: confidence interval; TIMI: thrombolysis in myocardial infarction.

other regimes, which gives it the highest probability of being the optimal therapy.

There were several small-scale studies directly comparing the antiplatelet effect directly of ticagrelor with prasugrel. In ACS patients with diabetes, ticagrelor presented a significantly higher platelet inhibition than prasugrel [21] and similar results were also found in ACS patients with high on-clopidogrel platelet reactivity [22]. However, other studies did not find the differences in antiplatelet effect between these new $P2Y_{12}$ receptor inhibitors [23,24]. A previous meta-analysis including TRITON-TIMI 38, PLATO, and DISPERSE-2 trials indicated the similar efficacy of prasugrel to ticagrelor, while ticagrelor was associated with a significantly lower risk of any major bleeding. Of note, this meta-analysis did not include the result from TRILOGY ACS. To our knowledge, there is no RCTs comparing the new $P2Y_{12}$ receptor inhibitors (e.g. prasugrel or ticagrelor) with novel oral anticoagulants (rivaroxaban or apixaban). It was required that large-scale RCTs directly comparing clinical value of these new antithrombotic agents were performed in order to achieve the sufficient power.

It has been reported that multiple medications may reduce patients' compliance and fixed-dose combination antihypertensive medication resulted in better compliance than the single agent [25,26]. In ALTAS ACS 2-TIMI 51, premature discontinuation of antithrombotic agents occurred in more than one fourth of patients in either rivoraxaban or placebo group [16]. However, the overall rate of drug compliance was 82.8% in PLATO using two antithrombotic agents [14]. Thus, oral anticoagulants in addition to DAPT may be a crowd for patients with ACS, who have already taken multiple medications [27].

It is no doubt that these new antithrombotic regimes are associated with reduced rate of recurrent ischemic events.

However, more potent platelet/factor Xa inhibition increases the risk of bleeding. In the current study, we found that rivaroxaban in combination with DAPT seemed likely to be the most efficacious in reducing MACE in ACS patients. However, the clinical benefit may be significantly offset by the increase in major bleeding events. This conclusion was confirmed by the recent meta-analysis, in which the administration of novel oral anticoagulant agents did not provide the net clinical benefit compared toplacebo in ACS patients, due to dramatic increase in major bleeding events [28]. Therefore, the target of antithrombotic therapies should be to inhibit platelet function or factor Xa, which may minimize the risk of ischemic and bleeding outcomes. This optimal range may be tailored to specific populations or clinical with different ischemic and bleeding risks [29].

Several limitations of this meta-analysis deserve comment. Firstly, in order to reduce heterogeneity, we included only phase 3 studies in our meta-analysis. Nevertheless, we conducted a sensitivity analysis by combining phase 2 studies with phase 3 studies, and we found the similar results to our original findings. Secondly, there was slight difference in baseline characteristics of enrolled patients in the meta-analysis due to different eligible criteria in the enrolled studies. Thirdly, although combining the major bleeding with the ischemic endpoints into a composite endpoint (net clinical benefit) has been widely used in contemporary trials [30–32], it may be associated with some pitfalls, such as lack of a proven link between lower bleeding rates and lower mortality rates [33]. Additionally, since this is a study-level meta-analysis, instead of patient-level meta-analysis, it was impossible to further analyze the effect of complex clinical factors, such as gender difference or the type of ACS.

Table 2. The odd ratios and the 95% confidence interval for all treatments relative to each other under the consistency model.

Odd ratios and 95% confidential interval for major adverse cardiac events (MACE)				
Apixaban	0.92 (0.63, 1.34)	0.87 (0.55, 1.35)	0.87 (0.56, 1.34)	0.88 (0.57, 1.35)
1.08 (0.74, 1.58)	**Prasugrel**	0.94 (0.64, 1.38)	0.94 (0.65, 1.37)	0.96 (0.67, 1.37)
1.15 (0.74, 1.81)	1.06 (0.72, 1.55)	**Rivaroxaban 2.5 mg b.i.d**	1.00 (0.73, 1.37)	1.01 (0.65, 1.56)
1.15 (0.75, 1.79)	1.06 (0.73, 1.55)	1.00 (0.73, 1.37)	**Rivaroxaban 5 mg b.i.d**	1.02 (0.67, 1.55)
1.13 (0.74, 1.74)	1.05 (0.73, 1.50)	0.99 (0.64, 1.53)	0.98 (0.64, 1.50)	**Ticagrelor**
Odd ratios and 95% confidential interval for TIMI major bleeding				
Apixaban	0.52 (0.09, 3.22)	1.35 (0.16, 11.05)	1.67 (0.20, 14.10)	0.40 (0.05, 3.33)
1.93 (0.31, 11.15)	**Prasugrel**	2.58 (0.41, 15.56)	3.24 (0.54, 18.99)	0.75 (0.13, 4.45)
0.74 (0.09, 6.21)	0.39 (0.06, 2.41)	**Rivaroxaban 2.5 mg b.i.d**	1.26 (0.29, 5.41)	0.30 (0.04, 2.38)
0.60 (0.07, 4.96)	0.31 (0.05, 1.86)	0.79 (0.18, 3.46)	**Rivaroxaban 5 mg b.i.d**	0.24 (0.03, 1.94)
2.52 (0.30, 19.94)	1.33 (0.22, 7.54)	3.36 (0.42, 25.52)	4.25 (0.52, 33.63)	**Ticagrelor**
Odd ratios and 95% confidential interval for net benefit				
Apixaban	0.89 (0.70, 1.13)	0.91 (0.68, 1.22)	0.96 (0.72, 1.28)	0.87 (0.67, 1.13)
1.13 (0.88, 1.43)	**Prasugrel**	1.03 (0.81, 1.29)	1.08 (0.85, 1.36)	0.97 (0.80, 1.19)
1.10 (0.82, 1.46)	0.97 (0.77, 1.23)	**Rivaroxaban 2.5 mg b.i.d**	1.05 (0.86, 1.28)	0.95 (0.74, 1.22)
1.05 (0.78, 1.40)	0.93 (0.74, 1.18)	0.95 (0.78, 1.16)	**Rivaroxaban 5 mg b.i.d**	0.91 (0.70, 1.17)
1.16 (0.89, 1.50)	1.03 (0.84, 1.25)	1.05 (0.82, 1.35)	1.10 (0.86, 1.42)	**Ticagrelor**

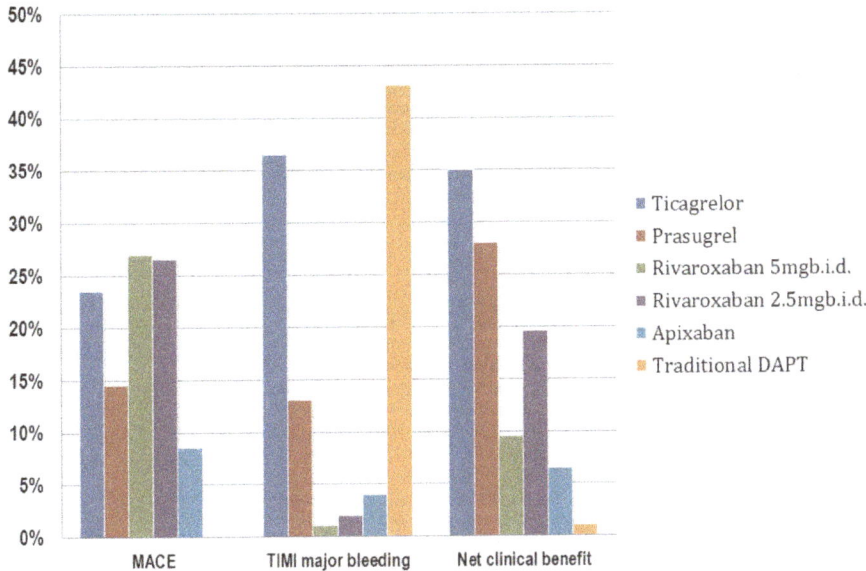

Figure 4. The cumulative probabilities of being among the two most efficacious regimes in reducing MACE, increasing TIMI major bleeding events and net clinical benefit. MACE: major adverse cardiac event. TIMI: thrombolysis in myocardial infarction.

Conclusion

New antithrombotic agents are associated with significantly reduced risk of MACE, as well as an increased risk of major bleeding, in comparison with traditional DAPT. Although no significant statistical differences were identified among these new antithrombotic regimes, there was a trend in net clinical benefit favoring the new P2Y$_{12}$ receptor inhibitor, ticagrelor. The findings may provide a support for ticagrelor plus aspirin to be an optimal antithrombotic regimen for patients with ACS.

Supporting Information

Figure S1   Risk of bias assessment.

Table S1   Major inclusion and exclusion criteria of the included studies. UA = unstable angina; NSTEMI = non ST elevated myocardial infarction; ACS = acute coronary syndrome; STEMI = ST elevation myocardial infarction; PCI = percutaneous coronary intervention; CABG – coronary artery bypass; NYHA = New York Heart Association.

Table S2   Medical history and medication of included studies. MI = myocardial infarction; CABG = coronary artery bypass; ACEI = angiotensin converting enzyme inhibitors; ARB = angiotensin II receptor blocker.

Table S3   The distribution of probabilities of each treatment being ranked at each of the possible 6 positions. DAPT = dual antiplatelet therapy; TIMI = thrombolysis in myocardial infarction.

Text S1   Search strategy (via EMBASE.com).

Author Contributions

Conceived and designed the experiments: YY SZ. Performed the experiments: YY HX YZ SZ. Analyzed the data: YY HX YZ XZ ZT SZ. Contributed reagents/materials/analysis tools: YY HX YZ SZ. Wrote the paper: YY HX YZ SZ.

References

1. Yusuf S, Zhao F, Mehta SR, Chrolavicius S, Tognoni G, et al. (2001) Effects of clopidogrel in addition to aspirin in patients with acute coronary syndromes without ST-segment elevation. N Engl J Med 345: 494–502.
2. Bellemain-Appaix A, Brieger D, Beygui F, Silvain J, Pena A, et al. (2010) New P2Y12 inhibitors versus clopidogrel in percutaneous coronary intervention: a meta-analysis. J Am Coll Cardiol 56: 1542–1551.
3. Oldgren J, Wallentin L, Alexander JH, James S, Jonelid B, et al. (2013) New oral anticoagulants in addition to single or dual antiplatelet therapy after an acute coronary syndrome: a systematic review and meta-analysis. Eur Heart J 34: 1670–1680.
4. Steg PG, James SK, Atar D, Badano LP, Blomstrom-Lundqvist C, et al. (2012) ESC Guidelines for the management of acute myocardial infarction in patients presenting with ST-segment elevation. Eur Heart J 33: 2569–2619.
5. Higgins JPT, Altman DG, Sterne JAC (2011). Assessing risk of bias in included studies. In: Higgins JPT, Green S, editors. Cochrane Handbook for Systematic Reviews of Interventions Version 5.1.0. Oxford: The Cochrane Collaboration. pp8.1–8.22.
6. Mantel N, Haenszel W (1959) Statistical aspects of the analysis of data from retrospective studies of disease. J Natl Cancer Inst 22: 719–748.
7. Higgins JP, Thompson SG, Deeks JJ, Altman DG (2003) Measuring inconsistency in meta-analyses. BMJ 327: 557–560.
8. Robert CP, Casella G (2004) Monte Carlo Statistical Methods, 2nd ed. New York: Springer-Verlag.
9. Dias S, Sutton AJ, Ades AE, Welton NJ (2013) Evidence synthesis for decision making 2: a generalized linear modeling framework for pairwise and network meta-analysis of randomized controlled trials. Med Decis Making 33:607–617.
10. Brooks SP GA (1998) General methods for monitoring convergence of iterative simulations. J Comput Graph Stat 7: 434–455.
11. Moher D, Liberati A, Tetzlaff J, Altman DG (2009) Preferred reporting items for systematic reviews and meta-analyses: the PRISMA statement. PLoS Med 6: e1000097.
12. Wiviott SD, Braunwald E, McCabe CH, Montalescot G, Ruzyllo W, et al. (2007) Prasugrel in patients with acute coronary syndromes. N Engl J Med 357: 2001–2015.
13. Roe MT, Armstrong PW, Fox KA, White HD, Prabhakaran D, et al. (2012) Prasugrel versus clopidogrel for acute coronary syndromes without revascularization. N Engl J Med 367: 1297–1309.

14. Wallentin L, Becker RC, Budaj A, Cannon CP, Emanuelsson H, et al. (2009) Ticagrelor versus clopidogrel in patients with acute coronary syndromes. N Engl J Med 361: 1045–1057.
15. Alexander JH, Lopes RD, James S, KiLaru R, He Y, et al. (2011) Apixaban with antiplatelet therapy after acute coronary syndrome. N Engl J Med 365: 699–708.
16. Mega JL, Braunwald E, Wiviott SD, Bassand JP, Bhatt DL, et al. (2012) Rivaroxaban in patients with a recent acute coronary syndrome. N Engl J Med 366: 9–19.
17. Cannon CP, Husted S, Harrington RA, Scirica BM, Emanuelsson H, et al. (2007) Safety, tolerability, and initial efficacy of AZD6140, the first reversible oral adenosine diphosphate receptor antagonist, compared with clopidogrel, in patients with non-ST-segment elevation acute coronary syndrome: primary results of the DISPERSE-2 trial. J Am Coll Cardiol 50: 1844–1851.
18. Alexander JH, Becker RC, Bhatt DL, Cools F, Crea F, et al. (2009) Apixaban, an oral, direct, selective factor Xa inhibitor, in combination with antiplatelet therapy after acute coronary syndrome: results of the Apixaban for Prevention of Acute Ischemic and Safety Events (APPRAISE) trial. Circulation 119: 2877–2885.
19. Mega JL, Braunwald E, Mohanavelu S, Burton P, Poulter R, et al. (2009) Rivaroxaban versus placebo in patients with acute coronary syndromes (ATLAS ACS-TIMI 46): a randomised, double-blind, phase II trial. Lancet 374: 29–38.
20. Wiviott SD, Antman EM, Winters KJ, Weerakkody G, Murphy SA, et al. (2005) Randomized comparison of prasugrel (CS-747, LY640315), a novel thienopyridine P2Y12 antagonist, with clopidogrel in percutaneous coronary intervention: results of the Joint Utilization of Medications to Block Platelets Optimally (JUMBO)-TIMI 26 trial. Circulation 111: 3366–3373.
21. Alexopoulos D, Xanthopoulou I, Mavronasiou E, Stavrou K, Siapika A, et al. (2013) Randomized assessment of ticagrelor versus prasugrel antiplatelet effects in patients with diabetes. Diabetes Care 36: 2211–2216.
22. Alexopoulos D, Galati A, Xanthopoulou I, Mavronasiou E, Kassimis G, et al. (2012) Ticagrelor versus prasugrel in acute coronary syndrome patients with high on-clopidogrel platelet reactivity following percutaneous coronary intervention: a pharmacodynamic study. J Am Coll Cardiol 60: 193–199.
23. Alexopoulos D, Xanthopoulou I, Gkizas V, Kassimis G, Theodoropoulos KC, et al. (2012) Randomized assessment of ticagrelor versus prasugrel antiplatelet effects in patients with ST-segment-elevation myocardial infarction. Circ Cardiovasc Interv 5: 797–804.
24. Parodi G, Valenti R, Bellandi B, Migliorini A, Marcucci R, et al. (2013) Comparison of prasugrel and ticagrelor loading doses in ST-segment elevation myocardial infarction patients: RAPID (Rapid Activity of Platelet Inhibitor Drugs) primary PCI study. J Am Coll Cardiol 61: 1601–1606.
25. Taylor AA, Shoheiber O (2003) Adherence to antihypertensive therapy with fixed-dose amlodipine besylate/benazepril HCl versus comparable component-based therapy. Congest Heart Fail 9: 324–332.
26. Dickson M, Plauschinat CA (2008) Compliance with antihypertensive therapy in the elderly: a comparison of fixed-dose combination amlodipine/benazepril versus component-based free-combination therapy. Am J Cardiovasc Drugs 8: 45–50.
27. Verheugt FW (2013) Combined antiplatelet and novel oral anticoagulant therapy after acute coronary syndrome: is three a crowd? Eur Heart J 34: 1618–1620.
28. Komocsi A, Vorobcsuk A, Kehl D, Aradi D (2012) Use of new-generation oral anticoagulant agents in patients receiving antiplatelet therapy after an acute coronary syndrome: systematic review and meta-analysis of randomized controlled trials. Arch Intern Med 172: 1537–1545.
29. Ferreiro JL, Sibbing D, Angiolillo DJ (2010) Platelet function testing and risk of bleeding complications. Thromb Haemost 103: 1128–1135.
30. Stone GW, McLaurin BT, Cox DA, Bertrand ME, Lincoff AM, et al. (2006) Bivalirudin for patients with acute coronary syndromes. N Engl J Med 355:2203–2216.
31. Fifth Organization to Assess Strategies in Acute Ischemic Syndromes Investigators, Yusuf S, Mehta SR, Chrolavicius S, Afzal R, et al(2006)Compar-)Comparison of fondaparinux and enoxaparin in acute coronary syndromes. N Engl J Med 354:1464–1476.
32. Lincoff AM, Bittl JA, Harrington RA, Feit F, Kleiman NS, et al. (2003) Bivalirudin and provisional glycoprotein IIb/IIIa blockade compared with heparin and planned glycoprotein IIb/IIIa blockade during percutaneous coronary intervention: REPLACE-2 randomized trial. JAMA 289:853–863.
33. Subherwal S, Ohman EM, Mahaffey KW, Rao SV, Alexander JH, et al.(2013) Incorporation of bleeding as an element of the composite end point in clinical trials of antithrombotic therapies in patients with non-ST-segment elevation acute coronary syndrome: validity, pitfalls, and future approaches. Am Heart J 165:644–654, 654.e1.

27

Periadventitial Application of Rapamycin-Loaded Nanoparticles Produces Sustained Inhibition of Vascular Restenosis

Xudong Shi[1⑨], Guojun Chen[2,3⑨], Lian-Wang Guo[1], Yi Si[1], Men Zhu[2,3], Srikanth Pilla[2], Bo Liu[1], Shaoqin Gong[2,3,4]*, K. Craig Kent[1]*

1 Department of Surgery, University of Wisconsin Hospital and Clinics, Madison, Wisconsin, United States of America, 2 Wisconsin Institutes for Discovery, University of Wisconsin, Madison, Wisconsin, United States of America, 3 Materials Science Program, University of Wisconsin, Madison, Wisconsin, United States of America, 4 Department of Biomedical Engineering, University of Wisconsin, Madison, Wisconsin, United States of America

Abstract

Open vascular reconstructions frequently fail due to the development of recurrent disease or intimal hyperplasia (IH). This paper reports a novel drug delivery method using a rapamycin-loaded poly(lactide-co-glycolide) (PLGA) nanoparticles (NPs)/ pluronic gel system that can be applied periadventitially around the carotid artery immediately following the open surgery. In vitro studies revealed that rapamycin dispersed in pluronic gel was rapidly released over 3 days whereas release of rapamycin from rapamycin-loaded PLGA NPs embedded in pluronic gel was more gradual over 4 weeks. In cultured rat vascular smooth muscle cells (SMCs), rapamycin-loaded NPs produced durable (14 days versus 3 days for free rapamycin) inhibition of phosphorylation of S6 kinase (S6K1), a downstream target in the mTOR pathway. In a rat balloon injury model, periadventitial delivery of rapamycin-loaded NPs produced inhibition of phospho-S6K1 14 days after balloon injury. Immunostaining revealed that rapamycin-loaded NPs reduced SMC proliferation at both 14 and 28 days whereas rapamycin alone suppressed proliferation at day 14 only. Moreover, rapamycin-loaded NPs sustainably suppressed IH for at least 28 days following treatment, whereas rapamycin alone produced suppression on day 14 with rebound of IH by day 28. Since rapamycin, PLGA, and pluronic gel have all been approved by the FDA for other human therapies, this drug delivery method could potentially be translated into human use quickly to prevent failure of open vascular reconstructions.

Editor: Xiaoming He, The Ohio State University, United States of America

Funding: This work was supported by National Heart, Lung, Blood Institute Grant R01-HL-068673 (to KCK) and a grant from National Science Foundation (DMR 1032187 to SG). The funders had no role in study design, data collection and analysis, decision to publish, or preparation of the manuscript.

Competing Interests: The authors have declared that no competing interests exist.

* E-mail: kent@surgery.wisc.edu (KCK); sgong@engr.wisc.edu (SG)

⑨ These authors contributed equally to this work.

Introduction

Over a million vascular reconstructions including more than 300,000 conventional open surgical interventions are performed in the USA each year to treat cardiovascular disease. Unfortunately a large number of these eventually fail due to the development of restenosis or intimal hyperplasia (IH). Despite our in depth understanding of this process and the development of inhibitors, treatments have lagged behind because of the lack of an effective method of drug delivery; this is particularly true for open vascular surgery where there are currently no clinically available methods to prevent recurrent vascular disease. Although systemic drug delivery has been attempted, toxicity has limited its success [1]. In addition systematic therapy cannot provide sufficient therapeutic drug levels at the target artery for a long time. To maintain effective drug concentrations without toxicity, local application is the optimal approach.

Advances in local drug delivery have been made for percutaneous vascular interventions. Both paclitaxel and rapamycin have advanced to clinical use and are currently applied *via* stents or balloons following percutaneous angioplasty. Although this approach has limitations including an increased risk of thrombosis, with the use of these stents, the rate of restenosis has diminished by at least 50% [2]. However, drug-eluting stents are not applicable in the case of open surgical procedures such as bypass, endarterectomy or dialysis access. For these procedures there currently are no viable clinical options for the prevention of restenosis. The result is an unmet clinical need for an effective method of drug delivery following open surgical revascularization. The absence of a technique for drug delivery following open surgery is surprising since the challenges of remote drug delivery following percutaneous angioplasty would seem more formidable than those for open surgery. At the time of open vascular reconstruction, the treated vessel is readily accessible making application of drug more direct and easily achievable. Periadventitial drug delivery has additional advantages, including minimized effect of the drugs on luminal endothelial cell growth due to the creation of a gradient resulting in diminished luminal drug concentrations.

Rapid progress in the field of nanomedicine in recent years offers new promising approaches to diagnose and treat many major diseases including cancers, vascular diseases, infections (*e.g.*,

HIV, malaria, tuberculosis), metabolic disease (*e.g.*, diabetes and osteoporosis), and autoimmune diseases (*e.g.*, glaucoma) [3–5]. Nanoparticles (NPs) encompass a variety of submicron colloidal nanosystems that may be inorganic, liposome-based, or polymer-based. Poly(lactic-co-glycolic acid) (PLGA) NPs are likely the most widely studied drug delivery NPs for the treatment of a broad range of diseases [4,6,7]. The popularity of PLGA NPs can be attributed to a number of factors. (1) PLGA has excellent biocompatibility and has been approved by FDA. (2) The biodegradability of PLGA and similarly, the drug release profiles of PLGA NPs can be conveniently engineered from weeks to months by controlling the chemical structure of PLGA (LA/GA ratio), its molecular weight, and the size of the NPs *etc* [8]. PLGA NPs can be used to encapsulate either hydrophobic drugs or hydrophilic drugs (*e.g.*, nucleic acids and proteins) using well-established emulsion processes. (4) PLGA NPs can provide local, site-specific, and sustained and controlled drug release. (5) PLGA NPs can enhance the cellular uptake of drug *via* endocytosis and may deliver drug to the target tissue/cell much more specifically *via* receptor-medicated endocytosis [6].

Originally used as an anti-fungal agent, rapamycin has been shown to be a potent anti-proliferative and anti-inflammatory drug which inhibits the mTOR-S6 Kinase 1 (S6K1) pathway [9]. Rapamycin also inhibits cell proliferation and inflammatory responses after angioplasty which are contributors to IH [10–12]. Intraluminal rapamycin-eluting stents are effective in suppressing IH, but detrimental late thrombosis develops due to the fact that locally released rapamycin also inhibits endothelial cells [13–15]. Moreover, patients treated with rapamycin-eluting stents still develop IH although to a lesser degree than bare metal stents. The potential use of NPs for the perivascular delivery of rapamycin to treat IH has not been fully explored. Rapamycin-loaded PLGA NPs (hereafter denoted as rapamycin-loaded NPs or rapamycin-NPs) may be potentially an ideal tool to provide sustained drug release to inhibit this process. Although several studies using animal models indicate that periadventitial application of rapamycin is a promising approach, currently there is no established method to provide sustained drug delivery after surgical procedures. Both rapamycin and PLGA are FDA approved, so it is relatively easy to translate these methods to clinical applications [12,14].

Using rapamycin as a model drug and PLGA NPs as the drug carrier, we have developed a drug delivery system that provides combined benefits of periadventitial local drug administration (convenient for application at the time of open surgery) and prolonged drug release resulting in improved efficacy. We found *in vitro*, that NPs were readily taken up by SMCs, allowing for more sustained release of rapamycin, and that rapamycin-loaded NPs produced a more sustained inhibition of S6 kinase than rapamycin alone. *In vivo*, in a rat carotid injury model, rapamycin-loaded NPs led to a more sustained inhibition of S6K1, SMC proliferation, IH and restenosis compared to rapamycin alone. Importantly, treatment with rapamycin-loaded NPs did not affect reendothelialization. Our studies thus suggest that periadventitial application of rapamycin-loaded NPs has a potential to develop into an improved therapeutic strategy for treating restenosis at the time of open vascular reconstructions.

Materials and Methods

Ethics Statement

The experiments involving animal use were carried out in strict accordance with the recommendations in the Guide for the Care and Use of Laboratory Animals of the National Institutes of Health. The protocol (Permit Number: M02273) was approved by the Institutional Animal Care and Use Committee (IACUC) of the University of Wisconsin-Madison. All surgery was performed under isoflurane anesthesia (through inhaling, flow rate 2 ml/min), and all efforts were made to minimize suffering. Animals were euthanized in a chamber gradually filled with CO_2.

Materials

Rapamycin was purchased from LC Laboratories (Woburn, MA). Chloroform (HPLC grade) was from Acros Organics (Fair Lawn, NJ). DMEM and fetal bovine serum (FBS) were from Invitrogen (Calsbad, CA). Poly(D,L-lactide-co-glycolide) (PLGA, 50:50, MW 40 to 75 kDa), poly (vinyl alcohol) (PVA, 95%, hydrolyzed, average MW 95 kDa), dimethyl sulfoxide (DMSO), Tween 80, paraformaldehyde, and FITC were from Sigma-Aldrich (St. Louis, MO). SDS gels (10% acrylamide) were from Bio-Rad (Hercules, CA). The FITC loaded NPs were a product from Phosphorex (Hopkinton, MA). The diameter of FITC-NPs is 220 ± 30 nm; the PLA:PGA ratio of NPs is 50:50. Kolliphor P407 (Poloxamer 407, a poly(ethylene oxide)-poly(propylene oxide)-poly(ethylene oxide) triblock copolymer) was kindly provided by BASF Corporation (Tarrytown, NY) and was used to prepare pluronic gel. Other reagents were purchased from Thermo Fisher Scientific (Fitchburg, WI) unless otherwise stated. TEM grids were purchased from Electron Microscopy Science (Hatfield, PA). The HPLC system is a product of Hitach High Technologies American, Inc. (Dallas, TX).

Rabbit anti-Ki67 antibody was from Abcam (Cambridge, MA); Rat anti-CD31 was from R&D Systems (Minneapolis, MN), antibodies to mTOR, phospho-S6 kinase-1 and S6 kinase-1 were from Cell Signaling Technologies (Danvers, MA); Alexa-468 conjugated secondary antibody was from Invitrogen (Carlsbad, CA). Fluorescence and bright field images were acquired using a Nikon Ti-U Eclipse microscope equipped with the Nikon Elements software packages. Microscopic images were processed and analyzed using the Image J software (NIH).

Preparation of Rapamycin-loaded NPs

Rapamycin-loaded NPs were prepared using a single emulsion (w/o) method as previously described [16,17]. Briefly, 12 mg of rapamycin and 65 mg of PLGA were added into a 100 ml flask. Subsequently, 6.5 ml of chloroform was added to the flask and stirred at 500 rpm at 40°C for 5 h. Thereafter, 26 ml of PVA water solution (3%) was added to the rapamycin/PLGA/chloroform solution followed by sonication using a probe sonicator (UP 100H from Hielscher) at 65% amplitude for 15 min. The resulting solution was stirred vigorously at room temperature for 6 days to evaporate the chloroform. Rapamycin-loaded NPs were collected *via* centrifugation at 22,800×*g* for 20 min at 4°C, and then freeze-dried and stored at −80°C in a desiccator. These rapamycin-NPs were found to be stable at least within a year. Blank PLGA NPs were prepared using a similar procedure without rapamycin.

Characterization of the PLGA NPs

The size distribution of the PLGA NPs dispersed in deionized water was measured using dynamic light scattering (DLS) (Malvern Zetasizer Nano-ZS90, 633 nm laser) at 25.0°C in triplicates. The morphology of the PLGA NPs was studied using transmission electron microscopy (TEM, Tecnai T12 G2) at 120 kV. The PLGA NPs were diluted with deionized water and then deposited on a copper grid coated with carbon. The NPs were negatively stained with 1% phosphotungstic acid solution and dried at room temperature.

Rapamycin loading level and its release rate from the rapamycin-NPs were measured by a high-performance liquid chromatography (HPLC) using ultraviolet (UV) detection at 278 nm. Rapamycin concentration in solution was quantified according to a standard curve established with known concentrations of rapamycin.

Localization of PLGA Nanoparticles in Cultured Vascular SMCs and in Injured Rat Carotid Arteries

Vascular smooth muscle cells (SMCs) were isolated from the thoracoabdominal aorta of male Sprague-Dawley rats based on a protocol described previously [18]. Cells were seeded in 4-well chamber slides with a density of 1×10^4 cells/well in DMEM containing 10% FBS and cultured at 37°C overnight with 5% CO_2 supplied. Then the culture media were changed to DMEM containing 2% FBS with 10 µg/ml fluorescein isothiocyanate (FITC)-loaded nanoparticles (FITC-NPs; 2% FITC loaded). The cells were then fixed by 4% paraformaldehyde at the indicated time points and imaged using fluorescence microscopy. For in vivo experiments, 1 mg of FITC-NPs was applied to the outside of the balloon-injured rat carotid artery as we have previously reported [19]. Carotid arteries were retrieved at the indicated time points and embedded in optimal cutting temperature compound (OCT); 5 µm frozen sections were prepared and imaged using a fluorescence microscope (200×).

In Vitro Rapamycin Release Study

To prepare 30% pluronic gel, 3 grams of Poloxamer 407 were dissolved in 10 ml PBS buffer by stirring overnight in the cold room. The in vitro rapamycin release profiles from either rapamycin-loaded NPs dispersed in pluronic gel (rapamycin-loaded NPs) or free rapamycin directly dispersed in pluronic gel (rapamycin) were determined in PBS (pH 7.4) containing 0.2% Tween 80 as described [20]. Three mg of rapamycin-loaded NPs or 300 µg of rapamycin in 15 µl DMSO/H_2O (v/v = 9/1) were dispersed in 300 µl of 30% pluronic solution contained in a microfuge tube on ice. The tube was then transferred to a 37°C incubator. After pluronic gel solidified at 37°C, 1 ml of PBS was added. At the indicated time points, microfuge tubes were spun at $22,800 \times g$ for 5 min to separate the supernatant from the PLGA NPs/gel mixture (recovery rate 99.6%); the supernatant was collected and replaced with fresh PBS buffer. The supernatant was filtered (membrane pore size 200 nm) to remove any uncollected NPs. The rapamycin concentration in the supernatant was then analyzed by HPLC. The drug release tests were conducted four times.

Western Blot

Rapamycin or rapamycin-loaded NPs (15 µg rapamycin for both) dispersed in 100 µl pluronic gel were placed in dialysis tubes with a molecular weight cut off (MWCO) of 10,000 Daltons (Thermo Fisher Scientific; Davenport, IL) that was capable of retaining NPs but not rapamycin. Dialysis tubes were then incubated with cultured smooth muscle cells. Cell culture media were replaced with fresh media every 24 h. Cells were retrieved at the indicated time points and lysed in RIPA buffer (50 mM Tris-HCl, 150 mM NaCl, 1% Nonidet P-40, 0.1% sodium dodecyl sulfate, and 10 µg/ml aprotinin). For in vivo experiments, carotid arteries were collected 14 days after surgery and treatment, and homogenized in RIPA buffer. Thirty micrograms of proteins from each sample were separated by SDS-PAGE on 10% gels and then transferred to nitrocellulose membranes. Protein expression was assessed by immunoblotting with rabbit anti-phospho-S6K1 or anti-S6K1 antibodies (Cell Signaling, Boston, MA). After incubation with horseradish peroxidase-conjugated secondary antibodies, specific proteins bands on the membranes were visualized by using enhanced chemiluminescence reagents (Pierce, Davenport, IL).

Cell Viability and Proliferation Assay

Cell proliferation was determined by modified 3-[4,5-dimethyl-thiazol-2-yl]-2,5-diphenyltetrazolium bromide (MTT) assay (Thermo Fisher Scientific; Davenport, IL). Rapamycin or rapamycin-loaded NPs (both 15 µg rapamycin) was mixed with 100 µl pluronic gel on ice, and then transferred into a microdialysis tube with a molecular weight cut off of 10,000 Dalton (Thermo Fisher Scientific; Davenport, IL). The dialysis media (1.5 ml) was collected (and stored) and replaced with fresh PBS buffer every day. Prior to rapamycin treatment, rat vascular SMCs were plated at 30–40% confluence on a 96-well plate and incubated overnight with 100 µl DMEM containing 10% FBS. Then 30 µl of the dialysis media collected at each time point was added to SMCs and cultured for 96 h. MTT solution (10 µl; 12 mM) in phenol red-free culture medium was added to each well and incubated at 37°C for 4 h followed by addition of 100 µl of the SDS-HCL solution. After incubation of the plate at 37°C for 4 h, absorbance was measured at 570 nm.

Rat Carotid Artery Balloon Injury and in vivo Drug Delivery

Male Sprague-Dawley rats (∼350 g) underwent carotid artery balloon injury. Briefly, after induction of anesthesia with isofluorane, a longitudinal incision was made in the neck. A 2-F balloon catheter (Edwards Lifesciences, Irvine, CA) was inserted through the left external carotid artery and inflated to a pressure of 2 atm to simulate the angioplasty procedure. Blood flow was re-established after injury. Rapamycin or rapamycin-NPs (100 µg rapamycin per 100 g body weight) was dissolved in 300 µl of 30% pluronic gel which remained as liquid on ice. The pluronic gel solution was then applied around the outside of the injured segment of carotid artery [19]. The gel solidified immediately after exposure to body temperature.

Tissue Processing

Animals were sacrificed and perfused with 4% paraformaldehyde at the pressure of 100 mmHg on day 14 or day 28 after surgery; then the carotid arteries were retrieved and processed for embedding and sectioning. Serial cross-sections were made at 50 µm intervals and used for histological analysis and immunostaining.

Immunohistochemistry (IHC)

Paraffin-embedded artery sections were immunostained with rabbit anti-Ki67 antibody (Cambridge, MA) and detected using goat anti-rabbit HRP conjugate IgG, developed in 3,3′ diaminobenzidine (DAB) solution, and followed by a counterstain of hematoxylin.

Immunofluorescent staining was performed on paraffin-embedded sections with rat anti-CD31antibpody (R&D Systems, MN; 1:400), signals were detected using donkey anti-rat Alexa Fluor 546 antibody (Invitrogen; Carlsbad, CA). DAPI was used to identify nuclei. Antibody controls included species-matched normal rabbit IgG antibodies.

Quantification of IHC Results

Five stained tissue sections from each animal were used. On each section images were taken from six different fields (magnification 200×). The Ki67 positive cells were manually counted. The number of Ki67 positive cells in each 200× image was defined as Ki67 positive (cells) per high power field (HPF). The data were pooled to generate the mean and standard deviation for each animal. The means from each of 5 animals were averaged, and the standard error of the mean (SEM) was calculated for each group.

For quantification of reendothelialization, previously published methods were used with minor modifications [21,22]. Briefly, the luminal perimeter and the percentage of this perimeter that stained for CD31 on serial sections (n = 5) were measured using NIH Image J. The percentage of reendothelialization was then scored from 1 to 5 (1: <20%; 2:20 to 40%; 3:40 to 60%; 4:60 to 80%; 5:80%–100%) and the scores were averaged.

Morphometric Analysis

Morphometric study was performed using H&E-stained paraffin sections of the carotid arteries. The areas enclosed by the external elastic lamina (EEL), the internal elastic lamina (IEL), and the luminal area were measured using the NIH Image J software as previously described [23]. Intimal area (IEL area minus luminal area) and medial area (EEL area minus IEL area) and their ratio (I/M ratio) were then calculated. Five sections per animal were used and a mean ± SEM was derived from at least three independent experiments. Data were analyzed by one-way analysis of variance (ANOVA). If significant, the ANOVA was followed by Turkeys multiple comparison test. P values less than 0.05 are considered statistically significant.

Results

Preparation and Characterization of Rapamycin-loaded NPs

Rapamycin was encapsulated in PLGA NPs *via* a single emulsion method. PVA was coated on the surface of PLGA NPs to enhance their solubility/dispensability in aqueous solutions. The rapamycin encapsulation efficiency and loading level in the PLGA NPs were of 69.1% and 11.6%, respectively. Figure 1A shows a representative transmission electron microscopy (TEM) image of the rapamycin-loaded NPs. The average diameter of the NPs was around 250 nm. The size distribution of the rapamycin-loaded NPs measured by DLS (Figure 1B) ranged from 220 to 350 nm with an average diameter around 265 nm, which was in agreement with the TEM analysis.

To evaluate the comparative release of rapamycin or rapamycin-loaded NPs *in vitro*, both were dispersed in pluronic gel to mimic our *in vivo* model. The amount of released rapamycin was determined by HPLC. For rapamycin dispersed directly in pluronic gel, the amount of drug released after 2, 4, and 5 days was 50.0%, 78.4% and 86.4%, respectively. In contrast, sustained drug release was observed for 28 days from the rapamycin-loaded NPs dispersed in pluronic gel (Figure 1C). In both studies, pluronic gel dissolved after 3–4 days. The release of rapamycin from the rapamycin-NPs-Gel system exhibited a well-defined tri-phasic profile [20]. The initial burst of release of rapamycin during the first 4 days is likely attributed to the release of rapamycin near the surface of the PLGA NPs (Figure 1C). During the second phase of rapamycin release (5 to 15 days), rapamycin was released slowly from the PLGA NPs *via* a diffusion-controlled process [24,25]. During the third phase (16 to 28 days), there was relatively rapid release of rapamycin again (16 to 21 days) likely attributable to the degradation and erosion of PLGA NPs [6,26,27], and then there was very minimal release of rapamycin after 21 days. These results demonstrate that rapamycin-loaded NPs dispersed in pluronic gel

provide drug release in a more sustainable manner than rapamycin directly contained in a pluronic gel.

Uptake of NPs by SMCs *in vitro* and After Periadventitial Application Around Injured Rat Carotid Arteries

To evaluate the cellular absorption and distribution of NPs *in vitro*, FITC-loaded PLGA NPs (FITC-NPs) were applied to cultured vascular SMCs as described in Methods. As is evident in Figure 2A, FITC-NPs were readily taken up by SMCs as early as 2 hours and NPs accumulated primarily in the cytoplasm. Punctate collections of nanoparticles were observed by 24 hours. We then investigated whether PLGA NPs could be readily dispersed into the arterial wall. FITC-NPs in pluronic gel were applied to the adventitia of rat carotid arteries immediately after balloon injury. We found at 24 h, FITC-NPs were localized around and within the adventitia of the injured carotid arteries (Figure 2B). At 72 h, after dissolution of the pluronic gel, FITC-NPs had migrated into the arterial wall as well as into the loose connective tissues that surround the artery (Figure 2B). Only a small portion of FITC-NPs was located in the arterial wall compared to the total applied amount, probably because of fast dissolution of pluronic gel, emphasizing the need to develop long-lasting gels in the future for *in vivo* applications.

Rapamycin-loaded NPs Produce Sustained Drug Release *in vitro* and *in vivo* in Balloon-injured Rat Carotid Arteries

After confirming uptake of NPs by SMCs *in vitro* and distribution into the arterial wall *in vivo*, we next examined the functional effect of drug release from rapamycin-loaded NPs on SMCs *in vitro* and on cells of the arterial wall. Previous studies have shown that rapamycin halts cell cycle progression by specifically targeting the mTOR pathway and inhibiting the phosphorylation of downstream S6K1 [9,28]. We first compared the inhibitory effect of rapamycin-loaded NPs with that of free rapamycin on S6K1 phosphorylation in cultured SMCs. Rapamycin or rapamycin-loaded NPs dispersed in pluronic gel were placed in a dialysis tube, capable of retaining NPs but allowing the release of rapamycin into the culture dish. Cells were seeded with a low density to allow their long term viability. Cell culture media were replaced with fresh media every 24 h. SMCs were then collected at the specified time points, and S6K1 phosphorylation was evaluated by Western blotting. Whereas free rapamycin inhibited S6K1 phosphorylation for only 3 days following treatment, rapamycin-loaded NPs significantly suppressed S6K1 phosphorylation for up to 14 days (Figure 3A, panels a and b). A similar pattern was observed regarding the effect of rapamycin-loaded NPs and rapamycin on SMC proliferation (Figure 3A, panels c and d). These results suggest that rapamycin-loaded NPs facilitated prolonged drug release which produced a sustained inhibitory effect on SMC function as evidenced by S6K phosphorylation.

Since the *in vitro* data indicated that on day 14 rapamycin-loaded NPs but not free rapamycin suppressed S6K1 phosphorylation (Figure 3A), we then assessed using that same time point whether perivascular application of rapamycin-loaded NPs provided prolonged drug release into the arterial wall compared to rapamycin alone (Figure 3B). We again used S6K1 phosphorylation as a surrogate for measuring rapamycin's functional effect. We placed rapamycin-loaded NPs or rapamycin alone in pluronic gel, which was then applied to the outside of balloon-injured rat carotid arteries. Arteries were retrieved 14 days after balloon injury and drug application. Proteins were then extracted and Western blotting was performed to examine S6K1 phosphorylation. Consistent with our *in vitro* findings, S6K1 phosphorylation

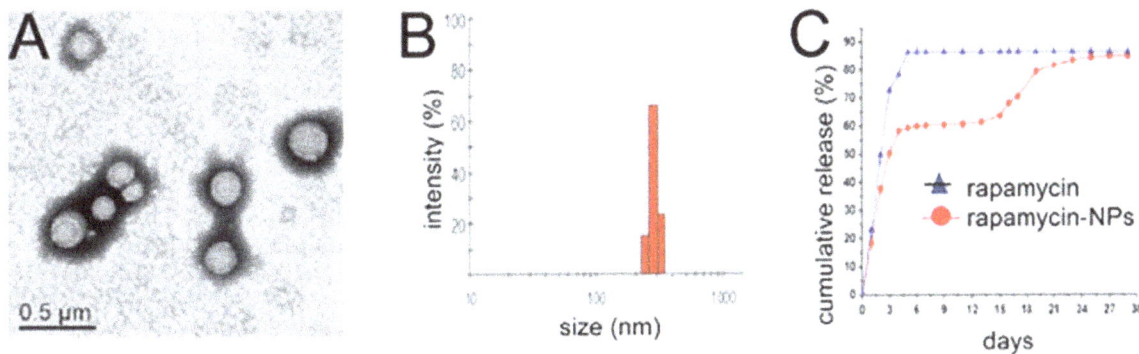

Figure 1. Characterization of rapamycin-loaded PLGA NPs (rapamycin-NPs) *in vitro.* (A). Transmission electron microscopy (TEM) image of rapamycin-NPs. (B). Size distribution of the rapamycin-NPs measured by dynamic light scattering analysis (DLS). (C). *In vitro* cumulative rapamycin release profiles from rapamycin-NPs (●, red) or free rapamycin (▲, blue), both encapsulated in pluronic gel immersed in PBS buffer. Data are presented as mean as mean). (C). ing analysis (DLS). (C.

on day 14 following treatment was reduced by ~70% in the rapamycin-NPs-treated group, however no significant effect was observed in the group treated with rapamycin alone (Figure 3B). Together, our data demonstrate that rapamycin-loaded NPs versus free rapamycin, provide sustained inhibition of S6K1 phosphorylation in SMCs both *in vitro* and *in vivo*. These findings suggest that a drug delivery strategy employing NPs can provide prolonged drug release with more sustained functional effects.

Periadventitial Administration of Rapamycin-loaded NPs Produces Sustained Inhibition of Intimal Hyperplasia (IH)

Encouraged by the observed sustained functional effect of rapamycin-loaded NPs compared to free rapamycin, we evaluated the comparative ability of both approaches to inhibit intimal hyperplasia in a rat carotid artery injury model. Rapamycin-loaded NPs or free rapamycin were placed in pluronic gel and applied around the carotid artery immediately following balloon injury. For controls, we applied the solvent for rapamycin (DMSO)

or unloaded NPs in pluronic gel. Arteries were retrieved 14 days or 28 days following treatment. As shown in Figure 4A at 14 days compared to both controls, intimal hyperplasia (measured by the I/M ratio) was markedly reduced and the arterial lumen was significantly greater in arteries treated with either rapamycin alone or rapamycin-loaded NPs. Thus, at 14 days both treatments were equally effective. Twenty-eight days after treatment there was sustained inhibition of IH and maintenance of lumen size in animals treated with rapamycin-loaded NPs. However, in animals treated with free rapamycin in pluronic gel, IH returned to a level similar to untreated controls with a corresponding diminution in lumen diameter (Figure 4B). These results suggest that sustained drug release from rapamycin-loaded NPs prolonged the inhibitory effect of rapamycin on IH leading to a durably patent vessel following arterial injury.

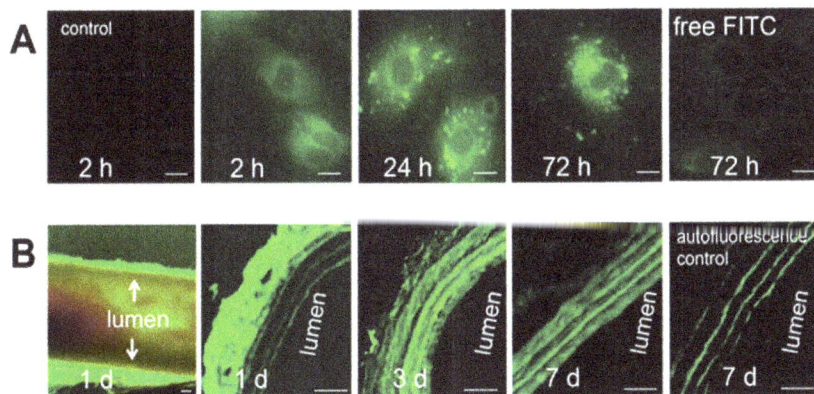

Figure 2. Accumulation of FITC-loaded NPs in cultured smooth muscle cells and in the arterial wall of the injured rat carotid artery after periadventitial application. (A). Representative fluorescence microscopic images demonstrate timein the arterial wall of the injured rat carotid arteµg FITC/ml) by cultured rat vascular smooth muscle cells (SMCs) (n = 3). Scale bar represents 10 µm. (B). FITC-NPs were applied around the rat carotid artery immediately after injury (see methods). Representative fluorescence microscopic images of carotid arteries demonstrate the in vivo distribution of FITC-NPs *(n = 3)* (1 mg FITC-NPs in 300 µl pluronic gel/artery). The first panel of B is a low-magnification longitudinal image of the artery showing perivascular application of NPs. Panels 2–4 are images of cross sections. The last panel shows the auto-fluorescence background of laminas. Scale bar represents 120 µm.

A *In vitro*

a. Rapamycin-NPs

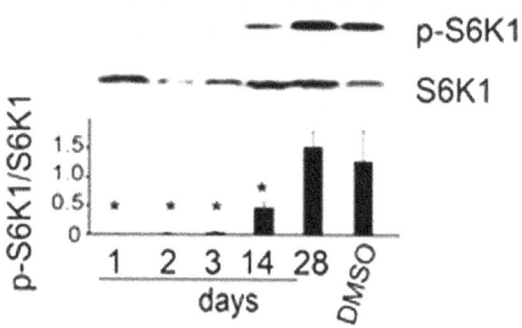

b. Rapamycin

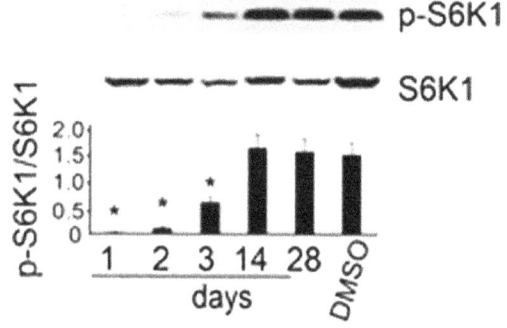

c. Rapamycin-NPs

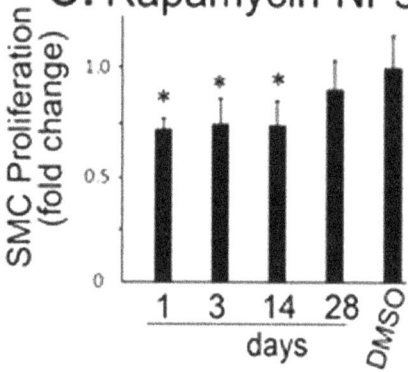

d. Rapamycin

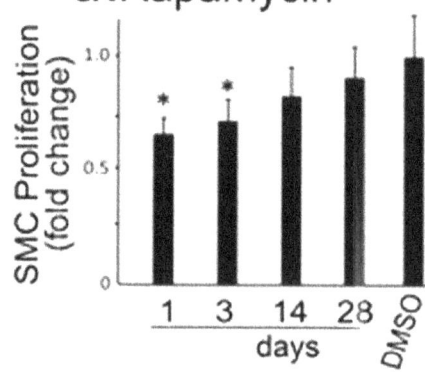

B *In vivo (14 days)*

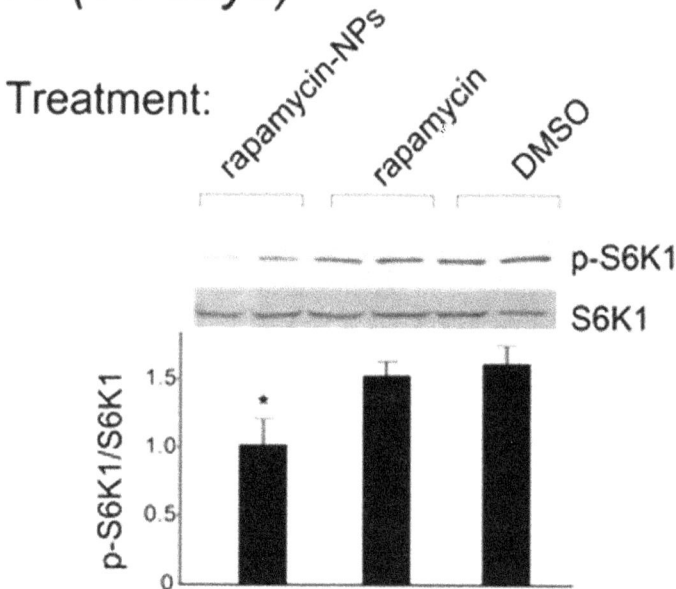

Figure 3. Prolonged inhibitory effects of rapamycin-loaded NPs on S6K1 phosphorylation *in vitro* and *in vivo*. (A). *In vitro experiments.* Treatment of SMCs with Rapamycin or rapamycin-NPs (15 μg rapamycin for both) is described in detail in Materials and Methods. Panels a and b show the effect of rapamycin-NPs and rapamycin on p-S6K, respectively. Proteins were extracted from SMCs at the indicated time points, and phosphorylated S6K1 (p-S6K1) and S6K1 were measured by Western blot analysis. Panels c and d show the effect of rapamycin-NPs and rapamycin on SMC proliferation (measured by MTT assay), respectively. Quantified data are presented as mean MC proliferation (measured by MTT (* P<0.05). (B). *In vivo experiments.* Following balloon angioplasty in rat carotid arteries, rapamycin or rapamycin-NPs (300 μg rapamycin for both) were dispersed in 300 μl pluronic gel and applied periadventitially to injured carotid arteries, as described in Methods. Carotid arteries were retrieved 14 days after surgery. Proteins extracted from carotid arteries were subjected to Western blot analysis for phosphorylated S6K1 (p-S6K1) and S6K1. Quantified data are presented as mean njured carotid arteries, as descri (* P<0.05).

Rapamycin-loaded NPs Provide Prolonged Inhibition of Cellular Proliferation in Media and Subintima of Injured Rat Carotid Arteries

Previous studies have indicated that rapamycin impedes IH at least in part by effectively inhibiting SMC proliferation [29]. In these studies we investigate the mechanism underlying the attenuation of IH by rapamycin-NPs. Using histological sections from the animals treated in the foregoing experiments, immuno-staining for Ki67 was performed to evaluate cell proliferation. Our data reveal that the proliferation or Ki67 index was substantially decreased (by ~50%) in both the free rapamycin and rapamycin-NPs treated groups compared to controls at 14 days following treatment (Figure 5, A and B). However 28 days after treatment, whereas the Ki67 index remained suppressed in the rapamycin-NPs treated group, the Ki67 index in the free rapamycin-treated group returned to the level of control (Figure 5, C and D). These results demonstrate that compared to rapamycin alone, the use of NPs to locally deliver rapamycin produced a prolonged inhibitory effect on cell proliferation in balloon-injured arteries likely accounting for the sustained inhibition of IH (Figure 4).

Rapamycin-loaded NPs Have no Effect on Reendothelialization of Injured Rat Carotid Arteries

It has been well demonstrated that rapamycin-eluting stents inhibit endothelial cell proliferation and thus delay reendothelialization, producing the adverse side effect of acute vascular thrombosis [30]. To evaluate the potential for periadventially applied rapamycin-loaded NPs to inhibit reendothelialization, we performed immunostaining for CD31 (a marker for endothelial cells) on carotid sections derived from animals treated with rapamycin-NPs, free rapamycin or controls. We found equivalent rates of reendothelialization in animals treated with rapamycin-NPs compared to controls (Figure 6). Moreover, the rate of reendothelialization was also not diminished in arteries treated with free rapamycin in pluronic gel. These findings were verified at both 14 and 28 days after injury. Thus rapamycin when applied to the arterial adventitia does not affect the regrowth rate of the endothelial layer.

Finally, we evaluated whether rapamycin-loaded NPs provide systemic toxicity to treated animals. We found that periadventitial application of either rapamycin alone or rapamycin-loaded NPs had no effect on weight gain (Supplemental Figure 1) or blood cell counts (Supplemental Tables 1 and 2) during the course of these experiments. Thus, local application of rapamycin externally to the artery wall, is a safe method for sustained drug release without systemic effects.

Discussion

Through periadventitial application of rapamycin-loaded NPs, we have achieved prolonged attenuation of intimal hyperplasia (IH) for at least 4 weeks while avoiding impairment of endothelialization. Our *in vitro* and *in vivo* experiments together indicate that NPs facilitate prolonged release of rapamycin. Persuasive evidence can be summarized as follows. Rapamycin-loaded NPs produce sustained drug release for up to 28 days compared to 3–5 days with free rapamycin. Rapamycin-loaded NPs produce prolonged inhibition of S6K1 phosphorylation (14 days) in cultured SMCs compared to rapamycin alone (3 days). It is well established that rapamycin inhibits mTOR leading to decreased downstream S6K1 phosphorylation, which is required for cell cycle progression and cell proliferation [10,31]. Thus, phospho-S6K1 is widely used as a valid functional marker for rapamycin bioavailability. Using phospho-S6K1 inhibition as an indicator, we found that rapamycin-loaded NPs applied periad-ventitially promoted prolonged release of rapamycin into the vessel wall compared to rapamycin alone. Finally, rapamycin-loaded NPs applied around the injured artery greatly outperformed rapamycin alone in durable inhibition of SMC proliferation and IH. These lines of evidence clearly show that NPs improve the durability of drug release and prolong the effect of rapamycin in impeding IH.

Currently the only clinically applied methods for treating IH are stents or balloons that release anti-proliferative drugs such as rapamycin or paclitaxel [1,32]. Drug-eluting stents have been successful in reducing the incidence of IH in patients treated with coronary artery angioplasty although there are limitations including the need for chronic platelet inhibition, the potential for stent thrombosis related to delayed endothelialization, as well as cost. Despite advances made over the past two decades in percutaneous angioplasty, thousands of patients each year are still treated with traditional open surgery. These procedures include lower extremity bypass both vein and prosthetic, coronary artery bypass and carotid endarterectomy (total up to 270 thousand cases per year) and vascular grafts placed for dialysis (~50 thousand cases per year) [33]. Unfortunately drug-eluting stents or balloons used following percutaneous angioplasty are not applicable for the patients undergoing open surgical procedures. There are currently no available measures to prevent the development of IH in these patients where the incidence ranges from 20–80%. Thus, there is a tremendous unmet clinical need for a clinically applicable technique to prevent IH in patients undergoing open vascular reconstructive surgery.

Since angioplasty is performed remotely, intraluminal drugs applied to the site of angioplasty must also be delivered remotely. Thus the challenges of drug delivery following a percutaneous intervention are substantial. Alternatively, drugs that inhibit IH can be directly applied to bypass grafts, anastomoses, prosthetic grafts, or endarterectomized arteries. The task of drug delivery following open surgery is conceptually less challenging since drugs can be directly applied to the arterial wall. In addition to the accessibility of the vessel at the time of surgery there are other distinct advantages of applying drugs to the arterial adventitia. Inhibitors of SMC proliferation also inhibit endothelial cell proliferation. Interestingly, rapamycin inhibits endothelial cells to a much greater extent than SMCs. Thus, rapamycin when applied intraluminally *via* a stent

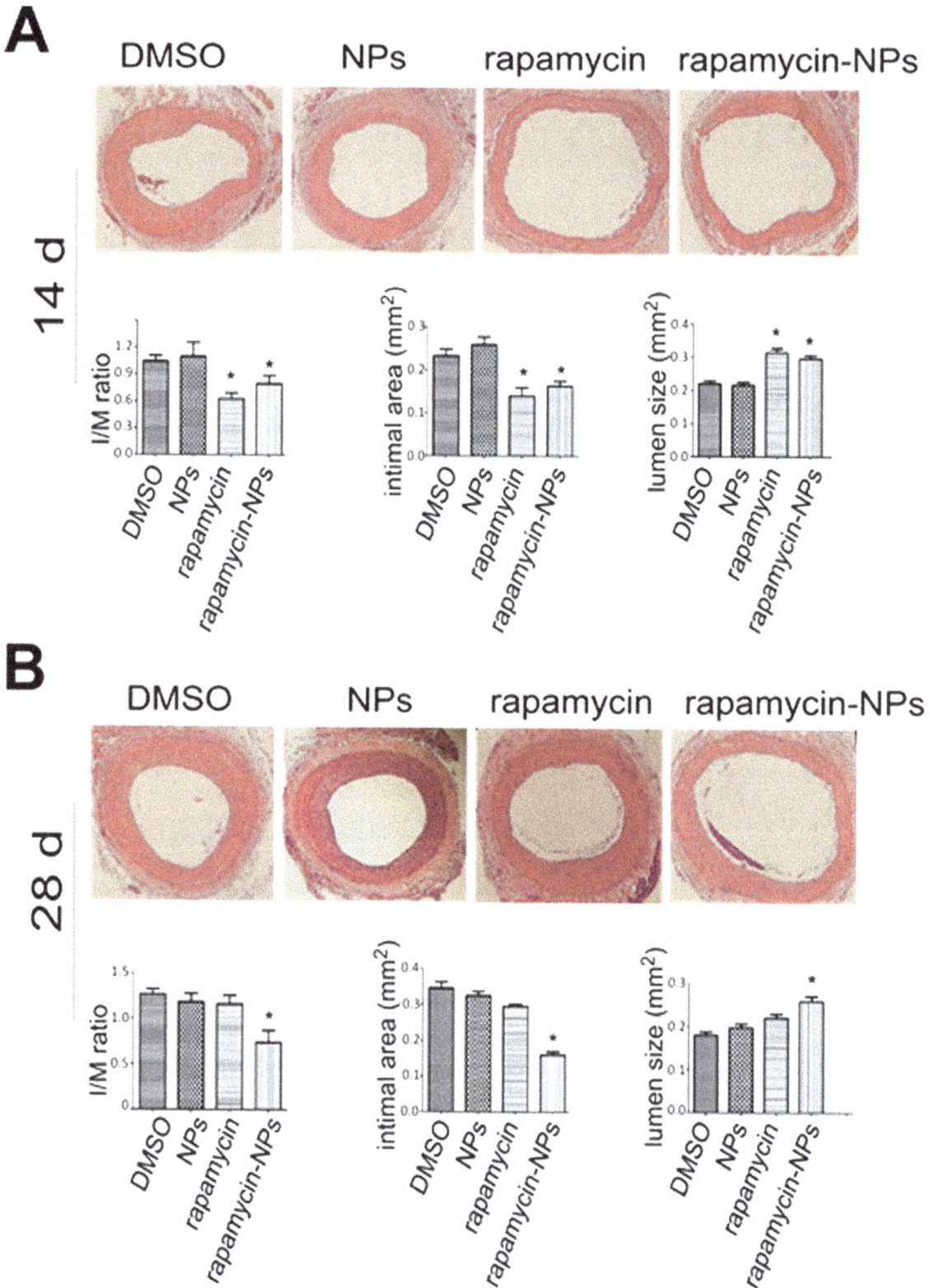

Figure 4. Sustained inhibitory effects of rapamycin-loaded NPs on intimal hyperplasia in balloon-injured rat carotid arteries. Balloon injury of rat carotid arteries was performed and rapamycin or rapamycin loaded NPs (300 µg rapamycin for both) dispersed in 300 µl pluronic gel was applied periadventitially immediately after vascular injury, as described in Methods. Solvent (DMSO) and NPs alone dispersed in pluronic gel were used as controls. Carotid arteries were retrieved 14 (A) or 28 days (B) after surgery. Sections were then prepared and H&E stained. Top panel shows representative microscopic images of carotid cross-sections from the indicated treatment groups. Bottom panel shows quantification of lumen size, intimal area, and intimal to media ratio (I/M). Data are presented as mean ± SEM from 5 animals in each group (*P<0.05 compared to DMSO control).

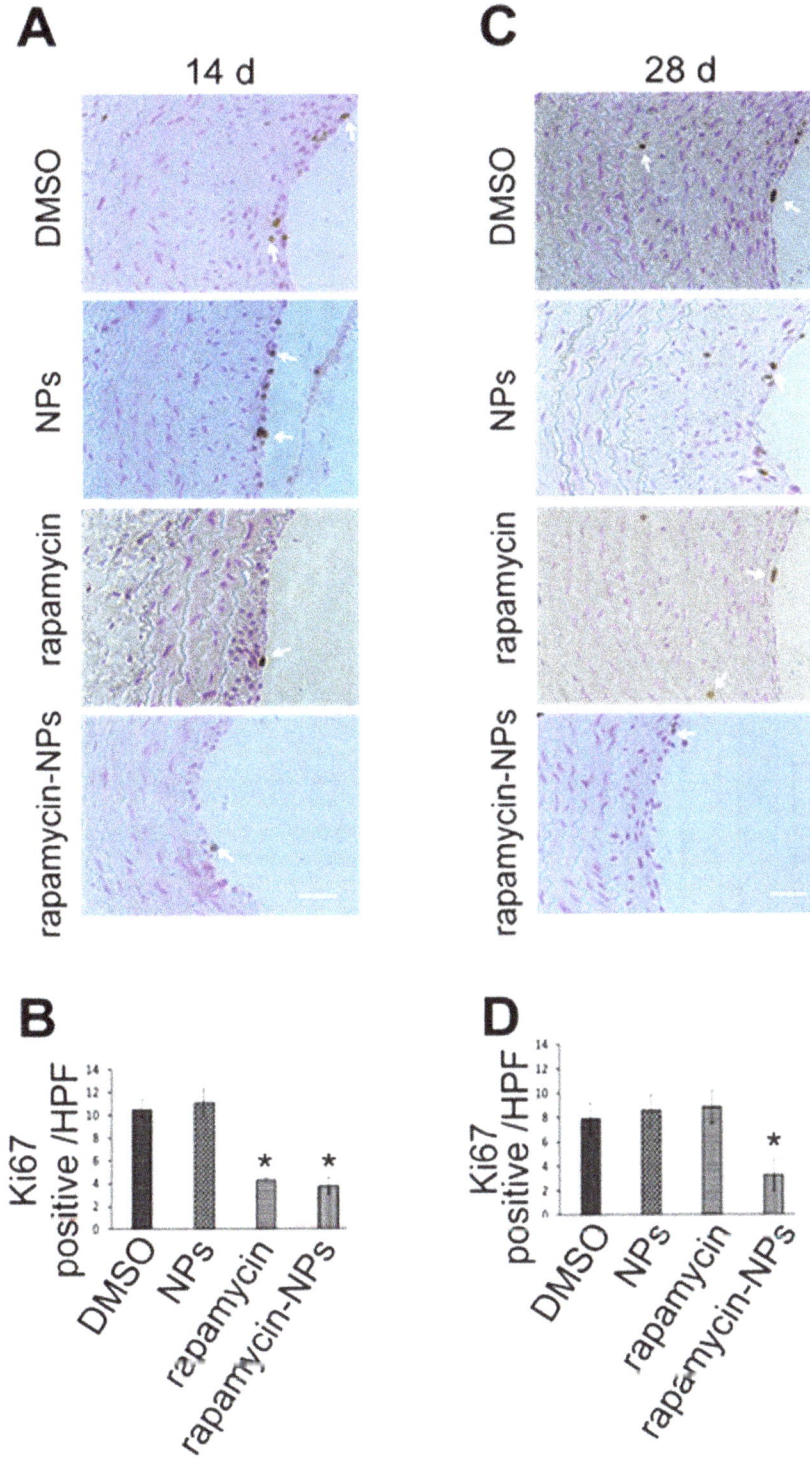

Figure 5. Sustained inhibitory effect of rapamycin-NPs on cell proliferation in balloon-injured rat carotid arteries. Rat carotid cross-sections were obtained from the same experiments as in Figure 4. Sections were immunostained for Ki67 as described in Methods. Representative microscopic images of Ki67 staining on arteries retrieved 14 days (A) and 28 days (C) after surgery. Arrows point to Ki67 positive cells. Quantification of Ki67 positive cell number per high power field (HPF) on sections retrieved 14 (B) and 28 days (D) after surgery (magnification is 200X). Each bar represents a mean ±SEM of 5 animals (* P<0.05 compared to DMSO control).

markedly inhibits endothelial cell proliferation leading to loss of the endothelial lining, the potential for acute vessel thrombosis and the need for prolonged platelet inhibition [1,34]. Periad-

ventitial application of rapamycin has the potential of creating a gradient so that the greatest concentrations of rapamycin influence the adventitia followed by the media and the

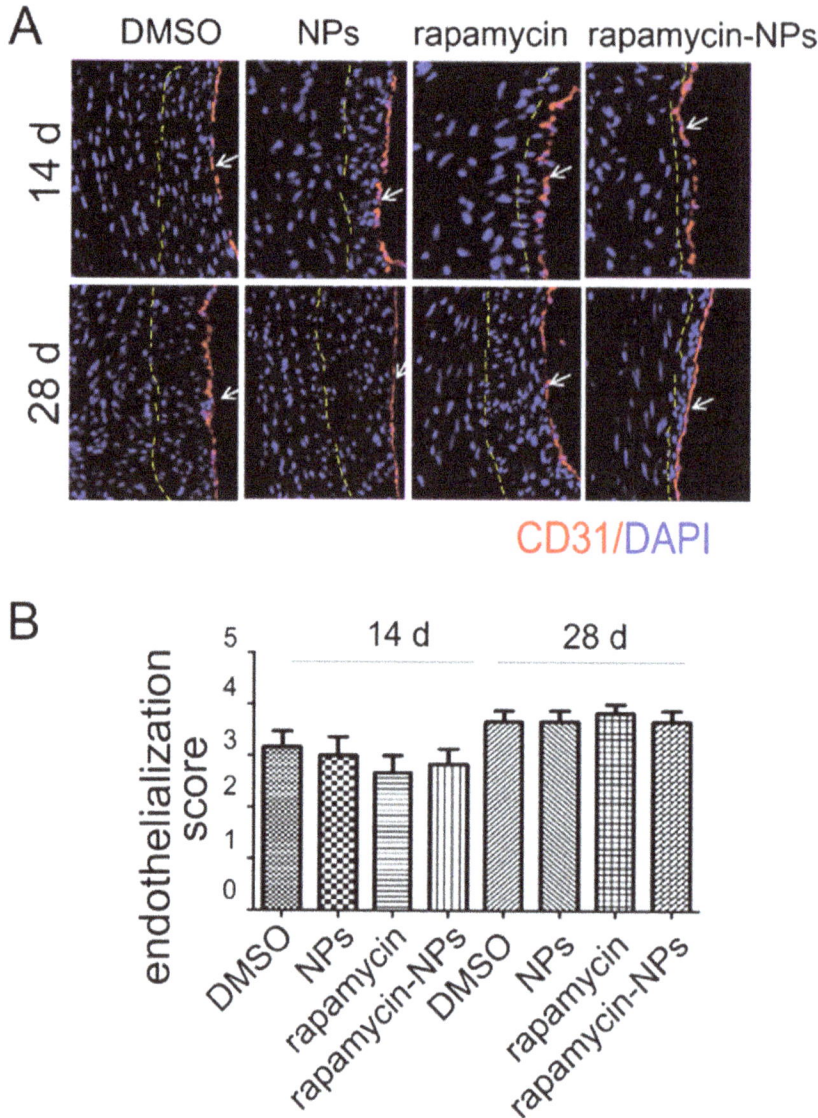

Figure 6. Periadventitial application of rapamycin-loaded NPs does not affect carotid artery reendothelialization after angioplasty.
Rat carotid cross-sections were obtained from the same experiments as in Figure 4. (A) Representative fluorescence microscopic images of CD-31staining (red, marked by arrows) of arteries retrieved 14 or 28 days after surgery. Blue dots are DAPI-stained nuclei. Dashed lines define internal elastic lamina (IEL). (B) Quantification of reendothelialization (CD-31 positive versus total perimeter) on sections retrieved 14 or 28 days after surgery. Each bar represents a mean ±SEM of 5 animals.

subintima with intimal endothelial cells exposed to the lowest concentration of drugs. To this end we studied reendothelialization in our model and found that when rapamycin was applied to the periadventitial tissue there was rapid endothelial regeneration without rapamycin's usual inhibitory effect. An additional theoretical advantage of periadventitial application of drugs that inhibit cellular proliferation is the ability of these drugs to influence cells in the adventitia. Myofibroblasts in the adventitia significantly contribute to neointimal hyperplasia. There is extensive data demonstrating that adventitial myofibroblasts migrate to the subintima and contribute to the formation of plaque [35,36]. Thus inhibition of adventitial myofibroblast proliferation may enhance the ability of drugs such as rapamycin to protect against IH. With an effective method of drug delivery, the potential to reduce morbidity and

mortality associated with recurrent disease, graft failure and vascular occlusion is substantial.

There is mounting evidence that prolonged drug delivery may be advantageous. There are various stimuli after vascular reconstruction that lead to the development of IH. Inclusive is vessel wall damage that accompanies manipulation and suture of a graft to the vessel wall. Veins used for bypass during harvest are exposed to trauma, desiccation, over-distention and *ex vivo* preservation. Endarterectomy produces direct trauma to the arterial media. Although these events are transient, the degree of injury can be profound leading to a protracted course of healing. A short burst of drug may be inadequate to completely block the maladaptive healing response that leads to IH. Moreover, some vascular reconstruction procedures are associated with an ongoing stimulus for IH. Following the creation of a bypass, "low pressure" veins are subject to arterial pressure, which provides a persistent (for the life of the bypass) stimulus for arterial remodeling that can lead to IH. Altered flow dynamics at the site of an anastomosis are persistent and likewise provide an ongoing hyperplastic stimulus. Grafts for bypass eventually reach a steady state of adaptive healing; however, this is likely not to be achieved for at least 3 to 6 months following the initial reconstruction. Thus prolonged delivery of drug over a several months period of time would seem advantageous.

Many of the pharmacological properties of conventional or "free" drugs can be improved through the use of NP drug delivery systems. First, NP drug delivery systems can significantly enhance the solubility of hydrophobic drugs in aqueous solutions. Encapsulating rapamycin in the PLGA NPs can significantly enhance its concentration in an aqueous solution [6]. Second, NPs provide controlled and sustained drug release profiles. Our in vitro data revealed that free rapamycin in pluronic gel was released over a period of 3 to 5 days whereas rapamycin in PLGA NPs was released over 3–4 weeks. Moreover, S6K1 phosphorylation and cell proliferation were effectively suppressed for at least 28 days in animals treated with rapamycin-loaded nanoparticles. It is likely that sustained release of rapamycin was a major factor that led to more durable inhibition of IH in our model. Another mechanism through which NPs can promote drug delivery is by enhancing the accumulation and absorption of drug by target cells or tissues. NPs can release rapamycin into the extracellular space and then free rapamycin can diffuse into cells of the arterial wall. NPs can also be taken up readily by cells via endocytosis, due to their relatively small size (~200 nm vs. SMCs being ~20 micrometers in size) [6]. In our in vitro system we observed that NPs were internalized by SMCs via endocytosis within two hours. The relative cellular uptake of free drug versus NPs varies and depends on the cell type, the nature of the drug, as well as the chemical, physical, and surface properties of the NPs (e.g., specific ligand-receptor interaction) [37]. In our system it is clear that rapamycin is able to enter the cell via both mechanisms. It is worth noting that once NPs are exposed to cell culture medium, proteins/peptides present in cell culture may coat the surface of the NPs, which later serve as a targeting ligand promoting cellular uptake of NPs [37]. Lastly, NPs prevent drug from premature enzymatic degradation in vivo. The in vivo half-life of free rapamycin is much shorter than in vitro. However, rapamycin encapsulated in NPs is protected from any enzymatic degradation until it is released from the NPs.

While many strategies involving NPs have been designed for the luminal treatment of restenosis, intraluminal approaches have the potential to cause undesirable inhibition of the inner endothelial protective lining [1]. A number of approaches for perivascular drug delivery of rapamycin have been employed but with varying success. These approaches include rapamycin-loaded microbeads, PLGA membranes, synthetic meshes, and non-constrictive cuffs [7,38,39]. Recently, periadventitial application of rapamycin-eluting microbeads (200 μm) was evaluated in a pig vein graft model. Low concentrations of rapamycin only partially inhibited IH whereas higher concentrations produced anastamotic disruption related to absent healing [40]. NPs have the advantage over these other approaches in penetrating the arterial wall allowing more direct cellular delivery.

Although our study has clearly demonstrated that perivascular application of rapamycin-loaded PLGA NPs is effective in the inhibition of IH, further research is needed to optimize this drug

delivery system. For example, we were not able to evaluate whether rapamycin-loaded NPs might affect IH beyond 4 weeks. A longer-term model of IH will be necessary to accomplish this evaluation. The current NP drug delivery system can also be improved through a number of manipulations. Pluronic gel was used to immobilize NPs in the periadventitial space. However, pluronic gel dissolves within 3–4 days after in vivo application. Using a long-lasting yet biodegradable temperature-responsive polymer gel to replace pluronic gel will further extend in vivo drug release from NPs. Moreover, NPs can be modified to meet specific needs for optimal drug release. Polymer chemistry and size of NPs can be altered to vary NP durability, and drug release profile. In addition, various ligands can be conjugated to the surface of the NPs to target specific cell populations overexpressing corresponding receptors in the hyperplastic vessel wall. Lastly, NPs are capable of encapsulating a mixture of drugs with complementary functions, which may further enhance the efficacy of drug-releasing NPs for treating restenosis. Further studies with new polymer gels, drug nanocarriers, animal models, and multi-drug administration regimens should be able to further improve the efficacy of drug delivery.

Conclusion

Our study shows that periadventitial delivery of rapamycin-loaded NPs is a promising approach for the development of a safer, more efficacious drug delivery system to treat IH. Using rapamycin as a model drug we have demonstrated that NPs extend drug release in vitro and in vivo. When applied outside the arterial wall, rapamycin-loaded NPs compared to rapamycin alone substantially prolonged inhibition of IH and maintained lumen patency in balloon-injured rat carotid arteries. Thus local drug delivery with NPs provides a useful template approach for future development of safe and efficacious drug delivery methods to treat IH and restenosis, particularly for patients undergoing open vascular reconstruction.

Supporting Information

Figure S1 Periadventitial application of rapamycin-loaded NPs does not affect body weight. Animal body weights were measured at the indicated time points after surgery. Data are presented as mean sents a mean ±SEM of 5 animals.CD-31s.

Table S1 Periadventitial application of rapamycin-loaded nanoparticles does not affect blood cell counts (14 days after Surgery). Hematological analysis from Sprague Dawley Rats 14 d after surgery. Results are expressed as mean ± SD, n = 5. RBC, red blood cells; WBC, white blood cells.

Table S2 Periadventitial application of rapamycin-loaded nanoparticles does not affect blood cell counts (28 days after Surgery). Hematological analysis from Sprague Dawley Rats 14 d after surgery. Results are expressed as mean ± SD, n = 5. RBC, red blood cells; WBC, white blood cells.

Author Contributions

Conceived and designed the experiments: XS GC LWG SG KCK. Performed the experiments: XS GC YS MZ SP. Analyzed the data: XS GC LWG SG KCK BL. Wrote the paper: XS GC LWG SG KCK.

References

1. Seedial SM, Ghosh S, Saunders RS, Suwanabol P, Shi X, et al. (2013) Local drug delivery to prevent restenosis. J Vasc Surg 57: 1403–1414.
2. Curcio A, Torella D, Indolfi C (2011) Mechanisms of smooth muscle cell proliferation and endothelial regeneration after vascular injury and stenting: approach to therapy. Circ J 75: 1287–1296.
3. Acharya S, Sahoo SK (2011) PLGA nanoparticles containing various anticancer agents and tumour delivery by EPR effect. Adv Drug Deliv Rev 63: 170–183.
4. Lü J-M, Wang X, Marin-Muller C, Wang H, Lin PH, et al. (2009) Current advances in research and clinical applications of PLGA-based nanotechnology. Expert Rev Mol Diagn 9: 325–341.
5. Martin-Banderas L, Durán-Lobato M, Muñoz-Rubio I, Alvarez-Fuentes J, Fernández-Arevalo M, et al. (2013) Functional PLGA NPs for oral drug delivery: recent strategies and developments. Mini Rev Med Chem 13: 58–69.
6. Danhier F, Ansorena E, Silva JM, Coco R, Le Breton A, Preat V (2012) PLGA-based nanoparticles: an overview of biomedical applications. J Control Release 161: 502–522.
7. Semete B, Booysen L, Lemmer Y, Kalombo L, Katata L, et al. (2010) In vivo evaluation of the biodistribution and safety of PLGA nanoparticles as drug delivery systems. Nanomedicine 6: 662–671.
8. Panyam J, Labhasetwar V (2003) Biodegradable nanoparticles for drug and gene delivery to cells and tissue. Adv Drug Deliv Rev 55: 329–347.
9. Fingar DC, Richardson CJ, Tee AR, Cheatham L, Tsou C, et al. (2004) mTOR Controls Cell Cycle Progression through Its Cell Growth Effectors S6K1 and 4E-BP1/Eukaryotic Translation Initiation Factor 4E. Mol Cell Biol 24: 200–216.
10. Zohlnhofer D, Nuhrenberg TG, Neumann F-JJ, Richter T, May AE, et al. (2004) Rapamycin effects transcriptional programs in smooth muscle cells controlling proliferative and inflammatory properties. Mol Pharmacol 65: 880–889.
11. Reddy MK, Vasir JK, Sahoo SK, Jain TK, Yallapu MM, et al. (2008) Inhibition of apoptosis through localized delivery of rapamycin-loaded nanoparticles prevented neointimal hyperplasia and reendothelialized injured artery. Circ Cardiovasc Interv 1: 209–216.
12. Daemen J, Kukreja N, van Twisk PH, Onuma Y, de Jaegere PP, et al. (2008) Four-year clinical follow-up of the rapamycin-eluting stent evaluated at Rotterdam Cardiology Hospital registry. Am J Cardiol 101: 1105–1111.
13. Abizaid A Costa JR (2010) New drug-eluting stents: an overview on biodegradable and polymer-free next-generation stent systems. Circ Cardiovasc Interv 3: 384–393.
14. Virmani R, Farb A, Guagliumi G Kolodgie FD (2004) Drug-eluting stents: caution and concerns for long-term outcome. Coron Artery Dis 15: 313–318.
15. Siqueira DA, Abizaid AA, Costa J de R, Feres F, Mattos LA, et al. (2007) Late incomplete apposition after drug-eluting stent implantation: incidence and potential for adverse clinical outcomes. Eur Heart J 28: 1304–1309.
16. Guzman LA, Labhasetwar V, Song C, Jang Y, Lincoff AM, et al. (1996) Local intraluminal infusion of biodegradable polymeric nanoparticles. A novel approach for prolonged drug delivery after balloon angioplasty. Circulation 94: 1441–1448.
17. Lutsiak MEC, Robinson DR, Coester C, Kwon GS, Samuel J (2002) Analysis of poly(D,L-lactic-co-glycolic acid) nanosphere uptake by human dendritic cells and macrophages in vitro. Pharm Res 19: 1480–1487.
18. Clowes MM, Lynch CM, Miller a D, Miller DG, Osborne WR, et al. (1994) Long-term biological response of injured rat carotid artery seeded with smooth muscle cells expressing retrovirally introduced human genes. J Clin Invest 93: 644–651.
19. Kundi R, Hollenbeck ST, Yamanouchi D, Herman BC, Edlin R, et al. (2009) Arterial gene transfer of the TGF-beta signalling protein Smad3 induces adaptive remodelling following angioplasty: a role for CTGF. Cardiovasc Res 84: 326–335.
20. Jhunjhunwala S, Raimondi G, Thomson a W, Little SR (2009) Delivery of rapamycin to dendritic cells using degradable microparticles. J Control Release 133: 191–197.
21. Brown MA, Zhang L, Levering VW, Wu J, Satterwhite LL, et al. (2010) Human Umbilical Cord Blood – Derived Endothelial Cells Reendothelialize Vein Grafts and Prevent Thrombosis. Arterioscler Thromb Vasc Biol 30: 2150–2155.
22. Tian W, Kuhlmann MT, Pelisek J, Scobioala S, Quang TH, et al. (2006) Paclitaxel delivered to adventitia attenuates neointima formation without compromising re-endothelialization after angioplasty in a porcine restenosis model. J Endovasc Ther 13: 616–629.
23. Tsai S, Hollenbeck ST, Ryer EJ, Edlin R, Yamanouchi D, et al. (2009) TGF-beta through Smad3 signaling stimulates vascular smooth muscle cell proliferation and neointimal formation. Am J Physiol Heart Circ Physiol 297: H540–H549.
24. Zhu W, Masaki T, Bae YH, Rathi R, Cheung AK, et al. (2006) Development of a sustained-release system for perivascular delivery of dipyridamole. J Biomed Mater Res B Appl Biomater 77: 135–143.
25. Kawatsu S, Oda K, Saiki Y, Tabata Y, Tabayashi K (2007) External application of rapamycin-eluting film at anastomotic sites inhibits neointimal hyperplasia in a canine model. Ann Thorac Surg 84: 560–567.
26. Makadia HK, Siegel SJ (2011) Poly Lactic-co-Glycolic Acid (PLGA) as Biodegradable Controlled Drug Delivery Carrier. Polymers (Basel) 3: 1377–1397.
27. Avgoustakis K, Beletsi a, Panagi Z, Klepetsanis P, Karydas a G, et al. (2002) PLGA-mPEG nanoparticles of cisplatin: in vitro nanoparticle degradation, in vitro drug release and in vivo drug residence in blood properties. J Control Release 79: 123–135.
28. Ding M, Xie Y, Wagner RJ, Jin Y, Carrao AC, et al. (2011) Adiponectin induces vascular smooth muscle cell differentiation via repression of mammalian target of rapamycin complex 1 and FoxO4. Arter Thromb Vasc Biol 31: 1403–1410.
29. Liuzzo JP, Ambrose JA Coppola JT (2005) Sirolimus- and taxol-eluting stents differ towards intimal hyperplasia and re-endothelialization. J Invasive Cardiol 17: 497–502.
30. Lüscher TF, Steffel J, Eberli FR, Joner M, Nakazawa G, et al. (2007) Drug-eluting stent and coronary thrombosis: biological mechanisms and clinical implications. Circulation 115: 1051–1058.
31. Rosner D, McCarthy N, Bennett M (2005) Rapamycin inhibits human in stent restenosis vascular smooth muscle cells independently of pRB phosphorylation and p53. Cardiovasc Res 66: 601–610.
32. Yang J, Zeng Y, Zhang C, Chen Y-X, Yang Z, et al. (2013) The prevention of restenosis in vivo with a VEGF gene and paclitaxel co-eluting stent. Biomaterials 34: 1635–1643.
33. Jim J, Owens PL, Sanchez LA, Rubin BG (2012) Population-based analysis of inpatient vascular procedures and predicting future workload and implications for training. J Vasc Surg 55: 1394–1399.
34. Inoue T, Croce K, Morooka T, Sakuma M, Node K, Simon DI (2011) Vascular inflammation and repair: implications for re-endothelialization, restenosis, and stent thrombosis. JACC Cardiovasc Interv 4: 1057–1066.
35. Si J, Ren J, Wang P, Rateri DL, Daugherty A, et al. (2012) Protein kinase C-delta mediates adventitial cell migration through regulation of monocyte chemoattractant protein-1 expression in a rat angioplasty model. Arterioscler Thromb Vasc Biol 32: 943–954.
36. Siow RCM, Mallawaarachchi CM, Weissberg PL (2003) Migration of adventitial myofibroblasts following vascular balloon injury: Insights from in vivo gene transfer to rat carotid arteries. Cardiovasc Res 59: 212–221.
37. Cartiera MS, Johnson KM, Rajendran V, Caplan MJ SW, Cartiera MS, Johnson KM, Rajendran V, Caplan MJ, et al. (2009) The uptake and intracellular fate of PLGA nanoparticles in epithelial cells. Biomaterials 30: 2790–2798.
38. Pires NMM, van der Hoeven BL, de Vries MR, Havekes LM, van Vlijmen BJ, et al. (2005) Local perivascular delivery of anti-restenotic agents from a drug-eluting poly(epsilon-caprolactone) stent cuff. Biomaterials 26: 5386–5394.
39. Chorny M, Fishbein I, Golomb G (2000) Drug delivery systems for the treatment of restenosis. Crit Rev Ther Drug Carrier Syst 17: 249–284.
40. Rajathurai T, Rizvi SI, Lin H, Angelini GD, Newby AC, Murphy GJ. (2010). Periadventitial rapamycin-eluting microbeads promote vein graft disease in long-term pig vein-into-artery interposition grafts. Circ Cardiovasc Interv. 3(2): 157–65.

Permissions

The contributors of this book come from diverse backgrounds, making this book a truly international effort. This book will bring forth new frontiers with its revolutionizing research information and detailed analysis of the nascent developments around the world.

We would like to thank all the contributing authors for lending their expertise to make the book truly unique. They have played a crucial role in the development of this book. Without their invaluable contributions this book wouldn't have been possible. They have made vital efforts to compile up to date information on the varied aspects of this subject to make this book a valuable addition to the collection of many professionals and students.

This book was conceptualized with the vision of imparting up-to-date information and advanced data in this field. To ensure the same, a matchless editorial board was set up. Every individual on the board went through rigorous rounds of assessment to prove their worth. After which they invested a large part of their time researching and compiling the most relevant data for our readers.

The editorial board has been involved in producing this book since its inception. They have spent rigorous hours researching and exploring the diverse topics which have resulted in the successful publishing of this book. They have passed on their knowledge of decades through this book. To expedite this challenging task, the publisher supported the team at every step. A small team of assistant editors was also appointed to further simplify the editing procedure and attain best results for the readers.

Apart from the editorial board, the designing team has also invested a significant amount of their time in understanding the subject and creating the most relevant covers. They scrutinized every image to scout for the most suitable representation of the subject and create an appropriate cover for the book.

The publishing team has been an ardent support to the editorial, designing and production team. Their endless efforts to recruit the best for this project, has resulted in the accomplishment of this book. They are a veteran in the field of academics and their pool of knowledge is as vast as their experience in printing. Their expertise and guidance has proved useful at every step. Their uncompromising quality standards have made this book an exceptional effort. Their encouragement from time to time has been an inspiration for everyone.

The publisher and the editorial board hope that this book will prove to be a valuable piece of knowledge for researchers, students, practitioners and scholars across the globe.

List of Contributors

Catriona Shaw
UK Renal Registry, Southmead Hospital, Bristol, United Kingdom
Department of Renal Sciences, Division of Transplantation Immunology and Mucosal Biology, Kings College London, London, United Kingdom

Dorothea Nitsch
London School of Hygiene and Tropical Medicine, London, United Kingdom

Retha Steenkamp
UK Renal Registry, Southmead Hospital, Bristol, United Kingdom

Cornelia Junghans
Department of Epidemiology and Public Health, University College London, London, United Kingdom

Sapna Shah
Department of Renal Medicine, Kings College Hospital, London, United Kingdom

Donal O'Donoghue
Department of Renal Medicine, Salford Royal NHS Foundation Trust, Salford, United Kingdom

Damian Fogarty
Department of Renal Medicine, Belfast Health and Social Care Trust, Belfast, Northern Ireland, United Kingdom

Clive Weston
Myocardial Ischaemia National Audit Project, College of Medicine, Swansea University, Swansea, Wales, United Kingdom

Claire C. Sharpe
Department of Renal Sciences, Division of Transplantation Immunology and Mucosal Biology, Kings College London, London, United Kingdom

Bronislava Bashinskaya
Massachusetts General Hospital and Department of Medicine (Cardiology Division), Harvard Medical School, Boston, Massachusetts, United States of America
Boston University, Boston, Massachusetts, United States of America

Brian V. Nahed, Brian P. Walcott and Jean-Valery C. E. Coumans
Massachusetts General Hospital and Department of Surgery (Neurosurgery Division), Harvard Medical School, Boston, Massachusetts, United States of America

Oyere K. Onuma
Massachusetts General Hospital and Department of Medicine (Cardiology Division), Harvard Medical School, Boston, Massachusetts, United States of America

Surya Dharma, Bambang Budi Siswanto, Isman Firdaus, Iwan Dakota and Hananto Andriantoro
Department of Cardiology and Vascular Medicine, Faculty of Medicine, University of Indonesia, National Cardiovascular Center Harapan Kita, Jakarta, Indonesia

Alexander J. Wardeh
Department of Cardiology, M.C. Haaglanden, The Hague, The Netherlands

Arnoud van der Laarse
Department of Cardiology, Leiden University Medical Center, Leiden, the Netherlands

J. Wouter Jukema
Department of Cardiology, Leiden University Medical Center, Leiden, the Netherlands
Interuniversity Cardiology Institute the Netherlands, Utrecht, the Netherlands

Vincenzo Jacomella, Kathrin Mosimann, Marc Husmann, Christoph Thalhammer and Beatrice R. Amann-Vesti
Clinic for Angiology, University Hospital Zurich, Zurich, Switzerland

Philipp A. Gerber Kaspar Berneis
Clinic for Endocrinology, University Hospital Zurich, Zurich, Switzerland

Ian Wilkinson
Clinical Pharmacology Unit, University of Cambridge, Cambridge, United Kingdom

Søren Lund Kristensen
Department of Cardiology, Copenhagen University Hospital Roskilde, Roskilde, Denmark
Department of Cardiology, Copenhagen University Hospital Gentofte, Hellerup, Denmark

Anders M. Galløe and Ole Havndrup
Department of Cardiology, Copenhagen University Hospital Roskilde, Roskilde, Denmark

Leif Thuesen
Department of Medicine, Aarhus University Hospital Herning, Herning, Denmark

Henning Kelbæk and Kari Saunamäki
The Heart Centre, Copenhagen University Hospital Rigshospitalet, Copenhagen, Denmark

Per Thayssen and Anders Junker
Department of Cardiology, Odense Universy Hospital, Odense, Denmark

Peter Riis Hansen and Ulrik Abildgaard
Department of Cardiology, Copenhagen University Hospital Gentofte, Hellerup, Denmark

Niels Bligaard
Department of Cardiology, Copenhagen University Hospital Bispebjerg, Copenhagen, Denmark

Jens Aarøe
Department of Cardiology, Aalborg University Hospital, Aalborg, Denmark

Jørgen L. Jeppesen
Department of Medicine, Copenhagen University Hospital Glostrup, Glostrup, Denmark

Jeffrey J. W. Verschuren
Department of Cardiology, Leiden University Medical Center, Leiden, The Netherlands

Stella Trompet
Department of Cardiology, Leiden University Medical Center, Leiden, The Netherlands
Department of Gerontology and Geriatrics, Leiden University Medical Center, Leiden, The Netherlands
Netherlands Consortium for Healthy Ageing, Leiden, The Netherlands

Iris Postmus
Department of Gerontology and Geriatrics, Leiden University Medical Center, Leiden, The Netherlands
Netherlands Consortium for Healthy Ageing, Leiden, The Netherlands

M. Lourdes Sampietro
Department Human Genetics, Leiden University Medical Center, Leiden, The Netherlands
Interuniversity Cardiology Institute of the Netherlands (ICIN), Utrecht, The Netherlands

Bastiaan T. Heijmans and P. Eline Slagboom
Molecular Epidemiology, Leiden University Medical Center, Leiden, The Netherlands
Netherlands Consortium for Healthy Ageing, Leiden, The Netherlands

Jeanine J. Houwing-Duistermaat
Department of Medical Statistics and Bioinformatics, Leiden University Medical Center, Leiden, The Netherlands

J. Wouter Jukema
Department of Cardiology, Leiden University Medical Center, Leiden, The Netherlands
Netherlands Consortium for Healthy Ageing, Leiden, The Netherlands
Interuniversity Cardiology Institute of the Netherlands (ICIN), Utrecht, The Netherlands
Durrer Center for Cardiogenetic Research, Amsterdam, The Netherlands

Marcella Maddaluno, Gianluca Grassia, Maria Vittoria Di Lauro, Antonio Parisi, Francesco Maione, Carla Cicala, Daniele De Filippis, Teresa Iuvone, Nicola Mascolo and Armando Ialenti
Department of Experimental Pharmacology, University of Naples Federico II, Naples, Italy

Angelo Guglielmotti
Angelini, ACRAF, S.Palomba-Pomezia, Rome, Italy

Pasquale Maffia
Department of Experimental Pharmacology, University of Naples Federico II, Naples, Italy
Institute of Infection, Immunity and Inflammation, College of Medical, Veterinary and Life Sciences, University of Glasgow, Glasgow, United Kingdom

Min-I Su and Cheng-Ting Tsai
Division of Cardiology, Department of Internal Medicine, Mackay Memorial Hospital, Taipei, Taiwan

Hung-I Yeh and Chun-Yen Chen
Mackay Medical College, New Taipei City, Taiwan

Luc Lorgis, Auré lie Gudjoncik, Carole Richard and Yves Cottin
Department of Cardiology, University Hospital, Dijon, France
Laboratory of Cardiometabolic Physiopathology and Pharmacology, INSERM U866, SFR Santé University of Burgundy, Dijon, France

Laurent Mock, Philippe Brunel and Damien Brunet
Department of Cardiology, Clinique de Fontaine-lés-Dijon, Fontaine-le`s-Dijon, France

Philippe Buffet, Jean-Claude Beer and Claude Touzery
Department of Cardiology, University Hospital, Dijon, France

Luc Janin-Manificat
Department of Cardiology, CH Beaune, Beaune, France

Luc Rochette and Marianne Zeller
Laboratory of Cardiometabolic Physiopathology and Pharmacology, INSERM U866, SFR Santé University of Burgundy, Dijon, France

Merete Osler
Research Center for Prevention and Health, Glostrup Hospital, Glostrup, Denmark
Institute of Public Health, University of Copenhagen, Copenhagen, Denmark

Solvej Mårtensson and Kathrine Carlsen
Research Center for Prevention and Health, Glostrup Hospital, Glostrup, Denmark

Eva Prescott
Department of Cardiology Y, Bispebjerg Hospital, Copenhagen, Denmark

Jinsong Xu, Yanqing Wu, Hai Su, Weitong Hu, Juxiang Li, Wenying Wang and Xiaoshu Cheng
Research Institute of Cardiovascular Diseases and Department of Cardiology, Second Affiliated Hospital of Nanchang University, Nanchang, Jiangxi, People' Republic of China

Xin Liu
Fuzhou Medical College of Nanchang University, Fuzhou, Jiangxi, People's Republic of China

Megan Coylewright and Henry H. Ting
Division of Cardiovascular Diseases, Department of Medicine, Mayo Clinic, Rochester, Minnesota, United States of America

Knowledge and Evaluation Research Unit, Mayo Clinic, Rochester, Minnesota, United States of America

Kathy Shepel
The Section of Creative Media at Mayo Clinic, Rochester, Minnesota, United States of America

Annie LeBlanc and Laurie Pencille
Knowledge and Evaluation Research Unit, Mayo Clinic, Rochester, Minnesota, United States of America

Erik Hess
Knowledge and Evaluation Research Unit, Mayo Clinic, Rochester, Minnesota, United States of America
Division of Emergency Medicine Research, Department of Emergency Medicine, Mayo Clinic, Rochester, Minnesota, United States of America

Nilay Shah
Knowledge and Evaluation Research Unit, Mayo Clinic, Rochester, Minnesota, United States of America
Division of Health Care Policy and Research, Department of Health Sciences Research, Mayo Clinic, Rochester, Minnesota, United States of America

Victor M. Montori
Knowledge and Evaluation Research Unit, Mayo Clinic, Rochester, Minnesota, United States of America
Division of Health Care Policy and Research, Department of Health Sciences Research, Mayo Clinic, Rochester, Minnesota, United States of America
Division of Endocrinology, Diabetes, Metabolism, and Nutrition, Department of Medicine, Mayo Clinic, Rochester, Minnesota, United States of America

Po-Chao Hsu
Division of Cardiology, Department of Internal Medicine, Kaohsiung Medical University Hospital, Kaohsiung Medical University, Kaohsiung, Taiwan
Graduate Institute of Medicine, College of Medicine, Kaohsiung Medical University, Kaohsiung, Taiwan
Faculty of Medicine, College of Medicine, Kaohsiung Medical University, Kaohsiung, Taiwan

Ho-Ming Su
Division of Cardiology, Department of Internal Medicine, Kaohsiung Medical University Hospital, Kaohsiung Medical University, Kaohsiung, Taiwan
Faculty of Medicine, College of Medicine, Kaohsiung Medical University, Kaohsiung, Taiwan
Department of Internal Medicine, Kaohsiung Municipal Hsiao-Kang Hospital, Kaohsiung, Taiwan

Hsiang-Chun Lee
Division of Cardiology, Department of Internal Medicine, Kaohsiung Medical University Hospital, Kaohsiung Medical University, Kaohsiung, Taiwan
Graduate Institute of Medicine, College of Medicine, Kaohsiung Medical University, Kaohsiung, Taiwan

Suh-Hang Juo
Department of Medical Research, Kaohsiung Medical University Hospital, Kaohsiung Medical University, Kaohsiung, Taiwan
Medical Genetics, Kaohsiung Medical University, Kaohsiung, Taiwan
Center of Excellence for Environmental Medicine, Kaohsiung Medical University, Kaohsiung, Taiwan

Tsung-Hsien Lin, Wen- Chol Voon, Wen-Ter Lai and Sheng-Hsiung Sheu
Division of Cardiology, Department of Internal Medicine, Kaohsiung Medical University Hospital, Kaohsiung Medical University, Kaohsiung, Taiwan
Faculty of Medicine, College of Medicine, Kaohsiung Medical University, Kaohsiung, Taiwan

Kasinath Viswanathan and Jakob Richardson
Vascular Biology Research Group, Robarts' Research Institute, London, Canada

Ilze Bot, Theo J. C. van Berkel and Erik A. L. Biessen
Division of Biopharmaceutics, Leiden/Amsterdam Center for Drug Research, Leiden, The Netherlands
University of Maastracht, Maastracht, The Netherlands

Liying Liu, Erbin Dai, Babajide Togonu-Bickersteth
Vascular Biology Research Group, Robarts' Research Institute, London, Canada
Department of Medicine, Divisions of Cardiovascular Medicine and Rheumatology, University of Florida, Gainesville, Florida, United States of America

Peter C. Turner, Jennifer A. Davids and Richard W. Moyer
Department of Molecular Genetics and Microbiology, University of Florida, Gainesville, Florida, United States of America

Jennifer M. Williams and Hao Chen
Department of Medicine, Divisions of Cardiovascular Medicine and Rheumatology, University of Florida, Gainesville, Florida, United States of America

Mee Y. Bartee
Department of Medicine, Divisions of Cardiovascular Medicine and Rheumatology, University of Florida, Gainesville, Florida, United States of America
Department of Molecular Genetics and Microbiology, University of Florida, Gainesville, Florida, United States of America

Alexandra R. Lucas
Vascular Biology Research Group, Robarts' Research Institute, London, Canada
Department of Medicine, Divisions of Cardiovascular Medicine and Rheumatology, University of Florida, Gainesville, Florida, United States of America
Department of Molecular Genetics and Microbiology, University of Florida, Gainesville, Florida, United States of America

Shang-Hung Chang, Chun-Chi Chen, Ming-Jer Hsieh, Chao-Yung Wang, Cheng-Hung Lee and I-Chang Hsieh
Second Section of Cardiology and Percutaneous Coronary Intervention Center Department of Medicine, Chang Gung Memorial Hospital and Chang Gung University, Taipei, Taiwan

Ana Lopez-de-Andres, Rodrigo Jimenez-Garcia, Valentin Hernandez-Barrera, Isabel Jimenez-Trujillo, Carmen Gallardo-Pino, Angel Gil de Miguel and Pilar Carrasco-Garrido
Preventive Medicine and Public Health Department. Rey Juan Carlos University. Alcorcón, Madrid, Spain

Farzin Fath-Ordoubadi, Magdi El-Omar, Douglas G. Fraser, Muhammad A. Khan and Ludwig Neyses
Manchester Heart Centre, Manchester Royal Infirmary, Manchester, United Kingdom

Erik Spaepen
SBD Analytics, Hertstraat, Bekkevoort, Belgium

Gian B. Danzi
Division of Cardiology, Fondazione IRCCS Ca`
Granda, Ospedale Maggiore Policlinico, Milan, Italy

Ariel Roguin
Department of Cardiology, Rambam Medical
Center, Haifa, Israel

Dragica Paunovic
European Medical and Clinical Division, Terumo
Europe, Leuven, Belgium

Mamas A. Mamas
Manchester Heart Centre, Manchester Royal
Infirmary, Manchester, United Kingdom
Cardiovascular Institute, University of Manchester,
Manchester, United Kingdom

Shiyan Ren, Xianlun Li and Peng Liu
Cardiovascular Center, China-Japan Friendship
Hospital, Beijing, People's Republic of China

Jianyan Wen and Wenjian Zhang
Clinical Research Institute, China-Japan Friendship
Hospital, Beijing, People's Republic of China

Judith Kooiman
Department of Thrombosis and Hemostasis and
Department of Nephrology, Leiden University
Medical Center, Leiden, Zuid-Holland, The
Netherlands

Milan Seth and Hitinder S. Gurm
Department of Internal Medicine, Division of
Cardiovascular Medicine, University of Michigan,
Ann Arbor, Michigan, United States of America

David Share
Blue Cross Blue Shield of Michigan, Detroit,
Michigan, United States of America

Simon Dixon
Beaumont Hospital, Royal Oak, Michigan, United
States of America

**Dongfeng Zhang, Xiantao Song, Shuzheng Lv, Fei
Yuan, Feng Xu, Min Zhang, Wei Li and Shuai Yan**
Department of Cardiology, Capital Medical
University affiliated Beijing Anzhen Hospital,
Beijing Institute of Heart, Lung and Blood Vessel
Disease, Beijing, China

**Ning Ma, Dapeng Mo, Feng Gao, Kun Gao, Xuan
Sun, Xiaotong Xu, Lian Liu, Ligang Song and
Zhongrong Miao**
Department of Interventional Neuroradiology,
Beijing Tiantan Hospital, Capital Medical University,
Beijing, China

Ziqi Xu
Department of Neurology, the First Affiliated
Hospital of College of Medicine, Zhejiang
University, Hangzhou, China

Tiejun Wang
Department of Neurology, the Daxing District
Hospital of Beijing, Beijing, China

Xingquan Zhao, Yilong Wang and Yongjun Wang
Department of Neurology, Beijing Tiantan Hospital,
Capital Medical University, Beijing, China

**Shakti A. Goel, Lian-Wang Guo, Bowen Wang,
Drew Roenneburg and K. Craig Kent**
Department of Surgery, University of Wisconsin,
Madison, Wisconsin, United States of America

**Song Guo, Gene E. Ananiev and F. Michael
Hoffmann**
Small Molecule Screening & Synthesis Facility, UW
Carbone Cancer
Center, Madison, Wisconsin, United States of
America

**Jennifer L. Bolton, Marlene C. W. Stewart, Niall
Anderson and Jackie F. Price**
Centre for Population Health Sciences, Medical
School, Teviot Place, University of Edinburgh,
Edinburgh, United Kingdom

James F. Wilson
Centre for Population Health Sciences, Medical
School, Teviot Place, University of Edinburgh,
Edinburgh, United Kingdom
MRC Institute of Genetics and Molecular Medicine,
University of Edinburgh, Western General Hospital,
Edinburgh, United Kingdom

Wen-Hsien Lee
Division of Cardiology, Department of Internal
Medicine, Kaohsiung Medical University Hospital,
Kaohsiung Medical University, Kaohsiung,
Taiwan
Department of Internal Medicine, Kaohsiung
Municipal Hsiao-Kang Hospital, Kaohsiung
Medical University, Kaohsiung, Taiwan

Po-Chao Hsu and Chun-Yuan Chu
Division of Cardiology, Department of Internal
Medicine, Kaohsiung Medical University Hospital,
Kaohsiung Medical University, Kaohsiung, Taiwan

Ho-Ming Su
Division of Cardiology, Department of Internal
Medicine, Kaohsiung Medical University Hospital,
Kaohsiung Medical University, Kaohsiung, Taiwan
Department of Internal Medicine, Kaohsiung
Municipal Hsiao-Kang Hospital, Kaohsiung
Medical University, Kaohsiung, Taiwan
Faculty of Medicine, College of Medicine, Kaohsiung
Medical University, Kaohsiung, Taiwan

**Chee-Siong Lee, Hsueh- Wei Yen, Tsung-Hsien
Lin, Wen-Chol Voon, Wen-Ter Lai and Sheng-
Hsiung Sheu**
Faculty of Medicine, College of Medicine, Kaohsiung
Medical University, Kaohsiung, Taiwan

**Xiang Xie, Yi-Tong Ma, Yi-Ning Yang, Xiao-Mei
Li, Xiang Ma, Zhen-Yan Fu and Ying-Ying Zheng**
Department of Cardiology, First Affiliated Hospital
of Xinjiang Medical University, Urumqi, P.R. China

Bang-Dang Chen and Fen Liu
Xinjiang Key Laboratory of Cardiovascular Disease
Research, Urumqi, P.R. China

**Yicong Ye, Hongzhi Xie, Yong Zeng, Xiliang Zhao,
Zhuang Tian and Shuyang Zhang**
Department of Cardiology, Peking Union Medical
College Hospital, Peking Union Medical College
and Chinese Academy of Medical Sciences, Beijing,
China

**Xudong Shi, Lian-Wang Guo, Yi Si, Bo Liu and
K. Craig Kent**
Department of Surgery, University of Wisconsin
Hospital and Clinics, Madison, Wisconsin, United
States of America

Guojun Chen and Men Zhu
Wisconsin Institutes for Discovery, University of
Wisconsin, Madison, Wisconsin, United States of
America
Materials Science Program, University of Wisconsin,
Madison, Wisconsin, United States of America

Srikanth Pilla
Wisconsin Institutes for Discovery, University of
Wisconsin, Madison, Wisconsin, United States of
America

Shaoqin Gong
Wisconsin Institutes for Discovery, University of
Wisconsin, Madison, Wisconsin, United States of
America
Materials Science Program, University of Wisconsin,
Madison, Wisconsin, United States of America
Department of Biomedical Engineering, University
of Wisconsin, Madison, Wisconsin, United States of
America

Index

www.ingramcontent.com/pod-product-compliance
Lightning Source LLC
Chambersburg PA
CBHW082046190326
41458CB00010B/3474